T0383341

Textbook of Pediatric Osteopathy

Senior Commissioning Editor: *Sarena Wolfaard*
Associate Editor: *Claire Wilson*
Project Manager: *Morven Dean*
Designer: *Charles Gray*

Textbook of Pediatric Osteopathy

Edited by

Eva Moeckel DO MRO MSCC

Noori Mitha DO MRO

Translated by David G Beattie, Mo Croasdale and Margaret Fryer

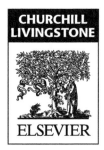

CHURCHILL LIVINGSTONE

ELSEVIER

Edinburgh   London   New York   Oxford   Philadelphia   St Louis   Sydney   Toronto 2008

CHURCHILL
LIVINGSTONE
ELSEVIER

An imprint of Elsevier Limited

© 2008, Elsevier Limited. All rights reserved.

This is a translation of Handbuch der pädiatrischen Osteopathie 1st Edition © 2005 Elsevier GmbH, Urban & Fischer Verlag Munchen. The translation was undertaken by the Publisher.

The right of **Eva Moeckel and Noori Mitha** to be identified as editor/s of this work has been asserted by him/her/them in accordance with the Copyright, Designs and Patents Act 1988.

No part of this publication may be reproduced, stored in a retrieval system, or transmitted in any form or by any means, electronic, mechanical, photocopying, recording or otherwise, without the prior permission of the Publishers. Permissions may be sought directly from Elsevier's Health Sciences Rights Department, 1600 John F. Kennedy Boulevard, Suite 1800, Philadelphia, PA 19103-2899, USA: phone: (+1) 215 239 3804; fax: (+1) 215 239 3805; or, e-mail: *healthpermissions@elsevier.com*. You may also complete your request on-line via the Elsevier homepage (*http://www. elsevier.com*), by selecting 'support and contact' and then 'Copyright and Permission'.

First published 2005 ISBN 3-437-56400-5
First published in English 2008

ISBN: 978-0-443-06864-5

British Library Cataloguing in Publication Data
A catalogue record for this book is available from the British Library

Library of Congress Cataloging in Publication Data
A catalog record for this book is available from the Library of Congress

Notice
Neither the Publisher nor the Editors assume any responsibility for any loss or injury and/or damage to persons or property arising out of or related to any use of the material contained in this book. It is the responsibility of the treating practitioner, relying on independent expertise and knowledge of the patient, to determine the best treatment and method of application for the patient.

The Publisher

ELSEVIER your source for books, journals and multimedia in the health sciences

www.elsevierhealth.com

Working together to grow libraries in developing countries
www.elsevier.com | www.bookaid.org | www.sabre.org

ELSEVIER   BOOK AID International   Sabre Foundation

The Publisher's policy is to use paper manufactured from sustainable forests

Transferred to Digital Print 2011

Contents

Contributors

Susannah Booth DO DPO (London)
Studied osteopathy at the British School of Osteopathy (BSO), UK, and graduated (DO) in 1988. She got her Diploma in pediatric osteopathy (DPO) 1998 from the Osteopathic Center for Children (OCC) in London. She has her own practice, and had a management position at the OCC until 2006. She lectures in pediatric osteopathy in London and at the Vienna School of Osteopathy.

Alison Brown DO, MSCC (London)
Studied osteopathy at the British School of Osteopathy (BSO), UK, and qualified (DO) in 1986. She has taught osteopathy since 1991, first at the BSO, then at the British College of Osteopathic Medicine. She now teaches mainly postgraduates with the Sutherland Cranial College (SCC) in the UK and in Germany. She has been the first chairperson of the SCC for many years and facilitates the SCC Osteopathic Education courses. She has her own practice in London.

Peter Cockhill BA (Hons)DO MSCC (Bath, UK)
Studied osteopathy at the European School of Osteopathy, UK, and graduated (DO) in 1980. He lectured at the ESO from 1980–1982. He was a member of the founding team of the Osteopathic Center for Children (OCC) in London. He has been a member of the faculty and board of the Sutherland Cranial College (SCC), UK, for many years. He lectures at SCC courses in England, Germany, Sweden and Australia. His practice is in Bath, England. He is particularly interested in the treatment of children.

Christine Conroy DO MSc (Ost) MSCC (Wales, UK)
Studied osteopathy at the British School of Osteopathy (BSO), UK, and graduated (DO Hons) in 1989. Received a Master of Science in Osteopathy (MSc Ost) from the University of Greenwich in 1997. She belongs to the faculty of the Sutherland Cranial College (SCC) in Great Britain, and lectures in England and Germany. She studied psychology and the human energy field at the Barbara

Brennan School, USA, and is particularly interested in the somatic effects of psycho-emotional conditions.

Manuela Da Rin DOYMSc (Ost) (Noosa Heads, Australia)
Studied osteopathy at the European School of Osteopathy (ESO), UK, graduating (DO) in 1993: received a Master of Science in Osteopathy (MSc Ost) from the University of Greenwich and the European School of Osteopathy in 2003. She was a member of the ESO faculty, lecturing in Europe until 2003. Her interest in pediatric osteopathy was developed primarily at the Osteopathic Center for Children in London. She has taught in children's clinics in Sri Lanka, Italy and Western Australia. She is a member of the faculty of the Biodynamics Program of Dr Jealous, lecturing in Australia, New Zealand and Europe and is now practising in Queensland, Australia.

Tajinder K. Deoora DO MSc Dipl. Phyt. (London)
Studied osteopathy at the British School of Osteopathy (BSO), UK, and graduated (DO) in 1983. Received a Master of Science in Immunology with Clinical Neuroscience from the University of Surrey in 1999. She is the author of 'Healing through Cranial Osteopathy' and co-author of 'Fundamental Osteopathic Techniques'. She is particularly interested in the treatment of children, and has for many years held a management position at the Osteopathic Center for Children, London. She is involved in the planning of training in pediatric osteopathy at the OCC. She runs two teaching outpatient clinics in pediatrics in Germany and Switzerland. Although she has her own practice in London, she also practises osteopathy for various projects in India several times a year.

Astrid Fischer (Hamburg)
Studied art and social anthropology, majoring in medical anthropology, in the USA and Hamburg. She has been a naturopathic practitioner (homeopathy and other naturopathic treatments and astrology) since 1989. Senior lecturer at the Arcana College of German Naturopathy Practitioners in Hamburg.

Maxwell Fraval DO MSc (Ost) (Kambah, Australia)

Studied osteopathy at the British School of Osteopathy (BSO), UK, and graduated (DO) in 1978. Subsequently he served as a member of the BSO's Board of Governors. He also served on the General Council and Register of Osteopaths (now the General Osteopathic Council), UK. He moved to Australia in 1983 where, as well as having his own practice, he is also a lecturer at the first university course in osteopathic training in Australia, at the Royal Melbourne Institute of Technology. He played a major part in developing Australia's first Master of Science course in pediatrics. Acquired his Master in pediatric osteopathy in 1998. He is a founder member of the Sutherland Cranial Teaching Foundation (SCTF) in Australia and New Zealand.

Dr. phil. Sigrid Graumann-Brunt (Hamburg)

Studied educational science and mathematics in Hamburg followed by several years' teaching. She got her doctorate in psychology from the University of Hamburg, followed by a period abroad and a postgraduate course in mathematics education; then taught the subject at tertiary level. She studied psychology and teaching the language-impaired, which led to involvement in the test construction and research into language in preschool children. She has had her own practice for language and developmental therapy for 15 years.

Sibyl Grundberg DO MSCC (London)

Studied literature at Brown University (USA) and osteopathy at the British College of Naturopathy and Osteopathy (now the British College of Osteopathic Medicine, BCOM), and graduated (DO) in 1986. Currently she teaches cranial osteopathy there. Since 1994 she has been on the faculty of the Sutherland Cranial College (SCC) and served on its board of trustees from 1996 until 2000. She has taught cranial osteopathy in England, Germany and Sweden. Her practice is in London and she has a particular interest in the treatment of women and children.

Dr. med. Dina Guerassimiouk DO (Hamburg)

Studied medicine at the Medical College of Pediatrics in St. Petersburg, followed by further specialist training in neurology and neuropediatrics. She received her Dr. med. in neuropediatrics in 1989 from the University of St. Petersburg. She was assistant professor of neurology and neuropediatrics at the Medical College in St. Petersburg for several years. The author of 17 publications, she

has been a pediatrician at the Center for Child Development, Hamburg, since 1993. She studied osteopathy at the Sutherland College, Hamburg, graduated in 2000 and received her diploma (DO) in 2003. She also has her own practice and lectures at the Sutherland College.

Prof. Dr. med. Dr. med. sc William Goussel (Hamburg)

Studied medicine at and awarded Dr. med. 1968 by the Medical College of Pediatrics in St. Petersburg. Conferral of a further doctorate, Dr. med. sc., in 1975. He spent two years as a private lecturer, then from 1978 until 1983 was assistant and from 1983 to 1994 full professor in pediatrics, pharmacotherapy and clinical pharmacology at the Medical College of Pediatrics in St. Petersburg. His scientific, clinical and pedagogic activity focuses on neurophysiology and neuropharmacology of the brain, epilepsy, infantile cerebral palsy and pharmacotherapy in pediatrics. Total of 140 publications. Pediatrician and consultant at the Center of Child Development, Hamburg, since 1994.

Giles Cleghorn DO MSc (Ost) MSCC (Bristol, UK)

Studied osteopathy at the European School of Osteopathy (ESO), UK, and graduated (DO) in 1984; then studied Chinese Medicine for 2 years, which is still a great interest. Later he also studied classical homeopathy, graduating in 1990. He acquired his Master of Science in pediatric osteopathy (MSc Ost) in 1997 from the Royal Melbourne Institute of Technology (RMIT), Australia. The following teachers are an important influence: Dr Viola Fryman, Dr Anne Wales and Dr James Jealous. For more than 10 years he has been on the faculty of the Sutherland Cranial College (SCC).

Elisabeth Hayden DO MSCC (Gloucestershire, UK)

Studied osteopathy at the British School of Osteopathy (BSO), UK, and graduated (DO Hons) in 1978. She is a founder member of the Sutherland Cranial College (SCC), and lectures in this capacity in England, Belgium and New Zealand. She a particular interest in pediatric osteopathy and is the author of 'Osteopathy for Children'.

Clive Hayden DO MSc (Ost) MSCC (Gloucestershire, UK)

Studied osteopathy at the British School of Osteopathy (BSO), UK, and graduated (DO) 1977. He gained his Master of Science (MSc Ost) from the University of Greenwich in 2001. He is on the faculty of the Sutherland Cranial College and in this capacity lectures in England,

Australia, the USA, France and Belgium. He has published a paper on his research into infantile colic. Pediatric osteopathy is one of the focal points of his practice.

Dr. med. dent. Ariane Hesse (Hamburg)

Doctorate in dentistry at Freiburg im Breisgau, followed by training as a specialist in orthodontics in Hamburg. She also trained in the Alexander technique, craniosacral therapy and qualified as a naturopath. For 3 years she trained at the School of Classic Osteopathic Medicine (SKOM) in Hamburg. Since 1994 she has been deeply interested in the functional associations between occlusion and the musculoskeletal system. Her practice is in Hamburg and offers further training in the interdisciplinary associations between osteopathy and orthodontics.

Teresa Kelly BSc Ost (Hons) DO (Cork, Ireland)

Registered nurse and midwife. She worked as a hospital and community midwife for 13 years and then studied osteopathy at the European School of Osteopathy, UK, graduating (DO) in 1996. She has her own osteopathic practice in Cork, where she treats mainly newborns, children and pregnant women. As part of the international faculty team of the ESO she teaches in Russia. She runs her own courses in obstetrics and pediatrics from the osteopathic perspective in Ireland, Great Britain, Germany and Italy.

Henry Klessen DO (Urbar)

Studied osteopathy at the Sutherland College in Hamburg until 1994 and received his diploma in 1999. He is a founder member of the Osteopathische Kindersprechstunde e.V. in Hamburg. He has lectured for 10 years in cranial and pediatric osteopathy to undergraduate and postgraduate level at the School of Classic Osteopathic Medicine (SKOM) in Germany and Switzerland. He is a member of the faculty of the Sutherland Cranial College, and in that capacity also lectures in Germany.

Dion Kulak DO Grad Dip (Osteo Paeds) (Melbourne, Australia)

Studied osteopathy at the European School of Osteopathy (ESO), UK, qualifying (DO) in 1985. Since then she has lectured in osteopathic pediatrics, first in England, then in New Zealand and Australia. She teaches osteopathy at the Royal Melbourne Institute of Technology (RMIT) and Victoria University of Technology (VUT), two universities in Melbourne that offer a university degree in osteopathy. She is a founder member of the Sutherland

Cranial Teaching Foundation (SCTF) in Australia and New Zealand, which has offered postgraduate courses in cranial osteopathy since 1991.

Kok Weng Lim DO MSc (Ost) MSCC (Norwich, UK)

Studied at the British School of Osteopathy (BSO), UK, qualifying in 1989. He received his Master of Science from the University of Greenwich and European School of Osteopathy in 2004. He has been involved in teaching undergraduates both at the BSO and at the British College of Osteopathic Medicine. He is also part of the international faculty of the European School of Osteopathy and the Sutherland Cranial College (SCC). He is a consultant osteopath at the Osteopathic Center for Children in Manchester and has a private practice in both London and Norwich.

Jens Peter Markhoff DO (Schleswig)

Studied biology in Hamburg, then trained as a physiotherapist and qualified in 1989. After completing his training as a manual therapist at the German Association for Manual Medicine in 1994, he studied osteopathy at the Sutherland College and qualified in 1999; he received his diploma (DO) in 2003. His osteopathic thesis dealt with disturbances in auditive perception in children. He has his own osteopathy practice in Schleswig.

Timothy Marris DO MSCC (Lake District, UK)

Studied osteopathy at the British School of Osteopathy (BSO), UK, qualifying (DO) in 1978. Since 1982 he has been regularly teaching osteopathy in the cranial field, first at the BSO and since 1993 at the Sutherland Cranial College (SCC). He is a founder member of the SCC, has a keen interest in pediatric osteopathy, and has his own practice in the Lake District.

Noori Mitha DO MRO (Hamburg)

Noori Mitha is a naturopath and osteopath. She qualified in osteopathy in 1996 at the School of Classic Osteopathic Medicine (SKOM) in Hamburg, and received her diploma in 2002. She taught at the SKOM, and since 1999 she and Eva Moeckel have offered postgraduate training in pediatrics. She is a member of the faculty of the Sutherland Cranial College, and teaches regularly in that capacity. She is a founder member of the Osteopathische Kindersprechstunde e.V. in Hamburg. She is one of the authors of the 'Leitfaden Osteopathie' (2002), and collaborated in the translation of Sutherland's texts into German (Sutherland Kompendium 2004).

Eva Moeckel DO MRO MSCC (Hamburg)
Studied at the European School of Osteopathy (ESO), UK, and received her diploma in 1991. She taught pediatric osteopathy to undergraduates for two years at the College Sutherland and for 10 years at the School of Classic Osteopathic Medicine. She is a founder member of the Osteopathische Kindersprechstunde e.V. in Hamburg. Since 1999 she and Noori Mitha have provided further pediatric training at postgraduate level. She is on the faculty of the Sutherland Cranial College, UK, and in that capacity lectures in the UK and Germany. She collaborated in the translation of Sutherland's texts into German (Sutherland Kompendium 2004).

Renate Sander-Schmidt (Hamburg)
She is a teacher, graduate in pedagogics and a naturopath. She has been practising as a body-mind psychotherapist for 19 years after qualifying in Gestalt body therapy and the imagination process. She has also qualified in regressive body work, in psychotherapy based on depth-psychology, ritual work and emotional Meridian work. For many years she has been involved in the treatment of prenatal trauma and its effects on feeling, thinking and acting. For several years she has also be a supervisor for body-mind psychotherapists, physical therapists, teachers and pedagogues.

Robyn Seamer DO MSc (Ost) MSCC (Noosa Heads, Australia)
Studied osteopathy at the British School of Osteopathy (BSO), UK, receiving her diploma (DO) in 1975. She received her Master of Science in osteopathy (MSc Ost) in 2003 from the University of Greenwich and the European School of Osteopathy. She held a leading position at the Osteopathic Center for Children in London and has taught in children's clinics in Sri Lanka, Italy and Western Australia. She is on the faculty of the Sutherland Cranial College (SCC), UK, and in that capacity lectured in England. She is also on the teaching faculty of the Biodynamics Program of Dr Jealous, lecturing in Australia, New Zealand and Europe and is now practising in Queensland, Australia.

Susan Turner DO MA MSCC (London)
Studied at the European School of Osteopathy (ESO), UK, graduated in 1979. She taught cranial osteopathy at the ESO for 20 years and was a co-founder of the ESO Children's Clinic, which she directed from 1989 until 2000. She was also a member of the founding team of the Osteopathic Center for Children in London, where she worked for 4 years. Since 1986 she has taught osteopathy in the Cranial Field at postgraduate level, first on the BSO faculty and subsequently with the Sutherland Cranial College. After studying in the USA with Anne Wales, DO, she has developed a course in Dr Sutherland's treatment of the whole body, based on the principles of Balanced Ligamentous Tension. She lectures internationally and since 1997 has been coordinating the cranial component of the ESO-run osteopathic training in Russia. She has been practising in London since 1979.

Stefan Wentzke (Ravensburg)
Studied medicine in Frankfurt am Main and Hannover. Trained as a surgeon under Dr Özbay, Garbsen. Studied osteopathy at the School of Classic Osteopathic Medicine in Ulm, qualifying in 2000. Since then he has been working as a physician and osteopath in Ravensburg. He teaches osteopathy at the German Workgroup for Manual Therapy, Isny-Neutrauchburg, under the leadership of the Philadelphia College of Osteopathic Medicine, USA. He is a lecturer at the Pedagogic Institute of Yoga and Health Education, Staig.

Preface

In our years of teaching, both of our own pediatric courses and on Sutherland Cranial College (SCC) courses in which we teach cranial osteopathy as part of a team, we have realised again and again just how much the constantly growing number of European osteopaths is interested in treating children. The more we know, the more we realise we still have to learn. And this is particularly true in pediatric osteopathy: a small patient's physiological circumstances change constantly as the child grows, and so we need a broad base of expertise in many different areas.

Practising osteopathy requires a special way of thinking and a special way of perceiving the people we face. A physical diagnosis is associated with the existing symptoms. The living anatomy and physiology under our hands shows us how it wants and needs us to support it in its constant striving for health and well-being.

The teaching of osteopathy has a strong verbal tradition – and there are many reasons for that. The main reason is probably because many of our learning processes are based on direct feedback. We do not learn the most by watching an osteopath at work, no matter how good he or she is (even though they may well inspire us), but rather by watching and assessing the patient's response. If we are in a supervised situation with the support of an experienced teacher, this can enhance the learning process even further. So we would urge you to seek out teachers who work 'hand in hand' with you – as advocated by Still – to support and refine the development of your palpatory perception. This applies in particular for cranial work, according to Sutherland. His courses included close support by tutors, with a ratio of four students to one tutor. This is the key that is used on SCC courses to create and maintain the optimum learning situation and maximize safety.

Osteopathy is by no means a collection of patent recipes, which could be the reason why there is so little literature on pediatric osteopathy. It is difficult to describe exactly what happens in an osteopathic treatment session. The main points of case history taking and examination can be described in a book on pediatric osteopathy; one must think about differential diagnoses and discuss significant influences during pregnancy and birth. Expert knowledge is essential: the more we know, the more fully we can include and acknowledge our patient's full history during treatment. This is the main topic in the first part of the book (Section 1, Chapters 1–10).

With regard to the actual treatment, the interaction with the living physical physiology, we soon realise that although we may begin with a specific treatment strategy, we must remain open to what the body requires of us in the way of support for the therapeutic process. The authors solve this dilemma – this challenge – of describing osteopathic treatments without falling into the trap of simply passing on 'recipes' by discussing basic treatment principles and the application of these treatments in regard to various pathologies. In Section 2 (Chapters 11–20) the authors offer suggestions, ideas and experiences regarding pathologies that usually occur frequently in pediatric osteopathy practice, illustrating them – where appropriate – with case descriptions.

It was also important to us that we provide relevant information on the subjects of orofacial orthopedics, logopedics and nutrition.

In this book we have concentrated mainly on working with Sutherland's treatment principles because we know from experience that they are particularly suitable for children. When used with respect, this treatment approach is non-invasive and very safe, especially for newborns, babies and toddlers. Techniques such as MET and functional techniques can also be used on older children from about 6 years of age. However, we advise against using manipulative techniques (HVT) on children younger than 8–10 years.

In early life children are almost entirely dependent on other people, their families, much more so than later on. The parents' health determines that of the growing, constantly developing child in many different ways, ranging from genetics and the emotional matrix of the family to diet. Experience has shown us that acknowledging these factors is essential when working with children. This can be achieved by supporting the family from the beginning, even before pregnancy. Quality of life and health in pregnancy and the decisions made regarding labor and delivery can have a significant effect on the birthing experience for all involved. The actual birth itself is usually an extremely memorable and emotional experience. New possibilities in reproductive technology and increasingly technical deliveries may lead to an increased need for osteopathy in newborns and children. What we want, however, is not to see osteopathy become a 'new baby treatment', but an all-encompassing form of care that is provided throughout childhood.

In this book we have tried, together with a large number of highly experienced osteopaths who work in pediatrics and a number of specialists from other areas, to provide and discuss a cross-section of what is happening in this extremely important area of osteopathy. *Textbook of Pediatric Osteopathy* is also intended to encourage the reader to think further, to research and to feel. Osteopathy is a living science. As Sutherland said, 'Dig on!' and 'To the dreamer who can work, and the worker who can dream, life surrenders all things' (Sutherland W: Contributions of Thought. 2nd edition, Sutherland Cranial Teaching Foundation, Stillness Press, Portland, Oregon, 1998).

Hamburg, September 2005
Eva Moeckel and Noori Mitha

Acknowledgements

First of all we would like to thank our editor, the Countess Dr von Pfeil, who encouraged us to write this book and played such an important part in its conception. Her enthusiasm for osteopathy and her experience as a former assistant doctor in pediatrics were of invaluable benefit in the production of this handbook. Special thanks for her revision of the clinical aspects and many other contributions in connection with her allopathic medical training.

Thanks also to the team at Elsevier-Verlag who were involved in the production of this book.

Many highly esteemed colleagues were also involved in the creation of this comprehensive book, and our thanks go to all of you; despite your numerous teaching commitments and practical work, you took the time to share your favourite subjects with us for this book, doing so with admirable and unfailing enthusiasm.

Being part of the Faculty at Sutherland Cranial College (SCC) is particularly important to both of us: we appreciate and value the inspiring and friendly atmosphere at our teaching events, where everyone is happy to share knowledge and experience. Which is why we would also like to thank all our colleagues at the SCC who, although not directly involved in the project, created the conditions for it; in particular Andria Marchant, Anette Schreiber, Nick Gosset and Nick Handoll.

Our thanks also go to our teachers, in particular Dr Carreiro, Dr Jealous, Dr Shaver and Prof. Willard, all of whom inspired us in their own unique way.

Midwife, journalist and author Bettina Salis provided active help and support in the chapter on childbirth, for which our warmest thanks go to her. Thanks also to midwife Kareen Dannhauer for her support.

Our thanks for the wonderful photographs go to photographer Karsten Franke and his assistant Andrea Lange, and to midwife Elske Rasenack and our colleagues Anette Jäger and Babett Rincke, who helped us to find children and parents to share in this project. Our warmest thanks to all the children who were so willing to be photographed: Alicia, Aurelian, Clara, Fabian, Finn, Hannah, Konstantin, Krabbe, Mak, Mathis, Paula, Selim and Suki and their parents.

And thanks, from the bottom of our hearts, to our families, who supported us with so much love – and so much patience – throughout this project.

Foreword

A few-month-old infant who has been crying inconsolably since birth becomes a happy contented baby. A newborn with a weak suck can now latch on and feed vigorously. A microcephalic child with irritability and uncontrollable seizures becomes seizure free and at ease. A normally developing 10-month-old who cannot crawl on all fours becomes able to do so. A young girl with a flattened and misshapen head from lying in an orphanage develops a lovely shaped head and face. These are some of the experiences I have had in my years of treating children with osteopathy in the cranial field. Some of these are common and expected results from osteopathic treatment. Others are hoped for, but more unpredictable, outcomes.

To help relieve the suffering of any person brings satisfaction to those of us who practice osteopathy, but to do so for a child has its own special reward. In many cases, osteopathy can help change the outcome of the life of a child, making the most of whatever potential is there.

In the very first course I attended on osteopathy in the cranial field, the lecturer for the pediatric session encouraged us all to go back to our practices and begin treating babies using the gentle decompressive techniques we were taught. We were reassured that we would do no harm and had the potential to do much good. That was my experience; despite my limited confidence and skill in those early days, much good was accomplished. I encourage all who have been trained to feel confident enough to treat the children who may come

to them using the gentle and respectful approach that is the hallmark of osteopathy in the cranial field.

With the ideal in mind that osteopathy in the cranial field be available to all children, *Textbook of Pediatric Osteopathy* is a great contribution. The editors, Eva Moeckel and Noori Mitha, are to be commended for the quality of the work they have produced. The book brings together in an organised fashion the knowledge, experience and insights of an impressive international array of osteopaths. Almost all the authors represented are long-standing practitioners and teachers of osteopathy in the cranial field with a great deal of pediatric experience among them. The other authors are respected experts in a variety of pertinent fields.

Textbook of Pediatric Osteopathy is valuable for all who treat children, whatever their level of experience. For most of those who practice osteopathy in the cranial field, children make up only a modest percentage of the patients they see. As a result, their experience and confidence in treating children comes more slowly than it does for adults. Even for experienced practitioners, there is a limit to the depth of knowledge they can have on such a broad array of topics. Therefore, we can all benefit greatly from the accumulated knowledge in *Textbook of Pediatric Osteopathy*.

Rachel E. Brooks, MD
Portland, Oregon

List of abbreviations

A.	arteria
Art.	articulatio
BFT	balanced fascial tension or balanced fluid tension
BLT	balanced ligamentous tension
BMT	balanced membranous tension
CNS	central nervous system
CS	cervical spine
ESR	erythrocyte sedimentation rate
BSO	British School of Osteopathy
CRP	Cross-reacting protein
CTG	cardiotocography
DO	Doctor of Osteopathy (USA), Diploma in Osteopathy (Europe)
DPO	Diploma in Pediatric Osteopathy
ESO	European School of Osteopathy
HVT	High Velocity Thrust (manipulation technique)
IM	involuntary motion
ICP	infantile cerebral palsy
ICS	intercostal space
CSF	cerebrospinal fluid
LS	lumbar spine
M.	muscle
MET	muscle energy technique
MSc	Master of Science
MSCC	Member of the Sutherland Cranial College, UK (a title that is currently only awarded to osteopaths who study osteopathy in GB)
N.	nerve
OCC	Osteopathic Center for Children
PBLT	point of balanced ligamentous tension
PDA	eridural anesthesia
PRM	primary respiratory mechanism
RTM	reciprocal tension membrane
SCC	Sutherland Cranial College
SBS	sphenobasilar synchondrosis/symphysis
TMI	traumatic membranous inertia
TS	thoracic spine
V.	vena
Vv:	venae

Section **1**

Introduction

Liz Hayden

HISTORY AND PHILOSOPHY

The potential for helping children with osteopathic treatment is enormous, and is one of the most rewarding and exciting aspects of osteopathy. There is a wealth of clinical experience among the profession in the pediatric field, but little written work. This book has been compiled by many experienced osteopaths and is an attempt to provide a reference source particularly for undergraduate osteopaths and osteopaths wishing to further their knowledge in this area.

Osteopathy has grown rapidly from its humble beginnings over 100 years ago in the USA. The vision of the founder of osteopathy, Dr Andrew Taylor Still, was profoundly inspired and his insight was way ahead of his time. His understanding was that there is an inextricable link between structure and function in the body, that the body has within it everything that is needed for healing and the maintenance of health, and that the whole person is a unit of function including mind, body and spirit. His emphasis in osteopathy was on the detailed study of living anatomy and physiology and the knowing application of palpatory skills to help the body to correct imbalances. This provides us with a rich framework to work with in osteopathy, and has tremendous potential for application in the pediatric field.

One of Dr Still's early students was Dr William Garner Sutherland. Sutherland graduated from the American School of Osteopathy in 1899. As a student he viewed a specially prepared and mounted skull and experienced a flash of insight in noticing that the cranial sutures were bevelled and articulated in such a way as to permit motion between the bones. The anatomical texts of the time stated that the sutures were fused, but the idea of the possibility of motion would not leave Dr Sutherland. He set out to prove that they could not move, but the more he studied the cranium the more convinced he became that not only did they move but that this motion, or lack of it, had profound effects on the health of the body. He spent most of his life studying the intricate cranial articulations, why they are present, and how they are intimately linked to the body as a whole. He developed the concept of 'cranial osteopathy', or 'osteopathy in the cranial field'. Based on Still's teaching of the link between structure and function, he studied how the effects of bending and warping of the cranial bones during the birth process influenced growth and development of the whole body.

One of Sutherland's observations was 'as the twig is bent so the tree inclines'. In other words, if the baby starts life with a distortion in the cranium from birth, then that pattern of distortion is reflected throughout the whole body. As the child grows, the distortion remains and may even become exaggerated, every structure in the body will be involved and the function of any part can be compromised as a result. It is rather like the way in which a tree growing in a prevailing wind grows into a bent and distorted shape.

Sutherland also stated that 'the little things are the big things in osteopathy'. One of the continual fascinations of osteopathy is that there is a constant need to pay attention to tiny, intricate details, but at the same time not lose sight of the whole picture. For example, a tiny disturbance of the condylar parts of the occiput at birth can have effects through the whole body, from digestive disturbances caused by irritation of the vagal nerve as it exits from the skull through the jugular foramen, to postural asymmetry or scoliosis caused by asymmetrical growth of the cranium that is reflected in the whole body. The treatment of a tiny area of dysfunction can have enormous benefits in the body as a whole.

Sutherland had a number of dedicated students of his work, all of whom had extensive experience of using the cranial concept of osteopathy in the treatment of both adults and children. Osteopaths familiar with the cranial approach to osteopathy will recognize the names of Dr Harold Magoun, Dr Beryl Arbuckle, Dr Harold Lippincott, Dr Rebecca Lippincott, Dr Rollin Becker, Dr John Harakal, Dr Alan Becker, Dr Viola Fryman, Dr Edna Lay, Dr Chester Handy and his wife Dr Anne Wales. Dr Wales (who passed away in 2005) was responsible for editing some of the writings of Sutherland, resulting in the publishing of *Teachings in the science of osteopathy* in 1990. These dedicated osteopaths, and many others, spent their whole lives studying Sutherland's approach to osteopathy and using it to help their patients. They were also devoted to passing on the legacy of Still and Sutherland's work in the education and training of future generations of osteopaths. After Sutherland died in 1954 the Sutherland Cranial Teaching Foundation (SCTF) was founded in USA to protect the teaching of his work. This organization is still thriving and active in ensuring that teaching is true to Sutherland's work. The SCTF in USA is affiliated to teaching organizations in Australia/New Zealand and in the UK.

In the UK there are two main organizations offering training in 'osteopathy in the cranial field'. The Sutherland Cranial College (SCC) offers an excellent pathway of postgraduate courses, and opens its courses to osteopaths from Europe. The pathway consists of 9 modules (one of which is in pediatrics) that encourage students to develop their understanding and skill using this approach. UK students (members of the General Osteopathic Council) who successfully complete the SCC pathway are eligible to become members of the SCC. The SCC also offers courses that are not part of the pathway, including further pediatrics training. The British School of Osteopathy also offers training in osteopathy in the cranial field, with a series of courses leading to an MSc in Osteopathy.

In the last 25 years the treatment of children using the cranial approach to osteopathy has grown enormously in popularity both among osteopaths and by demand from grateful patients and parents. There are now many very experienced osteopaths with special pediatric skills.

WHAT DO OSTEOPATHS TREAT IN CHILDREN AND WHY IS IT SO EFFECTIVE?

Children present to osteopaths with many types of problem; it is not possible to list them all here, but it is hoped that the reader will get an understanding of how apparently small problems early in life can have far reaching consequences many years later. It then becomes easy to understand how important early osteopathic treatment is in the prevention of many of these problems.

Unresolved birth trauma causes a common sequence of problems that begin in a young baby, and may persist throughout life. The following is just a example of the types of different problem that may arise and is intended as a guide, to demonstrate some of the main areas affected.

- A young baby may find feeding difficult, have digestive difficulties such as colic, and may cry excessively. This can lead to the development of poor sleep habits because the baby does not fall into deep restful sleep and wakes frequently. The baby may be fractious and demand to be carried around for much of the time.

- As the baby grows, he will generally grow out of the feeding and digestive difficulties, but the sleep disturbances may continue for many years and the restless behavior

continues. The child prefers to be on the move and often crawls and walks early because he is not relaxed and content to stay still.

- This continual craving for activity can lead to behavioural difficulties such as hyperactivity. A child may not develop the ability to concentrate on a single task for a period of time, because he is restless and always seeking to move around.

- This has implications when the child starts school, because he finds sitting still difficult and consequently has poor concentration. This can then slow his rate of learning.

- Sleep patterns often remain poor, with subtle signs of sleep deprivation such as irritability and poor concentration.

- The immune system is often depleted, with the child suffering many infections. Ear infections are common due to poor drainage of mucous from the ear, and underdeveloped nasal sinuses leads to chronic nasal congestion and mouth breathing. Asthma is more common if there has been delay or difficulty getting breathing established after birth.

- Headaches commonly start at about the age of 7 years if retained birth compression is severe because the bones of the skull are fully formed at this age and the compression reduces the ability of the skull to cope with the strain patterns.

- Hormonal problems can be caused due to poor function of the pituitary gland, which can be restricted by compression, and hence poor movement of some of the bones of the skull. This can result in problems such as delayed growth, delayed puberty, and irregular or painful periods in girls.

- Physical aches and pains, such as back ache due to poor postural development, may be related to the birth pattern.

- Unresolved birth compression can also cause restriction and asymmetry in the facial bones, causing crowding of teeth and bite imbalances. The correction of this with orthodontic appliances may impose further mechanical stresses on the head that can have far-reaching effects on the whole body and can have a significant detrimental effect on health. Regular osteopathic treatment concurrent with the orthodontic work can minimize these problems and reduce the time necessary for bite changes to take place.

- The child who is already having to cope with the effects of unresolved birth trauma will be unable to cope as effectively with other traumatic events later on in life, such as falls or accidents, illnesses or even emotional difficulties. This can be life long.

From this sequence it can be seen why osteopaths can help such a wide range of problems in children: because many of the problems have their origin in retained birth trauma. Osteopathic treatment can help young babies to become more contented and settled; improve behavior problems in toddlers, sleep problems, recurrent infections, learning difficulties and concentration difficulties, headaches, hormonal imbalances, and much more.

Osteopaths do not simply treat the symptoms, but aim to treat any structural imbalances in the whole body to help it to function more efficiently. Normally, many different symptom areas resolve, inducing a state of well-being or health in the infant or child, who usually becomes contented and relaxed in himself, and thus able to develop to his full potential in all ways. A relaxed and contented baby with no physical imbalances is in the best state to cope with the demands and challenges that life throws at him – not only normal developmental demands but also unexpected events such as accidents, falls, illnesses, or emotional trauma.

Many children benefit from regular osteopathic treatment during their developing years, particularly following the normal accidents and falls of childhood, to assist in the recovery from illnesses and help the immune system become more effective at preventing illness, or during times of emotional stress. These can cause more problems in a the child who is already having to cope with unresolved birth trauma than in a child who was fully healthy before the accident.

Osteopathic treatment is particularly beneficial at times of major change such as puberty. Puberty is a time of massive growth and postural change which can leave the muscles and ligaments relatively weak and vulnerable for a time, as concurrently great hormonal and emotional changes are taking place. Osteopathic treatment can help maintain physical and emotional balance during these developmental changes.

During growth and development many systems are changing and what is normal at one stage may not be normal a few months or years later. For example the axes of the legs change from being bow-legged at birth to straight at 2 years, to being knock-kneed to being straight again at about 6 years.

FEATURES OF PEDIATRIC OSTEOPATHY

Pediatric osteopathy is a specialist area requiring considerable dedication and study to develop the necessary knowledge and skills. Osteopaths wishing to work in this field need a full understanding of the physical, sensory and emotional development of a child. This includes:

- Embryological and fetal development, because prenatal events may affect the health and vitality of the fetus, making him more vulnerable to birth trauma (see Ch.4, Influences in prenatal experience).

- The birth process and how different presentations affect the baby (see Ch.5 Normal labor, and p.59 Dysfunctional labor).

- The specialized anatomical features of the newborn that allow babies to tolerate and even benefit from the highly compressive forces of a normal birth (see Ch.5).

- The enormous physical changes that take place as the child grows, and the stresses that this can place on the body at critical times.

- How the child perceives the world, and how this changes with maturity (see Ch.9, A child's world).

- How emotional trauma has a physical effect on the child throughout life. Even a newborn infant can suffer from emotional trauma from a difficult labor or issues that have arisen in pregnancy. Some children are more vulnerable to emotional tension and trauma throughout life, and this is reflected in their physical development (see Ch.9, Diagnosing and treating emotional factors).

- Family dynamics – infants and children are emotionally intimately linked to the parents, particularly the mother, so this needs to be taken into consideration. It is beneficial to treat the mother before birth to prepare her body for labor, and to help her body to recover after the birth. The baby will pick up on tension in the mother and it is often necessary to treat the mother in order to help the infant to relax and become more settled (see Ch.3).

- Normal development – a thorough understanding is essential in order to be able to recognize when a child is not achieving expected milestones (see Ch.6).

- The constant evolution of all systems of the body, particularly the nervous system. An osteopath must be able to assess whether the development is normal and appropriate for the age of the child, or whether there is some neurological damage (see Ch.6; Ch.7, pp 99–149; Ch.16, Developmental delay)

- The dangerous 'red flag' situations that necessitate immediate referral to a medical specialist (see Ch.7, Warning signs and differential diagnoses). All osteopaths, whether treating adults or children, must always be able to recognize these. This is particularly important with children because serious situations can arise rapidly. It may still be appropriate to offer the child osteopathic treatment to complement the medical approach. For example, a newborn infant with a heart problem such as a murmur or 'hole in the heart' obviously should be seen by a pediatrician. However, an osteopath may consider how the change over of the fetal circulation at birth may have been disrupted, and, using appropriate gentle treatment approaches, help the umbilical connections, heart and lungs to integrate those changes more fully.

TREATMENT

Techniques used for children are extremely gentle, coaxing a response from the tissues rather than using strong techniques to force a response. Often the biggest challenge for the osteopath is learning to treat a child 'on the move'. This can be difficult at first, but with a little practice it becomes possible to remain focused on the involuntary mechanism no matter what the child is doing or how much he is moving.

Children can be effectively treated at any age, but obviously the younger the better since many of the later problems can be avoided by early correction of the underlying problem.

Children are all different. Some are robust and healthy, with few health problems. Others benefit from regular osteopathic treatment during their growing years to help them to maintain optimum health and emotional well-being as they meet the challenges of life. Particular key times when treatment may be beneficial are in the first 2 years of life, around 5 to 7 years when the child's personality is emerging, and at puberty. Puberty is a time of rapid growth, with many social, emotional and hormonal changes for the teenager to cope with. Osteopathic treatment at this time can help maintain whole body balance, and help the child.

In general, children respond very quickly to treatment, because the problems have not been present for as long as in an adult. Some of the problems that we see in adults also have a direct link to their own unresolved birth trauma, which can be difficult to treat simply because it has been present for so long. It is never too late to treat, but the earlier the better.

2 The pediatric osteopathic practice

Eva Moeckel

Treating children in osteopathic practice is different in many ways from treating adults. As practitioners we have to allow for this different treatment situation.

Children's needs are often different from those of adults; for instance, children like playing, they don't like keeping still for long, and so on. We need to work with the child to establish what level of cooperation is feasible and necessary in any particular situation for the treatment to be as beneficial as possible for all involved.

Children are usually brought to the practice by their parents, which means that the consultation becomes a three-way event. Parents are often concerned and need lots of information, especially during the initial examination and first treatment session. They want to know exactly what osteopathy is and whether it can help their child. It is right and fair that as much time as necessary is taken to address their concerns. Children will often be looked after by a whole team of practitioners, especially if there is a delay in their development or they are seriously ill. It is important that there is a good flow of information to help the different treatment approaches work together successfully.

ORGANISING THE PRACTICE

External factors also play a part in creating a relaxed examination and treatment situation; these are described in detail in the following.

Waiting time

Before the first consultation it is often a good idea to give children a little extra time to arrive at the treatment center and to settle down. This could be in the waiting room or even the treatment room, if it is already vacant. The waiting time, which could be spent reading or playing, should however not exceed 10 minutes, as otherwise it could affect the child's cooperation during the subsequent examination and treatment.

Child-appropriate practice

A child-appropriate layout and interior of the practice will help parents, children and practitioner to relax. This should include childproof sockets, furniture with no sharp edges, no trailing cables, and a sturdy shelf of toys. The shelf must not tip if a toddler tries to pull itself up by it. The waiting room should include a corner with books and toys, but also an area for relaxing and cuddling. A large bean bag is ideal as it is also a good place for parents to safely lay down babies or bigger disabled children. The waiting room should also be suitable for breastfeeding.

A changing table is also important, and should ideally be positioned in the bathroom. Changing a baby's nappy in the waiting room may bother other people, and changing it on the treatment couch costs time.

In the treatment room there should also be a safe play area, somewhere where the child can move about freely while you are talking to the parents. Things can happen quickly when there are children about. I remember one particular situation: I had just finished the treatment and was talking to the baby's mother as we left the room. The older brother, who had been perfectly happy until then, had managed to find my stamp pad and was now happily 're-decorating' the freshly painted walls with his hands. Fortunately, it was washable ink.

Toys

It is a good idea to have special toys in the treatment room as they can also be important for diagnosis and treatment. Different kinds of toys can be particularly appealing on the treatment couch and will help to keep the child entertained while lying supine for a half-hour treatment session. Depending on the age, suitable toys are small puppets, rattles, coloured beakers that stack together, simple puzzles and small cars. A selection of books with choices for different ages is essential for reading to the child. A mobile over the couch may also be helpful.

It is also a good idea to have a range of objects within easy reach of the treatment couch as a 'playful' aid to obtaining diagnostic information on perception:

- a small bell to test the child's hearing and response

- a small torch to test pupil reaction and to encourage the eyes to follow the light

- a small tin for putting objects inside to observe how far the child's neurological development has progressed

- objects of different sizes to observe how the child grasps (e.g. with her whole hand, using pincer movements), and whether she wants to put the items in her mouth (hand–mouth coordination).

Clothing

Children usually prefer the osteopath to wear cheerful, bright clothing, rather than black or white. When working with babies, practitioners who wear colourful necklaces or glasses also seem to have an advantage. Despite that, though, I usually remove my glasses for the treatment session as I find I am then more relaxed and receptive for osteopathic palpation.

Children who have spent a lot of time in hospital may not like a white paper cover on the treatment table. In this case the solution is to work on the coloured couch cover without the paper a few times. The situation usually changes gradually as the child becomes more familiar with the relaxed examination and treatment situation. Another solution is to ask the parents to bring a large colourful towel that the child is particularly fond of with them.

PARENT INFORMATION

Case history taking is a triangular situation. Depending on the level of development, the talk will take place partly with the child and partly with her parents. It is important to make sure that no one talks over the child's head – make the conversation as inclusive as possible. During case history taking the parents should be discouraged from making negative statements about a child who is present in the room. In some cases it may be better to talk to the parents alone after the examination and treatment, perhaps by telephone. The initial contact made with the child and parents during case history taking will usually have created favourable conditions for the physical examination and treatment that now follow.

As the responsible adults, it is very much in the parents' interests to know what exactly is happening to their child during the examination and treatment. An initial explanation of what to expect during an osteopathic examination and treatment will probably be given during the telephone conversation when the appointment is first made. It is very important to make sure that enough time is taken to answer parents' questions during the initial consultation. If the findings during osteopathic examination indicate that the child will benefit from treatment, then this diagnosis should be explained to the parents and the child using appropriate terminology.

Getting the child to cooperate is essential; but it is equally important to tell the parents exactly what is being done and why. They need to have an idea of why this form of treatment may work, because – especially with younger children – they are the ones who decide whether they think this form of treatment will benefit their child. An important tip: do not try to give the parents detailed explanations about osteopathy while you are still treating the child. Children react very quickly when they realize they no longer have your full attention. They become agitated, and you may soon find that the treatment process has been disturbed. So try to give the parents as much information as possible during case history taking, but without taking longer for it than necessary. Here too, remember not to try the child's patience to the limits.

It is worth telling the parents that you need to concentrate on the child during the physical examination and treatment session and will not really be able to talk to them during this time. Ask them to make a mental note of anything they want to talk to you about so you can address these matters after the treatment. Children are usually more relaxed then too; they no longer feel they are the focus of what is happening, will rest or simply occupy themselves for a while. This is the ideal time to explain what may be achieved with osteopathy in this situation. If detailed talks with the parents mean the first few treatment sessions have to be shorter than normal, this just has to be accepted – unless the child's symptoms are very serious. Experience has shown us time and again just how important it is that the parents feel they have been given all the information they want and need.

One way of giving parents an insight into what you are doing during the treatment, and why, may be by talking to the child. 'I'm now helping your rib cage to relax, which will make it easier for you to breathe. And then the lymph will be able to drain from your head more easily, and that will help to make your sniffles go away.' You can also address a baby or toddler like this; you are still getting your message across, and most children like to be talked to during treatment.

Of course, parents and children may also be given leaflets on osteopathy and/or other subjects, and in specific cases will be recommended or lent additional literature. But this should never be a substitute for your own answers to the most frequently asked questions: What exactly are you doing? Why does it work?

CHILDREN AS PATIENTS

Whereas the parents' understandable interests and concerns can be addressed during case history taking and after the treatment session, the child should be the center of attention during the physical examination and treatment session. Proceed with tact and understanding to establish the best way of creating contact with the baby, child or young adult. To the child or young adult, both the examination and osteopathic treatment may be an unaccustomed and unusual physical and psychological experience.

Babies

A baby is usually examined and treated lying on her back, or sometimes in a prone position. Most babies are happy to lie on the treatment couch and respond well to being spoken to softly and gently. Try to change the position of your hands as little as possible. After the required orthopedic or neurological tests you will usually perform a caudal to cranial examination with slow and relaxed contact, using the involuntary motion to establish where treatment is required and provide it as necessary (see Ch.8, An osteopathic approach to the newborn and infant). As always when using the involuntary motion, it is important to match the patient's inner tempo. If you are pushy or move too fast, you may irritate the child.

Babies and children love people who radiate a deep inner peace. The calmer and more centered you are during treatment, the more the child will relax. That is why it is so important to look after yourself. Everything that can make the treatment situation pleasant for those involved may be relevant (see Ch.9, Unexpected interactions).

If a baby is hungry and unsettled you may be able to treat while the mother is breastfeeding. Also a child who is generally irritable will often be calmer if given a pacifier or the mother's breast. It is sometimes easier to treat a colicky baby in a 'reverse cradle hold': place the baby stomach-down along your forearm with her head near the crook of your elbow and legs straddling your hand (see Fig. 8.61 for a variation of the reverse cradle hold). A song by Mummy or Daddy or playing a musical toy can buy you precious minutes for the treatment.

A baby who is already able to turn over may not always be willing to lie on her back for the 20 to 30 minutes usually required for examination and treatment. Talking to the child may make a big difference. It can also help if the baby has a squeaky toy or rattle to play with.

It can be of tremendous benefit to work with four hands on children of this age, with one person working with contact on the pelvis and the other on the thorax or head, as – amongst other advantages – this will encourage the child to stay on her back. The person working on the pelvis then also has better eye contact, which makes it easier to talk to and keep the child entertained. If working alone, then the accompanying parent should always have a hand close to the child in order to prevent the risk of a fall from the couch in the event of a sudden movement.

Crying during treatment

- Crying is one of the ways a baby communicates with us; it can express hunger, a reluctance to do something, fright, sadness, anger, etc. As with any other type of communication, the child wants to be acknowledged and respected, though it is not always easy to establish just why a baby is crying. Treating a crying baby is far from pleasant for everyone; it is extremely stressful. It is difficult to concentrate. As an osteopath, it is also difficult to make a correct diagnosis because you too are stressed – as would be anyone who can hear a baby crying. Parents become nervous and upset if they hear their babies cry and feel they can't pick them up. Therefore a crying baby should only be given a treatment as a last resort, if you are sure you are not overstepping the baby's boundaries in any way, and you have the consent of the parents. If a baby starts to cry during treatment, try to establish why. What is the baby trying to tell you? Common causes are:

- The palpatory approach may be too intensive and too overbearing. Perhaps too much testing is being done, and this is stressing the baby.

- You may be moving too quickly.

- You have started to explain something to the parents, and in doing so have moved away from the child and are no longer centered when palpating.

- The child may be hungry.

- The child may have a tummy ache or headache. Of course, acute or chronic illness can also be a reason for continuous crying.

- Sometimes a child that had been completely relaxed will suddenly start crying when you reach a 'hot spot'; for instance an occipital compression that restricts the expression of the body's physiology significantly. This type of crying is evident from the fact that it starts as soon as the compression starts to release. The child will soon calm down again if picked up and soothed by the mother or father. I believe in this case the child may be processing a memory.

If the child usually cries most of the time (see Ch.11, Irritable infants and colic), and this is the reason for the consultation, then it may be necessary to carry out treatment while the crying persists. If the above suggestions do not help, then short, intensive treatments may be necessary, but could then be carried out more often, for example two 15-minute sessions a week. If there are times throughout the day when the baby cries less or not at all, then it is advisable to treat at those times.

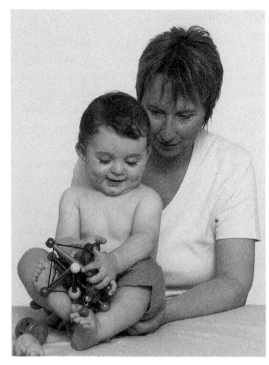

Figure 2.1 Treating the pelvis with the child sitting. With permission, Karsten Franke, Hamburg

Infants

Infants that have just learnt to stand and walk may not want to lie down during the day. Before stressing everyone present by expecting the child to lie still on her back for 20 to 30 minutes, try treating with the child sitting. Feet, legs, pelvis and thorax can all be treated equally well with the child in this position (Fig. 2.1). The child sits on the treatment table with the mother on a chair in front of her. Have a small box of toys close by to entertain the child for a while. You may sit on a stool behind the child.

Although it is possible to treat the cervical spine and head when a child is sitting, it can be more tiring because the child usually moves her head around more in this position, making it more difficult to find a relaxed fulcrum for the hands. Still, sometimes you will have no choice, and with a little practice you will manage well. However, in my experience a small child is often happy to lie down for 5 to 10 minutes at the end of the treatment session. In a firm but friendly manner tell the child that you would now like her to lie on her back for a few moments. Both the practitioner and the parents should avoid saying 'Would you like to lie on your back now?' to the child because if she then says 'No', there is really nothing you can do.

Also remember that even very small children differ tremendously in temperament. Well-balanced children are usually happy to go along with anything, whereas shy or nervous

children will need more time for every stage of the physical examination and treatment.

Older children

It is important to tell a child of nursery school age, and more especially one of school age, why you want to examine and treat her. After a certain age a child may be embarrassed at undressing down to underwear. In my experience, it is usually possible to overcome this problem by explaining that you have to look at her back to make sure it is nice and straight, and that the T-shirt can be put back on again for treatment. It may not always be necessary for the child to remove trousers or tights on the first visit. However, in such cases remember to perform a complete visual examination during a later treatment session when you have built up more trust with her.

During the examination, remember Still's words: 'To find health should be the object of the doctor. Anyone can find disease.' Stay positive and emphasize the positive aspects of your findings. We are all aware of the phenomenon that causes us to remember negative statements about ourselves more firmly than positive ones. I remember Susan Turner describing a finding along the following lines: 'This pelvis would like to be able to express itself more freely.' She has never told a patient that, 'This pelvis is restricted.' This is an excellent example of osteopathic thinking.

In line with this approach, emphasize the positive in your examination and only tell the child and parents the main areas that need to be treated. Even a small child will understand that her head, which she has fallen on several times, may need to be treated.

Adolescents

Adolescents aged approximately 12–18 years are not quite children any more, but also not yet young adults. Their needs may be individually different, and may also vary from session to session.

According to Buddeberg (2004), we should remember that patients of these ages will tend to 'overrate, play down or deny their symptoms. So we should establish clearly during case history taking just what the young person has observed in his or her body and how this change is being considered'.

Puberty

During puberty adolescents may suffer from hormonally induced changes in mood, increased irritability and oversensitivity. It is not unusual for them to be moody when they arrive for their treatment (Buddeberg 2004). In my experience, youngsters can be very silent when dealing with adults and will give short, monosyllabic answers to questions. You, however, will be expected to provide detailed information before any physical contact is permitted, even though this may not be immediately apparent.

Therefore it is advisable to explain exactly what you are doing during the osteopathic examination and treatment and why. Understandably, an adolescent will only come for osteopathic treatment if he or she believes it is going to be worthwhile. In case of doubt they may give us a few chances to prove ourselves. So as with an adult patient, the treatment plan, duration of treatment and potential success need to be explained thoroughly.

There is often a degree of embarrassment during the examination, which may be due to the fact that the adolescent is not yet accustomed to his or her changing body. This must be taken into account, especially if the practitioner and patient are of different gender. In some cases it will suffice if only some items of clothing are removed, and a light cover should always be available.

Parental presence

With older children it is a good idea to ask whether they want their parents to stay in the room during the treatment. Parents can provide a feeling of safety, especially during the initial consultations, but their presence may also keep the child in a state of tension and prevent a deep level of relaxation or sleep during the treatment, e.g. by conversing. If there is any tension between parent and child then it is undoubtedly of benefit for the mother or father to wait outside, at least for part of the treatment. Often, adolescents aged 14 to 16 will want a parent to read to them or just wait quietly in the room with them. I find it is more relaxing if the parents either read out loud or to themselves, as I then do not feel that I am being observed.

If neither parent is present for the treatment, then there may be a risk of the physical contact that occurs during the examination and/or treatment appearing threatening, especially if you and your patient are of different genders, and particularly if you are male. 'Distortions in the perception of a relationship occur more frequently with adolescents than with adults, since subconscious fantasies play a major role in their thoughts and experiences', according to Buddeberg (2004). He believes that explaining actions emphasizes reality and prevents the fear of sexual transgression. So the pros and cons of parental presence need to be balanced carefully. It may be of benefit if one of the parents is present for the treatment.

Young adults

Young adults of 17 or 18 years of age can appear to be quite grown up. It may well be appropriate to use a more formal tone. Except for the case history taking, parents are not normally present for the treatment, but the above does, of course, also apply in this case.

COOPERATION WITH DOCTORS AND OTHER PRACTITIONERS

Children, especially if they are seriously ill or disabled, are often treated by a whole team of practitioners. Osteopathy is usually compatible with simultaneous allopathic treatment. Physiotherapy and homeopathic or herbal treatments also go well together with osteopathy. I would advise against any other form of manual treatment being done simultaneously unless the treatment plan is carefully balanced to not cause conflict. Because the body needs a certain amount of time to integrate a manual treatment, and another form of treatment may well be given on a very similar level, it could easily result in overtreatment. In my experience too much treatment may cause certain achieved changes to regress.

It is also important not to schedule too many treatment sessions in the same week to prevent overloading the child. Ideally, no other therapy should be planned for the same day as the osteopathic treatment unless there is a very good reason for it.

Communication

You should ask the child's parents to revoke the right to confidentiality to enable you to exchange information about the child with doctors or other practitioners. It is advisable to arrange for the document to be signed during the initial consultation.

A brief report is a matter of professional courtesy on referral of a child and should not be omitted for reasons of time. It contains a diagnosis, a brief osteopathic diagnosis and treatment plan, and may be kept very short and handwritten on a preprinted form (see p.12).

A detailed report is written to give interested doctors or other practitioners more detailed insight into the osteopathic treatment plan, to justify it to the health insurer or as a final report.

Your own notes from when you took the case history, initial examination and subsequent examinations and treatments will serve as the base for brief or detailed reports. They contain the patient's or parents' view of what is happening, the results of the examination including any special tests, and your osteopathic diagnosis; that is, the understanding of the interrelationship between structure and function. You need to record your visual diagnosis, noting the mobility of individual joints, together with the findings obtained with palpation of involuntary motion. Bear in mind that the file is to be made available to the patient or parents on request, that a copy may be requested by the health insurer, and that it may well be used by a colleague who is covering for us. It should therefore be precise, well laid out and easy to read with minimum abbreviations. A list of abbreviations may be produced or attached.

But how do you write down what you are feeling before, during and after the treatment? Taking notes of your subjective perceptions during the therapeutic process of the treatment session may help you to remember. This will probably not be of interest to other practitioners who, in my experience, prefer to be informed of clinical changes. The easiest and most objective solution is to describe the osteopathic diagnosis of the tissue restrictions before and after every treatment. What dysfunctional areas do we believe to affect the relevant symptoms? What tissue mobility parameters changed as the result of treatment, and to what extent?

Personal talks can also be a good way to obtain feedback and exchange information. What information has really come across? Something that strikes the osteopath as completely self-explanatory may not be so to the medical doctor. The reverse may also be true: the doctor may assume that the osteopath knows something that is in fact unknown to him or her (Philippi 2004).

It may sometimes also be helpful, especially when dealing with health insurers, to explain the associations between structure and function and to include references to studies and/or literature in the report.

The following are some samples:

Brief report for the pediatrician

Dear Dr. Rose,
Thank you for referring Jara M., born 8.11.04.

Diagnosis: Asymmetrical head shape and torticollis.

Osteopathic finding: initial examination on 08.01.05. Jara turns her head predominantly to the right and her whole spine prefers a right-concave curve. There is a marked flattening at the back of her head. Osteopathic examination revealed restrictions in the bones of the pelvis and restrictions of the spine at L5/S1, T4-T8, C2/C3 and C1/C2. In the cranial area, a intraosseous rotation dysfunction of the occipital bone is particularly evident. The cause may be assumed to be the protracted labor and delivery.

Treatment plan: A series of 6–8 treatments every 3 weeks has been agreed with Jara's parents.

Concluding report to the GP

Dear Dr. Wild,
As agreed, a concluding report on the progress of the osteopathic treatment of Julia W., born 27.11.93.

Diagnosis: hip dysplasia

Case history taking: Julia first came to my practice on 2.12.01 at the age of 8. Her parents told me that since the age of 4 she has been intoeing, more the left side than the right. At the age of 6 she was diagnosed as having hip dysplasia in both hips with an angle of the acetabular roof on the right of 23º, on the left 20º. The orthopedic consultant prescribed physiotherapy with the idea of possibly operating when she was 18. Julia's parents wanted to know whether osteopathy could help.

Osteopathic finding: The osteopathic examination revealed an increased internal rotation of the two hip joints and bilateral genua valga. The back- and leg muscles were slightly hypotonic. There were restrictions of the spine in the upper cervical area with compensatory mal-tension of the pelvis. Cranially, there was a compression of the base of the skull and a general increase in tissue tension, possibly the result of this compression.

Ossification of the bony pelvis does not progress fast until puberty; before then the positioning of the bones in the pelvic region may react in a positive way to osteopathic treatment as it releases asymmetrical tension patterns in muscles and related tissues.

Asymmetrical tension patterns in tissues may also result in increased proprioceptive input into the nervous system (known as 'chatter'), which can interrupt normal coordinated function in both the motor and the sensory field. Conversely, breaking down asymmetrical tension patterns throughout the body can lead to better muscle coordination and improved muscle tone.

Treatment: We agreed a series of 12 treatments for 2002 to see whether Julia's condition could be improved. During these treatment sessions, the main focus was on influencing the tendency towards internal rotation of the hip joints. A positive change was brought about both by treating the local intraosseous and fascial dysfunction patterns in the hip region and by treating the restrictions around the cervical spine and the base of the skull. A check-up X-ray in December 2002 showed the following improvement: angle of acetabular roof on the right approx. 15º, on the left approx. 13º. Five further osteopathic treatments were carried out in 2003 and four in 2004 in order to ensure that the gained symmetry was maintained even during growth spurts. In a further check-up X-ray towards the end of 2004, the results were again as good as they had been at the end of 2002. There was no doubt that Julia's increased interest in sports had contributed towards this stabilization; she has now been playing volleyball regularly for 18 months.

Treatment plan and prognosis: Until Julia finishes growth, I advise carrying out three or four balancing osteopathic treatments a year in order to maintain the improvement.

Please do not hesitate to contact me should you require any further information.

Report to the health insurer

Name: Elsa F., born 07.10.03

Diagnosis: functional torticollis with resulting plagiocephaly.

Case history taking: Elsa was first brought to my practice on 28.3.04. There was a slight delay in development, found at developmental check-up no. 5, and increased flattening of the back of her head. Elsa faces predominantly to the left, but her head will turn to the right both actively and passively.

Elsa was born 5 weeks before the calculated date of birth. Labor lasted 20 hours and a caesarean section was performed when labor stopped.

Osteopathic finding: The examination revealed no indication of dysfunction of the sternocleidomastoid muscle itself, but there was a functional torticollis. Restrictions in spinal mobility were particularly evident around C0/C1, C1/C2, T4/T5, L4/L5 and L5/S1. Cranially, there was a disturbance of the symmetry of the base of the skull with intraosseous dysfunctions of the occipital bone and the left temporal bone The pelvis had a disturbance of symmetry with intraosseous compressions of the sacrum and increased tone in the left psoas muscle.

Reason for the proposed osteopathic treatment: As the body is still soft, during labor it adapts perfectly to the birth channel by molding. Normally the child unfolds after delivery without outside help, aided for example by breathing and the increase in pressure brought about by crying. However, this process may be prevented by certain factors, the results of which cause restrictions in the muscular and other connective tissue, which usually disturb the body symmetry. As muscular restrictions are controlled neurologically, they may be resolved or helped by a gentle form of manual therapy such as osteopathy. Fascial asymmetries also respond well to osteopathy. One frequent cause of a disturbance in symmetry is a birth which is too quick or delayed, especially if delivery is then brought to an end with vacuum extraction, forceps or a Caesarean section. Premature babies such as Elsa seem to be less able to process the normal compressive forces of birth easily, possibly because their tissue is generally softer and more malleable.

Treatment plan: We propose a series of 10 osteopathic treatments at intervals of 2 weeks in order to rectify the disturbances in the symmetry of the cervical spine. I would also expect an improvement of the plagiocephaly.

Report to the physiotherapist

Dear Ms. Neuberg,

I am pleased to report the following regarding our patient, Theo M., born 13.07.02.

Diagnosis: Myopathy, developmental delay.

Case history taking: Theo was first brought to my practice on 11.08.04. His parents told me there was a myopathy and delay in development. They wanted to know whether osteopathic treatment would be a useful addition to the treatment Theo was already receiving. As you are treating Theo currently you know his case history well.

Osteopathic finding: The first examination revealed a longitudinal compression pattern of the spine with a marked asymmetry in the area of C0/C1 and C1/C2. Cranially, there was a superior strain pattern of the base of the skull; i.e. a functional asymmetry of the cranial bones between the front and back areas, the effects of which could be felt through to the thorax. Such asymmetrical tension patterns in the tissue can result in increased proprioceptive input into the nervous system (known as 'chatter'), which can interrupt normal coordinated function in both the motor and sensory field.

Treatment: Osteopathic treatment in combination with physiotherapy is often very effective in children with functional delays in development. When the delay is caused by a pathology, success is usually based on the functional proportion of the disease, which can be extremely difficult to estimate. Thus it will usually take a few treatment sessions to establish whether the functional patterns of the fascia are balancing and an improvement in the muscle tone follows.

The first treatment addressed the longitudinal compression pattern of the spine specifically in areas L5/S1, C1/C2 and C0/C1. In the second and third treatments, more attention was given to the treatment of the cranial asymmetries.

Progress: Theo is now trying to reach out more, and his overall muscle tone has improved somewhat. The fascial tension patterns are beginning to balance out.

Prognosis: These small steps would indicate that it is worth giving Theo osteopathic care in addition to physiotherapy. I would assume that there will be some further improvement in tone. I suggest one treatment per month, initially for 10 months, and then check-ups at longer intervals.

Please do not hesitate to contact me should you require any further information.

Bibliography

Buddeberg C: Psychosoziale Medizin. 3rd issue, Springer, Berlin 2004
Philippi H: Aspekte des Dialogs zwischen Kinderarzt und Osteopath. Deutsche Zeitschrift für Osteopathie 2, 2004: 24–25

3

Accompanying the mother before, during and after pregnancy

Noori Mitha

BASIC ASPECTS OF PREGNANCY

Pregnancy is a very special time in the life of a woman and her unborn child. The pregnant woman is very sensitive to environmental influences; she feels the changes in her body clearly, her perception is heightened and she experiences impressions more intensely.

The progression of the pregnancy is of particular importance in the development of the unborn child and for the delivery. Pregnancy must be seen as a natural process, not as an illness. In some parts of Germany, 60–80% of all pregnancies are classed as high-risk, often because the mother is aged 35 or over, and therefore monitored more closely (Schönberger 2001). Because of the increasing employment of technical devices in modern pregnancy care and the many possible antenatal check-ups which may be done in order to rule out potential disabilities in the child, parents-to-be are confronted with possible pathologies. They need to decide whether to undergo particular tests and what advantages and disadvantages they offer mother and baby. Although these tests can go a long way towards calming some parents' worries, others find the added responsibility of them hard to bear. A relaxed, worry-free and positive pregnancy, however, reduces the risk of a premature birth and complications in labor.

Because of the range and variety of available information, many questions and doubts arise that often cannot be addressed adequately by the GP because of a lack of time or because the mother does not dare ask them. Midwives have more time for the antenatal checks, and are often able to answer questions more thoroughly. Furthermore, these antenatal checks are usually performed in a relaxed atmosphere. The best model has proved to be the one where midwife and doctor work closely together, with the midwife providing the primary care and the doctor being called in as required.

However, this type of antenatal care is not available everywhere, and pregnancy issues are often raised in the osteopathic practice. We are able to help the mother-to-be by offering treatments and time to talk, and help her to deal with her anxieties.

The importance of psychological equilibrium

The psychological equilibrium of the mother-to-be during pregnancy and labor is extremely important. Furthermore, how the pregnant woman copes with stress will influence the way her child deals with it in later life (Nathanielsz 1999).

The adrenergic system plays a key role in the physical response to stress and worrying or threatening situations. As the stress level rises, the body produces more cortisol. The placenta is able to block and deactivate certain amounts of cortisone, but if the level becomes too high, maternal cortisone will cross the placenta and be transmitted to the unborn child. This has a significant affect on the activity level of the fetal adrenergic system for the rest of the child's life, and he may develop a low stress threshold (see p.34).

Osteopathic support for the unborn child

The development of an embryo is a highly complicated process that is subject to many factors, most of which are still not researched fully. In my experience, the best way to help the unborn child is by giving the mother appropriate expert care and helping her enjoy a pregnancy that is as pain-free and physically pleasant as possible.

I do not believe it is safe to treat the embryo directly and intervene in an extremely fragile balance. Nearer the time of birth it may become necessary to treat the mother – and her uterus in particular – perhaps in order to turn the baby into the desired position or to prevent the weight of the baby from compressing organs or vessels, and thereby also ensuring better fetal care.

Antenatal checkups

Modern medical care during pregnancy has helped to achieve a significant reduction in the mortality rate of mothers and babies. Deformities can be identified early, complications anticipated and the appropriate preparations made; for example arranging a planned caesarean section if the mother or baby is at risk.

These days, antenatal checkups include ultrasound screening, blood tests and genetic tests on samples taken from the mother, the embryo or the amniotic fluid.

These tests do bring with them various risks, which are explained below, and the stress factor experienced by parents while waiting for the results of these tests must not be underestimated. None of these tests is 100% reliable, and there is a risk of an incorrect diagnosis causing further concern during the pregnancy or even leading to an unnecessary abortion.

Pregnancy is a natural event and should be treated as such. Modern medical diagnostic possibilities can encourage us to monitor a pregnancy as closely as possible and even pathologize it. The tests and antenatal checkups are done in a doctor's surgery or hospital. The principle of high tech-low touch often dominates. According to an investigation by the WHO in 1996, there is a tendency to be too quick to classify a pregnancy as high risk.

The Association of German Midwives has made the following suggestion: 'Prenatal diagnostics need to be dissociated from antenatal care, and should only be undertaken for good reason and after extensive information has been provided. The combination of prenatal diagnostics and antenatal care is one of the main sources of fear during pregnancy.'

It is important that parents decide before these tests are carried out what action they will take if the results indicate a pathological finding.

Ultrasound scan

In Germany, three ultrasound scans are routinely carried out during pregnancy. In high-risk pregnancies this number may rise to 12. There is currently much discussion as to whether ultrasound poses any risk or not.

During the 10th to 12th week of pregnancy, the date of delivery is calculated and the folds of skin on the back of the neck are measured (nuchal fluid). This fluid is usually absorbed during the 13th week, but until then it is extremely prominent in children with Down syndrome. However, it may also remain in healthy children. If the results indicate thickened folds, then further tests will usually be suggested.

During the 19th to 22nd week the organs will be screened by ultrasound. This screening calls for considerable experience and should therefore be carried out in a specialist clinic to prevent the risk of a false diagnosis. The third screening is carried out during the 29th to 32nd week.

False diagnoses often happen in ultrasound screening. According to a November 1992 report in Ärztezeitung, a German medical journal, in only 5% of all women who were referred to a specialist because a malformation was suspected during an ultrasound was this found to be true. In the publication Raum und Zeit (1996), Schmidt reported on five studies in Scandinavia and the USA involving a total of 30,000 pregnant women that showed that routine ultrasound screening did not improve the outcome of the pregnancy.

Serum testing

In this blood test, the mother's serum is tested for the quantity of fetal α-fetoprotein, maternal β-hCG and oestriol. The statistical risk of the child being disabled is calculated using these results, the details of the pregnancy duration and the mother's weight and height. If the results are positive, amniocentesis will be advised.

The diagnosis is not reliable and often leads to false-positive results. Furthermore, 40% of children with Down syndrome are not identified in this test (Weigert 2001).

Amniocentesis

Amniocentesis (amniotic testing) is carried out between the 15th and 17th weeks; a sample of fetal cells is taken from the amniotic fluid for chromosomal testing.

For the amniocentesis a needle is inserted through the abdominal wall and into the uterus, and approximately 10–20 ml of the amniotic fluid drawn off; the process being monitored by ultrasound. The cells are taken from the amniotic fluid and cultivated. The cell nuclei are then separated and the chromosomes isolated and analysed.

Deformities and genetic defects can then be identified. Although diagnosis is generally reliable, there is a 0.5–2% risk of miscarriage following the procedure. The often weeks of waiting for the results are a major concern for the parents. Research is still being carried out to establish whether the procedure has any further negative consequences for the child.

Chorionic villus sampling

Chorionic villus sampling, or biopsy, is carried out after the 10th week of pregnancy. It involves taking a tissue sample from the chorion, the tissue that envelops the embryo and amnion. The sample is taken either through the abdominal wall or transvaginally. Again, the cells are analysed genetically.

The risk of miscarriage with this procedure is about 1% higher than in amniocentesis, but the result is also less reliable. As extra-embryonic tissue is taken, the sample may also contain maternal cells, which could cause the diagnosis to be unclear. If the biopsy is carried out very early on, there is a higher risk of deformity of the embryo.

PREPARING FOR PREGNANCY

If possible, it is a good idea to treat a woman osteopathically before conception. This will ensure that she has optimum energy available, a balanced autonomic nervous system, and that from a bio-mechanical point of view the pregnancy will be as unproblematic as possible. Treatment of the pelvis will enable it to adapt better to the changes in the woman's weight and posture during her pregnancy. It is a good idea to release lesions of the cranial base and the reciprocal tension membrane in order to support the function of the pituitary gland and thus facilitate the release of hormones.

The osteopathic treatment should include improvement of the arterial and venolymphatic flow, especially in the area of the abdomen and pelvis. Good blood circulation is one of the main requirements for healthy development of the child and the mother's optimum adjustment to the pregnancy. The lower thoracic spinal cord segments are of particular significance as they control the arterial and neurological supply of the uterus.

Any abdominal scarring caused by previous infections or surgery, e.g. on the Fallopian tubes or appendix, should be treated in order to aid conception and to prevent growth restrictions in the uterus during pregnancy.

TREATMENT DURING PREGNANCY
General aspects

During pregnancy, the mother-to-be has to adapt to major changes in a very short period of time. This adjustment is supported by hormones that are produced in greater quantities and which result in greater sensitivity to external influences. This must be borne in mind when we treat a pregnant woman. It is also important to give her the opportunity to talk about her feelings and her situation, and to take her concerns and questions seriously.

We must be extremely empathic during the treatment session. Also bear in mind that it is very easy to over-treat. Ask the patient for feedback during treatment, and remember not to crowd the involuntary mechanism. My experience has shown me that gentler techniques such as used in cranial osteopathy are then particularly effective. Personally, when treating mothers-to-be, I prefer to work with the involuntary mechanism according to the principles described in Chapter 8, Diagnosis and treatment with the primary respiratory mechanism.

The general idea is to make pregnancy and childbirth easier and to create the best possible environment for the development of the unborn child.

Treatment during the first trimester

Pregnancy can be divided into three stages, during each one of which specific areas of the mother-to-be's body require particular attention.

During the first trimester, which is from weeks 1 to 12 of the pregnancy, the focus is on the changes in the mother. She has found out that she is pregnant and now must get used to this new situation and think about her future. Depending on her environment and circumstances, it can be a wonderful time – or it can cause uncertainty and fear. She will also experience major physical changes. Her body is now looking after two people. It will secrete more hormones such as estrogen and progesterone, which maintain the pregnancy and help her body adjust to it. At the same time, this can also cause symptoms such as mood swings and water retention.

Estrogen causes the uterine musculature and blood vessels to grow in order to maintain the oxygen supply to the wall of the uterus. It also makes the pelvic ligaments more flexible and stimulates the development of the milk ducts in her breasts. Progesterone helps the embryo to embed itself in the uterus, and will later prevent the uterus from overactivity and the associated risk of early labor.

Half of all pregnant women will now experience varying levels of nausea and vomiting (emesis gravidarum). We do not know entirely what the purpose of this nausea is. It could be a warning mechanism that has evolved over millennia and is intended to make us aware of the new and delicate situation (Rockenschaub 2001). However, the maternal organism also has to work and detoxify for two, which can put quite a strain on the liver. Osteopathic techniques that improve the blood supply to the liver and liver drainage can be of benefit. The mother's psyche can also play an important part in these symptoms. If she is able to share her anxieties and concerns and is able to look forward to her pregnancy and the prospect of motherhood in a more relaxed way, the nausea often disappears by itself. From an osteopathic point of view, this process can be helped by treating the autonomic nervous system. This can be done by addressing possible irritations of the fibres and ganglions of the sympathicus and parasympathicus. Frequent snacks can also often help to calm the mother's stomach. If, however, the nausea becomes severe, she should consult a psychologist. In some cases the nausea can become so severe (unstoppable vomiting, hyperemesis gravidarum), that the mother-to-be has to be admitted to hospital to ensure that she and her child receive the proper nourishment. In cases such as this it is important to include the whole family in finding ways to make the mother's daily life easier.

Constipation may occur during the first trimester and continue throughout the entire pregnancy. However, it can usually be dealt with by the correct diet and drinking plenty of liquids. Treatment of the viscera, the pelvic floor and the associated parietal and neurological areas can be of benefit.

It is advisable to treat any existing lesions, especially those of the musculoskeletal system, during the first trimester. The woman is still mobile enough to be treated in any position and able to lie on her back for long periods of time. Pay attention to the psoas major muscle. It acts as a slide during birth for the baby, guiding it into the minor pelvis during labor. It is also important in assuring lumbar spinal stability.

Mobility limitations of the pelvis should be addressed, as they can cause pain during pregnancy and obstruct the birth. In siblings similar cranial patterns are often evident if the mother has a particular malposition of the pelvis which may mold the shape of the babies' heads.

The sacrum and coccyx should be free from lesions by the time of delivery. During labor, the apex of the sacrum moves dorsally up to 2 cm in order to create enough space for the baby's head. The coccyx also has to be able to move dorsally so as not to obstruct the birth canal. The pelvic floor can also be considered in association with the coccyx and there should be an even tone throughout the pelvic floor. Uneven tension, changes due to scarring or highly or insufficiently toned pelvic muscles may cause problems during delivery. During labor, the baby uses the pelvic floor as a fulcrum for its head as it makes the necessary rotation when leaving the birth canal. The pelvic floor needs to be elastic so it is not damaged during delivery and is then able to return to its previous shape afterwards.

Other problems during the first trimester can include frequent micturition, tender breasts, slight pains in the lower abdomen and mood changes. These symptoms are not significant and usually disappear in later stages of pregnancy.

Treatment during the second trimester

The physical changes become evident during this time. During the first trimester the mother-to-be will have put on at least 3 kg, and during the second trimester she will put on a further 5 kg. Of this, 6 kg will be due to the physiological water retention in her tissue and blood. If she puts on much more (over 16 kg), this can often be due to venolymphatic congestion, which can be treated osteopathically.

As most of the weight increase is around her abdomen, the woman's posture will change. The lordoses of the spine are accentuated. Normally our center of gravity when we stand upright runs through the third lumbar vertebra. As her girth and weight increase, the mother-to-be will lean back more and more to compensate. The center of gravity then runs eventually through the eleventh thoracic vertebra. The musculoskeletal system has to adjust to this new position. This can be painful, as the strain on the lower thoracic vertebrae and the dorsolumbar area increases. These areas need to be particularly observed as lesions here can affect the uterus. Viscerosensitive and visceromotor fibres run between the lower thoracic segments and the uterus. Mobility in the dorsolumbar area is

important for the action of the diaphragm, and thus for the breathing and oxygen supply both to the mother and her baby.

The growth of the uterus stretches the ligaments of the uterus considerably. These ligaments are the lig. teres uteri and lig. latum uteri, which stabilize the uterus. The lig. latum uteri runs down from the side of the outer wall of the uterus to the inner wall of the minor pelvis. The lig. teres uteri is a thin fibrous strand that runs from the fundus uteri through the inguinal canal to the labia major (Fig. 3.1). Stretching of these ligaments can be painful; this can be treated by considering the pelvis as a whole and using a balanced ligamentous tension approach (BLT). The uterus can also be treated with the principles of BLT, but with maximum consideration for the life contained therein.

The growing of the uterus pushes the surrounding organs aside. The bladder is compressed, which may cause the mother-to-be to feel a frequent need to urinate.

Bladder infections may occur more frequently. This is not only due to the position of the bladder, but also to dietary and hormonal changes. Mothers-to-be with recurring bladder infections may be helped by osteopathic treatment of the bladder. Special attention is to be paid to the tone of the pelvic floor, position, blood supply and autonomic innervation of the bladder and its sphincter musculature. The uterus should be free to move upwards and compress the bladder as little as possible. The diaphragm should be flexible and mobile and the abdominal organs as free from restrictions as possible to make room for the growing uterus. The mother-to-be may also find reducing her sugar consumption and avoiding carbohydrates in the form of refined white flour helps. Too much sugar encourages the growth of bacteria in the bladder and creates an acidic environment on the mucous membranes. This can also cause an overproliferation of yeast spores such as *candida albicans* on the vaginal mucous membranes. Furthermore it is very important to drink plenty (approx. 2–3 l/day during pregnancy) to flush through the kidneys and bladder and prevent urinary tract infections.

Varices occur more frequently because the absorption of liquid by the maternal system, the loosening effect of estrogen on tissue and the repositioning of the abdominal organs hamper the venolymphatic return. Varicose veins are most common on the legs, but may also occur in the genital area, which can be quite alarming. In order to prevent phlebitis and edema, the mother-to-be should put her legs up as often as possible, make sure her digestive system is in order and perform specific exercises to encourage venolymphatic return. Osteopathic venolymphatic techniques are helpful, as is treatment to rectify restrictions of the veins and especially their passages through the diaphragm.

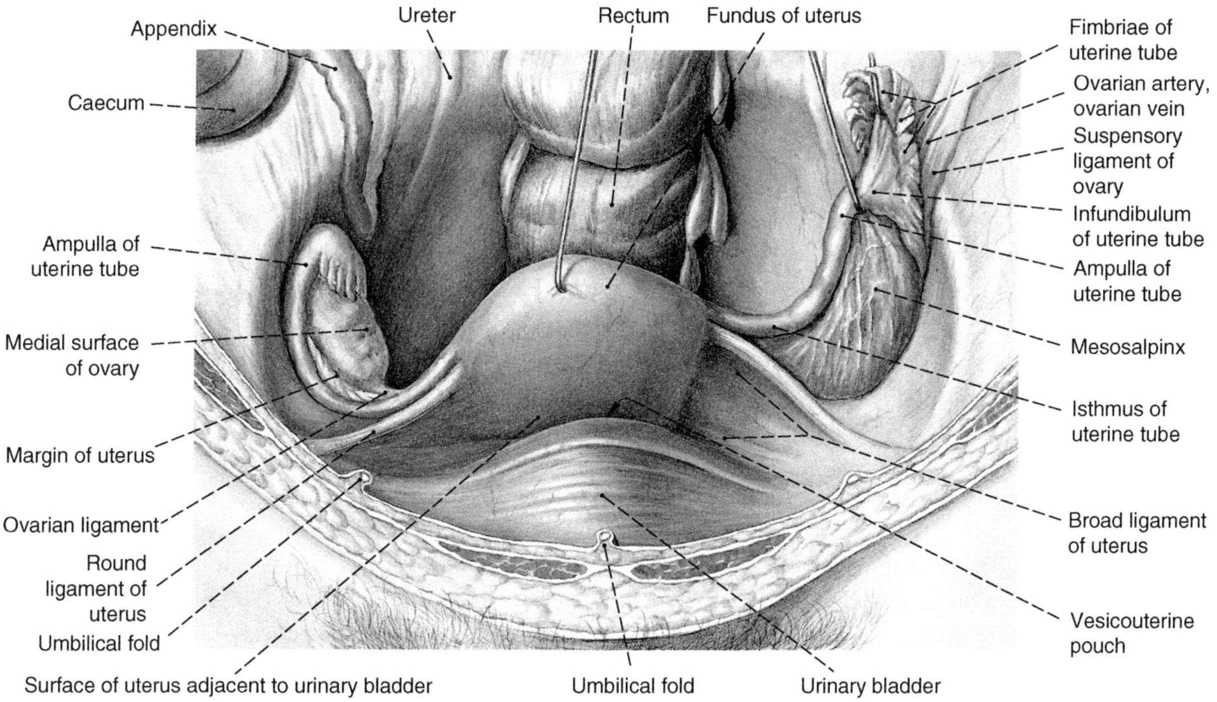

Appendix
Ureter
Rectum
Fundus of uterus
Fimbriae of uterine tube
Caecum
Ovarian artery, ovarian vein
Suspensory ligament of ovary
Infundibulum of uterine tube
Ampulla of uterine tube
Ampulla of uterine tube
Medial surface of ovary
Mesosalpinx
Margin of uterus
Isthmus of uterine tube
Ovarian ligament
Round ligament of uterus
Broad ligament of uterus
Umbilical fold
Vesicouterine pouch
Surface of uterus adjacent to urinary bladder
Umbilical fold
Urinary bladder

Figure 3.1 Course of the ligaments of the uterus (ventral view).
With permission, Sobotta: Atlas der Anatomie des Menschen. Publisher: R. Putz and R. Pabst, 21st edn. Elsevier/Urban & Fischer, Munich/Jena 2000

Treatment during the third trimester

The size of the woman's body increases dramatically during the third trimester. Many women now find it uncomfortable to lie on their backs because the fetus presses against the inferior cava vein, which can soon make her feel unwell. The mother-to-be can be treated while lying on her side or sitting down.

To treat the uterus or perhaps turn the baby into the desired position, the woman may also find it helpful to rest on all fours, with the osteopath placing her hands around her abdomen to treat her from the side. This position gives the baby maximum freedom of movement and is most likely to convince it to change its position, as long as there are no restrictions such as the cord being wrapped around the baby's neck or being too short.

Edemas are also more likely during the last trimester. The increased production of relaxin and estrogen prepares the mother's pelvis for the birth. They loosen the tissue, especially the symphysis pubis joint, and make the musculature more flexible; but this also can reduce the venolymphatic return; they also encourage water retention in the tissue. Congestion appears not only in visible places as edema in the legs, but happens also in the pelvis and abdomen. Hemorrhoids are common and congestion in the abdominal cavity can cause obstipation. There is also the possibility of vasomotoric instability (Fig. 3.2). This manifests itself when

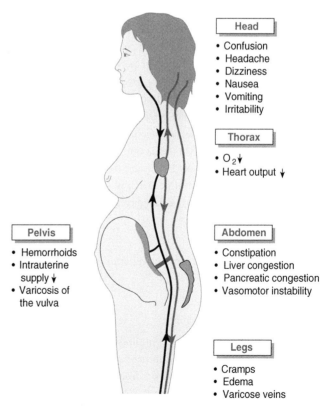

Head
• Confusion
• Headache
• Dizziness
• Nausea
• Vomiting
• Irritability

Thorax
• O_2↓
• Heart output ↓

Pelvis
• Hemorrhoids
• Intrauterine supply ↓
• Varicosis of the vulva

Abdomen
• Constipation
• Liver congestion
• Pancreatic congestion
• Vasomotor instability

Legs
• Cramps
• Edema
• Varicose veins

Figure 3.2 Signs of venous congestion during the third trimester.
With permission, Henriette Rintelen, Velbert

the mother-to-be changes position as dizziness, nausea and disturbed vision. Abdominal organs such as the liver and pancreas may be congested, which will impair their function.

The venous return may also become more difficult. This can cause symptoms such as headaches, dizziness, nausea and vomiting, irritability and, occasionally, confusion. Congestion in the thorax may cause breathlessness and weakness of the heart. It is therefore important not to just treat a particular area or organ, but to bear this complex problem of potential congestion in mind. Freedom of movement of the diaphragm is of tremendous importance. The diaphragm functions like a venolymphatic pump for the lower extremities; it supports heart action and breathing, and the function and drainage of the abdominal organs.

Other passages for vessels and nerves such as the cranial base, thoracic inlet and pelvic floor should also be freed of any restrictions. It is especially important that the cranial base is able to move freely to assist the optimum release of hormones at the time of birth.

The mother may develop iron deficiency (anemia) but she can treat this by increasing her consumption of beetroot, dark green vegetables, parsley, meat, dark grape juices and special herbal teas. Vitamin C aids iron absorption; black tea, phosphates and additives in convenience food reduce it. Iron supplements may cause constipation and should only be taken if other measures do not have the desired effect.

It is important to ensure that the mother's-to-be digestive system works efficiently, since bowel peristalsis stimulates and exercizes the uterus. Mobility of the pelvis should be checked to ensure that the bony structures 'give' more easily in labor. The psoas major should be relaxed on both sides to help guide the baby into the small pelvis during labor. A baby will be able to pass through an average bony pelvis without any difficulties. It is usually the fascia and muscles of the small pelvis that create resistance. If they are free from restrictions, and if the mother's autonomic nervous system is balanced, then the outlook is good for a straightforward birth.

Contraindications

Relative contraindications for osteopathic treatment during pregnancy are:

* early contractions
* bleeding of unclear origin.

In my experience, these contraindications are relative. If the cooperation between mother-to-be and osteopath is good, the osteopath takes feedback from the patient seriously and treats her involuntary mechanism with respect, then osteopathic treatment can be extremely beneficial in these situations. However, the symptoms need to be clarified and

treated if necessary using conventional medicine. Osteopathy may then be considered as a supportive measure.

Complications in pregnancy
Premature delivery

Modern medicine has been able to improve the care of mother and baby during pregnancy and labor and achieve a significant reduction in mortality rates. However, it has not yet been able to reduce the number of premature births. In Germany the rate of premature births is approx. 6% (Schönberger 2001), and the rate is increasing. From the 25th week of pregnancy onwards, babies have a good chance of survival, but it does leave many (approx. 30%) with serious disabilities. The high level of medical care that is required, such as respiration, treatment with drugs, examinations, and in particular the fact that the conditions in which 'premmies' are kept are completely different from those inside the womb and can often cause permanent damage (see Ch.5 Prematurity and associated complications).

Medically, the underlying reasons for premature birth are largely unknown. Possible risk factors for premature delivery include:

* existing conditions in the mother such as diabetes mellitus, kidney disease, hypo- or hyperthyrosis
* anomalies of the uterus, uterus myomatosus
* uterine bleeding during the pregnancy
* previous deliveries of ≤2500 g, previous stillbirth
* underweight mother (BMI ≤ 18)
* multiple pregnancy
* polyhydramnios
* EPH gestosis, HELLP syndrome
* early contractions
* incompetent cervix
* problems with the baby's position
* infections
* premature rupture of the membranes

As yet it is not possible to influence the risk of a premature delivery with orthodox medicine (Weigert 2001). However, there have been reports from doctors and midwives that indicate the possibility of influencing the high rate of premature delivery by other means.

Munich-based Doctor Paluka is of the opinion (Weigert 2001) that a threatened premature delivery is the result of excessive demands on the mother; she is under too much pressure or stress. She also believes that during this important time women should learn to take their needs seriously and respect their limitations. Rockenschaub (2001) believes that an increase in stress factors results in premature delivery.

Gynecologist Dr. Edith Bauer has been running a successful prenatal clinic in Bremen since the early 80s. Mothers-to-be are cared for by the doctor herself plus a highly qualified psychologist and a midwife. As Dr. Bauer explains: 'From our initial contact early in the pregnancy, we aim to support and encourage mothers-to-be in understanding and taking their own sensitivities and their needs seriously.' They also provide nutritional advice, inform mothers of their rights at work, and are generally a place for mothers to go with their questions. In the 90s, although the number of patients increased, there were no premature deliveries in mothers who had been looked after by the practice.

Many surveys have confirmed that women who are able to express and talk about their anxieties and concerns during pregnancy have fewer complications during delivery than others who largely ignore their fears or are unwilling to confront them (Weigert 2001).

Our job as osteopaths is to answer questions, put fears into perspective, ensure that the mother has as few physical complaints as possible and, if necessary, to encourage her to visit midwives, therapists and doctors.

Early contractions

Early contractions and dilation of the cervix may result in an early delivery. The symptoms include pains in the abdomen, hardening of the abdomen, a downward drag and general exhaustion. There may also be a shortening of the cervix. When there is a threat of premature delivery, the cervix may start to dilate.

When early contractions start, the remedy is usually rest and relaxation, possibly combined with hospitalization. Drugs (tocolytics) are also given, although there is some question as to the wisdom of this because of the side-effects for mother and baby. These may include minimal brain damage to the baby, and tachycardia and tremor in the mother. The positive effect is questionable, since despite widespread use of these drugs there has been no reduction in the incidence of premature labor (Kitzinger 1984).

As already mentioned, there have been some successful attempts to reduce premature labor. Bauer, Schulz-Züllich and Linder agree that premature labor is an indication that the mother is under stress. In their therapeutic approach the mother is encouraged to express her fears in talks, and to find a way to relieve the stress she feels. The important aspect is to sensitize the perception of the mother for factors which may be stressing her and to find a way of helping her to deal with it in a way that is appropriate to her circumstances.

This course of action has significantly reduced the incidence of premature labor and birth to less than 1% in their practices.

When there is a threat of premature labor, osteopathic treatment to balance the autonomic dystonia may be advisable. However, compression of the fourth ventricle (CV4) is contraindicated because it could stimulate contractions. For the reasons outlined above, it is essential to talk to the mother-to-be. These conversations should not focus on her problems, but rather give her mental support and help increase her pleasure in her pregnancy and her baby.

Gestosis

Gestosis (gestational toxicosis) is one of the most frequent pathologies in pregnancy. Osteopathic treatment can be useful, and also help to prevent long-term consequences.

Gestational toxicosis is a condition in which the mother's metabolism gets derailed. Toxicoses may also appear outside pregnancy; these symptoms are similar to those of gestational toxicosis. Toxicosis is not caused by the actual pregnancy, but is the result of the organism being overloaded. During pregnancy this overload and stress is called 'maternal distress.'

The symptoms differ according to the time at which they occur. During the first trimester it is known as early gestosis. The symptoms affect mainly the gastrointestinal tract and the liver, and include hyperemesis gravidarum and heartburn. The mother's metabolism is so stressed that it is unable to perform its excretory functions sufficiently. Symptoms such as nausea and vomiting appear, and later they may include signs of kidney stress such as proteinuria and hypertonia.

Late gestoses which appear during the third trimester include EPH gestosis with edema (E), proteinuria (P) and hypertonia (H; the main symptom), also known as pre-eclampsia. If the gestosis increases, CNS symptoms such as headaches, ringing in the ears, disturbed vision, somnolence, nausea, vomiting, hyperreflexia, hemoconcentration and oliguria will occur. There is a serious risk of eclampsia (spasmophilia). A spasm of the brain vessels may cause tonic-clonic spasmophilia (eclampsia).

An unusual form of pregnancy-induced hypertonia is HELLP syndrome, which includes hemolysis (H), elevated liver enzymes (EL) and a low platelet count (LP).

Because the mother's metabolic output is impaired in late gestoses, the supply to the child is at risk. As the gestosis increases so too does the risk of an early labor, and a spontaneous delivery is often no longer possible. In many cases a caesarean section is necessary.

With regard to osteopathy, it is definitely possible to positively influence gestosis. The first consideration has to be to watch carefully for the early warning signs. Vomiting that continues beyond the first few weeks of pregnancy must be observed closely. Talk to the mother-to-be about how she can relax more and encourage her to accept help from others.

A woman's blood pressure should not exceed 140/90 mmHg during the last trimester. In a normal case her blood pressure should reduce during pregnancy because of the hormonally induced reduction in muscle tone and the consequent expansion of her blood vessels. Higher readings indicate that her organism is stressed. Proteinuria ($\geq$0.3 g/l/day) must always be seen as a warning sign that her kidneys are overworking.

The mother may be given osteopathic treatment to support her metabolism. As already mentioned earlier, the venolymphatic drainage is of significant importance in detoxifying and draining the interstitium. The passageways of the diaphragm need to be clear to allow this. Treatment via the 12th rib, diaphragm and venolymphatic drainage techniques are appropriate. Encourage excretion via the liver and kidneys and the blood circulation to these organs. There must be optimum circulation in the brain in order to prevent seizures. To achieve this, it is necessary to encourage free movement of the cranial base, to check whether there are any restrictions of the dura and treat them if appropriate so that the blood supply to the brain and venolymphatic drainage can occur without hindrance. Sutural restrictions of the cranium should therefore also be treated.

Helping the mother to relax is preferable to resorting to medication.

TREATMENT DURING LABOR

Osteopaths are sometimes asked to assist during labor. This is an opportunity that should not be missed, as it is an unforgettable learning experience. The mother usually knows what kind of help she requires. She will probably not ask for gentle techniques, but instead will want to have specific trigger points massaged. If the baby's head has descended into the small pelvis then pressure on the base of the sacrum will help it move on through that area. Should the contractions become weaker, or even stop altogether, then compression of the fourth ventricle (CV4) may stimulate them.

TREATMENT AFTER DELIVERY

After the delivery it is a good idea to check the baby and the mother and treat them if and as necessary. Mothers tend to put themselves in the background and do everything to ensure their baby's well-being before thinking of themselves. However, it is very important that the mother is well-balanced and happy, as this will help her to cope with the challenges of life with a new baby. When mothers bring their babies to my practice, I always ask them how they are and how the delivery was for them. It can often be helpful and desirable to give the mother osteopathic treatment after treating her baby.

Case history and treatment approaches

In case history taking it is important to ask about the pregnancy and delivery. Earlier stress situations, illnesses or problems during pregnancy, the progress and duration of labor, any medication given during the pregnancy and birth, the baby's position and type of birth and any surgical interventions during or after the birth are of particular interest. With regard to the period after delivery, if appropriate, ask how her scars have healed, whether the uterus has returned to its normal size, whether she is generally able to cope and whether she has symptoms of any kind. If she had any problems during pregnancy, check whether the body system in question requires any further support.

The progress and duration of the birth provide information on possible stresses of the musculoskeletal system. It can usually be assumed that a woman who gives birth for the first time will deliver within 24 hours, and within 12 hours for subsequent deliveries. If the delivery is too quick (precipitate delivery or very short delivery of just a few hours), then the ligaments, fascia and musculature of the pelvic floor may have undergone considerable stress. A very long delivery will weaken the mother overall, and again there may be excessive traction on the soft tissue.

Any medication that is given during the delivery may also affect the mother. Suppositories given to stimulate contractions and relax the cervix (active ingredient: prostaglandin; see p.56) may induce side effects including nausea and pain. Oxytocin is given as an infusion, and causes severe contractions that the mother will usually find more difficult to handle than naturally induced contractions. Pethidine is often given to help her cope with the pain; this makes both mother and baby tired, reduces the mother's ability to cooperate, and can cause symptoms such as nausea, vomiting and disorientation. This in turn could make it more difficult for mother and baby to bond after birth.

Drugs given during labor may take some time to leave the mother's system, so it is a good idea to check liver and lymphatic drainage and stimulate them if necessary.

Sometimes the waters are broken to stimulate contractions. Without the protection provided by the amniotic fluid around the baby's head, the mother – and presumably the baby – find the contractions far more painful.

Epidural anesthesia is given in almost every fifth labor (WHO 2005; see p.57). According to the WHO, such anesthesia is used with inappropriate frequency. A local anesthetic is injected into the epidural area at LV2/3. With modern technology it is possible to give the correct dosage to anesthetize the mother from the waist down. Despite this, she often does not have enough feeling to be able to bear down and help push the baby out. The epidural reduces her muscle tone, which means the baby's head does not have the resistance from the pelvic floor to rotate out of the birth channel. This often leads to mispositioning, and the use of vaginal operative intervention such as vacuum extraction (ventouse) and forceps to complete the delivery increases fivefold (Kitzinger 1984). The mother often spends too much time in a position that may be unfavourable for her pelvis without being able to perceive pain as a warning signal. This can lead to long-term lesions of the pelvis and sacrum. Side effects of the epidural, such as headaches and backache may occur; the etiology of these symptoms, from an osteopathic point of view, will be explained later in the text.

It may be possible to establish the cause of any lesions in the mother from the position of the baby during delivery:

- Generally, spontaneous delivery with the occiput anterior does not cause any significant lesions in the mother. However, the position, mobility and tone of the tissue of the sacrum, coccyx and surrounding tissue should be checked and treated if necessary.

- In an occiput posterior delivery, where the baby's face is facing the pubis, or with face presentation, the final stage, which normally does not take longer than 30 minutes, takes much longer. It can take 3 hours or more, which can cause major stretching of the mother's pelvis and pelvic floor.

- A breech presentation may also take a long time to deliver.

If there is a failure to progress in labor, necessitating the use of vacuum extraction (ventouse) or forceps, there can also be significant stress on the mother's pelvis. The Kristeller maneuvre (named after its inventor) is often used in Germany, although not in the UK, and it involves the obstetrician exerting pressure on the fundus of the uterus by pressing on the abdomen to augment the contraction. This increases the pressure on the mother's pelvis significantly, and her soft tissue is damaged more often and usually more severely than if she were delivering without use of the Kristeller maneuvre (Hebammenforum 2002) (see p.60).

It is also important to establish whether an episiotomy was performed and how it has healed. An even tone of the pelvic floor musculature is extremely important for the mother's posture. Correct functioning of this area is essential for fecal and urinary continence, but also for the woman's general well-being and sex life.

Today, a caesarean section is carried out in 20.6% of all deliveries (WHO 2005; see p.64). It is important to find out whether this was planned or not, how the mother felt about the intervention and how her scars have healed. If a caesarean section is planned, then the mother is able to prepare herself for it. However, an emergency caesarean section may leave some mothers feeling they have 'failed' in their ability to give birth; others feel they have been injured without having given their permission. I often see women in my practice in whom these suppressed feelings rise to the surface during the treatment of their caesarean scar. These women usually feel much better after treatment. The scars can also cause unpleasant tension around the pelvic area and abdomen.

Some patients say they feel as if the lower part of their bodies no longer belongs to them. The scars usually respond very well to fascial techniques.

The mother's state of mind is essential for successful bonding between mother and child. If she is exhausted, the mother will be irritable, soon feel overwhelmed by life, and be less able to respond to her child's needs. This condition is often not only the result of a lack of sleep but also due to changing biomechanical factors that are initiated by giving birth. Often, as the baby leaves the mother's pelvis, it exercizes a strong pull on the pelvic floor and sacrum. If the body is unable to compensate for these forces, the mother is often left with two lesions which Sutherland calls 'fascial drag' and 'sacral sag,' a downwards pull on the fascia and a dropped sacrum. After the birth, the base of the sacrum is often left in a position that is fixed to the anterior and inferior. As the baby is pushed out, the apex of the sacrum is pushed dorsally by the baby's head, and the whole sacrum pulled inferiorly by delivery. This position of the sacrum creates a drag via the dura and other fascias to the cranial base, and in particular the tentorium cerebelli. The cerebellum may be pushed down caudally, closing in on the fourth ventricle and the cisterna magna and the fluctuation of the cerebrospinal fluid may be impaired. This fascial drag may also restrict the mobility of the thoracic inlet, the diaphragm and the pelvic floor. The venolymphatic return is inhibited, and the mother feels weak and tired. This condition may even lead to postnatal depression. The motility of the spinal cord and the brain may be restricted because the mobility of the lower attachment of the surrounding dura at S2 is impaired by the dropped sacrum.

Treatment approach

The following treatment approaches were developed by Sutherland and are designed to support the body to release fascial drag. In my opinion it is not generally advisable to follow a pre-assigned plan in treatment. However, the following treatment approaches are an exception, and are particularly effective in the sequence suggested here. Typical problems ranging from tiredness, exhaustion and a lack of drive to depression, poor concentration, backache and pelvic floor instabilities can be relieved most satisfactorily by this sequence of lifts. Usually a single treatment of the mother is sufficient, but it can be repeated as required until the mother is feeling well again.

Anterior sacral lift (Fig. 3.3)

To perform the diagnosis, palpate the patient's sacrum with her in a supine position, and check its movement with the primary respiratory mechanism (PRM). If the sacrum is fixed in an anterior and inferior position it cannot rise upwards cranially during the inhalation phase. This causes significant restriction of the movement of the sacrum with the PRM.

The patient should then sit on the couch; sit in front of her on a stool with your knees lateral to her knees. The patient's lower arms rest on your shoulders.

Place your hands firmly around the patient's iliac crest, carefully palpating around the spina iliaca anterior superior (SIAS) medially with the thumbs in the direction of the alae ossis sacri.

Ask the patient to lean forward, keeping her back straight, and to shift her weight onto your shoulders. This emphasizes the lesion of the sacrum, releasing it somewhat from the clasp of the ossa ilia.

The patient then relaxes her back while leaning on you in order to position the base of the sacrum in the direction of your thumbs and relax the fascia of the pelvis and the spine. You could ask the patient to take several long, deep breaths to support this procedure.

There should now be a discernible change in the tension of the ligaments of the sacrum. The sacrum starts to correct its position, and to our palpating hands it appears as if the sacrum is trying to move upwards slightly. At this point ask the patient to inhale deeply and to straighten up vertebra by vertebra; she should remove her hands from your shoulders and sit up straight. Meanwhile, hold the SIAS medially in order to keep the ossa ilia a little apart dorsally. At the same time, press the patient's knees together with your knees to support the procedure. Accompany the sacrum upwards with your thumbs. Then slowly release the contact. Ask the patient to lie down again and check the mobility of the sacrum once more.

Pelvic lift (Fig. 3.4)

Ask the patient to lie on her side with her legs flexed. Sit or stand behind her and place your fingers gently and medially to the ischial tuberosity. Exert slight pressure on the fossa ischiorectalis in a cranial direction on exhalation. Maintain the position of your fingers on inhalation. Your fingers, wrist and lower arm are aligned.

In Sutherland's words, performing this technique feels as if the pelvic floor is 'being drawn over the fingers like a glove'. Layer by layer the tone of the pelvic floor tissue is balanced.

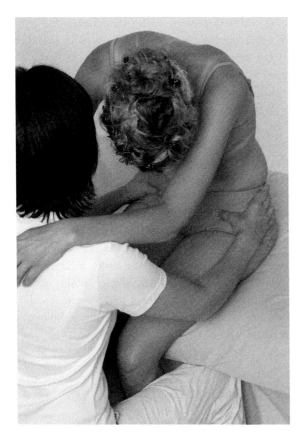

Figure 3.3 Anterior sacral lift.
With permission, Karsten Franke, Hamburg

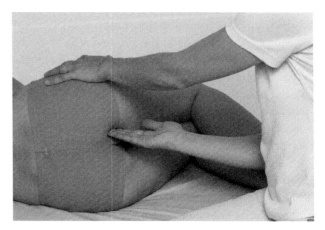

Figure 3.4 Pelvic lift.
With permission, Karsten Franke, Hamburg

Gently release the pressure once the pelvic floor is soft and malleable again and feels evenly toned. It is a good idea to treat both sides, starting on the right as this side is usually softer. The left side tends to be more tense because of the position of the sigmoid colon.

Diaphragm lift (Fig. 3.5)

The patient lies supine with her legs flexed at the knees, you stand at the head of the treatment couch. The patient places her hands on her lower ribs and then you place your hands on top of hers. Ask the patient to breathe deeply.

As she breathes in, follow the movement of the ribs with both hands; as she breathes out follow the upward movement of the diaphragm's central tendon. This supports the doming of the diaphragm. Follow the patient's breathing in this manner until the diaphragm ceases to give way cranially.

Now ask the patient to exhale deeply and then hold her breath, then to expand her ribcage as if she were inhaling deeply but without actually breathing air. Follow the movement of the diaphragm. Hold this position until the patient has to inhale again.

Manubrium lift (Fig. 3.6)

The patient lies on her back with you standing beside her. Place both your hands on the patient's manubrium sterni with your fingers pointing cranially. The lower hand palpates; the upper hand induces the movement. The contact is very gentle, leaving a good distance to the thyroid.

Then induce a very light movement, usually slightly dorsally and superior, until the ligamentary connections of the manubrium to the ribs and the pericard are engaged as in a BLT approach. Wait until the manubrium starts to feel as if it

were 'floating' and a still point usually occurs. The lift results from the renewed swelling of the involuntary motion after the still point. The manubrium rises slightly cranially and ventral. The fascias of the mediastinum are raised upwards via the fascial connection to the manubrium sterni, and the fascial drag that often occurs during labor is reduced.

Parietal lift (Fig. 3.7)

Gradually release the contact once the manubrium is again moving evenly with the rhythm of the Primary Respiratory Mechanism.

A lift of the parietals is helpful at the end of this lifting sequence in order to release the tentorium cerebelli from its caudal position and support the circulation of the cerebrospinal fluid. In order to achieve this, the two parietals need to be released from the squama of the temporals and the mastoid portions.

The patient lies in a supine position on the couch. Sit behind the patient and use a vault hold with crossed thumbs.

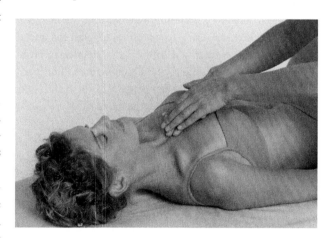

Figure 3.6 Manubrium lift.
With permission, Karsten Franke, Hamburg

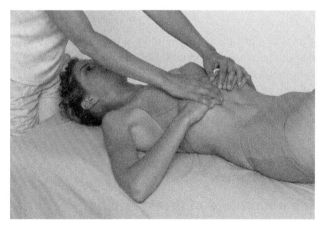

Figure 3.5 Diaphragm lift.
With permission, Karsten Franke, Hamburg

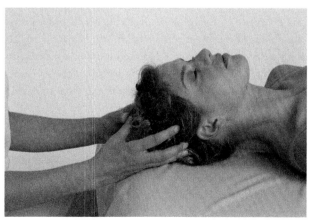

Figure 3.7 Parietal lift.
With permission, Karsten Franke, Hamburg

Position your fingers lightly along the parietals to include the mastoid angle. Your thumbs do not touch the head, as that might irritate or compress the sagittal suture.

Perform a very light medial compression of the parietals on the squamous margin to release it from the temporals and balance the sutural membrane according to balanced membranous tension (BMT). Then wait for the activity of the fluids, a spontaneous fluid drive of the body, which lifts the parietals. Leave your hands lying softly on the patient's head until the correction has taken place and the involuntary mechanism expresses itself well, including the lateral expansion.

After the lift a spread of the sagittal suture may be necessary in order to ensure that the inhalation and exhalation phases are in balance.

Treatment after epidural anesthesia (Fig. 3.8)

After an epidural, many women suffer from long-term diffuse problems such as exhaustion, headaches and back problems. These problems are not usually associated directly with the epidural, as local symptoms rarely occur at the injection point. They are more likely to be associated with the added daily stress of life with a new baby. In my experience, problems such as these can often be relieved or even eliminated by a careful specific osteopathic treatment, as they can be the consequence of dural restriction. The explanatory model is derived from palpatory findings.

The dura normally has a certain elastic feel to it, and moves with the expression of primary respiration in inhalation and exhalation. This movement guarantees motility of the CNS as described by Sutherland. The fulcrum around which the reciprocal tension membrane (RTM) – i.e. the dura – moves is situated near the sinus rectus in an ideal case. If an epidural was given, the dura often feels as if there is a restriction at the site of injection, creating a false fulcrum, which impairs the movement of the dura around its physiological fulcrum. This may be caused by microinjuries from the needle or local irritations caused by the injected medication. Palpation reveals as a loss of mobility of the RTM, and locally a difference in the quality of the dura tissue. It feels dry and more brittle; its elasticity is reduced. Such a restriction of the dura may cause irritations and pain in the nervous system.

The patient lies supine for the treatment; you stand at her side. First put one hand under the sacrum to check the mobility of the dura from here. Then place your two middle fingers under L2 (one finger on top of the other, with the finger touching the patient palpating and the other inducing the movement). Often it is possible to feel the exact point of injection from the change in the quality of the dura, although it may also vary by one vertebra in either direction.

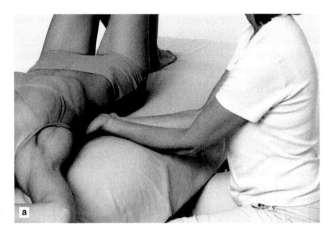

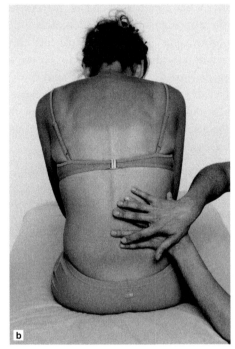

Figure 3.8 Treatment after epidural anesthesia. With permission, Karsten Franke, Hamburg

Using the principle of BMT, find a position where the tension of the dura is balanced in all directions. Wait until a still point occurs, the tissue quality changes and the involuntary motion can be clearly palpated once again. To compare, check the mobility of the dura again from the sacrum.

OSTEOPATHIC SUPPORT WHEN BREASTFEEDING

The importance of breastfeeding

Breastfeeding is important for mother and baby, for many different reasons. It strengthens the bond between them and provides the baby with the optimum nutrition and protection against illnesses and allergies.

The baby is normally put to the breast immediately after birth, and the sucking and nearness stimulates the mother's breastfeeding reflexes. These consist of nipple erection, the production of milk and letdown. Milk production and letdown are controlled by hormones. The baby's suckling releases prolactin and oxytocin which stimulate milk production. Oxytocin also helps the uterus to return to its normal size.

The newborn smells his mother and feels her warmth whilst lying in her arms, and this gives him a feeling of safety and comfort. This helps the baby come to terms with the birth process and his arrival in the world outside the uterus.

This contact with the mother also gives the baby some of its first bacteria, which are essential for intact intestinal flora. Streptococci and lactobacillus pass from her to the baby's intestines, which are still sterile at birth. The baby will have received other useful bacteria while passing down the birth canal. The intact intestinal flora that is created in this way forms the first barrier against pathogens, and therefore an essential defence mechanism. Also the mother's milk is tailored perfectly to her baby's requirements. Her high level of immunoglobulin A (IgA) protects the baby against infections. The IgA in the mother's milk also helps to prevent foreign proteins from penetrating the baby's intestines, making it less susceptible to allergies.

Much is done, both in hospital and in post-delivery care at home by the midwife, to encourage the mother to breastfeed her baby. Mothers who have had a caesarean section or were unable to have their baby with them after birth because of an infection or prematurity are often still able to breastfeed. And yet we still see mothers who find the process difficult. As is described in the following, osteopathy can help in many cases to give the mother the help and encouragement she needs. Sometimes it is simply a matter of correcting a false assumption. Sometimes it is decided, too quickly, that the mother 'is not producing enough milk' or that 'the milk does not agree with the baby,' and the switch is then made to formula. Once the baby has got used to a bottle it may be difficult to introduce the breast again.

Reasons for poor feeding and breastfeeding difficulties

It is advisable to put the baby to the breast as soon as he is born to encourage lactation.

There are several reasons for poor feeding in newborns. Any drugs given during labor, such as pethidine, may make them sleepy for the first 12 hours and less inclined to suckle. Jaundice may also make babies tired and apathetic.

Weak sucking can also be due to an irritation of cranial nerves IX and XII at the cranial base after a strenuous birth with excessive extension of the baby's cervical vertebrae. Poor muscle tone, perhaps due to genetics or a trauma during delivery, may also make it more difficult for the baby to suck.

If the newborn has an asymmetrical cranium or a restriction of the upper cervical vertebrae, he will find some positions uncomfortable. He may be fidgety while feeding, maybe cry and arch his back, which makes it very difficult for mother and baby to relax. It helps to explain the reasons for this behavior to the mother and for her to try nursing in different positions (e.g lying on her side while feeding her baby or feeding the baby when it is held in front of her). If necessary, suggest an osteopathic treatment for the baby.

When to feed

Today's preference is to feed on demand (ad libitum). However, many mothers wish to feed regularly, and are surprised if their baby wants to feed more often than is thought usual.

It is therefore a good idea to explain the reasons for possible changes in her baby's feeding pattern. Babies experience a growth spurt between the 10th and 14th days of life, after 4 to 6 weeks, and again around the age of 5 months, when they require more nourishment. At these times the mother could easily assume she is not producing enough milk. Frequent feeding stimulates milk production to satisfy the baby's requirements. Often she will find it impossible to keep to the advised 2-hour interval between feeds.

In warmer weather, the baby will feed more frequently, but for shorter periods of time, to quench his thirst. The feed starts with a more watery milk, which provides a baby's liquid requirements. A baby suffering from an infection, with a raized temperature and diarrhea, may also wish to feed more often.

Mothers are deluged with information about the frequency of feeding, how much her baby should feed and how much weight it should put on. However, stress and pressure reduce the amount of milk she produces because sympathicotonic stimulation increases the production of epinephrine (adrenaline). Epinephrine suppresses oxytocin. Vagotonic stimulation is the prerequisite for milk production (Rockenschaub 2001). If the mother starts to worry that she is not producing enough milk for her baby, she could soon find herself in a vicious circle. She can encourage milk production by keeping up her own intake of liquids and making sure she gets enough sleep. Many mothers do not take the time during the day to lie down when the baby is sleeping, which would be a good opportunity to catch up on the sleep they are missing at night.

28 3 Textbook of Pediatric Osteopathy

Mastitis

Mastitis may be caused by stress. Stress lowers the immune response, and if there is not enough time to feed the baby properly, milk gets congested in the breast. The mother is more sensitive to bacteria such as stapyhylococci that can enter her body through microscopic injuries to the nipple. Milk congestion increases the pressure in the alveoli of the breast. These may then tear, and protein escaping into the tissue can activate the mother's immune system, which causes an increase in body temperature.

We must take the time to find out the reasons if there are difficulties in the feeding relationship and help the mother by giving her specific information, putting her in touch with midwives or breastfeeding advisors, and by giving osteopathic treatment.

In the osteopathic treatment it is important to use venolymphatic techniques to stimulate the lymphatic flow. The thoracic fascia should be free from restrictions to facilitate circulation and venous drainage in the breasts and reduce tightness in them. A CV4 to prevent infection is often useful. An approach to the autonomic nervous system should also be included, because mastitis can be unsettling and very painful for the mother and could easily lead to a general sympathicotonic situation.

I often see mothers in my practice who breastfeed their babies with the active support of their midwives for the first few weeks. As the babies get older, there is less contact with the midwife, and mothers may become less willing to persevere with breastfeeding. Talking to a mother at the right time can easily encourage her to continue – especially if the baby is given an osteopathic treatment and becomes calmer and more balanced.

Case study

S. had already come to me for treatment several times during her pregnancy. She was expecting her first baby and was nervous and insecure. There was little support in her relationship because the father was living in a different town. She often came with questions and anxieties, but was also easy to calm down.

Three weeks after the birth she brought the baby for a check-up. She told me that she had had a milk congestion and was developing mastitis; her midwife had advised her to wean the baby. The baby was thriving, was happy and generally easy to handle. On further questioning it transpired that her midwife had in fact suggested she try

massaging her breasts but had not shown her how to do it. S. had massaged her nipples a few times, but soon gave up because it was too painful. She had been unable to use a milk pump. All in all, she was feeling helpless and unable to cope. I showed her how to spend a few minutes encouraging the milk down to the areola and release it from the 'pools' in the milk ducts, before finally the milk flow set in. After some initial discomfort, she soon felt relief. I advised her to express some milk several times a day and to wrap her breasts in raw cabbage leaves, which are known to be antiphlogistic when applied externally.

During the osteopathic treatment, I took great care to optimize the venolymphatic return and balance the thoracic fascia. I also performed a CV4 to reduce infection and then worked on the autonomic nervous system to help her overcome her stress.

Her baby continued to develop well, is now 11 months old, and is still breastfeeding in the morning and evening.

Bibliography

Kitzinger S: The experience of childbirth. 5th edn. Penguin, London 1984

Kroth C: Stillen und Stillberatung. Ullstein Medical, Wiesbaden 1998

Kuchera ML, Kuchera WA: Osteopathic considerations in systemic dysfunction. 2nd edn. Ohio Greyden, Columbus 1994

Linder J: Psychosomatische Aspekte der drohenden Frühgeburt. In Janus L, Haibach S: Seelisches Erleben vor und während der Geburt. LinguaMed, Neu-Isenburg 1997

Moll R, Schain-Emmerich U: Allergiekost für Mutter und Kind. Econ und List, Munich 1998

Nathanielsz PW: Life in the womb – the origin of health and disease. Promethean, New York, Ithaca 1999

Rockenschaub A: Gebären ohne Aberglauben – Fibel und Plädoyer der Hebammenkunst. 2nd edn. Facultas, Vienna 2001

Schönberger P: Schwangerenvorsorge durch die Hebamme. Hebammenforum, März 2001

Stadelmann I: Die Hebammensprechstunde. 5th edn. Ingeborg Stadelmann Eigenverlag, Ermengerst 1996

Sutherland W: Teachings in the science of osteopathy. SCTF, Fort Worth, Texas 1990

Sutherland W: Contributions of thought. 2nd edn. SCTF, Fort Worth, Texas 1998

Weigert V: Bekommen wir ein gesundes Kind? Pränatale Diagnostik: Was vorgeburtliche Untersuchungen nutzen. Rowohlt, Reinbek bei Hamburg 2001

WHO: Betreuung der normalen Geburt – Ein praktischer Leitfaden. Geneva 1996

4

The world of the unborn child

Eva Moeckel

BEHAVIOR AND LIVING SPACE OF THE UNBORN CHILD

Our knowledge of the behavior of unborn babies has increased dramatically in recent years, especially due to the use of ultrasound. It is excellent for observing the baby's motor system, but also for understanding its sensory perceptions. Perceptions of any kind are usually associated with responsive movements. Therefore the behavior of the unborn child often reveals an interaction with her environment, because her development depends also on what she experiences. From the first signs of growth to birth and thereafter we live in a constant flow of nourishment and sensoric experience. The dynamic response to that determines our development and being. 'The function exists before structural development is finished' (Relier 1996). Thus the growth of the unborn child depends not only on genetic background but also on environmental factors and the baby's response to them.

The movements of the unborn child

Most mothers first notice their baby moving ('quickening') between the 18th and 20th weeks, although sometimes it may not be until week 25. Fetal movements indicate that the fetus is healthy. A reduction in movements or complete immobility, and in rare cases a significant increase in motor activity, can be an indication of fetal distress.

Using ultrasound, prenatal researchers have been able to record slow, minor and unspecific movements from as early as the 6th week of pregnancy. Isolated movements of the embryo's legs and arms are observed from week 7, and from week 8 it is possible to see how she stretches her head back or turns it, moves her hand to her face or even sucks her thumb. Bending the head forward is observed from week 10 onwards (Krüll 1997).

The first primary circuits develop at the same time as the muscle and nerve cells. 'A neuroblast is already a nervous apparatus with central apparatus, afferent and efferent signal transmission. Here too, the same developmental principle applies both for the peripheral and for the central sections of the nervous system: the creation of an organ is already the beginning of its subsequent performance' (Blechschmidt 1989).

It appears that the first tactile receptor cells develop together with the motor system. Repeated stimuli help to develop the system further. Neurological associations are created with the aid of the baby's sensory perception and motor responses, and are stabilized through repetition. It is possible that over the course of the embryonic development the first motorneurons or receptor cells in the skin regularly absorb recurring impulses, such as contact with the wall of the uterus or a touch on the arm. This creates impulse patterns between the interneurons in the developing brain, some of which stay the same while others continue to differentiate as more nerve cells participate in this interplay with impulses. These patterns of stimuli within the interneurons work reciprocally on the activities of the muscle fibres and sensory cells. 'This central control network integrates every newly created muscle or sensory cell of the embryonic body in a fantastic interplay' (Krüll 1997). Thus the central nervous system gradually develops in an interaction between genetically controlled development of the nerve cells, own action and own perception.

More movements will constantly be added over the coming weeks. At 10 weeks, for instance, it is possible to see how the fetus moves her hand towards her face, yawns, opens her mouth and moves her tongue. At 12 weeks she can be seen to move her fingers.

Depending on the source, after week 8 or 10 a healthy, unborn baby can be observed making breathing movements which at first are irregular and occasional. As the pregnancy progresses, they become more frequent and 'exercise' the breathing function. Reflex centers for these breathing movements already develop in the 2nd month (Blechschmidt 1989). In these fetal breathing movements, however, the ribcage is drawn inwards and the abdomen curves outwards. Prechtl, a leading researcher into the prenatal period, believes that this regular flushing of the lungs with amniotic fluid also aids their normal development (Piontelli 1996). The development of many organs, including the lungs, depends not only on genes but also on their activity. Nathanielz (1999) quotes studies that have shown that animal fetuses that failed to breathe adequately before birth were born with smaller lungs.

Sucking and swallowing movements are evident from weeks 10–11, as the baby swallows amniotic fluid. This may play a part in controlling the volume of amniotic fluid.

At 15 weeks the fetus has developed almost her entire repertoire of movements and is on a par with a newborn; only the quality of the movements that effectively take place underwater is different. Everything happens more slowly and less frequently. With ultrasound it is possible to observe how the baby moves her whole body, moves to the side or turns somersaults, both backwards and forwards, and how she touches herself, moving hands to mouth or genitals. Twins can be seen touching each other.

It can be assumed that these prenatal activities and changes in position are all part of the development of the nervous system and help to develop the musculoskeletal system. 'Prolonged physical inactivity, as in congenital myopathia and various neural dysfunctions, leads to physical anomalies such as joint contractures, deformations of the face and skin, impaired growth and lung hypoplasia' (Piontelli 1996).

At the beginning of the pregnancy in particular, the unborn child has plenty of room to move around in her underwater world and can perform many different movements. From the 7th month, when the fetus is much bigger, there is less room in the uterus. Now the baby can mostly only move the arms, legs and head.

Sensory perceptions of the unborn child

It is not easy to determine when the human sensory organs start to function. Sensory perceptions can only be tested from the outside when they lead to a motor response. According to Relier (1996), chemical perceptions such as smell and taste develop first in humans and in other mammals, then skin sensation, vestibular perception, hearing and, finally, the eyes.

Certain senses, especially proprioception and the sense of balance, play a major role in the development and coordination of the CNS. The fact that they develop so early can be seen as an indication of how important perception of our environment is for growth and quality of the CNS.

Sense of taste and smell

These two forms of perception develop at the same time, presumably stimulated by the composition of the amniotic fluid. The composition and thus the flavour of the amniotic fluid, which is a plasma filtrate, fluctuates according to the mother's hormone balance and diet. According to Piontelli (1996), the fetus drinks the amniotic fluid and then excretes it, which also changes its composition. The oxygen content also affects the composition of the amniotic fluid. In hypoxia there is an increase in the amount of metabolic waste. It is assumed that the change in the flavour of the amniotic fluid stimulates the formation of the taste buds.

By weeks 13–15 the taste buds are so well developed that the baby can take in information through her mouth. Tests have shown that if sweetened amniotic fluid is injected, the unborn child will swallow more frequently; if the amniotic fluid is bitter she will drink less and grimace as she does so.

The olfactory nerve is developed from week 7; the olfactory bulbs are evident from week 8–9. The unborn child has more sensory cells in its nose than an adult does, and they also work in a liquid environment. Not only can the fetus taste the composition of the amniotic fluid, but she can also smell it (Relier 1996).

Relier believes the sense of smell and taste is a fundamental biological base for communication between the mother and her child not only before birth, but also afterwards. After the birth, the baby recognizes the mother immediately by her smell and the smell of her milk.

The skin as a sensory organ

Our biggest and most versatile sensory organ is our skin, which has receptors for pressure and touch, pain and temperature. As already mentioned, the first tactile responses to touch can be observed from about the 6th week – the same time as the first movements occur. In the 1960s, Hooker (1952) and Humphrey (1964) proved that 6-week-old human embryos responded to a touch on the skin of their face by moving of their whole body. They found that the mouth is the first part to become sensitive, followed by other areas of the face, which are sensitive by week 7. Around this time, the palms of the hands, soles of the feet and the genital area also start to become sensitive to touch – the parts of the body that also have lots of receptors later on. These findings have been confirmed by modern ultrasound techniques (Krüll 1997).

In the uterus there are plenty of opportunities for the child to make tactile contact with her surroundings, such as touching or licking the umbilical cord or placenta. She will also touch parts of her own body, such as her thumb or genitals. Of course, she is also in contact with the amniotic fluid. 'Perception via the skin is so highly developed that the amniotic fluid will almost seem like a skin to the fetus, from which it will be separated at birth' (Relier 1996). Once the baby is bigger and fills the uterine space, she is in constant contact with the walls of the uterus.

Perception of pain and temperature

The perception of pain seems to develop at the same time as the response to skin contact. Corresponding reflex responses

The world of the unborn child   4   31

in the uterus have been observed when, for instance, the fetus has been accidentally pricked during an amniocentesis.

Because the temperature in the uterus remains more or less the same, it is possible that this sense does not develop quite so much in utero.

Perception of movement and space

The organ of equilibrium of the inner ear consisting of the sacculus, utriculus and the three semicircular canals, registers and controls every change in the position of our body. The sacculus and utriculus develop before the 5th week, the canals by the 8th week. So we can probably perceive changes in position and our first independent movements from a very early age using our vestibular system, and save them as patterns. Krüll (1997) indicates that the unborn child begins to make turning movements at the same time as the canals form; that is, the part of the system that records three-dimensional turning movements. She believes this supports the assumption that the movements are not only perceived and registered but also stimulate the development of the organ of equilibrium. The perception of movement and space is constantly stimulated and exercised by the baby's own movements and those of the mother. The child also learns not to respond to every movement the mother makes.

We know that the inner ear reaches the size it will have when adult size at about the middle of the prenatal period. As this is not the case with any other organ, it does indicate that the ear is of particular importance to human beings both as an organ of equilibrium and for hearing.

Perception of sound

The cochlea, our hearing organ in the inner ear, grows out of the sacculus from the 7th week and is fully formed by the 10th. The receptor cells (corticells) are situated at the bottom of the spiral, the hairs of which move in the fluid within the space with sound oscillations. Corticells are able to differentiate between the frequencies of perceived sounds. Tones with high frequencies are perceived at the entrance to the spiral, low frequencies at the tip. Because there are more corticells at the entrance, more cells are stimulated by high tones than by low ones. These cells also develop first, so the baby will perceive high frequencies earlier than low ones, which means the human voice can be heard by the fetus at a very early stage. The receptor cells at the tip of the spiral are not fully formed until the 5th month.

According to Krüll (1997), the amniotic fluid filters low frequencies so that the baby probably does not hear noises such as the mother's heartbeat and digestive noises, which are lower in frequency, but is more likely to perceive them as vibrations. The baby probably hears the mother's voice more often than anything else.

Many trials have confirmed that babies like to listen to stories that their mothers also read to them before they were born. There is also literature to confirm that the baby will recognize, or like listening to, music heard during pregnancy.

In tests with acoustic stimulation, unborn babies responded with a motor response; namely faster movements and an increase in heartbeat, after weeks 22–24. Piontelli (1996) describes trials that were set up so the mother was unable to hear the acoustic stimulation in order to be sure that the baby was responding directly, and not indirectly via a placental transfer of the mother's messenger substances.

A number of environmental factors, either alone or in combination, may interrupt hearing development by damaging the cochlea. These include infections, ototoxic medication, drugs and noise.

The eyes

The eyes develop late in the embryonic period. The rod and cone receptors are fully formed by the 10th week. The eyelids grow over the eyes at the same time. The baby's eye movements are observed for the first time in weeks 16 to 18. The rapid eye movements of REM sleep occur beginning from weeks 23 to 24. What does an unborn child dream of? Unborn children obviously also have experiences that they integrate while they are sleeping.

The baby's eyelids gradually start to open again from the 5th month onwards, and they are fully open by the 7th month. There is however not much to see in the darkness of the uterus. It is assumed that it may be very slightly brighter in the uterus when the mother is outside in the sun – perhaps the baby can even see the colours red and orange. The ability to see does not develop fully until after birth.

What makes a human being human?

If we think about the prenatal period of our lives and any traumatising events that may have occurred during this time, then we cannot help but wonder from which time onwards a trauma is actually perceived as such – when does a human start to become aware, and to perceive, whatever form that may take? A chemical-toxic trauma or stress resulting from a lack of oxygen does not, of course, require any kind of perception by the child – it will have an affect on her anyway; what we are talking about here is emotional and psychological traumatization.

When does our consciousness begin, and from what time onwards are we able to perceive? Often consciousness is considered to be on a par with communication and memory.

A person who is in a coma is not conscious and cannot talk to us. But can she hear us? Is she 'there' or not? At what point is an unborn person wholly present?

Some writers believe that a person is fully present when the embryonic development of the CNS is complete; that is, once we possess the mental capacities that are typical of humans as the cerebral cortex develops. Blechschmidt (1989) showed in his human-embryonic research that embryonic humans absolutely do not develop from animal stages, as used to be believed, but that we are human from the beginning. According to his research there is no single point in our development that could justify the belief that a person is not a person until a particular time. 'It is not called human development because an atypical bundle of cells gradually becomes more and more of a person as it develops, but because a person only ever develops from one single essentially human egg cell. ... So we cannot talk of a life that is developing ... Development is not an accidental adding-to from one stage to the next in the sense of progression from something simple to something complicated, but the differentiation of what is already a uniform whole.'

According to Blechschmidt, it is wrong to assume that personality only forms with the development of the cerebral cortex. If we reduce the existence of a person to the development and functioning of the cerebral cortex, then anyone who loses their mental faculties through ageing or illness would no longer be a person. Blechschmidt is clear on this point: 'Human-embryonically, the peculiarity of human development can be proven from the time of conception onwards. If it is the spirit-soul that sets us apart from all other life forms, then it has to be assumed that this is present from the time of conception.' Even from the very point at which one single cell can still split to grow into two people, that person exists as a person. He adds: 'Who can actually prove that twins do develop only at day 4, and do not already exist as anlage at conception? The fact that hereditary twins occur indicates a very early predestination.'

This is a very interesting comment, because the fact that after a few days still more than one embryo may develop from a blastocyte, and no individual is evident at first sight, gives rise to the ethical argument that a blastocyte may be used to obtain stem cells.

There are reports in prenatal psychology that speak of memories from the time before development of the cerebral cortex. Is this possible, or is it fantasy? It's certainly highly imaginative if we assume that memory only occurs in the CNS. Does our entire perception happen there or is there another, possibly cellular, form of perception and memory? From my own experience I would guess that a multilayered, also emotional traumatization is possible before the cerebral cortex has formed even if we are as yet unable to understand the physiological associations.

INFLUENCES IN PRENATAL EXPERIENCE

The development of the unborn child on an organic and emotional level is obviously dependent on many factors. From the medical point of view, we often are accustomed to consider mainly harmful influences. The following paragraphs are therefore also intended to provide information on the positive aspects of prenatal experiences. Emotional and social security for the mother are particularly important prerequisites for healthy development, but so are a good diet and plenty of oxygen. In general it can be said that the child quite literally needs plenty of room to develop in every respect. If this space is restricted, we must accept that there will be consequences.

Harmful influences can be physical, psychological, hormonal or chemical in nature. The child's environment is determined above all else by the mother's physical health and life situation. By the same token, the mother may be exposed to environmental influences such as chemicals or rays that affect her child as well as her. Obviously, the effects of a potentially harmful substance are also determined by the time in the child's development at which they occur. Thus, for instance, malformation may occur at the time the organs are developing, whereas disturbances in the growth or development of the CNS are more likely in the 2nd and 3rd trimesters. The Greek word 'teras' means star, mark of the gods, miracle or amazing appearance. That is why factors or substances that are potentially harmful and cause deformations are called teratogens. There have been many investigations into their harmful effects on unborn children. In particular, there are records of extreme consequences such as premature births and obvious malformation, such as growth disturbances, microcephalus, etc., that are found either before or shortly after delivery. Research is underway into long-term consequences such as learning disabilities, changed social behavior and the predisposition towards certain diseases such as diabetes mellitus.

The list of potentially harmful influences ranges from trauma and infections to all sorts of drugs and harmful materials. This is obviously a very broad subject. For further information please refer to the bibliography.

What many of these harmful influences have in common is that they can disturb the expression of 'the potency in the tide'. Hayden (2004) comments: 'Something may have suppressed the expression of inherent health or potency. It may have happened at any point between conception to birth. It can affect the expression of health for life. It undermines health in many ways; these are the patients whose mechanisms never seem to spark up, it is difficult to get a good expression of the tide from within, … and they don't get better quickly or maintain themselves well … They become our chronic patients. I refer here to all age ranges from babies to adults.'

If we assume that a good expression of primary respiration is an important homeostatic factor that is always available to us and helps us to heal ourselves, then we can understand why it can be so important to consider the child's earliest life circumstances.

Diet

Nutrition an extremely important factor in pregnancy. At the time of fastest growth between weeks 32 and 34, the baby's weight increases by 250 g every week. It is therefore essential that the mother's diet includes plenty of protein and vitamins. Nathanielz (1999) tells us that a poor diet, especially one that is low in protein, will cause stress for the mother and may increase the cortisol level in her blood – and that of the fetus. This is partly due to the fact that if the mother's diet is deficient in protein, the placenta, which normally protects the fetus against the transfer of cortisol, is smaller than normal.

Folic acid is extremely important for embryonic development, cell division and cell growth, and the mother's diet must contain a sufficient quantity of it. Studies have shown that there is a correlation between adequate levels of folic acid and correct closure of the neural tube. Other studies have shown a significant reduction in the risk of a cleft palate and in the rate of congenital malformation of the major blood vessels and urinary tracts (Kelm-Kahl 2004). According to Kelm-Kahl, folic acid taken as a preventative measure around conception or during the early stages of pregnancy is generally undervalued; in Germany it is only taken in 3.4% of all pregnancies.

By contrast, iron is prescribed in 50%, and other minerals in 80% of all pregnancies. However, if the mother makes sure she has an adequate diet then there should be no need for mineral supplements.

Oxygen

Lack of oxygen causes functional disturbances in energy metabolism and may lead to structural changes of the parenchyme. Cells are particularly vulnerable at times of frequent division because they need plenty of oxygen, amino acids, vitamins and glucose at these times. Since oxygen cannot be stored, there must be a constant and plentiful supply of it. It is essential that the placenta is large enough and well vascularized so that it is able to perform its important task

until the end of the pregnancy. Poor vascularization of the placenta as the result of early disturbances may cause fetal distress later on.

There is a correlation between constant psychological stress on the mother's part and a reduction in the oxygen supply to her unborn baby (Relier 1996). All kind of stress factors may impede deep and relaxed breathing by the mother, and this in turn may affect the supply of oxygen-rich blood to the placenta. One of the aims of osteopathic support in pregnancy is therefore to optimize the oxygen supply. This can be achieved, for example, by treatments that ensure the free mechanical movement of the thorax, and influence and balance the autonomic nervous system. It may also be necessary to help the mother-to-be establish what she can do to reduce the stress in her life.

According to Nathanielz (1999), an unborn child that is growing under suboptimal conditions in the uterus will protect the main organs that are essential to its survival at the expense of other growing tissues. This compensatory mechanism, in which the volume of blood is redistributed regionally if the unborn child is receiving insufficient oxygen or nutrients, comes to the fore in the second half of the pregnancy, as soon as the heart and blood vessels are controlled by the baby's brain. If specialized cells in the unborn baby's brain realize that the oxygen level in the blood is dropping, then it will reduce the blood supply to less important organs such as the skin, muscles and liver. The supply to the heart, brain, adrenal glands and placenta is increased. If this compensation has to be maintained for long, it will impair growth and possibly, later on, the function of the undersupplied organs. In order for the organs to function well in later life, it is important that there is an adequate expansion of the vascular system. If an organ contains too few blood vessels, this may have a long-term detrimental effect on it.

If these suboptimum conditions persist, the compensatory mechanism of redistributing the blood flow will tire. Continuing poor oxygen supply may therefore lead to damage to the CNS, the extent depending on the degree of insufficiency. The cause of disturbances in sensory perception and processing, and partial performance may well lie here (see Ch.16, Sensory integration disorders, Specific learning difficulties, Attention deficit hyperactivity disorder).

The endocrine role of the pancreas in the growth of the unborn child is also interesting. In contrast to the newborn and baby, whose growth is controlled mainly by growth hormones and thyroxin, the pancreas, or rather its insulin production, plays a major role in the unborn child. Insulin adjusts the absorption, storage and processing of glucose and amino acids, and thus energy metabolism and protein development. The extent and speed of cell growth before birth are probably determined by the efficiency of the pancreas. Animal trials in sheep have shown that deactivating pancreatic function two-thirds of the way through pregnancy stops growth almost entirely, unlike removal of the hypophysis. Because a long-term shortfall in oxygen will also affect the pancreas, the result may be a general reduction in growth (Nathanielz 1999).

Oxygen supply and smoking

Studies have shown that the absorption of nicotine immediately reduces the supply of maternal blood to the placenta. Furthermore, the carbon monoxide in the smoke binds with the hemoglobin in the mother's and the baby's blood, thus inhibiting the ability of the red cells to transport oxygen. So smoking leads directly to a restriction of the oxygen supply to the unborn baby. Verny (1988) quotes an interesting study by Liebermann, who found that the unborn baby responds to every single cigarette smoked by the mother with an increased heart rate. Furthermore, Liebermann also found that unborn babies started to respond in the same way if the mother even only thought about smoking a cigarette. Verny believes this may well give rise to an anxious psychological disposition later on, since the fetus could never know when to expect the next attack. 'It puts him in a chronic state of insecurity and fear. He never knows when this unpleasant physical condition will occur again, and how painful it will be; he only knows that it is going to happen again. This type of experience leads to a deep-rooted, pre-programmed anxiety.'

Babies born to mothers who smoke weigh an average of approximately 440 g less (Charlton 1996) than those born to non-smoking mothers. Women who smoke often have damaged arteries – the uterine artery may even be damaged before pregnancy. This may also reduce the blood flow to the child to some extent. A good supply of oxygen is essential for the development of the child's tissue. Even the father's smoking appears to have an affect on birth weight.

Prenatal orientation of the stress response level

Although the mother and her unborn child each have their own nerve and blood systems, they communicate at neuro-hormonal level. This usually starts with the mother and runs across the axis brain–hypothalamus–hypophysis–adrenal glands. If, for instance, a woman experiences a strong emotional stress-stimulating response such as fear or excitement, the cortisol level in her blood will increase in order to mobilize her reserves for the fight-or-flight response. In our society, stress factors are usually psychoaffective and psychosocial in nature, but physical and diet-related stress may also increase the level of adrenal hormones during pregnancy. Animal trials

have show that a low-protein diet, for instance, increases the cortisol level both in the mother and in the fetus (Nathanielz 1999). Cortisol affects the function of the heart, blood vessels and immune system. If the cortisol level in the pregnant woman's blood flow increases as the result of stress, the cortisol passes to the baby via the placenta. The placenta does its best to protect the unborn baby by deactivating maternal cortisol on its way through the placenta. Obviously, a small or under-functioning placenta can be a significant disadvantage here.

If the level of maternal cortisol is very high it cannot be neutralized to the same extent and will pass to the child's bloodstream. If this occurs frequently it may affect the child's developing control of its hypothalamus, endocrine system and autonomic nervous system. If the stress-induced stimulation continues; for instance if the mother is constantly worried or upset during her pregnancy, the baby's brain–hypothalamus–hypophysis–adrenal gland axis may be permanently set incorrectly. Animal tests have shown that the feedback system that suppresses cortisol production during stress is interrupted in such a scenario (Nathanielz 1999). So it is possible that a mother with a constantly raised level of adrenal gland hormones may well produce a child with a tendency to hyperactivity of the adrenal glands. This could be one reason why babies are nervous, restless and without appetite, suffer from poor digestion, sleep badly and cry a lot (see Ch.11, Irritable infants and colic). As such a child is particularly sensitive to irritation, this, combined with other factors, may set the scene for subsequent hyperactivity or behavioral problems (see Ch.16, Attention deficit hyperactivity disorder).

Janus (2001) speaks of prenatal stress syndrome. Postnatally, these prenatally stressed babies present with increased irritability and a lower resistance to stress-causing factors, so when treating such children with osteopathy, it is important to remember that they may initially find it a problem to relax. Feeling relaxed is unusual, may be confrontational and therefore causes stress. This means that an osteopath working with one of these children, who starts to relax physically, may find that the child becomes stressed and starts to cry. Under some circumstances, prenatal stress syndrome may have far-reaching consequences in a permanently altered readiness to respond to stress, and thus increased susceptibility to illnesses that are associated with stress-causing factors.

Because our immune system is impaired by our response to stress factors, many of the symptoms and illnesses experienced in childhood can be associated with prenatal stress. Relier (1999) quotes several studies that confirm a link between emotional stress on the mother's part during pregnancy and increased susceptibility to typical childhood diseases such as digestive problems, otitis media and bronchitis in one- to three-year-olds (Stott 1973, Choquet 1985, Richard 1990).

It is of key significance that cortisol, which is produced by the adrenal glands, if released in response to stress factors inhibits growth and cell division. In a dangerous situation, growing is not the most important thing. If the cortisol level remains high for long it could have a significant impact on the development of the fetal circulation, liver and brain (Nathanielz 1999).

Studies into the influence of stress in pregnancy on the development of the CNS have also addressed the effects of extreme stress. A much-quoted Finnish study (Huttune and Niskanen 1978), for instance, looked at the potential effects of the sudden death of the father before or after the birth. Obviously, the loss of her partner is a major stress situation for the mother, and that may be then transmitted to her baby. The researchers were particularly interested in establishing whether it mattered if the event was before or after the birth. The histories of the now adult children revealed a much higher rate in psychiatric illness in those individuals who had suffered this traumatic loss before birth; which led to the conclusion that psychological trauma and a biological disturbance in the development of the CNS both followed. The 2nd trimester is of particular relevance, the time when the neurones move massively in the direction of the cortex, and the period between the 3rd and 5th months of pregnancy, when the thalamus organizes itself as the center for emotions (Verny 1988, Relier 1996).

By contrast, Verny (1988) believes moments of minor stress during pregnancy probably encourage the development of the fetus. 'Being excited, upset or confused by noisy messages is an uncomfortable experience, so he kicks, he squirms, he gradually begins devising ways of getting out of the way of anxiety – in short, he starts erecting a set of primitive defense mechanisms'.

Teratogens

Harmful external influences include well-known teratogens such as nicotine, some medications, alcohol, drugs (e.g. cocaine and heroin, but also marijuana), heavy metals, solvents, X-rays, etc. The risks of professional exposure to chemical and physical influences must not be underestimated.

According to Schaefer, the director of the embryo-toxicological advisory center in Berlin, every pregnancy carries with it the so-called background risk; that is, in 2–3% of all pregnancies there is the risk of structural anomalies that become obvious at birth. Most teratogens will double or treble this background risk, but this still means that 90% of all children will be born healthy.

Schaefer estimates that a maximum of 1–4% of all malformations in newborns can be proven to be due to medication, drugs or other harmful substances. He believes that the mother's alcohol consumption plays a major role in malformation. 'It harms more children than any medication.'

Some chronic diseases in the mother, such as diabetes mellitus and epilepsy, are associated with potential adverse effects on the baby. A number of infections can also harm the unborn child, including HIV, rubella, syphilis and chickenpox. Toxoplasmosis, a common parasitic disease that is almost always without symptoms can, if contracted in pregnancy, cause significant harm to the child.

According to Schaefer (1998), modern medical science indicates that the causes of congenital developmental disorders are as follows: hereditary causes 20%, chromosomal aberrations 5%, uterine factors such as twin pregnancy, oligohydramnios, anatomic anomalies 3%, medication and stimulants 3%, maternal disease and infection 3%, unknown cause 66%. It should be noted that these figures refer to obvious malformations. However, materials with toxic potential for the unborn child or diseases often lead to more subtle impairment of the organism. Malformations and obvious pathologies are probably the tip of the iceberg.

The week or month in which the potentially harmful influence occurred (Fig. 4.1) is always of interest. Minor illness

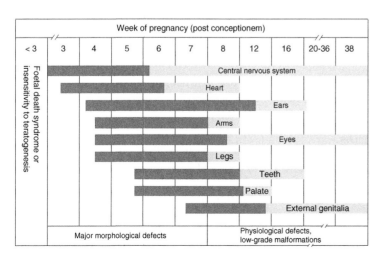

Figure 4.1 Organogenesis and sensitive phases (*dark*: very sensitive, *light*: moderately sensitive).
With permission, Gerda Raichle, Ulm, in association with the series Klinik- und Praxisleitfaden, Urban & Fischer.

of the mother is usually well compensated for during pregnancy, especially if she is in good physical and mental health.

Medication

Medication is taken more often during pregnancy than is widely believed. There are more and more highly effective medicines, which may also have proportionate side effects. 'Today, the side effects of medication are the cause of 5–10% of all hospital admissions. The side effects of medications are the most common cause of disease' (Müller-Oerlinghausen 1998).

In a prospective investigation into the taking of medication during pregnancy, the PEGASUS study, which was carried out in Munich in 1995, it transpired according to Kelm-Kahl that approximately 20% of pregnant women had taken analgesics. Some 20% had also been prescribed systemic antibiotics. Other medications that are often prescribed in pregnancy include antiemetics, antiasthmatics and antihypertensives; hyptertonia occurs in 6–8% of all pregnancies. According to Müller-Oerlinghausen little is known about the safety of many medications. In an inventory taken 10 years ago it was shown that 70% of some 1500 medicines available in Germany contained no detailed information of the possible prenatal toxic risk. Sufficient data was provided for less than 10% of the medication. Little has changed since then.

If a chronically ill patient has a planned pregnancy, her constant medication may be a well-known product with few side effects. However, it is also possible that a woman taking medication suddenly finds she is pregnant. This is why women who might become pregnant should only ever get prescriptions of medicines that have been proven for many years. Even 'medication that is not known to have any toxic effects is not necessarily safe' (Müller-Oerlinghausen 1998).

Medications that are known to have a teratogenic effect include: anticonvulsants such as valproic acid, phenytoin or carbamazepine, diethylstilbestrol, lithium, phenobarbital, tetracycline, thalidomide, warfarin and high doses of vitamin A. According to Schaefer (2001), the risk of teratogenic damage is greatest between the 15th and 60th days of conception.

Alcohol

Drinking alcohol during pregnancy can cause major growth disturbances in the child, especially during the early development, which may be before the mother knows she is pregnant. Alcohol probably has an inhibitory effect on cell division and migration. Studies with pregnant sheep have shown that alcohol reduces the bloodflow in the fetal brain (Nathanielz 1999).

Fetal alcohol syndrome (FAS) is the extreme consequence of drinking alcohol while pregnant. According to Rossi (1989), FAS is as common as Down syndrome, namely 1:700 newborns. Children with FAS are normally small and thin. They are typically slow to grow, and even with a good diet fail to put on weight ('thrive'). This is probably due to the generally reduced number of cells, as alcohol inhibits early cell division. According to Rossi, there is microcephalus, and mental and motor retardation in about 90% of cases. Characteristic growth abnormalities of the face such as mandibular hypoplasia are common. Heart defects are found in 40%. Behavioral disturbances and hyperactivity are also symptoms of FAS. It is not clear whether there are 'safe' limits for alcohol consumption in pregnancy. Even with a low alcohol consumption of 1–2 units a week, there is believed to be a correlation with restlessness in newborns and babies.

Fertility treatment

Fertility problems are common. Up to 15% of all couples in Germany remain childless despite wishing for a child. The WHO speaks of sterility if pregnancy has failed to occur after a year, despite the desire for a child and regular sexual intercourse.

Fertility has declined in our culture over the last 30 years. There are probably many reasons for this. One is that many women wait, or are unable, to start a family until later in life, when their fertility is physiologically less than it was when they were in their twenties. One frequent organic cause is a blockage in the tubes. Hormonal problems or myomas can make conception difficult, and there appears to be a correlation between endometriosis and childlessness.

However, there are also many factors that can impair the man's ability to reproduce. Various studies have shown that stress can also affect sperm quality. Sperm function can be impaired by pesticides, solvents or estrogens in foods. It is therefore recommended that the parents-to-be detoxify in order to achieve optimum general health.

Fertility treatment (artificial insemination or in-vitro fertilization, IVF) has been possible since the mid-1980s, and has become commonplace. 'The number of attempts at artificial insemination has increased consistently in recent years. 66,000 German couples used IVF in 2000. Four years before that, it was just half that number; 14 years before less than one-tenth' (Spiewak 2002).

In Germany today, 1–2% percent of newborns are conceived outside the mother's body. Children's practices, including osteopathy clinics, are seeing more and more children who were conceived by IVF or ICSI (intracytoplasmatic sperm injection).

In-vitro fertilization (IVF) and embryo transfer (ET)

In IVF, the woman's natural hormone production is deactivated so that the cycle can be controlled externally with drugs, and to prevent premature ovulation. Drugs are then used to stimulate the ovaries so that, ideally, 6–10 follicles ripen in a cycle, thereby increasing the chances of success. Once ovulation has been stimulated chemically, the follicles are harvested using a vaginal probe (follicular puncture). The partner's sperm is prepared. Egg cells and spermatazoa are then placed in an incubator in a nutrient solution and cultivated. Pre-nuclei are visible after 16–20 h, and 12 h later the egg cell begins to divide. 40–72 h after harvesting, the embryo consists of between two and six cells, and can be implanted in the uterus. This is called embryo transfer (ET). In Germany, a maximum of three embryos can be implanted in one cycle. Two or three embryos are passed into the uterus lumen via a special transfer catheter, and with any luck will implant in the normal way.

In 3% of successful IVF attempts, all three embryos will continue to develop. Although implanting several embryos increases the success rate, a multiple pregnancy brings with it its own risks – especially in the event of triplets. Because there is an increased risk of disability in triplet births, it is estimated that in Germany about 150 abortions, euphemistically termed 'reductions,' are carried out every year (Spiewak 2002). One solution is to implant only two embryos.

Blastocyst transfer (BT)

In this procedure, the embryo is not implanted into the uterus until the 5th or 6th day. For this, the most developed blastocyte with the best 'look' is selected. This procedure is more labor-intensive and more expensive, but it is also more successful. In Germany, BT is not possible due to the embryo protection laws: because no more than three embryos may be cultivated at once, not enough blastocytes are available from which to choose.

Embryo protection law in Germany

Once the egg is fertilized, that is to say the sperm has penetrated the egg and there are two cell nuclei, called pronuclei, each with half a set of chromosomes, it may be selected or discarded. These fertilized early-stage egg cells may also be frozen and used later for IVF. The chances of becoming pregnant are then lower, but the woman needs less hormonal stimulation and there is no follicular puncture.

However, once the two nuclei have combined after 24–48 h then it is an 'embryo', and they are protected in Germany. The embryo protection law is intended to prevent, for ethical reasons, the production of embryos for other than reproductive purposes.

Pre-implantation diagnosis (PID)

PID has been used in various countries such as Belgium and Great Britain since the beginning of the 1990s. In 2002 there were an estimated 1000 PID children all over the world, but this form of diagnosis has now increased significantly. In PID, before it is implanted, a cell is extracted from the embryo by biopsy and its chromosomal and genetic quality checked. Certain genetic defects can be identified, and the corresponding selection is made. In some countries, however, this procedure is also used for gender selection.

PID is banned in Germany under the embryo protection law.

Intracytoplasmatic sperm injection (ICSI)

In ICSI the sperm is injected directly into the cytoplasm with the help of a microscope. It was invented in 1991, almost by accident. A researcher in a fertility clinic at the Free University of Brussels accidentally penetrated the membrane of an egg cell as he was depositing a sperm in front of the egg cell using a pipette. When, to the amazement of all, the damaged egg cell developed into an embryo, the procedure was followed up. The first ICSI baby was born in 1992. Since then the method has been used many times.

ICSI is used when there are andrological factors and the sperm are unable to fertilize the egg cell for some reason. The reasons may be a low sperm count, poor motility, a high level of malformed sperm, or a combination of all these factors. ICSI fertilization can also be promising if, for instance, the husband suffers from a systemic disease or if frozen sperm are used following treatment for testicular cancer.

Stimulation and egg harvesting are the same as in IVF.

The egg cell is then released from the surrounding cells using enzymes, and mechanically from the surrounding corona radiatio. A single sperm is aspirated using a microneedle and carefully flushed into the cytoplasm of the egg cell.

Consequences of IVF/ICSI for the parents

Attempts at conceiving a child by means of IVF or ICSI cause much inner conflict, and are therefore emotionally and psychologically trying. According to Zuber-Jerger (2002), IVF is the next most stressful life event after the death of a close family member. There is much criticism of the fact that fertility treatment mostly concentrates exclusively on the rectification of organic disturbances and/or overcoming them by means of extracorporeal fertilization. There is little in the way of psychological support when it fails.

It is estimated that some 50% of women still fail to conceive despite repeated attempts at IVF. Another point to bear in mind is that pregnancy does not necessarily result in a child.

Only in 10–13% of all cases can the partners expect a successful pregnancy and the birth of a child after IVF or ICSI (Telus 2001, Spiewak 2002). This is the realistic baby take-home rate for each cycle of hormonal stimulation that is commenced. And yet information brochures from fertility clinics often quote a success rate of 25–35% per attempt.

The treatment risks for the woman include ovarian hyperstimulation syndrome, the develoment of cysts on the ovaries, possible injury or infection when the eggs are harvested, an increased rate of multiple pregnancy, a miscarriage rate of 25% as opposed to 15% in natural conception, and a high rate of depression.

Consequences of IVF/ICSI for the baby

Research into the effects on the babies have until now invariably focused on the results immediately after delivery. Babies born after IVF or ICSI often have a lower birthweight than after normal conception. This is usually ascribed to the parents' infertility.

The research also sought to establish whether the rate of congenital malformation was higher after ICSI than after natural conception. A German study found major malformations in 8.6% of all ICSI/IVF pregnancies compared with 6.9% in natural pregnancies. An Australian study found a malformation rate of 8.6% compared with 4.2% in the control group. The research addressed the question whether this was due to the method of obtaining the egg cells/sperm, the in vitro culture or other factors such as the age of the parents (Schuh 2004). New studies have shown that there is no increased risk of malformation when women of the same age are compared. In the first-mentioned studies the ICSI women were much older than the control group who conceived naturally. So it would appear that a higher rate of malformation is only due to the increased age of the parents and has nothing to do with the method of conception.

However, some fertility centers recommend amniocentesis and potential selection. There have not yet been any major studies that also address the long-term consequences of artificial insemination.

An osteopathic examination of children conceived with ICSI-IVF using the involuntary movement often shows a lack of orientation to the mid-line. It is then difficult to feel a strong, regular expression of involuntary motion when palpating; the system feels chaotic. The treatment of biomechanical problems is more successful if this condition is addressed first.

The importance of affection, ambivalence or rejection by the parents

Children, even before they are born, appear to have a kind of emotional radar. Verny (1988) speaks of 'sympathetic' communication. We know that physiological communication occurs between the mother and her child via hormones;

I also believe that a form of perception exists on a soul level that cannot be explained by a physiological-medical model.

The main concern for children is that their will to live is acknowledged. Babies' chances of survival are much better if they are accepted by their parents. In his article 'Isolation, rejection and communion in the womb,' Verny (1988) offers the theory that psychological, social and developmental damage is more likely in children who were rejected before birth than in the control groups. He refers to several studies. One, by Coker at the University of South Carolina 1994, shows, for example, that the probability of death in the first year of life is more than twice as likely in babies from unwanted pregnancies than in babies who were wanted. The group used in the investigation consisted of married women with good medical care and no financial concerns.

Janus quotes a 1974 study by Rottman that differentiated between three groups of mothers: those who looked forward to their babies, those who were ambivalent and 'catastrophic' mothers who rejected their child. After the birth the ambivalent and catastrophic mothers had a higher rate of babies with hyperactivity and vomiting, and among the rejecting mothers there were more babies who alternated between apathy and excessive crying. The fathers' roles were not included in the study.

Of course, not all parents are instantly delighted about a pregnancy. Sometimes their relationship is too uncertain to offer a safe base; sometimes life plans have to be questioned and the parents-to-be have to adjust. Fortunately, most are able to adjust happily to the new situation and accept the child. According to Findeisen (1994), such a situation is an injury to the baby, but it can and will heal if the baby is loved after birth. However, if the rejection continues then the disturbance deepens. Fleeting ambivalence during pregnancy is undoubtedly normal, and should not be given too much consideration. According to Verny: 'Occasional negative feelings or stress will not have a negative influence on intrauterine bonding.'

Sometimes the mother also withdraws internally from the baby, perhaps because she is ill or if she is grieving for a loved one. In certain circumstances this may lead to feelings of rejection in the unborn child, since babies perceive everything in relationship to themselves. Verny believes this may be a cause of later depression.

The following observations quoted by Chamberlain (2001), which were made often in association with amniocentesis, are interesting in relation to communication and perception by the unborn child. After all, the main question with amniocentesis is: Do we want you? Are you good enough? 'When the fluid has been taken for amniocentesis, some fetuses freeze as if frightened or in shock; their heart rate increases and then drops again. … In some studies the fetus's breathing movements dropped dramatically, occasionally even taking several days to return to the former frequency. Doctors do not know why the loss of such a small amount of liquid leads to these reactions, especially as amniotic fluid forms particularly quickly.'

Bonding before and after the birth

Obviously the child's well-being before and after birth depends directly on the mother and father. The best way of supporting the baby prenatally and during development is by supporting the mother and father during pregnancy. The greater the parents' well-being, the better it is for the baby.

The first pregnancy and delivery are particularly liable to bring fears and depression to the surface – or to reopen psychological wounds about a parent's own family history. When a child is brought to the practice, the osteopath automatically observes the interaction between the mother and child or father and child. How relaxed are they? Are they able to relax with their child? What is communication between the three like? Are the mother or father so involved in their own stress that they fail to acknowledge their child properly? In cases such as these it may be more important to treat the parent than the child.

It is not about making sure that the mother is always happy after the birth and is a 'good mother'. Her presence and acknowledgement are much more important for the baby. So it may be important to support the mother in acknowledging what and how she is – even if she is sad and not the blooming, socially recognized, radiant mother-to-be or new mother.

Compensation through postnatal contact and care

Back in the 1950s, the researcher Levine was the first to demonstrate in animal tests that increased contact and stroking after birth had a significant effect on improving life-long susceptibility to stress. Several other studies have been carried out since then, all of which show that early life experiences, especially maternal care, can change the setting of the brain–hypophysis–adrenal gland axis in its response to stress. Contact and stroking are of particular importance. Animal trials confirmed that increased contact raised the number of receptors for the adrenal gland hormones in the hippocampus, and thus reinforced the feedback mechanism.

Conversely, Nemeroff showed that baby rats who were separated from their mothers for 6h a day between days 2 and 20 responded to stress with a higher cortisol level in later life (quoted in Nathanielz 1999).

If these findings are transposed to humans, it follows that the more attention, caresses and contact a human being has

in early life, the less susceptible she will be to stress in later life. Janus (2001) also writes of compensation through postnatal circumstances, especially skin contact. 'However, it is widely agreed … that unfavourable pre- and perinatal circumstances can be corrected by favourable postnatal conditions, but that unfavourable postnatal conditions will keep the early trauma alive and have a negative effect on subsequent conflict situations.'

Relier (1999) writes thus on the subject of prenatal stress: 'The mother can not only screen her baby from most of these "environmental influences", but she also plays a major role in the healing capacities that … lead to a complete return to normal bodily functions, thanks to the adaptability that characterizes almost all [the baby's] organs during this stage of development. … This ability to recover is … influenced markedly by the quality of the bond with the mother.' He quotes his colleague Godfrey: 'Love, whose impact cannot yet be measured, undoubtedly represents the peripheral or environmental stimulation that is most important to ensure the growth and harmonious equilibrium of the infant.'

The effect of prenatal physical or emotional trauma

What does it mean for the baby to experience physical or emotional stress prenatally? How does her body respond, and how can we help the child with osteopathy?

According to Perry (1998), trauma throws the organism off balance; it responds in turn with regulatory compensation mechanisms. This compensation results in turn in a new but less flexible state of balance. However, this new homeostatic condition needs more energy than the previous one did and does not adjust so well to new circumstances; it will therefore be less flexible when responding to a new trauma. 'Trauma induced homeostasis consumes more energy and is maladaptive compared with "normal" homeostasis. By inducing this expensive homeostasis and compromising full functional capacity, trauma robs the organism. It has survived the traumatic experience, but at a cost.'

Prenatal experiences probably determine to a large extent how a child experiences the perinatal stage and may process a trauma during birth. When examining children osteopathically, we see frequently that some children come out of birth quite well, with no major structural or functional restrictions, even if the birth was traumatic. The reason for this may be that these children experienced an exchange with their environment intrauterinely and postnatally that gave them everything they needed. Their bodies and souls suffered no trauma before birth, and still possess their full ability to compensate. According to Hayden (2004), here the potency is expressed well in involuntary motion; the organism is able to respond, regulate and correct itself optimally. Either these children need no osteopathic support to unfold after birth or, if we do treat them, the asymmetries soon correct themselves.

Other children may have experienced in utero a discrepancy between that which they needed and what they actually got, but were able to bear it. They got what they needed most; growth and development follow the original plan. The potency is probably somewhat limited, but still able to function through health. Hayden (2004) quotes F. Lake on this topic: 'The conditions are not perfect, but good enough for the basically secure self to "go along with it". These individuals are used to having to make the best of situations, and may be better placed to cope with later troubles than those for whom their development has been "ideal".'

This is an interesting point. Something not perfect can even be positive, because this stimulates our own innate activity which will help us adapt to difficult situations later in life. How comforting, because circumstances are often far from ideal!

There is of course a flowing transition between that which is not perfect on the one side, and trauma on the other. Our body responds in a number of different ways to trauma of any kind. Our brain also responds and attempts to integrate the threat. That is why unborn and small children whose brains are still developing are particularly vulnerable with regard to traumatic experiences. For adults, most new experiences are only partly new; all they really do is modify neurological patterns that are already being used. In a child, this experience may be the first one, the one which everything else builds on. That is why early experiences are so formative.

These primary experiences determine the basic organization and homeostatis of the neurological key systems. 'Experience in adults alters the organized brain, but in infants and children it organizes the developing brain....the experiences of early childhood create patterns of neuronal activity that will become the template neural networks and patterns against which all future experience will be sensed, processed, and internalized' (Perry 1998).

Depending on the extent of it, a trauma will reach or exceed the boundaries of our ability to compensate. The organism always responds with the best possible compensation, but this requires strength, and it makes the organism less flexible when it then needs to respond to a new trauma. This is a good answer to the question of why some babies have difficulties in compensating even minor birth-related asymmetries after an apparently untraumatic birth, to say nothing of the complicated patterns that result from a difficult birth. In such cases the primary respiratory mechanism does not respond so well to our treatment; the expression of potency is restricted or suppressed by an experienced trauma. Extreme trauma may even render the mechanism unable to act.

In our treatment we work with the existing expression of potency in the tide. We respect the experienced trauma without focussing on it. This often enables the mechanism to orientate itself to the pre-traumatic expression of the potency, and the vitality in the mechanism is improved.

Understanding the reason for a restriction can help in treating it. In such a multidimensional topic as this, we are often left to surmise. We rarely deal in black-and-white scenarios. For that reason, it should also be emphasized that only in rare cases will we verbalize our diagnosis to the parents. It would mostly only cause feelings of guilt or put us in a situation for which we do not have the correct psychological training. Nor is there any desire to be seen as clever experts in prenatal trauma. Evaluation often leads to devaluation.

Rather, we need to achieve acceptance, to create a safe environment for the child – but also for the parents. The ultimate objective is that what was experienced is allowed to exist, and the effort and the battle are also acknowledged and honoured. Often no words are necessary.

The discussion concerning prenatal influences is designed to encourage further study in this area. This helps us to see what support, but also what challenges, the surrounding world offers already to the unborn baby.

POSSIBLE QUESTIONS IN CASE HISTORY TAKING

(see also Ch.7, Case history)

With regard to possible fears or unchanged ambivalence on the part of the mother and/or father, it is worth asking the following questions during case history taking:

- Was your baby planned or a surprise?

- Was your partner also pleased about the pregnancy, or did he have to get used to the idea?

- Satisfaction in the partnership: How are you as a family able to cope with the changes that having a child brings? Do the parents feel they mutually support each other?

- Do those around you, e.g. grandparents, support you? Did they do so during the pregnancy too?

- Did you undergo hormone or fertility treatment before pregnancy (IVF, ICSI)?

Any illnesses or accidents on the part of the mother, stress at work, in the family or as the result of moving house, deaths and so on are also relevant during pregnancy.

Bibliography

Blechschmidt E: Wie beginnt das menschliche Leben: Vom Ei zum Embryo. 6th edn. Christiana, Stein am Rhein 1989

Chamberlain D: Woran Babys sich erinnern. 5th edn. Kösel, Munich 2001

Charlton A: Tobacco and Health. British Med Bull 52, 1996: 90–107

Choquet M, Ledoux S: La valeur prognostique des indicateurs de risques precoces. Etude longitudinale des enfants a risque a 3 ans. Arch F Pediatr 42, 1985: 541–546

Choquet M, Facy F, Laurent F, Davidson F: Les enfants a risque en age prescolaire. Arch F Pediatr 39, 1982: 185–192

Findeisen B: Kein Baby sollte unerwünscht sein. In: Häsing, Janus: Ungewollte Kinder. Rowohlt, Hamburg 1994

Fishel S: Pregnancy after intracytoplasmatic injection of spermatids. The Lancet 345, 1995: 1641–1642

Groβ U, Roos T, Friese K: Toxoplasmose in der Schwangerschaft. Dt Ärzteblatt 98, 2001: A3293–3300

Hayden L: Factors affecting conception and pregnancy that influence the potency of the mechanism. Lecture, pediatric course at Sutherland Cranial College UK 2004

Henderson C: Prenatal and birth trauma patterns: what to look out for in the treatment room. The Tide, Journal of the Sutherland Society UK, Autumn edn. 1998

Hooker D: The prenatal origin of behaviour. University of Kansas Press, Lawrence, Kansas 1952

Humphrey T: Some correlations between the appearance of human fetal reflexes and the development of the nervous system. Brain Research 4, 1964: 93–135

Huttunen R, Niskanen P: Prenatal loss of father and psychiatric disorders. Archives of General Psychiatry 35, 1978: 429–431

Janus L, Haibach S: Seelisches Erleben vor und während der Geburt. LinguaMed, Neu-Isenburg 1997

Janus L: Die Psychoanalyse der vorgeburtlichen Lebenszeit und der Geburt. Psychosozial, Giessen 2000

Janus L: The enduring effects of prenatal experience. Mattes, Heidelberg 2001

Kelm-Kahl I: Arzneimittel in der Schwangerschaft. Hebammenforum 8, 2004: 548

Krens I, Krens H: Grundlagen einer vorgeburtlichen Psychologie. Vandenhoek und Ruprecht, Göttingen 2005

Krüll M: Die Geburt ist nicht der Anfang. 4th edn. Klett-Cotta, Stuttgart 1997

Kuemmerle H, Brendel K: Clinical pharmacology in pregnancy. Thieme, Stuttgart 1984

Lackmann G, Salzberger U, Hecht S, Töllner U: Rauchen während der Schwangerschaft. Dt. Ärzteblatt 96, 1999: A2080–2083

Müller-Oerlinghausen B: Arzneimittel in der Schwangerschaft und Stillzeit. Dt Ärztebl 95, 1998: C957–960

Nathanielsz P: Life in the womb – the origin of health and disease. Promethean, New York 1999

Perry B, Pollard R: Homeostasis, stress, trauma and adaptation – a neurodevelopmental view of childhood trauma. In: Stress in children. Baylor College of Medicine, Texas 1998

Piontelli A: Vom Fetus zum Kind: Die Ursprünge des psychischen Lebens. Klett-Cotta, Stuttgart 1996

Relier J: Importance of fetal perceptions in the organization of the mother–fetus interactions. In: Biology of the neonate. 69, 1996: 165–212

Relier J: Influence of maternal stress on fetal behaviour and brain development. Biology of the neonate. 79, 1996: 168–171

Relier J: Liebe und Stress im pränatalen Leben. lecture, 3rd European Osteopathy Symposium, Fraueninsel Chiemsee, February 1999

Richard S: Influence du vecu emotionnel de la femme enceinte sur le temperament et la sante physique du nourrisson. In: Relier J: Progres en neonatologie 10, 1990: 202–223

Rossi E: Pädiatrie. 2nd edn. Thieme, Stuttgart 1989

Schaefer C, Koch I: Die Beratung der Schwangeren und Stillenden zum Medikamentenrisiko. Dt Ärztebl 95, 1998: C1874–1876

Schaefer J, Spielmann H: Arzneiverordnung in Schwangerschaft und Stillzeit. 6. edn. Urban & Fischer, Munich/Jena 2001

Schuh H: Roulette in der Retorte. Die Zeit, 9th June 2004

Spiewak M: Wie weit gehen wir für ein Kind? Eichborn, Frankfurt 2002

Stott H: Follow-up study from birth of the effects of prenatal stresses. Developmental Medicine and Child Neurology 15, 1973: 770–787

Telus M: Reproduktionsmedizin – Zwischen Trauma und Tabu. Dtsch Ärztebl 51–52, 2001: A3430–3434

Verny T: The secret life of the unborn child. 2nd edn. Dell Trade, New York 1988

Verny T: Isolation, rejection and communion in the womb. International Journal of Prenatal and Perinatal Psychology and Medicine 8, 1996:287–294

Zuber-Jerger I: Zu hohe Risikobereitschaft. Dtsch Ärztebl 19, 2002: A617–619

5

Birth and treating the baby

Liz Hayden, Eva Moeckel

'The osteopath who succeeds best does so because he looks to Nature for knowledge and obeys her teaching. ... one asks how we may know the normal' (Still 1910).

For optimum treatment, it is important to have a clear idea of how labor usually progresses, of the most frequent complications and medical interventions. That makes it easier to understand the forces that the child we treat may have been exposed to during the birth process. These influences can vary tremendously: they can be mechanical, stress-related, psychological or metabolic-toxic if drugs are used. An understanding of the birth process also makes it easier to communicate with parents, midwives and doctors.

Children's antenatal health on every level plays a key role in determining how their systems handle the forces they are exposed to at birth. The environment into which a child is born is also important. Often we find that children are well able to compensate for a very stressful delivery if their living conditions, and especially the emotional environment, are optimum. So we are dealing with a large puzzle of different influences before, during and after birth.

If the pregnancy and labor go well, there will be a good, vital expression in the tissues when assessing joint mobility and palpating tissue expression using involuntary motion in the newborn. Then there is often nothing, or only a little to treat; perhaps just a little support for the child's normal process of unfolding after birth. However, the stress patterns that may occur after a lengthy delivery or the use of forceps or ventouse do usually require osteopathic treatment. In our postnatal examination it is also important to establish whether the vitality of the child's tissues is likely to facilitate self-correction after delivery. Any drugs or anesthesia given during labor may hinder this process.

Apart from physical strains, there may be psychological birth patterns that stay with us for life, such as those experienced by babies who are born by caesarean section (English 1997). Nor can physical birth patterns always be dissolved. Usually, the sooner any strains or restrictions of motion that are caused by birth are treated, the more successful treatment will be. And yet experienced practitioners are still amazed at how stubbornly birth-related dysfunctions can persist. Many of our colleagues therefore like to see

children they have already treated once a year for follow-up treatment.

It can be helpful both for treatment and prognosis to have an idea what influences may have caused the functional impairments in the child's system. To make labor and delivery possible, many factors come together in the most wonderful way. Even today we still do not fully understand what they all are and do. The psychological and physical condition of a mother-to-be and child definitely both play a large part in determining what the birth will be like.

Osteopathic treatments can benefit the mother both before delivery and afterwards to support the physical and emotional changes that becoming a parent and being a mother bring – and fathers can also benefit from treatment (see Ch.3, Preparing for pregnancy, onwards). Osteopathic treatments will also help the newborn in the process of adapting. The actual birth, though, is a very private matter. Michel Odent, a well-known French obstetrician who is based in London, was quoted thus by his colleague Gordon: 'The more people there are around, the longer it takes. And if practitioners such as osteopaths and acupuncturists are around too, it takes even longer!' (Personal message 1991).

NORMAL LABOR

Eva Moeckel

In labor, mother and child cooperate. The opening of the bony and the soft tissue birth canal is determined by the mother, as are the contractions; and not for nothing is the process known as 'labor.' The child positions and molds himself to adapt to the passage through the birth canal, and plays an important part in starting the contractions.

The birth canal

Mechanism of labor

The baby's head normally fits perfectly inside each part of the small pelvis. Seen from above, the pelvic inlet, which is level with the promontory of the sacrum and the upper edge of the symphysis, forms a distinct transverse oval. The head engages transversely in order to position itself optimally in the pelvic inlet (Fig. 5.1a).

The pelvic cavity below that is almost round. This is where both the narrowest and widest parts of the pelvis are to be found. The narrowest part is at the level of the ischial spines, and it can be widened using the thigh as a lever if the woman closes her knees during the first stage of expulsion (Steffen 2002). In order to pass through the pelvic cavity the head flexes (chin on chest) and rotates by 90º (Fig. 5.1b, c).

The pelvic outlet between the coccyx and the lower edge of the symphysis is a longitudinal oval (longer from front to back). It may extend by approximately 2 cm during the birth as the baby's head pushes the coccyx back. The symphysis is used to support the back of the head while the head is born by deflexion (Fig. 5.1d). So one after the other the back of the head, forehead, face and chin appear over the perineum.

While the head is born through the longitudinal oval of the pelvic outlet, the shoulders fit exactly in the transverse oval pelvic inlet. During passage through the pelvic cavity, the baby then rotates by 90º, usually back into the original position (Fig. 5.1e), so first one and then the other shoulder can be born (Fig. 5.1f).

The hormones estrogen and relaxin, which are produced by the mother's corpus luteum during pregnancy, help to loosen the iliosacral joints and the symphysis, which is known as adaptation of the pelvis. This enables the pelvic girdle to enlarge to some degree to assist the passage of the baby.

Position of the mother

The mother's position during birth has also an important influence on the diameter of the pelvis. If, for instance, the mother spends a lot of time lying down during the first stage of labor, the uterus and its contents will press against her spine: the angle of descent of the baby's head will be changed. The head presses against the lower part of the uterus with each contraction and less efficiently against the cervix. This can slow down labor (Fig. 5.2a).

However, if the mother leans forward, gravity will take the uterus so far forward that the baby's head will adjust properly to the pelvic inlet and push directly against the cervix as desired (Fig. 5.2b).

It certainly helps if the mother keeps moving during labor. Certain positions may have a positive influence on the progression of labor. The midwife's awareness and knowledge of what the head has to do next is important. Thus, for instance, if the mothers legs are bent as in squatting, then the symphysis shifts cranially and the longitudinal diameter of the pelvic outlet may extend by up to 2 cm. This makes it easier for the head to emerge. Other positions may

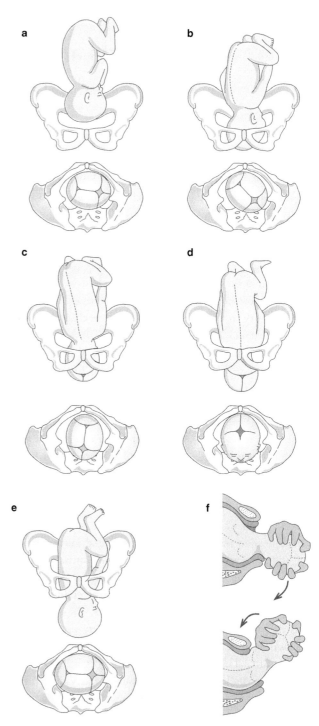

Figure 5.1 Mechanics of labor. **a:** Head entering into the pelvic inlet. **b:** Rotation of the head in the pelvic cavity. **c:** Head against the pelvic floor. **d:** Head being born via the perineum. **e:** External rotation of the head. **f:** Birth of the shoulders.
With permission, S Adler, Lübeck

also be beneficial, such as resting on all fours – which also opens the pelvis – or active hanging positions during the second stage, which protect the pelvic floor. At this stage the mother should avoid sitting with a rounded back, as the

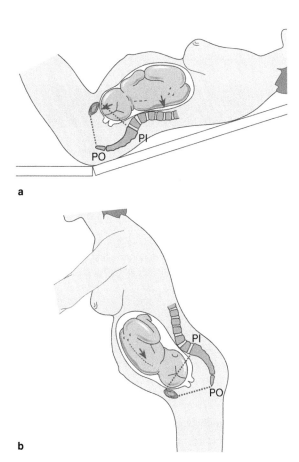

a

b

Figure 5.2 Positions of the mother during the first stage of labor. *PI* = pelvic inlet, *PO* = pelvic outlet. **a:** Lying on her back is less advantageous. **b:** Supporting herself while leaning forward is better. With permission, Henriette Rintelen, Velbert

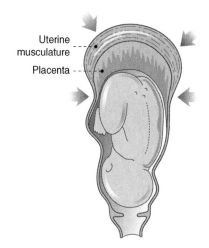

Uterine musculature

Placenta

Figure 5.3 Functional division of the uterus during labor into an upper active and lower passive section. With permission, Henriette Rintelen, Velbert

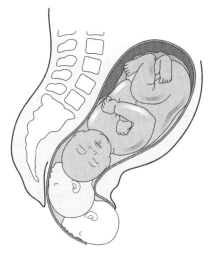

Figure 5.4 The 'birth axis'. With permission, Henriette Rintelen, Velbert

coccyx is then unable to move. Nor will the pelvis open properly if she is lying on her back; lying on the side is more advantageous.

The musculature

The uterus has two different areas of function during labor. The upper part contracts concentrically, which pushes the baby down. The lower part is more passive and opens gradually with the cervix (Fig. 5.3). The lower segment of the uterus and the cervix have a rich supply of sympathetic fibres; they may possibly not open easily if there is a raised sympathetic tone.

The so-called muscular birth canal, through which the baby is pushed by the contractions, consists of the lower part of the uterus, the cervix, the vagina and the musculature of the pelvic floor, which is normally about 4 cm thick but changes into a long tube of about 15 cm during the second stage. The levator ani muscle has an important mechanical function in labor: it guides the baby downwards towards the pelvic outlet, and supports him as he rotates.

Birth axis

As he moves down during the birth, the baby rotates on an axis that runs from the navel of the mother to the coccyx (Fig. 5.4). This means that the anus becomes very thinly stretched at a certain point. Only once the head has moved far enough below the symphysis does it move down along a vertical axis, and then forwards.

Physiological contractions before birth

Contractions are the periodic contractions, or movements, of the uterine muscles during pregnancy and labor.

Pregnancy contractions (Braxton Hicks)

From early in the pregnancy these occur as uncoordinated contractions. The woman generally does not notice them during

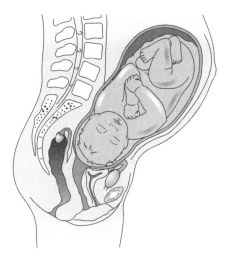

Figure 5.5 Due to physiological contractions, 'false labor' or 'lightening,' the baby lowers in the last few weeks before delivery. With permission, Henriette Rintelen, Velbert

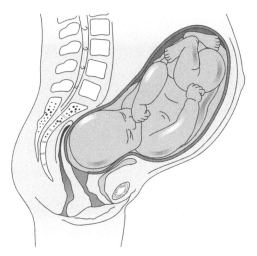

Figure 5.6 Position of the child during the first stage of labor. With permission, Henriette Rintelen, Velbert

pregnancy, or if she does then only as a slight tightening in her lower abdomen. A normal average is 30–40 contractions a day. They probably aid blood circulation and the development of the myometrium.

'False labor' or 'Lightening'

Physiological contractions which occur about 4 weeks before the due date are called 'false labor' or 'lightening.' The mother usually notices these contractions as a hardening of the abdomen. Their task is to help the lower segments of the uterus to open out. The baby can then move further down towards the pelvic inlet (Fig. 5.5), allowing more room for the mother's diaphragm, her breathing to become easier and relieve the pressure on her stomach. However, there is now less room for her bladder, as the result of which she has a more frequent urge to urinate.

The head moves over the pelvic inlet so that the sagittal suture is transverse or at a slight angle. It is still in a neutral position, with the neck neither flexed nor extended. Usually only when labor starts does the head move into the pelvic inlet for the first stage of labor, which is called 'engaging'. Sometimes the head engages several weeks before the onset of labor, which may restrict further growth and/or produce some degree of intraosseous compression or distortion in the cranium before the onset of labor.

Premonitory pains

Premonitory pains usually occur in the last weeks or days of a pregnancy, are quite noticeable or even painful, and may therefore be confused with the first stage of labor. These contractions stretch and soften the cervix.

Stages of labor

Labor is a carefully graded physiological process that every woman experiences differently – and presumably every baby too.

First stage

The first stage usually begins after some irregular contractions with regular contractions every 3–6 minutes or with the mother's waters breaking. It lasts between 3 and 30 hours. There are massive differences in the frequency of contractions: in some women they follow each other closely, whereas others may have long breaks in between. The first stage ends when the cervix is fully dilated at approximately 10 cm.

The baby's head is pushed into the funnel-shaped pelvic inlet during the first stage. Now it gradually opens the cervix. 'The neck of the womb … is folded in such a way that the canal easily extends from 5 mm to 100 mm provided there are no spasms or scars to hinder it …. The fibrous system of the cervix is pleated so that all it has to do for the cervix to dilate fully is unfold; there is no stretching of this fibrous system. The same applies for the vagina' (Rockenschaub 2001). The baby moves down towards the dilating cervix. In order to adapt better to the circular pelvic cavity, he bends and begins to rotate at the same time (Fig. 5.6).

Transitional stage

This is often the most strenuous time, and can last up to several hours. With his head down, the baby moves out of the uterus deep down into the maternal pelvis and into the birth canal (Fig. 5.7). The contractions are now more frequent and usually perceived as painful. Intra-amniotic pressure increases to 50–60 mmHg.

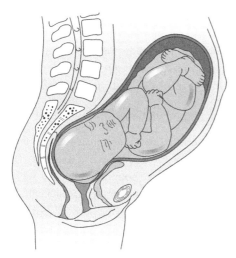

Figure 5.7 Position of the child during the transitional stage of labor.
With permission, Henriette Rintelen, Velbert

The mother often feels extremely emotional during this stage; her feeling is: I can only go forwards; there's no going back. And I've got to have this baby all by myself. Odent (2001) describes a sudden change in the woman's hormone level at this time, which is expressed as fear, anger or euphoria. Odent uses this change in behavior to also define the beginning of the second stage of labor. Between the transitional and second stages the contractions may often, but not always, stop for up to 10 minutes.

Second stage

The contractions slow down slightly in the second stage, and they are different. Many women find them easier to bear. Now the cervix is no longer opening; the baby is being pushed out. In a maximum of 3–4 bearing down pains /10 minutes, the mother may push – 'bear down' – two or three times per contraction.

Due to the contractions during the second stage the uterus lengthens. This elongation happens because the muscular body of the uterus gets tighter during contractions. Both uterus and baby stretch towards the cervix. The baby which, curled up before birth, measured 24–26 cm from vertex to coccyx, now extends another 8–10 cm to about 34 cm (Fig. 5.8a). These 8–10 cm equate to the distance that the head needs to move down to get from the pelvic inlet to the outlet.

The baby's head also continues rotating to complete the 90º turn, and arrives at the pelvic floor in the correct position for passage through the pelvic outlet. As the opening it needs to pass through is a longitudinal-oval gap; the head moves through it most easily if the sagittal suture is lined up with the longitudinal diameter of the opening. The baby usually rotates so that his face is towards the mother's back. The

baby's head then follows the birth canal, which is directed anteriorly, in an arch around the symphysis. The head also extends in a movement that is known as deflexion.

In order to pass through the pelvic floor, there is now an additional surge of muscle power in the form of abdominal press, which is activated by a reflex. As the baby's head pushes against the pelvic floor with a contraction, the abdominal muscles contract in reflex.

A sudden increase in epinephrine (adrenaline) seems to be important for strong, effective contractions in the actual expulsion of the baby, unlike in the earlier stage of labor when high levels of epinephrine may inhibit the contractions. The intervals between contractions are usually longer during expulsion. This could be because the women now needs all her strength to push, and so she is given little breaks to recover. The baby also needs time to recover between contractions, because the oxygen supply is physiologically reduced during contractions. Whether this hypoxemia has any detrimental effect depends on the possibilities for compensation offered during the aforementioned intervals between contractions. If contractions are forced during the second stage and there are no adequate rests between contractions there is a risk of a lack of oxygen. The same may happen if the placenta is small or for some other reason not working to its full capacity.

Even if the hypoxemia is not so severe that it leads to permanent neurological damage, it does obviously stress the child. Due to the temporary lack of oxygen generalized 'shock patterns' may result, which can be palpated by the trained osteopath.

Because the occipital bone of the baby's cranium uses the pubic symphysis as a pivot point during the second stage of labor (Carreiro 2004), if the second stage is long it may encourage intraosseous dysfunctions of the occipital bone. Sergueff (1995) is also of the opinion that the occipital bone can be subjected to high pressure at this stage (Fig. 5.8b).

Once the head has appeared, the baby's body has to turn back in order for the shoulders to be born using the more favorable anteroposterior diameter (Fig. 5.8c). Once the shoulders have been born, the rest of the body slides out smoothly.

Pressure during labor

One question that never fails to fascinate osteopaths who work with children using Dr. Sutherland's approach is: what pressure is the baby's cranium subjected to during birth, and what may be the consequences of that?

Depending on the stage in labor, the pressure of a contraction can be 20–60 mmHg. This is illustrated more clearly in the following: the pressure exerted by the contractions on the baby's cranium in the first stage is the same as at

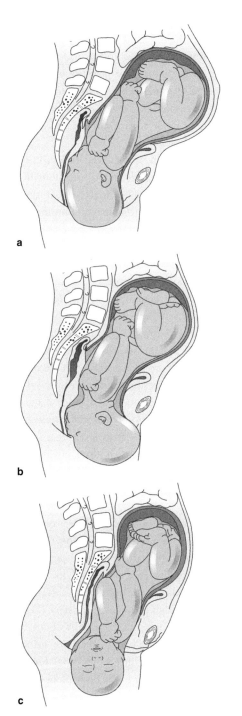

Figure 5.8 Position of the baby during the second stage of labor. **a:** The baby extends towards the cervix. **b:** The occipital bone uses the pubic symphysis as a pivot point. **c:** The shoulders are born through the more favourable anteroposterior diameter of the pelvic outlet.
With permission, Henriette Rintelen, Velbert

Montevideo units (MU). MU not only include the strength of the contraction, but also the frequency (contractions/ 10 min × average pressure in mmHg). A value of 100 MU is considered normal at the beginning of labor, increasing to approx. 250 MU at the end of the first stage of labor.

Contractions and circulation

The pressure during labor has no direct effect on fetal circulation, but it does on the circulation of the uterus. This can be reduced temporarily at the point of the highest wave surge. A healthy fetus with a well-functioning placenta will usually not suffer from a lack of oxygen during normal labor.

However, the physiological reduction in uterine circulation at the peak of the contractions may lead to decompensation of a latent acidosis in the baby if, for instance, the mother's vessels have been affected by diabetes mellitus or smoking, or if the gaseous exchange in the placenta is unsatisfactory because of placental insufficiency.

Third stage of labor

This is the period between the cutting of the baby's cord and expulsion of the placenta. More contractions occur between a few minutes and up to half an hour after the birth as the uterus contracts over the placenta and it detaches. The placenta is then produced with a contraction.

Afterpains are contractions that occur once the uterus is completely empty and which serve to stem the blood flow and help the muscles return to normal. They usually continue until the mother's milk comes in.

Length of labor

The first stage usually lasts between 3 and 24 h, although it may on occasion continue for more than 30 hours.

In a primagravida the transitional and second stage last usually a total of 1–2 h, in a multigravida between 20 min and 1 h. In a hospital delivery, a second stage of up to 2 h with constant contractions is deemed acceptable. According to Weiss (1994), a second stage lasting up to 3 h with fetal monitoring will have no negative effects on the child. Longer times have been described as normal for a home delivery. Epidural anesthesia will almost double the length of the second stage. There is an increased risk to the child if the second stage lasts less than 15 min. 'Systematic computer tomographic examinations of mature newborns have revealed that cerebral hemorrhage occurs almost entirely in babies whose second stage of labor lasted less than 10 minutes' (Weiss 1994). In a so-called 'precipitate delivery' the baby's head is unable to adapt sufficiently.

Progressive molding of the baby's head during labor causes cerebrospinal fluid (CSF), and to some extent venous

80 cm under water, and during the second stage is the same as 160 cm under water (Weiss 1994). The pressure on the baby is distributed equally on all sides, so it is mechanically gentle. The work relatively of the uterus is often given in

blood, to pass out of the cranium into the body, thus reducing its volume. If this alteration of the intracranial fluid balance is not permitted, such as in a very rapid delivery, then the compression of the body of fluid against the membranes can result in 'traumatic membranous inertia' (TMI). In this condition there is usually little evidence of external molding, but fluctuation of the CSF is reduced and the membranes are unable to express motion. The baby usually cries excessively, sleeps poorly and is generally very cranky.

The child moves further down with each increasingly strong contraction. If the contractions are very strong (that is, if the mother is given drugs to speed them up, or if the delivery is taking too long because the cervix is opening too slowly), then the baby's longitudinal axis may be compressed. After delivery, these compressions are most easily detected in the spine. Most frequently affected are the sacrum with an intraosseous compression, the region of L5 and S1, the dorsolumbar transitional area and the thoracic spine. On osteopathic examination, these areas should all be checked carefully after delivery to ensure that the body has decompressed in its long axis. Of particular importance may be unresolved compression in the region of the transition from the cervical spine to the head. Motion restrictions and asymmetries in this region and their effects are these days often termed 'kinematic imbalances due to suboccipital strain', or KISS. As long ago as 1946, in Des Moines, Sutherland taught his students about asymmetrical strains to the occipital bone and C1 and their effect on body physi-ology; his student Magoun went on in 1951 to write extensively on the subject in 'Osteopathy in the Cranial Field'.

The child during labor

The baby adapts to the birth canal by molding, changing position and rotating. Arbuckle (1994) also speaks of adaptation by a shifting of fluids: 'Due to the forces of labor, and to facilitate delivery, the cranial capacity is reduced by the blood and cerebrospinal fluid being forced out of the cranium …'

In about 96% of all deliveries, the baby's head presents first. 'The living human head is a remarkable structure at birth, when you come to think about it. At this age it is easy to see it as a soft-shelled egg, or a modified sphere, while later in life it is harder to visualize it as such. All these parts of bones are held together by the dura mater functioning as an interosseous membrane. Because of this the newborn head can hold together and adapt so as to allow a safe passage through the birth canal. Think of it!' Here, Sutherland (1990) is describing the head as a modified globe; the head is not absolutely round. The baby's cranium is usually long and slender, tapering towards the occipital bone. In order for

it to pass through the birth passage with the smallest possible diameter presenting, it goes into flexion.

The neurocranium is able to mold because of the membranous connections between the individual bones or parts of bones. Molding means changing shape to adapt to the birth channel. The strong pressure that the muscular tube of the birth channel exerts by its contractions onto the baby's head cause the cranial bones to shift. According to Mändele (1997), the head circumference reduces by 0.25–0.5 cm, and to Martius (1979) by up to 1 cm. The bones of the cranium do not truly slide over each other under physiological conditions.

In a delivery with cephalic presentation, the 'soft-shelled egg' of the head is well protected by the sickle shaped folds of the dura. Beryl Arbuckle (1994) first mentioned them in osteopathic literature as 'dural stress bands.' We know from preparations done by Willard, Wa, Grasso, Hagiopian and Trafeli in the early 1990s at the New England College of Osteopathic Medicine that the anterior dural girdle (anterior transverse septum) is extremely pronounced at delivery (Fig. 5.9). At this time, it is about eight times stronger than the tentorium cerebelli. This provides excellent protection for the part of the head that usually leads during delivery. If the birth has been strenuous, it may then be necessary to treat and rebalance this anterior dural girdle osteopathically.

Sutherland used to work a lot with the dura to resolve intraosseous dysfunctions caused by birth. 'Consider some trauma, either from adaptation to the birth canal or from falls later on in life. Visualize a pull on "mother dura" that pulls the bones out of their normal position or relations. It is necessary to utilize the membranes in order to bring these little bones back to their normal' (Sutherland 1990).

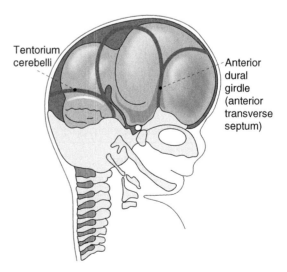

Figure 5.9 The front dural band protects the presenting part of the head during birth.
With permission, Henriette Rintelen, Velbert

Magoun wrote in 'Osteopathy in the cranial field' (Magoun H, 1st edition 1951) of the enveloping dural membrane of the cranium, into which the parts of the bones are inserted like reinforcements and which, together with the activity of the fluid, restore the cranium after delivery.

The shoulder girdle, which has an average circumference of 35 cm, has to adapt a lot during birth. Here too, there are often asymmetries found after delivery that not only influence the mechanics of the body but may also hinder the lymphatic return under the collarbones at the venous angle.

The trunk is also malleable. When the head is rotated, the trunk and pelvis remain behind. The forces of torsion not only commonly affect the occiput and C1-C3, but the entire trunk and the pelvis. This can particularly affect the diaphragm, contributing to problems such as reflux, difficulty in bringing up wind, and colic in the baby. That is why torsion patterns may also be palpable after delivery in areas apart from the base of the cranium if the body's own homeostatic mechanisms are unable to resolve the asymmetry in the bodies fascias.

Apgar score

The Apgar score, which is named after pediatrician Virginia Apgar, assesses the heart rate, respiration, skin color, muscle tone and reflexes 1, 5 and 10 min after birth on a scale with between 0 and 2 points, resulting in a maximum of $5 \times 2 = 10$ points. If the figure is below 7 points after 10 min, the baby needs some medical assistance; if it is lower than 5 then a lot of help is needed (Table 5.1).

Neurohormonal regulation of labor

The hormonal control of the contractions is effected primarily by local regulatory mechanisms that are initiated just before labor commences, continue during it and then break down again. They are subject to complicated neuroendocrine control mechanisms and thus also to psychological influences. According to Enning (2003), two factors have to concur – hormonal induction of contractions and a safe birthing environment – for the activity of the contractions to commence. 'Within a specific window of time peculiar to her species, any female can delay giving birth using hormonal adaptation … until the safest possible time.'

Progesterone

The placenta already begins to produce progesterone early on in pregnancy. It is absorbed into the uterus by the placenta and prevents contractions during pregnancy by means of what is known as the 'progesterone block.' As the uterus grows, the size of the placenta decreases in relation to the inside of the uterus and the contraction-inhibiting effect gradually reduces. Progesterone also stimulates prostaglandin synthesis. Prostaglandin contributes to the formation of contractions at the end of the pregnancy.

Estrogen

Estrogen is produced by the placenta, but in a smaller quantity than progesterone. The counterpart to progesterone, it encourages the uterus to contract. Its level is relatively low at the beginning of the pregnancy, increases over time, and eventually overcomes the inhibiting effects of progesterone. Estrogen encourages the formation of oxytocin receptors (OTR) in the uterus. The efficacy of the contraction hormone oxytocin, which is formed later, is determined by the number of receptors intended for it. It also increases prostaglandin synthesis. As the estrogen level increases, a protein called connexin is also formed by the cells in the uterine musculature that facilitates coordinated contractions during delivery.

Prostaglandin

Prostaglandins stimulate contractions and are produced in the uterus itself.

Table 5.1 Apgar score for the assessment of neonatal adaptation

Criteria	0 points	1 point	2 points
Appearance (skin color)	Pale, cyanotic (blue)	Trunk pink, blue at extremities	Pink
Pulse (heart rate)	None	≤100/minute	≥100/minute
Grimaces during suction	None	Pulls a face	Cries
Activity (muscle tone)	No spontaneous movement	Some flexion of extremities	Strong, active movements
Respiration (breathing)	None	Slow, irregular	Regular, no dyspnea, strong crying

The different types of prostaglandin are produced during the last trimester in the endometrium and amnions, and during labor in the myometrium. This tissue hormone initiates the production of collagen-degrading enzymes on the cervix. This enables the neck of the uterus to soften, expand and finally open.

Oxytocin

Oxytocin is produced in the hypothalamus and stored in the posterior pituitary, from where it is released. It reduces the membrane potential of the myometrium and increases therefore the excitability of the uterus. In turn, the efficacy of oxytocin is determined by the number of oxytocin receptors (OTR) in the tissue. From around mid-pregnancy onwards, there is a constant increase in OTR, and the amount increases dramatically just before the beginning of birth. The development of the OTR is of extreme importance for the commencement and continuation of labor. The prostaglandins make the OTR in the myometrium receptive to the oxytocin. So the activity of the contractions depends on the direct effect of oxytocin on the uterus, but is linked to the presence of sufficient amounts of prostaglandins. This effect is also used to start labor by applying a prostaglandin-based gel to or into the cervix. Directly after birth, the increased level of oxytocin plays an important part in encouraging the bonding between mother and baby (Odent 2001).

Corticotropin releasing hormone, ACTH and cortisol

Before birth the baby's hypothalamus starts to release corticotropin releasing hormone (CRH). This leads to an increased production of adrenocorticotropin hormone (ACTH) by the hypophysis and thus to an increase in cortisol by the fetal adrenal cortex, which encourages the baby's lungs to mature.

So what causes the increased production of estrogen by the placenta, encouraging the uterus to prepare for the birth? In the 1980s, endocrinologists found that messengers produced by the fetus use the shared circulation to influence the mother's organism. We now know that CRH is also produced by the placenta, which is actually one of the baby's organs, in gradually increasing amounts from the 12th week. Thus CRH, and then the ACTH from the fetal hypophysis, stimulate the baby's adrenal glands to produce dehydroepiandrosterone sulfate (DHEA-S) which the placenta converts to estrogen. As already mentioned, estrogen in turn stimulates the production of prostaglandins, which cause the cervix to soften and support the uterine contractions. So once CRH, estrogen, prostaglandins and possibly certain other factors exceed their critical thresholds, the changes that allow delivery to take place commence in the uterus and at the cervix.

The placenta's hormonal response to distress is interesting. 'In unfavorable conditions that cause distress, the placenta will produce increased amounts of CRH, which in early pregnancy can lead to miscarriage and later on can accelerate fetal maturity. In plants this stress response is known as "premature ripening"' (Enning 2003).

Role of the autonomic nervous system

The autonomic nervous system has an additional task in the gradual opening of the cervix. Sympathetic nerve endings encase the myometrium fibres; the lower and cervical parts of the uterus are more richly innervated. Norepinephrine (noradrenaline) on the α-receptor of the muscle fibres appears to stimulate uterine contraction. However, epinephrine's (adrenaline) main affinity is with the β-receptors, and stimulation of them inhibits excitement. If the epinephrine level is too high, for example if there is fear, this can severely delay the opening of the cervix. This may be an old survival mechanism of the 'fight or flight' response. If in danger, it may be better to flee than to give birth.

The uterus is a system that works subtly. The pregnant organism often responds to open or hidden concerns and fears with contraction anomalies.

Role of the neocortex

The neocortex probably suppresses the production of all the hormones that are important when giving birth. At the time of labor there is a reduction in activity in this part of the brain. 'This is why women, from a particular point in a normal physiological birth onwards, seem to shut themselves off from everything around them, also from their birthing assistants, and seem to move to a different planet. Their level of consciousness changes' (Odent 2000). Light stimulates the neocortex, which is why soft light or darkness is better for labor.

Another reason for this change in consciousness could be the production of endorphins. Endorphins are morphine-like substances that are produced in greater quantities if the physiological birthing process continues without interruption. It changes the perception of place, time and pain. During the birth the baby also produces endorphins, so both mother and baby have large amounts of these hormones in the hour after delivery. Together with the increased level of oxytocin, they create the physiological foundation for this very special time of bonding, an extremely important stage in the whole process of mutual bonding.

Birth assistance

'Birth is an involuntary process. Considered from this angle, it is obvious that it is not possible to give a woman active support when she is giving birth. The more important task is to protect her from any unnecessary disturbances' (Odent 2001).

Michel Odent, a well-known obstetrician from France who now lives and works in London, researched the subject of home deliveries in industrial countries on behalf of the WHO. He believes that there is least disturbance to the deep experience of giving birth if the mother's private sphere is protected. The care given by midwives and birth assistants should be unobtrusive and not obvious.

He also researched what type of environmental factors may inhibit labor. Interestingly, animal tests revealed that the following factors make delivery more difficult: moving the contracting female to an unfamiliar place and giving birth in a transparent glass cage. Odent is convinced that women would experience a more relaxed birthing process if they are in a small, dark room and do not feel they are being watched. 'Removing all fears and thereby avoiding the dangers and complications that these fears bring is one of the main duties of those caring for a mother in labor' (Rockenschaub 2001). That is why the support of a midwife and, if necessary, a doctor, who care for the mother before, during and after delivery is ideal. Under such circumstances a relationship of trust can develop as the basis for the subsequent delivery.

In hospitals, a midwife may have several mothers to look after at the same time, or a mother may be cared for by several midwives if she is there when shifts change. One mother told me that her labor stopped altogether when she was being cared for by a midwife that she didn't like. Finding herself with a friendlier midwife after a change in shifts, she was able to give birth.

If the mother-to-be feels safer giving birth in hospital, she may be able to take her own midwife with her, or perhaps meet the hospital midwives and doctors beforehand.

Birth assistance is a balancing act between too much and too little support; there is a constant risk of the physiological birthing process being pathologized. 'Most birth assistants could not even imagine how a birth would go if it were not controlled and monitored' (Odent 2000).

Unfolding of the child after birth

In order to pass through the cylindrical birth passage, the baby undergoes a process of molding; that is, he changes his position, folds together and possibly even shifts body fluids from the cranium to the body to be compressed in a physiological way (Fig. 5.10). If the normal physiological limits are not exceeded, the baby will gradually unfold during the days following delivery in a gradual process.

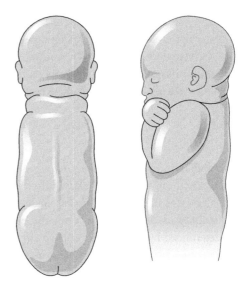

Figure 5.10 Molding of the baby as it adapts to the birth canal. With permission, Henriette Rintelen, Velbert

Unfolding of the thorax: 'first breath'

The thorax has to expand after birth and the lungs begin to breathe air. The diaphragm begins to practice moving from the 3rd month of pregnancy, and the fetus breathes amniotic fluid. After birth this water in the lungs is reabsorbed by the lymphatics, the pulmonary alveoli unfold, and the baby takes his first breaths of air. The osteopath Robert Fulford, a student of Sutherland, studied the importance of these first breaths in newborns in depth. He wrote: 'For many, birth is the first major trauma. The baby's body takes on a compact form for delivery, and after a gentle birth, as the baby swallows a healthy first breath of air, the body is reassembled, unfolded. Unfortunately, this process doesn't occur properly in many births, and the body never fully expands, making it predisposed to imbalance and distortion' (Fulford 1996).

This changeover of circulation and activation of the lungs, which is so important for further unfolding of the whole body, is commonly termed by osteopaths 'The first breath,' although it obviously does not just happen over a single breath.

So what has to happen in order for the baby to experience this change from intrauterine oxygen supply via the umbilical cord to obtaining his own supply via the lungs using thoracic respiration? The thorax has to be able to expand fully, and regular respiratory movements will also help other body parts such as the cranium and pelvis to unfold. This first major step in adaptation obviously not only includes the unfolding of the lungs, but also the adjustment of the blood circulation in the lungs and the efficiency of the breathing musculature.

The lungs are assisted in their expansion by a recoil effect of releasing the compression of the thorax that has been present during the delivery. Occasionally a baby makes a respiratory effort after delivery of the head and before the body is delivered. The thorax is unable to expand because that part of the body is still in the birth canal, and this can significantly limit the ability of the baby to fully expand the lungs. This can contribute to asthma and respiratory problems later on. Stimuli such as change of temperature, sensory stimulation through skin touch, and exposure to gravity are all stimuli for the initiation of respiratory breathing.

Contractions play an important role in ensuring this changeover of circulation and respiration takes place. The contractions bring about a massive increase in catecholamines in the fetus, which are produced by the adrenal medulla. This increased catecholamine level is the perfect preparation for this extremely important change directly after birth. The catecholamine level in the blood of babies born by C-section, if there has not been much contraction activity before delivery, is one-third that of babies born normally, and they are at far greater risk of respiratory distress syndrome. Any drugs (e.g. opiates) given during labor and which pass to the baby via the placenta can also impair this first expansion of the thorax.

A disturbance can also be caused by non-physiological stress or fear, experienced by the baby during labor (Janus and Haibach 1997). We all know that fear can restrict our breathing.

While the baby changes to lung breathing, it is also important to give the umbilical cord sufficient time to stop pulsating. This ensures that the newborn is still safely supplied with oxygen via the umbilical cord in the first few seconds and minutes after birth, and can slowly get used to breathing air. If there is a lack of patience or under certain medical conditions such as a C-section, or if the baby has the cord around his neck or if there is a problem with the mother's and baby's blood groups, the umbilical cord is cut straight away. This can lead to shock and dysfunctions in the newborn's umbilical region (see p.219).

Something else to bear in mind is that being born is like coming onto dry land after being underwater. Jealous (2001) wrote thus on this topic: 'There is a lot happening with the newborn, when you think about it. It has been suspended in a fluid field, so it is relatively buoyant, it weighs a lot less inside the uterus than it does outside the uterus … so this child is born, it comes out … into a gravitational field, and there is a lot more to deal with. The child's body actually must feel a lot heavier. So we need to have more power, more voltage.'

So we are more or less suddenly exposed to gravity. If there is a C-section this happens quite unexpectedly, and Carreiro (2004) speaks of the 'rebound,' a shock-like contraction of the entire body tissue. This is probably why a water birth is so relatively gentle for the baby. Out of water the baby comes

into water and then emerges gradually directly to the mother's breast. Water is also the ideal place for the fascial system to correct itself (Enning 2003).

Unfolding of the entire body

In an ideal situation the molding and asymmetry present in the cranium and body at birth will remodel over a period of 1 to 3 weeks. So what forces ensure that this normal process of unfolding not only takes place in the thorax, but all over the baby's body, and especially in the cranium and pelvis?

The baby's movements, for instance when kicking, definitely play a part. Thoracic breathing works all over the body. Crying increases intracranial pressure and thus assists the molded cranium to unfold. But not all babies cry a lot and still their heads unfold, so there must be another effective factor.

Sutherland (1990) writes thus on this topic in 'Teachings in the Science of Osteopathy': 'It is instructive to consider what is at work in accomplishing such a change. The baby's crying and suckling function in many ways to realign the bones and the parts of bones. Then there is the regular breathing that contributes to the fluctuation of the cerebrospinal fluid. The hydraulic lift that the cerebrospinal fluid gives in the infant head from within is smooth and powerful. Its service is enhanced by the baby's crying. The problems that are prevented by these natural processes are understood only when conditions limit their effectiveness.' So Sutherland sees a regulatory influence that is brought about by secondary respiration, and especially crying, onto the fluctuation of the cerebrospinal fluid; and he also comments that this 'process (of crying) fluctuates the cerebrospinal fluid. Then the membranes go to work and pull the bones into position.' Both the fluctuation of the liquor and the motility of the reciprocal tension membrane are two important factors in the expression of the involuntary motion as an effect of primary respiration. The expression of primary respiration as 'involuntary motion', a slow rhythmic shape change, which was first described by Sutherland, works 24 hours a day, 365 days a year to support our body in its constant striving for homeodynamic balance. This involuntary motion, which is also present in utero, gradually gains in strength in the first hours and days of life. This may be described as the first breath in relation to primary respiration. According to Jealous (2001), after birth there is a synchronization of primary respiration and respiration of the lungs that integrates all systems under these new conditions. 'The pulmonary, the visceral, the psychological and the postural systems need to integrate and to become one homeostatic shift, one movement with a new beginning … So the child, the whole body of the child is going to expand, the whole lungs and primary respiration, and this whole thing: the tent, cranium, the diaphragm, the pelvic diaphragm, the whole organism in all three dimensions, it's just going to breathe in, and if we synchronize the inhalation of thoracic respiration with the inhalation of primary respiration we end up with a crescendo that then creates the foundational synchrony through which that organism will then go on throughout life.'

These are the forces that, under optimum conditions, ensure that the child adapts to his new environment. After a normal delivery, the body then uses these forces to compensate or resolve any asymmetries, distortions or restrictions of motion that may have occurred, either by itself or with osteopathic help. As Sutherland (1990) wrote: 'There is great importance, therefore, in examining newborn babies with care and precision. At that time it is easy to assist the powers in the primary respiratory mechanism, already in action, so as to establish normal positions and relations among cranial bones, especially among the four parts of the occiput.'

Osteopathic support for unfolding

Osteopathic diagnosis of the newborn using involuntary motion usually reveals quite clearly how the child's self-correction is progressing. In a diagnosis with subsequent treatment from caudal to cranial, there are often certain zones that need support in order for the child to release the molding patterns.

Failure to unfold or partial unfolding after birth is usually expressed as varying degrees of reduced involuntary motion. The visible unmolding of the cranium that occurs in the first few days and weeks of life is primarily due to remodelling of the vault bones. It is always necessary to examine the cranial base carefully: if excessive compressive forces have caused significant intraosseous distortion of the incompletely ossified cranial base bones, such as the parts of the occiput, within the temporal bone, or between greater wings and body of the sphenoid, then these commonly persist beyond the first few weeks of life.

If the baby's system is unable to correct itself – with or without osteopathic assistance – permanent compression patterns may remain in the cranium, thorax and pelvis that could lead to reduced expression of the body's physiology.

It is often necessary to treat the sacrum first to secure sufficient fluctuation of the cerebrospinal fluid and body fluids. The unfolding of the thorax may be supported osteopathically by treating the diaphragm, ribs, sternum and thoracic spine (see pp.195–200). This is then generally followed by treatment of the upper cervical spine and the cranium. If the cranium is very compressed and irritated it may be advantageous to treat the sacrum and thorax in the first treatment until the CSF starts to move as described by Sutherland

(1990). By the time of the next treatment, often, the fluid and membranes will have improved the situation of the cranium, and treatment of the cranium can now continue without irritating the system unnecessarily. For further information on the subject of treating a newborn: see Ch.8, An osteopathic approach to the newborn and infant.

Bibliography

Arbuckle B: The selected writings of Beryl Arbuckle D.O. American Academy of Osteopathy, Indianapolis 1994

Carreiro J: Pädiatrie aus osteopathischer Sicht. Urban & Fischer/Elsevier, Munich/Jena 2004

English J: Physische und psychosoziale Aspekte der Kaiserschnittgeburt. In: Seelisches Erleben vor und während der Geburt. LinguaMed, Neu-Isenburg 1997

Enning C: Wassergeburtshilfe. Hippokrates, Stuttgart 2003

Fischer H: Die Logik der Gebärhaltungen. Die Hebamme, Hippokrates, Juni 2002

Fulford R: Dr. Fulford's touch of life. Simon and Schuster, New York 1996

Geisel E: Tränen nach der Geburt. 4th edn. Kösel, Munich 2000

Hofmann H, Geist C (publ.): Geburtshilfe und Frauenheilkunde. Lehrbuch für Gesundheitsberufe. de Gruyter, Berlin/New York 1999

Janus L, Haibach S (publ.): Seelisches Erleben vor und während der Geburt. LinguaMed, Neu-Isenburg 1997

Jealous J: The ignition system. Audiotape produced by Robert Trafeli 2001

Kimbrough H: Dr. Arbuckle's stress bands. Sutherland Cranial College Newsletter, Spring 2002

Mändele C, Opitz-Kreuter S, Wehling A: Das Hebammenbuch. Lehrbuch der praktischen Geburtshilfe. 2nd edn. Schattauer, Stuttgart 1997

Martius G: Hebammenlehrbuch. 3rd edn. Thieme, Stuttgart 1979

Odent M: Geburt und Stillen. 2nd edn. Beck, Munich 2000

Odent M: Die Wurzeln der Liebe. Walter, Düsseldorf 2001

Rockenschaub A: Gebären ohne Aberglauben. 2nd edn. Facultas, Vienna 2001

Sergueff N: Die Kraniosakrale Osteopathie bei Kindern. Wühr, Kötzting 1995

Smith R: Das Timing der Geburt. Die Uhr in der Plazenta. Spektrum der Wissenschaft 4 2002

Steffen G: Babys werden nach hinten geboren. Leitfäden zur Mechanik der Geburt. Hebammenforum, January 2002

Sutherland W: Teachings in the Science of Osteopathy. Sutherland Cranial Teaching Foundation, Stillness Press 1990

Weiss P: Sectio caesarea und assoziierte Fragen. Springer, Vienna 1994

DIFFICULT DELIVERY

Eva Moeckel

There are situations when the baby is unable to complete the normal self-correction or unmolding process after birth; for instance if the mechanics of a complicated birth process, drugs or medical intervention are more of a challenge to the baby's physiology.

A 15-year study of childbirth involving more than one million cases was concluded in Lower Saxony, Germany in 1999 (Schwarz 2002). It revealed a distinct increase in the technicalization of childbirth and a constant increase in the use of drugs. In 1999 2% of all deliveries were home births, 98% hospital births. Of these 98%, only 4% of women delivered their babies without any medical intervention such as induction, oxytocin drips, epidural or epidural anesthesia or other analgesic medication, forceps, vacuum extraction, caesarean section or episiotomy.

According to Schwarz (2002), every 5th birth in Lower Saxony is now induced by medication. In 32% of all hospital deliveries, the mother is put on an oxytocin drip to aid contractions. In 15 years, the number of episiotomies has increased from 27.7% (1984) to 52.1% (1999). Caesarean sections increased to 21.9% over the same period. This means that every 5th baby is now born with the help of an operation. The frequency of an epidural is now between 15.9% (low risk deliveries) and 23.6% (high risk deliveries). Of course every medical intervention may be both necessary and sensible, but it usually also has its price.

At this point it needs to be emphasized that there is no such thing as birth trauma per se. However, there are many different ways a trauma can occur at the time of birth. The effect of the trauma in the body's tissues may be palpable to the trained osteopath's hands as reduced and/or asymmetrical motion of the head or body on osteopathic examination. Osteopathic treatment may then help the child to process the trauma he experienced and to compensate better for it.

The following is intended to demonstrate what effects a difficult delivery may have on the structure of the body. In particular drugs and other medical interventions may have a strong influence on the body's ability to process the birth.

Induction and augmentation of labor

Induction is an initiation of labor with medication, augmentation the further stimulation of labor that has begun spontaneously.

We can assume that almost every fifth delivery in Germany is now induced. Interestingly, the Lower Saxony study mentioned above (Schwarz 2002) showed that in 1984 only every ninth labor was induced (12.5%); by 1999 this figure had increased to 18.1%. Probably in most western countries there has been a similar development.

Causes of induction

Labor may be induced with medication if the mother has gone beyond her due date or if the membranes have ruptured.

Post-term birth

We talk of a post-term birth or prolonged gestation when the mother has been pregnant for 42 weeks or 294 days. The occurrence of post-term birth ranges from 4% to 14% (MIDIRS 2004), depending on which study you read. However, the 'natural occurrence' of post-term birth is difficult to calculate because of the frequent interventions in modern obstetrics. Labor will usually be induced if it has not occurred spontaneously by the 14th day after the calculated due date. In practice, though, impatience or forensic pressure often leads to labor being induced 10 days after the calculated due date.

The estimated date of delivery will be calculated with the help of the first ultrasound screening in early pregnancy (see p.16). Studies have shown that the exclusive use of menstrual dates for calculating the due date often result in the pregnancy being calculated as further along than it actually is. However, if 3 days are added to the calculation based on the menstrual dates, the result is just as reliable as ultrasound (MIDIRS 2004).

The main cause for a post-term birth is poor excitability of the uterine musculature. Whether an extended pregnancy is actually detrimental to the well-being of the unborn child can be established using cardiotocography (CTG) and a sonographic calculation of the amount of amniotic fluid. 'According to scientific research, after 41 weeks of pregnancy (290 days), calculated using ultrasound data, there is a probability of labor commencing spontaneously within the next 3 days in 60% of cases, and within 7 days in 90% of cases – assuming that there is no other indication for an elective induction. So if the mother decides to wait, then she can safely be told that her labor will almost certainly commence before the end of the 42nd week of her pregnancy' (MIDIRS 2004).

The risks of a post-term birth are placental insufficiency and a marked increase in perinatal mortality (it increases steadily from 0.2% after 40 weeks to 0.3% by the end of the 42nd week, and to 0.4% by the end of the 43rd week). There also appears to be a slight increase in birth complications such as an extended labor and the need for surgical intervention. There is also a moderately increased risk of a low Apgar score and meconium aspiration.

Premature rupture of the membranes

Premature rupture of the membranes is defined as a loss of amniotic fluid resulting from rupture of the amnion before commencement of the first stage of labor. Contractions then usually commence spontaneously, so if the membranes rupture very early on then delivery may be premature.

Possible causes include: premature contractions, polyhydramnios, multiple pregnancy, infections, after amniocentesis or amnioscopy.

The most dangerous complication of premature rupture of the membranes is an infection of the baby (amnionic infection syndrome, neonatal sepsis) or of the mother. There is also a risk of a prolapse of the umbilical cord if the baby's head is relatively high or if there is a misalignment.

There may also be a gradual loss of amniotic fluid, which could – if the rupture occurs very early on and labor does not commence at the same time – lead to oligohydramnios. This may lead to position-related intraosseous dysfunctions, and also, due to the baby not being able to move enough in utero, to delays in motor development later on.

Oxytocin

Since 1948 oxytocin has been given intravenously to induce labor or to augment it if labor slows down (uterine inertia). Weiss (1994) quotes several studies that show that fetal distress and the need for a caesarean section are more common if oxytocin is used to induce labor. It does seem to make a difference, though, if oxytocin is given because there are no contractions at all or if there is some contraction activity and it is given to help labor along, as augmentation. If uterine inertia is only treated later, when the cervix has already dilated to approximately 3–4 cm, then the rate for C-sections is not increased.

Early in the 1990s it could be shown that the body produces oxytocin in a pulsatile manner, with the number of pulses increasing between the beginning of the first stage and delivery. One study showed that if oxytocin is supplied in a pulsatile rather than continuous manner, in other words there is a therapeutic imitation of the normal physiological process, the dose of oxytocin could be halved (Weiss 1994).

If given in the case of a non-contracting uterus, oxytocin leads usually to a much higher contraction pressure than when given when there are already contractions present. If the cervix is not soft and expanding ('ripe') when oxytocin is given, a caesarean section becomes necessary in 50% of all cases, as either the myometrium does not respond to the oxytocin or the increase in contractions coincides with resistance in the lower area of the uterus. This is the reason why prostaglandins may also be given to ripen a cervix as a so-called 'priming'. However: 'There is a strong association between priming or induction and CTG alterations, which in turn lead to the diagnosis of intrauterine asphyxia' (Weiss 1994). Intrauterine asphyxia itself brings with it a 30–40% increased likelihood of a caesarean section.

One major disadvantage of intravenous oxytocin for the mother is the need to be on a drip. Due to the resulting impairment in mobility, it will be more difficult for her to adopt useful birthing positions (see Ch.5, Normal labor). Also these effectively unphysiological contractions are often far more painful and difficult to handle, which in turn often leads to an epidural being administered.

Prostaglandin

Prostaglandins have been used in childbirth since the 1970s, and are applied locally, as otherwise far-reaching systemic side effects may occur. They are applied to the cervix as a suppository or endocervically as a gel. They offer the added advantage of both ripening the cervix and inducing labor. However, it is difficult to get the dosage right; it cannot be adapted to the actual progression. The results are therefore not as easy to control as on an oxytocin drip. One advantage over induction with oxytocin is that the mother's mobility is maintained.

Other methods of assisting contractions

Some midwives and birth assistants are more patient and will accept periods of less activity as they are a chance for mother and baby to recover. It is possible to continue stimulating and supporting the contractions by the mother moving around, bathing, and with essential oils, Bach Flower Remedies or homeopathy. Sometimes castor oil or an enema will be given to stimulate bowel function and, indirectly, the uterus.

Complications

Giving prostaglandin and oxytocin at the same time can often lead to overstimulation, and Martius (1979) advises against it. However, also giving just one of the drugs by itself can overstimulate contractions. If the contractions are very strong with reduced placental and fetal blood flow, the result may be hypoxia of the fetus. Orthodox medicine treats this with amniotomy (rupturing of the membranes), thereby reducing intrauterine pressure, or by giving the mother a betamimetic drip.

Possible consequences from an osteopathic viewpoint

If you are told during case history taking that labor was induced using oxytocin or prostaglandin, then ask how strong the contractions were. In my opinion, this is something mothers are usually very good at estimating. After medical induction contractions are usually much stronger, especially if there was no activity beforehand; in 40% of instances they are more than 300 MU. To compare: a value of 100 MU is considered normal at the beginning of labor, increasing to about 250 MU at the end of the first stage (see p.48).

On osteopathic examination of the baby after birth, even in a normal delivery there is often an axial compression along the longitudinal axis of the spine to be found. Restriction of motion is then particularly common in the sacral area and around L5, the thoracic spine and C0/C1. After very strong contractions these patterns are usually very noticeable. Cranial asymmetries may also be more common (see Ch.5, The birth process and its effect on the infant cranium).

There may also be psychological consequences if the labor has been induced with drugs. Normally, the birth process is initiated by a subtle hormonal interplay between child and mother. An induction or speeding up of the process interrupts the natural rhythm of birth. The child is exposed to feelings of confusion, fear, interruption or being taken over, which according to Emerson (1997) can become deeply entrenched as induction shock. According to Emerson, birth memories or experiences may be activated later in life by events that somehow correspond symbolically to a birth; this is called symbolic activation. Another form of activation is recapitulation. This is when events are staged unconsciously in a particular way to bring a past experience into the present and potentially release oneself from it.

Anesthesia and analgesics during labor

It can generally be assumed that almost every kind of drug that is given to the mother during labor will pass to the baby. Most types of anesthesia and analgesics can easily cross the placental barrier. Orthodox medicine discusses primarily the directly measurable side effects on the mother and baby; for example respiratory depression after the administration of opiates. However, it can be assumed that other, more subtle side effects may also occur in a pre-pathological 'grey area' whenever any medication is given. The different developmental processes in the body after birth, the commencement of lung breathing and the coordination of primary respiration with all the systems, which is also known as 'first breath,' can be obstructed by drugs given during labor as well as by mechanically induced stress patterns.

As long ago as 1948 Beryl Arbuckle (1994) discussed the possible traumatic effects to the baby's cranium as the result of birth mechanics or drugs. 'The earliest result of birth injury that may be witnessed is the possible failure of the infant to breathe. The newly delivered baby has a medulla much less irritable than that later in life. This excitability of the medulla in the newborn may be decreased by drugs given the mother, but mechanically it may also be reduced by pressure of the medulla against the anterior rim of the foramen magnum'.

Psychotherapists have observed many other effects of drugs that are given during labor (Emerson 1997, Chamberlain 2001). Emerson found that the bonding behavior in babies who had been born without any anesthesia was far superior to that of children where it had been used. The loss of consciousness during anesthesia impaired their 'desire and/or ability to enter into contact with the mother'. According to Emerson, the sudden dose of anesthesia can even lead to psychic shock which can result in babies being more inclined to respond to sudden events with shock. However, he also points out – and he believes that this applies to all forms of assisted labor – that the 'most traumatising experiences are reduced somewhat if the baby is genuinely in serious danger during the birthing process. In such cases, the feelings of assistance, of being saved and protected, are stronger than those of disturbance, being overpowered and controlled.' Chamberlain also reports that on one level, children know very well whether a medical intervention was really necessary or if they would have survived without it.

Analgesics

Opiates may be given when the labor pains are very strong. Most cross the placenta. The most frequently used one is pethidine which is given intramuscularly. Some of the noted side effects include respiratory depression or an impairment of the neuroadaptive behavior of the baby. 'One practical consideration is an impairment in the sucking behavior of newborns whose mothers had been given pethidine to help with contractions' (Frölich 2000). Other opiates such as pentazocine or tramadol are also used.

During the first stage the pains are mainly the result of the contractions of the uterus and the dilation of the lower uterine segment and the cervix. The pain impulses are conducted by visceral afferent fibres, which can easily be blocked with opiates. During the second stage, pain occurs as the pelvic floor, vagina and perineum dilate; these pains are transmitted via somatic nerves and are more difficult to block using drugs (Fig. 5.11). That is why one favoured alternative is to combine opiates with a local anesthetic. 'Satisfactory analgesia of labor pain using opiates alone … can only be achieved in the first stage of birth. During the second stage an … opioid has to be combined with a local anesthetic for an adequate analgesic effect to be achieved' (Frölich 2000). Most local anesthetics are also transmitted to the baby to a certain extent, but they do not seem to have the same side effects as opiates and barbiturates.

Epidural anesthesia

For epidural anesthesia the lig. flavum is punctured to reach the extradural space between the ligament and the spinal dura mater. Then a local anesthetic is injected via an epidural catheter, usually combined with an opiate.

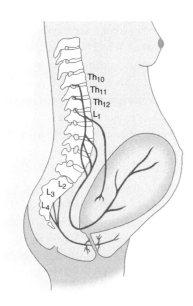

Figure 5.11 Conduction pathways for labor pains. First stage: segments Th10L16   cond stage:p lus S2–S4. With permission, SAd ler, Lb eck

It used to be common practice to inject only a local anesthetic, but this caused problems with the mother's blood pressure and severe motor restrictions in her legs. These days a local anesthetic combined with an opiate results in analgesia with hardly any motor impairment, which means that the mother can move around relatively freely. The drugs pass through the dura into the CSF, and from the CSF into the spinal cord and to the intradural nerve roots. In the extradural space they reach the nerve roots as they exit through the intervertebral foramen.

Several studies have confirmed that an epidural causes the second stage to last longer (Weiss 1994, Frölich 2000). Acute complications of an epidural due to the toxicity of the local anesthetic or the effect on the autonomic nervous system may be: a drop in blood pressure, urine retention or restriction of the motor function of the legs. Arterial hypotonia – a reduction in the systolic blood pressure of more than 25% – is caused by the effects on the sympathetics and the resulting loss of tone in the venous vessels. A vasopressor such as ephedrine may be given as a preventive measure. In the event of hypotonia, bradycardia of the fetus may result from impaired blood circulation in the uterus. Paresthesias are fairly frequent; the needle is then repositioned to avoid permanent damage. Insufficient anesthesia occurs in 2–6% of cases. Dura perforation may be a complication in 1–4% of cases (Frölich 2000).

Longer-term complications include post-punction headache and backache. Frölich assumes that a dura perforation hole leads to a loss of liquor and thus a change in the position

of the brain in relation to the cranium, and a meningeal irritation. I believe this may explain the headache directly after an epidural if there was a perforation. After an epidural, in many cases a restriction of the reciprocal tension membrane (RTM) can be found on osteopathic examination in the vicinity of the injection site, which may result in a marked reduction in the normal mobility of the membrane system (see Ch.3, Treatment after delivery) and may be a cause for long-term headache or backache.

Absolute indications for an epidural are pregnancy-induced hypertonia or heart disease in the mother, as an epidural will lower the blood pressure. An epidural will also usually be chosen if the mother suffers from diabetes mellitus as it can often reduce the acidosis that may occur in the second stage.

Spinal anesthesia

Spinal anesthesia (SA) may be used in an emergency or elective caesarean section, but also to help with labor pains. Spinal ganglions, nerves and spinal cord are blocked directly with a combination of a local anesthetic and an opiate. Following the subarachnoidal injection, the anesthetic spreads out slightly cranially and caudally. As far as the anesthetist is concerned, the advantage of a spinal block is that the drugs are positioned directly at the site where they are to work, and are not dependent on the diffusion barriers of the extradural space. 'SA produces a more reliable block without the risk of segmental gaps' (Frölich 2000). Also here a side effect may be hypotonia. SA is given during the second stage, when delivery is in sight, or during the first stage and in combination with epidural anesthesia if the labor pains are strong. As the effects of SA wear off after about 2 hours, an epidural 'top-up' is given at this time. A continuous SA may be given if the labor has been classed as high-risk.

In the osteopathic examination using the involuntary motion, similar restriction patterns in the RTM are found after an SA as after an epidural.

Inducing anesthesia, sedation

Barbiturates such as thiopental or methohexital may be given to induce anesthesia. Propofol is also given to induce anesthesia and may also be used as a sedative with SA. They all quickly pass into the baby's system.

Inhalation anesthetics

These are used to keep the mother anesthetized during a C-section and easily cross the placental barrier. 'A long period of time between starting the caesarean section and cutting the baby's cord with the patient under general anesthetic … is … associated with lower Apgar scores' (Frölich 2000).

Muscle relaxants

These only pass the placental barrier to a limited extent.

Dysfunctional labor (dystocia)

Dystocia or dysfunctional labor is labor that does not progress normally. Nowadays, labor is often considered protracted if it lasts for longer than 12 hours. There has been, however, a 'marked reduction in the patience of birth assistants. In older obstetric books the acceptable time limit for a normal labor was reduced from one issue to the next. The exaggerated expectations regarding duration of labor are evident from the fact that an average accepted time of delivery of 15 hours in the 1950s had dropped to 7 hours by the 1960s, the dawning of the oxyctocin era' (Weiss 1994).

Dysfunctional and protracted labor may be the result either of ineffective uterine expulsive forces like with uterine inertia or spastic dystocia, especially of the lower uterine segment, an abnormal lie, presentation or position on the part of the baby or more rarely a disproportion between the size of the baby and the mother's pelvis.

Uterine inertia – hypotonic uterine contractions

Primary uterine inertia usually occurs in a primagravida at the beginning of the first stage of labor. Secondary uterine inertia is defined as an interruption occurring after initially normal progressing labor. There may be many reasons for this, including psychological ones. I remember a story I was told by a midwife who had been working on a delivery ward with five women in labor. When one of the five mothers was moved for an emergency C-section, the contractions of the other four stopped for a while – presumably because they were concerned to see whether they too were about to experience an emergency. As mentioned before, ineffective, hypotonic uterine contractions may also be caused by conduction anesthesia or excessive sedation. If the effect of a sedating drug is allowed to wear off, normal labor patterns will usually resume.

Orthodox medical practitioners speak of an arrest of dilatation if a period of 2 hours or more passes in the first stage without progress in cervical dilatation and arrest of descent if for more than 1 hour the presenting part of the baby fails to move forward. If there is no fetal malposition, hypokinetic contractions may be stimulated with oxytocin, but also by moving around, homeopathy, etc.

Uterine spasm – hyperkinetic uterine contractions

Hyperkinetic contractions, and especially a spastic lower uterine segment, may impede the baby's head positioning itself in the transverse position at the entry to the small pelvis. If the sagittal suture is anteroposterior the head cannot descend this way. It may be possible to correct the baby's position if the mother changes her position; the use of a spasmo-analgesic such as pethidine or an epidural may also be considered. Oxytocin should obviously not be given. If the diagnosis persists, a caesarean section will be performed – this is quite a common cause of the operation. According to the Graz caesarean section analysis, this abnormal presentation is more common after induction of labor, and also with heavy babies (Weiss 1994).

According to Martius (1979), another result of a functional disturbance in the lower uterine segment may be asynclitism. This is a variation in the transverse course of the sagittal suture to ventral or dorsal as the baby's head engages in the small pelvis. A small deviation anteriorly before labor commences and posteriorly after it has done so is physiological.

Asynclitism may be corrected if the mother changes her position, otherwise a dose of pethidine or an epidural may be tried.

Presentation and position

Presentation is defined as that part of the baby that first enters the maternal pelvis; most commonly the head is the leading part, which is called cephalic or vertex presentation.

The way the baby enters is defined as position. This is named according to the position of the fetal occiput in relation to the maternal pelvis (Fig. 5.12). We differentiate between left occiput anterior (LOA; the fetal occiput approximating to the left anterior part of the mother's pelvis) and right occiput anterior (ROA), where the fetal occiput is oriented to the right anterior part of the mother's pelvis. Positions other than occiput anterior are considered abnormal. In cases of abnormal position there is usually an unfavourable relationship between the leading (presenting) part of the baby and the mother's pelvis, leading to difficulties with dilatation or descent of the baby.

The head of the baby descends and engages into the mother's pelvis in a transverse position (see Fig. 5.1). It then rotates to an occiput anterior position, either LOA or ROA, or, in a small percentage of cases, to a more unfavourable occiput posterior position (OP).

Occiput anterior (OA) positions

The LOA position is the most common (70 % of all head presentations) and most favourable cephalic presentation. This is the position adopted by the baby in most vertex presentations.

The ROA position is also favourable and occurs in about 10% of all deliveries. With both left and right occiput anterior

Right side of mother   Pubic bone   **left side of mother**

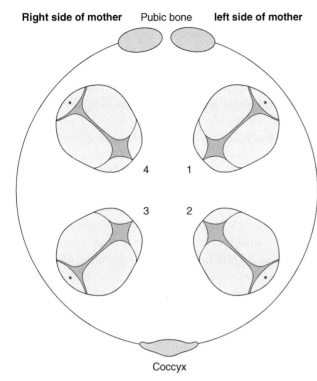

Coccyx

Figure 5.12 The cephalic presentations are named according to the position of the baby's occipital bone (marked with an *) in relation to the mother's os pubis. In position 1 the head is in the left anterior, in position 2 in the left posterior, in position 3 in the right posterior and in position 4 in the right anterior vertex presentation.
With permission, from EC Carreiro, Biddeford; courtesy of the Willard and Carreiro Collection

positions, the baby turns through about 90°, to be born facing the mother's sacrum (see Fig. 5.1).

Occiput posterior (OP) positions

Generally, during its descent into the maternal pelvis, the baby's head rotates from the transverse position into an OA position. According to Bashore and Hayashi (2004), even if the head is initially in an OP position (see Fig. 5.12), most babies will spontaneously rotate to an OA one during birth, either with a long or a short rotation (see pp.70–71 for further discussion and common osteopathic findings after long or short rotation).

Transverse position and transverse arrest

In a small number of cases, the baby's head will enter the pelvis in a transverse position, but fail to flex and rotate so the sagittal suture points in the advantageous anteroposterior direction. Being held in this transverse position is usually due to secondary uterine inertia. Also 'this position may be caused by cephalopelvic disproportion … an android pelvis,

or a relaxed pelvic floor, brought about by epidural anesthesia or multiparity' (Bashore and Hayashi 2004). Because the large occipitofrontal diameter is now the leading part, further descent becomes very difficult. If this situation persists, with descent stopping for an hour or longer, it is called transverse arrest (see p.71 for further discussion and common osteopathic findings after transverse arrest).

Depending on how far the baby's head has come, either a caesarean section will be performed, or if it has come down low enough, a midforceps delivery (see p.82) with rotation, or a ventouse delivery may be feasible. If the cause is secondary uterine inertia this may be treated by the mother changing her position and lying on the side of the child's occiput, support for the labor activity, a pudendal block or an epidural. According to Martius (1979), in a low transverse position attempts may also be made to flex the baby's head using the 'Kristeller maneuvre' (See Ch.3, p.23). Often, after the Kristeller technique (which is sometimes used in Germany) has been employed in labor, it is possible to see corresponding compression patterns in the baby, especially in the cervical area. It is also of note that pressure inside the brain can increase significantly if great pressure is exerted on the baby's head. This can result in hemorrhage with all its neurological consequences. The use of this technique often also has a negative effect on the mother's tissues (see Ch.3, Treatment after delivery).

Vertex presentation (parietals leading)

In some cases in a cephalic presentation the parietals will be the leading part (Fig. 5.13 vertex presentation). This involves minimal extension and may be a useful adaptation in the case of a brachycephalic head. As long as mother and baby are well, positioning of the mother can change the scenario. However, ventouse or caesarean section are common with this presentation.

Brow presentation

Brow presentation (see Fig. 5.13) occurs when the leading part of the baby's head is between the eyes and the anterior fontanelle. It is rare, the incidence is about 1 in 1400 deliveries (Moore 2004). It is the least favorable of all cephalic presentations, because the presenting part is the supraoccipitomental diameter, which is the largest diameter possible of the head, and is larger than the size of the pelvic outlet. The head cannot be delivered without resolving into either a face presentation through extension, or vertex presentation through flexion. Then it can get born vaginally, otherwise a caesarean section is necessary. It is a lot more likely that labor is both prolonged and dysfunctional (see p.72 for

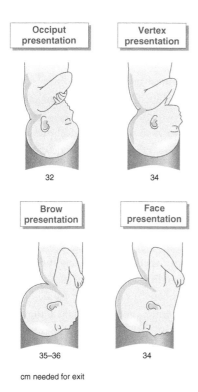

Figure 5.13 Flexion and extension positions of the head as it enters the pelvis.
With permission, SAdᵢler, Lübeck

further discussion and common osteopathic findings after brow presentation).

Face presentation

Face presentation (see Fig. 5.13) occurs when the baby's head enters the pelvis in hyperextension, with the child's face, between the chin and eyes, as presenting part. According to Moore (2004), the incidence is about 1 in 500 deliveries.

In the majority of cases of face presentation, the chin leads the way and the baby is born with his face towards the mother's pubic bone (mentoanterior position). This is a very difficult birth presentation for the baby because the face is poorly designed to resist the forces of delivery. It is inevitable that the baby is left with severe intraosseous restrictions of the face and cranium. The face as the presenting part is less effective at dilating the cervix, so delivery invariably takes longer. Often a caesarean section is performed (see p.71 for further discussion and common osteopathic findings after face presentation).

Breech position

Breech position occurs when the baby's pelvis or lower extremities are the presenting part. The incidence is 4% of all deliveries (Moore 2004). Since the 1970s babies in breech presentation have increasingly been delivered by caesarean section.

In Germany, the rate of C-sections is currently approx. 90%; internationally it varies between 5 and 95%. The reason for this is that a vaginal breech delivery is more difficult. With a well-trained and experienced birth assistant, it should however be possible to deliver an uncomplicated breech position vaginally (Martius 1979, Rockenschaub 2001). In a Californian study in 1990, Weiss (1994) compared the 'outcome of babies in 1240 breech deliveries after C-section and vaginal delivery. The study analyzed birth complications and maternal injuries, and complications in the baby such as asphyxia, craniocerebral injury, neonatal fits, brain damage and developmental delay up to the age of 4. After joint evaluation of all the parameters, the results after spontaneous delivery were better than after a C-section.' Based on his years of experience as the director of the Graz Obstetric Clinic, he concludes: 'At least two-thirds of breech positions at every stage of gestation can safely be delivered vaginally without any risk.'

There is an increased rate of perinatal morbidity and mortality following breech deliveries, regardless of whether delivered vaginally or by C-section. According to Martius (1979), this is probably due to a larger number of breech babies having had problems before labor, such as placental insufficiency, malformation and infectious or toxic embryopathies, with a reduction in fetal movement which may also be a cause of the breech position. 'Perinatal mortality and morbidity of breech babies is determined by a range of different factors, of which the birth method is just one … Breech position is more often associated with prematurity, malformation, twin births, premature rupture of the membranes with amnion infection, premature placental separation, trauma due to assistance at delivery and umbilical complications during the second stage of labor' (Martius 1979). This may be one reason why children born in a breech delivery have problems more often than vaginally delivered babies. Cerebral hemorrhage is no more common after term breech deliveries than in children born in cephalic presentation, but it is in breech babies born prematurely.

A caesarean section is always advised for breech positions if any of the following apply:

- premature babies (prematurity before the 28th week of pregnancy)
- very large babies (≥ 4500 g)
- footling positions
- additional risks, such as diabetes mellitus in the mother

Osteopathic findings

In a breech baby delivered vaginally, there are invariably intraosseous compression patterns within the sacrum and the three parts of the innominate as the pelvis is not designed to be the presenting body part in delivery. In my experience, these patterns can be very stubborn, and it is often a good idea to continue treating the growing child at increasing intervals. As the baby is coming out first with one hip and then the other, there may be also a marked lateral flexion of the lumbar spine. The cranium is not able to progressively mold during delivery, and the forces work from below up instead of the other way round. There is generally a circular compression pattern around the head, from the occiput to the zygomatic arches, from compression during the delivery of the head, with intraosseous dysfunctions in the face as well. As the body's fluids are pressed into the head rather than out of it in this type of delivery, fluid is forced upwards into the cranium from below, giving it a classic 'over-inflated' feel. TMI may be present due to the rapid delivery of the fluid-filled head (see p. 68).

A breech delivery that results in a caesarean section often not only causes the usual C-section patterns, but also a compression of the pelvic ring if the baby's pelvis had already engaged with the mother's pelvis.

For more findings in osteopathic diagnosis see also see p.72.

Surgical intervention

If labor stops during the second stage due to uterine inertia, or if the mother is getting tired, or there is fetal hypoxia, then the delivery will often be finished using vaginal surgery, either using forceps or with vacuum extraction (ventouse). In a cephalic presentation this can only be done if the cervix is fully dilated and the baby has moved down far enough (the maximum head diameter must be at least on the interspinal level, better still on the pelvic floor). Otherwise a caesarean section will be carried out.

Forceps delivery

With forceps, traction and/or rotation of the baby's head can be provided. Depending on how far down the birth canal the baby has moved, a forceps delivery is differentiated between pelvic outlet, low forceps and mid-pelvic forceps extraction. The pelvic outlet forceps are used most often. As the name implies, in this case the baby's cranium is already at the pelvic floor. With the low forceps the baby's head has already passed the interspinal line.

With the mid-pelvic forceps the baby is further up, at the level of the ischial spines. Ideally forceps are used with precision rather than with excessive force, but the reality is that a tremendous pulling force may be applied with the forceps. There is an increased risk of morbidity and mortality of the baby with a mid-pelvic forceps extraction. Perineal anesthesia

is required for a forceps delivery. According to Frölich (2000), the success rate of a pudendal block (block of the pudendal nerve proximal to its branch to the dorsal nerve of the clitoris and perineal nerve) is only 50%, which is why an epidural or a combined spinal and epidural anesthesia are used more and more frequently.

In a forceps delivery, an unphysiological pressure is always exerted on the baby's cranium that is determined by the degree of urgency when they are applied and the distance the baby still has to travel. The blades of the forceps are not always applied symmetrically.

Osteopathic findings

The prolonged time spent in labor has inevitably already led to increased molding and asymmetries of the cranium. It should be remembered that the forceps are applied when the baby's head is stuck, and has reached the limit of its physiological molding. As such any extra pressure applied by the forceps causes further intraosseous strains and asymmetries, depending on where they were placed. As the two blades of the forceps are usually positioned in the region of the greater wings of the sphenoid, often a superior strain of the cranial base can be found. This may be asymmetrical, depending on how the head was grasped. According to Hayden (2005), an alternating lateral component can occur here if the head is pulled first in one direction and then in the other. Intraosseous strains between the greater wings and body of the sphenoid are common. The motion of the temporal bones may also be restricted by intraosseous strains.

Sometimes the use of forceps can cause a facial nerve paresis or tear the ear. The forceps may have been positioned on the face, causing a local compression in the area of the zygomatic bone. Children who have been delivered by forceps often also display a marked tension in the area of the diaphragm, possibly as a reaction to the strong pull or due to the stressful circumstances that are associated with this delivery.

Vacuum extraction (Ventouse)

Today, vacuum extractions (VE, ventouse, suction cup) are more common than forceps deliveries. One reason for this could be that more manual skill is required for a forceps delivery. Studies have shown that both methods carry the same risks. However, a well-performed forceps extraction may well be gentler than a VE. It is certainly quicker when there is an acute risk.

For VE, a metal suction cup is attached to the cranium with a vacuum of 450–700 mmHg. This creates a bulge of the head that fills the cup. Then a chain in or beside the tube system is used to pull the child, always at the same time as a contraction, parallel to the axis of the birth canal. It is not uncommon for the suction to suddenly break and the cup fall off. It is actually quite a violent way to make your entry into the world.

Possible osteopathic diagnosis

As with a forceps delivery, here too the extended labor may have caused asymmetries of the head with additional strain patterns induced by the use of the vacuum extractor. On osteopathic examination there is almost always a displacement within the fluid field. It feels as if the head and upper part of the thorax are full to bursting, whereas the lower part of the body feels 'empty'. In my experience, the intraosseous dysfunctions in the cranial region caused by the suction cup can be addressed a lot more efficiently if this fluid imbalance has been treated before. The strong suction will probably also cause an imbalance of the membranes and a distinct pull in the body's fascias. This can usually be felt down to the feet. According to Hayden (2005), this pattern often has a fulcrum a few centimeters above the head. If the suction cup pulls off during the procedure, the recoil effect causes extra membranous and fluid shock.

When choosing either a forceps or a vacuum extraction, one prerequisite is that the child must have been stuck for some time and therefore have been in distress. Therefore, the cranium will have molded as much as it can, and have withstood quite an amount of compression. Afterwards it will be difficult for the child to resolve the body patterns created by the additional force vectors without help. Often, the prolonged labor will have caused a marked compression along the longitudinal axis of the body.

Caesarean section

Depending on when a caesarean section (C-section) is performed, we talk of an elective or planned section if it is carried out before or just as labor starts, and of an emergency section if it is carried out during labor.

Planned caesarean section

According to the latest statistics (Schücking 2004), the most common medical reasons for a planned/primary section are:

- breech position
- previous caesarean section (if the previous delivery was by C-section, it will be repeated in approx. 50% of cases).
- relative misproportion between the baby's head and the mother's pelvis
- pathological CTG

- transverse position of the baby
- placenta praevia
- premature placental separation
- serious illness of the mother
- eclampsia
- prematurity.

In Germany approximately 6–7% of today's caesarean sections are elective. A planned caesarean section is usually carried out with an epidural (see pp.57–58), which has several advantages over a C- section with endotracheal anesthesia. No anesthetic passes over to the baby; however side effects such as a possible drop in blood pressure are of relevance. The father, midwife or other familiar person can stay with the mother, helping to calm her and thus her baby. Both parents are able to experience the birth consciously. Once the cord has been cut, the newborn can be placed next to the mother's head, or held in her arms, and the two can say 'hello'. 'If mother and baby are not separated, this has a positive effect on both. As she greets her child, the mother can ignore more easily what happens behind the screen. The baby experiences the proximity of both parents in the first few minutes of his life. He already knows them, and so is able to deal with the stress of being born more easily' (De Jong 2003).

Emergency (unplanned) caesarean section

An emergency or unplanned caesarean section will be performed if there is, for example:

- prolonged or arrested labor
- certain presentation or position anomalies (see p.60)
- risk of asphyxia of the baby
- prolapse of the umbilical cord.

As speed is generally essential, endotracheal anesthesia is used more often if an epidural is not already in place. The abdomen is opened horizontally, the longitudinal abdominal muscles are pushed aside, the bladder pushed out of the way, and the lower part of the uterus opened horizontally with a cut of approximately 15 cm. Then the baby is lifted out. The incision is quite small; the baby needs to be liberated as in a vaginal delivery. The entire procedure takes about 5–10 minutes. The umbilical cord is cut and frequently the baby is suctioned. In the best scenario, the baby will now be welcomed by his father. A pediatrician will attend if the child's condition is poor. The mother is then given more anesthetic, the placenta removed, the uterus undergoes curettage, and the uterus and abdomen are stitched. This takes another 30–40 minutes.

Since 1994, much use has been made of the Misgav-Ladach method in Germany. Cutting is kept to a minimum, and the fascia, abdominal muscles and uterus are separated and pulled apart with the fingers. Although it sounds somehow violent, this method does have the advantage of less bleeding and less stitching; fewer analgesics are required, and usually fewer intraabdominal adhesions develop. The duration of the operation and thus of the anesthetic is shortened to about 20 minutes (De Jong 2003).

Rate of caesarean sections

It is not easy to talk about C-sections as such and their consequences, as there are so many reasons for them. A caesarean section can save a life, but it can also be an unnecessary intervention after a number of manipulations of the normal birthing process. Every child has his own story, which we need to acknowledge when we enter into therapeutic contact.

There has in recent times been an increase in the number of mothers-to-be deciding for an elective section. At the moment, this is the case in 6–7% of all caesarean sections in Germany, and the tendency is still increasing. It is possible that well-known personalities from the world of TV and cinema are setting this trend. There are probably many sociological reasons for it – not the least of which being the desire to control what is an uncontrollable archaic procedure in one's own body.

So a caesarean section is a different birth experience that is starting to become normal – if you consider normality on a par with frequency. In Germany the rate for caesarean sections is currently 22% (Federal Office of Statistics Wiesbaden 2001). In the USA the figure has been 23% for many years. Just why there should be this constant increase in the number of caesarean sections is a topic that is much discussed. This is important, because it is a fact that not all caesarean sections are necessary. In a study quoted by De Jong (2003) undertaken at a clinic in Chicago, a tighter attitude towards indications reduced the number of caesarean sections by one-third, from 18% to 11%, over 2 years without affecting the mortality or morbidity of either mother or baby.

Weiss (1994) finds: 'A lack of patience is ... one of the main reasons for the inappropriately high rate of caesarean sections. A number of spontaneous deliveries are prevented by a caesarean section, supposedly because of dystocia. The lack of patience is not only a matter of personal temperament on the part of the obstetrician, but can also be due to uncertainty resulting from a lack of experience. Furthermore, the willingness to take responsibility and remain physically present for a long period of time if required varies among individuals. By making the decision for a caesarean section ... the obstetrician is released from psychological stress.'

Another reason for the increase in the rate of caesarean sections can be today's often impatient use of oxytocin and prostaglandin to induce labor. The use of an epidural is also associated with a higher rate of C-sections. Also premature amniotomy (rupture of the membranes before the cervix has dilated to at least 3 cm) often leads to umbilical complications, CTG changes and abnormal presentations, and is associated therefore with an increased rate of C-sections (Weiss 1994).

The WHO (World Health Organization) calls for a guide figure of a maximum of 11% caesarean sections.

Possible consequences for the mother

Because caesarean sections are now so commonplace, the possible complications are often played down. A C-section is major abdominal surgery that can lead to septic wounds, bleeding from damaged blood vessels, peritonitis, ileus, thrombosis, pulmonary embolism or even cardiovascular failure. In 1994 the Bavarian perinatal census into maternal complications during and after a C-section reported between 2.8 and 38.8%, depending on the clinic. Figures regarding these complications were not published in the survey of 2001 (De Jong 2003). One side effect of C-section that often occurs but is rarely mentioned is unwanted sterility (Weiss 1994). This is probably due to post-operative adhesions. De Jong quotes a meta-analysis involving 22 studies that showed that in 21–84% of all cases after a secondary C-section sterility occurred.

Because a C-section can leave parts of the uterus in the abdominal area, it may be a possible cause of endometriosis.

A C-section also increases the risks in a future pregnancy. The risk of premature separation of the placenta is increased to 67%, and there is also an increased risk of placenta praevia. It is also often assumed that the maternal rate of mortality in a caesarean section is the same as in a vaginal delivery. What is certain is that the mortality rate has reduced generally in the past 30 years. It is also possible that pregnant women die because of the individual cause for the caesarean, but there is also a definite risk of dying from anesthetic accidents or as the consequence of infection. According to Weiss (1994), in the USA, for instance, there are between 0.6 and 5.9 deaths for every 10,000 C-sections (depending on the state), and in women with additional risks such as pre-eclampsia between 2.2 and 10.5 per 10,000. 'This number may appear small, but still it means that in the USA with an estimated 475,000 unnecessary C-sections every year, between 28 and 100 women die needlessly.'

Possible consequences for the baby

For the unborn child, normal labor activity means stress and stimulation. The child's large adrenal glands are prepared to produce large amounts of catecholamines. The trigger for this, and the baby's production of oxytocin and endorphins, seems to be largely dependent on the contractions – without experiencing them the baby's catecholamine level is much lower. Catecholamines are a great help in adapting to the new demands that the transition from fluid surroundings to the outside world, with its influence of gravity, places on all systems at birth.

About 6% of all babies born by caesarean section suffer from respiratory distress directly after delivery (De Jong 2003). This may be because in a planned caesarean section the stimulating effects of the contractions are not experienced. Therefore some clinics try not to perform planned C-sections until the mother has been in labor for a few hours. Another cause may be because the baby has not been pushed through the birth canal and had the amniotic fluid pushed out of his lungs. Yet another reason may be the suddenness of the birth, which exceeds the baby's ability to adapt. It only takes a few minutes to pull the baby out in a caesarean section. There is no rhythm of effort and rest as there is in a vaginal delivery.

So a fully developed respiratory distress syndrome may be actually only the tip of the iceberg. From my own clinical experience I know that almost every baby born by C-section that comes into our practice has some kind of problem with the integration of lung and primary respiration (see p.52).

With an endotracheal anesthesia, the baby is delivered within 5 to 10 minutes. And yet some of the anesthetic still passes to the baby. This reduces his vitality, and the ability to resolve compression patterns, for example after a prolonged labor followed by a secondary C-section, is usually impaired.

It can be assumed that hardly any drugs pass to the baby when a C-section is performed with an epidural. As mentioned before, there may be some side effects, such as a sudden drop in the mother's blood pressure, which may affect the child.

Possible osteopathic findings

Clinically, osteopaths often find compression patterns of the cranium and entire body in babies born by caesarean section. One typical symptom of cranial compression that may be recounted during case history taking is that the child does not like any pressure on his head (for instance wearing a hat or being touched on the head), or conversely that the child actively seeks pressure, such as by burrowing his head into a pillow. The cranial compression pattern becomes obvious when palpating using involuntary motion.

It could be assumed that C-sections are mechanically gentler for the head and would be easier for babies than having to twist and turn their way out of the birth canal. But that is not the case. In a caesarean section the opening through

which the baby is manually extracted is also relatively small. The baby is packed tight in the uterus, is slippery and needs to be grasped firmly – and quickly because of the anesthetic, or maybe because it is an emergency. Significant manual pressure is exerted on the cranium and the whole body. Peter Weiss (1994), who published an interesting monograph on caesarean sections after 30 years' experience of them, and in which he not only records the Graz C-section analysis but also evaluates hundreds of clinical studies on the subject, writes thus: 'Whereas the pressure of contractions is distributed evenly over the baby's cranium first by the amniotic fluid when the amniotic sac is intact, and then by the soft tissue tube once the waters have ruptured, the pressure in a caesarean section is intermittent and subject to quicker changes in pressure. In order to mobilize an object, the circumferential pressure of the hand on a dry object needs to be 60% over and above the weight of the object being moved, but on a wet and slippery object it needs to be at least 100% over and above that weight. So in a caesarean section of a baby weighing 1000 g, assuming the best case and assuming that the liberation continues without any resistance from the constricted spatial conditions, a force of approx. 20 N needs to be exerted on approx. 10 cm^2 of cranium. This equates to the pressure exerted underwater at a depth of 2 m, and is thus higher than the natural pressure of contractions at delivery. Furthermore this pressure is one-sided, intermittent and unsteady. So delivery by caesarean section may be far more traumatic than a vaginal delivery.'

In addition, if the head is well descended into the pelvis it may be difficult to lift it up out of the pelvis and require significant whole body manipulation for delivery by caesarean. Forceps are sometimes used to assist delivery of the head.

This throws new light on the fact, long known by osteopaths, that children that are born by C-section often display generalized compression patterns of the cranium. Presumably this high pressure leads to a recoil reaction of the entire cranium, and particularly a stress reaction of the membranes. But as the cranial vault is extremely adaptable, after a while it may appear as if the compression is primarily in the base of the cranium, especially if the strain was not so severe.

Extensive compression patterns in the body are also often found after a C-section; commonly there is a restriction in the thoracic area resulting from a failed integration of the 'first breath'. As already mentioned, labor causes strong hormonal stimulation. This facilitates a better integration of all systems after delivery, especially breathing, and thus more power for unfolding after delivery. A lack of integration of the 'first breath' is more common in elective C-sections, but may also occur after an emergency C-section, perhaps because of the speed of the delivery.

So how does a lack of integration of the 'first breath' show on osteopathic examination? The quality of the expression of the Breath of Life as involuntary motion is held back in all the body's tissues, it is as though the system has not been 'kick started' with potency. Involuntary motion seems so delicate that it sometimes appears as if it is not there at all. If this motion, which rhythmically pumps the body fluids, is reduced in the child, after a while the typical compressive feeling of the whole head and body appears.

Further stress in the thoracic area may be caused by suctioning the baby. Babies born by C-section usually need to be suctioned, possibly because the lack of contractions means that the amniotic fluid has not been pushed out of their lungs. Supporting the integration of the 'first breath' by osteopathic treatment of the thorax with the aid of the primary respiration often leads to significant improvements in the quality of involuntary motion. In children with delayed development there often follows a noticeable leap in development.

Babies born by caesarean often also have asymmetrical tissue tension in the neck. The baby is pulled out of the uterus fast – and with a firm grip because he is very slippery. The traction forces can cause reactive tension and symmetry disturbance in the neck area. If in an emergency C-section the baby had already been compressed along his longitudinal axis during delivery, then the neck will have experienced both: compression and traction.

A further observation is that babies born with an elective caesarean with no prior labor often compensate for the traumatic forces they experienced less well than those who have had the benefit of the stimulation of some labor contractions. The mechanisms of babies born by elective caesarean are often quite fluid, but with no sense of engagement or direction of the bony membranous system. Later on, these children do not seem to be able to deal very well with the effects of physical trauma such as impacts on the head.

Stress

An emergency caesarean section is usually extremely stressful both for the baby and mother and for the obstetricians. Even a planned C-section can be associated with lots of fear and worries, especially if the baby is premature and his very survival is at risk. Just how this stressful situation is processed by the baby and parents varies tremendously between individuals. In my experience, it makes a lot of difference if the mother feels well looked after by the surgical team and believes she is in safe hands.

It is normally babies that start labor off, when they want to be born. In a planned caesarean section without labor, the baby may be so surprised by his own birth that the initiation of the 'first breath' suffers.

Psychological consequences

Emerson (1997) writes of a psychological shock in caesarean section deliveries that is the result of the speedy – lasting just a few minutes – liberation of the baby. One indication of this may be that the baby is easily startled; for example if there is a sudden noise. Tactile rejection, when the baby tenses or becomes rigid on being touched, is another pointer. If it cannot be integrated and processed, a shock like this may be activated in response to certain situations for the rest of the person's life. According to Emerson, the sudden intervention also leads to an invasion or control complex with a wide range of consequences.

English (1997) spent a long time studying the characteristics of babies born by C-section, and especially those who were born without contraction activity. She finds there are typical characteristics which, although they are of course also present in other people, are often more marked in these babies. They include different perception of space and difficulties in identifying boundaries, including their own. 'During a vaginal delivery the contractions show the baby boundaries; they tell it where its place is and where it should go' (De Jong 2003). Watch the children in your practice, and see if the ones who keep testing the boundaries are also more likely to have been born by C-section.

Long-term consequences

As far as I am aware, there have not yet been any long-term studies that compare children born by vaginal delivery with those born by caesarean section. Because babies born by C-section will often have had a medical problem before or during labor, it is difficult to find suitable groups. Comparison would be easiest with the increasing number of elective C-sections. Based on my clinical experience I think that there are symptoms that may be associated with the generalized compression patterns of babies born by C-section. I have noticed that many older children who were born by C-section not only have marked tension in the cranial region, but also often have a restriction of the entire spine, a loss of mobility that is inappropriate to their age. I believe that this may be a long-term consequence of restrictions in the body including the cranium as discussed earlier. If further emotional or physical traumas are added, it can be difficult for the body to compensate. One further observation is that children with generalized compression patterns like to compensate with very active, wild behavior. This ties in with the observation by English (1997), who found that children who were born by C-section often test the ability of their environment to set boundaries for them. Mothers may have a latent guilty conscience if they have given birth by C-section. A mother who is subconsciously in a defensive mode will often have difficulties setting boundaries for her child. As a practitioner, it is therefore important to discuss our findings and describe the need for osteopathic treatment with sensitivity.

How the mother feels about her C-section, and how she copes with it, varies very much from person to person. It may be helpful for the mother to reflect and process her birth experience in a self-help group or with therapy. This in turn will benefit her child.

Compensating for a difficult birth

I have noticed that the child's compensation for a long, difficult birth, or deliveries that end with vaginal surgery or a Caesarean section, can vary tremendously. There are children who have had a very difficult birth but osteopathic diagnosis reveals good mobility and free expression of involuntary motion. In other cases, the case history taking may cause you to think that things were not so bad, but then the diagnosis is really striking.

In my personal experience, two things are particularly important for helping a child to process what may have been a traumatic birth: a good time before birth, and a good time afterwards! Birth is potentially very memorable, but by the same token it is also only a moment in our life. A child that has had an good time while in the uterus will approach his individual birth experience strengthened in many aspects(see Ch.4). Family circumstances after birth are equally helpful: the more relaxed and happy they are, the better is usually the compensation for the physical consequences of the C-section. I think that a feeling of deep safety and a family where the child is happy and peaceful are very important for successful compensation.

Bibliography

Albrecht-Engel I, Albrecht M: Kaiserschnitt-Geburt. Rowohlt, Hamburg 1995

Arbuckle B: The selected writings of Beryl Arbuckle D.O. American Academy of Osteopathy, Indianapolis 1994

Bashore R, Hayashi R: Uterine contractility and dystocia. In Hacker, Moore, Gambone (eds) Essentials of obstetrics and gynecology. 4th edn. Elsevier, Philadelphia 2004

Chamberlain D: Woran Babys sich erinnern – Die Anfänge unseres Bewusstseins im Mutterleib. 5th edn. Kösel, Munich 2001

De Jong T, Kemmler G: Kaiserschnitt. Wie Narben an Bauch und Seele heilen können. Kösel, Munich 2003

Emerson W: Geburtstrauma – psychische Auswirkungen geburtshilflicher Eingriffe. In: Seelisches Erleben vor und während der Geburt. LinguaMed, Neu-Isenburg 1997

English J: Physische und Psychosoziale Aspekte der Kaiserschnittgeburt. In: Seelisches Erleben vor und während der Geburt. LinguaMed, Neu-Isenburg 1997

Frölich M: Geburtshilfliche Anästhesie und Intensivmedizin. Springer, Vienna/New York 2000

Hayden E: Personal communication 2005

Hofmann H, Geist C (publ.): Geburtshilfe und Frauenheilkunde. Lehrbuch für Gesundheitsberufe. de Gruyter, Berlin/New York 1999

Knobloch-Neubehler C: Kristeller-Technik. Eine prospektive Untersuchung. Hebammenforum, Dec. 2000: 524–526

Mändele C, Opitz-Kreuter S, Wehling A: Das Hebammenbuch. Lehrbuch der praktischen Geburtshilfe. 2nd edn. Schattauer, Stuttgart 1997

Martius G: Hebammenlehrbuch. 3rd edn. Thieme, Stuttgart 1979

Midwives Information and Resource Service MIDIRS: Informierte Entscheidung für Profis: Übertragung. Hebammenforum October 2004

Moore T: Multifetal gestation and malpresentation. Hacker, Moore, Gambone: Essentials of obstetrics and gynecology. 4th edn. Elsevier, Philadelphia 2004

Odent M: Die Wurzeln der Liebe. Walter, Düsseldorf 2001

Qualitätsbericht 2000 – Außerklinische Geburtshilfe in Deutschland. Bund deutscher Hebammen, Bund freiberuflicher Hebammen Deutschlands

Rockenschaub A: Gebären ohne Aberglaube. 2nd edn. Facultas, Vienna 2001

Schücking B: Primäre Sectio – bessere Wahl oder unnötige Qual. Hebammenforum, July 2004: 465–468

Schwarz C: Wie häufig kommt eine 'normale' Geburt heute in der Klinik vor? Bericht über die Niedersächsische Perinatalerhebung 1984–1999. Die Hebamme 3, 2002: 127–131

Schwarz C, Schücking B: Adieu, normale Geburt. Dr. med. Mabuse 148, March/April 2004

Silver L, Wolfe M: Unnecessary Caesarean sections – how to cure a national epidemic. Public citizens' health research group. Washington DC 1989

Weiss P: Sectio caesarea und assoziierte Fragen. Springer, Vienna 1994

THE BIRTH PROCESS AND ITS EFFECT ON THE INFANT CRANIUM

Liz Hayden

Molding of the cranium before and during labor

Molding is a combination of the:

- **movement between** the bones of the cranial vault

- **bending** of the vault bones and, to a limited extent, the bones of the basicranium

- **buckling** or hinging of the cartilagenous junctions of the bones of the basicranium.

The vault bones, which are ossified in membrane, distort fairly easily during labor and also unmold and reorganize themselves readily, usually in the first few days after delivery. The bones of the basicranium, which are ossified in cartilage, take greater forces to cause them to mold and distort, and are more difficult to release after birth. They are often sites of retained compression. Head shape improves naturally in the first few weeks of life as the activity of the reciprocal tension membrane causes the bones of the cranial vault to remodel, assisted by the infant crying, suckling and yawning. The natural unmolding process can continue for up to 2 weeks after birth.

The shape of the head and amount of molding depends on a combination of factors including:

• in utero molding
• presentation
• maturity of the fetus (suppleness of bones and degree of ossification)
• length of labor
• maternal position in labor
• shape of the maternal pelvis, and the ability of all parts of the pelvis to expand during labor.

Traumatic membranous inertia (TMI)

Progressive molding causes CSF, and to some extent venous blood, to pass out of the cranium into the body, so the head circumference is reduced slightly. If this alteration of the intracranial fluid balance is not permitted, such as in a very rapid delivery, then the compression of the body of fluid against the membranes can result in traumatic membranous inertia. In this condition there is usually little evidence of external molding, but fluctuation of the CSF is reduced and the membranes are unable to express involuntary motion. The baby usually cries excessively, sleeps poorly and is generally very irritable (see Ch.11, Irritable infants and colic).

Molding in utero

Molding of the fetal head often begins in pregnancy, especially if the fetus is large and the mother small, if there is asymmetry of the uterus present, as in myoma, or there is a reduced amount of amniotic fluid (oligohydramnios). If before birth the fetal head is in contact with a bony part of the pelvis for any length of time, it will begin to mold to that shape.

Babies who lie in a breech position with the head tucked up under the maternal ribs often have little room to move, and the head can take on quite marked molding.

Maturation of the lower segment of the uterus as well as lack of space for the growing fetus within the maternal abdomen cause the head to descend or engage into the mother's pelvic bowl. If this happens fairly early on, it may be another cause of intrauterine molding.

Also, if the placenta is low, the space for the head is reduced and intrauterine molding occurs more readily.

Molding at birth

A number of factors may influence the degree of molding during labor:

• baby's presentation (the part that enters the mother's pelvis first)
• diameter of the baby's head (straight, in flexion, etc.)
• size of the mother's pelvis
• length of labor
• possible intervention and surgery during delivery (e.g. vacuum extraction, forceps).

In the following text we will refer to the two main stages of labor (see p.46). The first stage begins when the uterus is contracting regularly and lasts until the cervix has dilated to approximately 10 cm. This is usually the longest part of the labor. The second stage of labor begins when the cervix has dilated fully and ends with the birth of the baby.

In normal labor the baby is usually in an OA presentation (see Fig. 5.12). LOA is, with 70% of all head presentations, more common than ROA with about 10%. During labor, the child normally follows the line of least resistance through the pelvis. He is subjected to strong uterine contractions which focus pressure on the cranium as it meets the resistance of the soft tissues and bony contours of the pelvis.

The forces on the infant will vary depending on whether the amniotic membranes are intact. If they are intact, under ideal circumstances pressure is distributed over the whole body of the fetus, which reduces some of the focal pressure on the fetal head. If the membranes have already ruptured, then the fetal head is subject to the full pressure of contractions (see p.47) as it resists the dilatation of the cervix.

First stage of labor
(see p.56)

In the first stage of labor the head flexes, which reduces the diameter of the presenting part, the head, because any ovoid body being pushed through a tube will tend to adapt its long diameter to the long axis of the tube. It is also interesting to note that the occipital condyles are slightly posterior; that is, nearer to the occiput than to the forehead. The cervix and pelvic floor resist axial pressure of the body on the condyles. The long arm of the lever meets more resistance, so the head is tipped forward on the fulcrum of the condyles (Fig. 5.14).

As the head continues to descend into the pelvis, it continues to flex. The occipito-atlantal complex therefore needs to be particularly well protected, which is why structurally it is

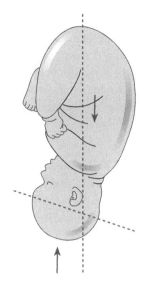

Figure 5.14 The baby's head is tipped forward with the condyles as the fulcrum.
With permission, Henriette Rintelen, Velbert

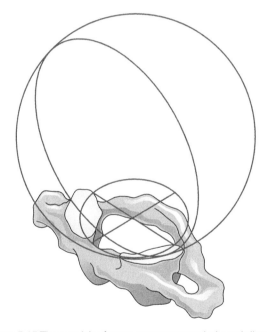

Figure 5.15 The condylar facets converge anteriorly and diverge posteriorly, a safe arrangement to resist compression at birth.
With permission, Henriette Rintelen, Velbert

arranged as a 'cone within a cone'. The shape of the condyles of the occipital bone that converge anteriorly, diverge posteriorly and face laterally form a cone shape; the configuration of the articular facets of the atlas form the other cone shape. Mechanically, the strongest shape to be able to resist compression is this cone within a cone (Fig. 5.15).

When descending into the pelvis, the child's head meets the sacrum of the mother. Passive resistance of the maternal sacrum creates a drag on the side of the vault approximated to the sacrum, while the other side of the vault is relatively free to progress into the anterior soft tissues of the pelvis. In LOA presentation the left side of the vault (i.e. the left parietal and left frontal) is closer to the sacrum, and their descent is restricted. Therefore the right parietal bone begins to override the left. In a typical molding situation, in about 60% of cases, the right parietal overrides the left parietal, frontal and occipital squama. However any variation is possible.

During the first stage of labor uterine contractions exert compressive forces down the long axis of the infant. This compression can often be palpated after birth as a whole body compression down the length of the spine from pelvis to head. In particular the occiput and condylocervical junction is subjected to constant pressure throughout the first stage of labor. This is a combination of the head being driven into the cervix by forces from the body of the fetus, and the passive resistance of the muscular cervix.

Second stage of labor
(see p.47)

When the baby's head is deep in the pelvis, the left frontal bone (in LOA presentation) comes into contact with the gutter formed by the pelvic floor muscles; this provides a pivot or fulcrum for rotation of the head. The head continues to descend in the direction of least resistance, which is usually to internally rotate through 90° (the occiput rotates internally towards the midline of the maternal pelvis). This turns the long diameter of the fetal head into an anteroposterior direction, and allows it to pass between the ischial spines of the maternal pelvis. The face is now facing the maternal sacrum. This internal rotation is aided by the spiral nature of uterine muscle fibres, which rotate the baby slightly during contractions.

During the second stage the cranium is subjected to further molding. Internal rotation further compresses the left frontal and parietal bones. The left frontal acts as a compression pivot for the internal rotation, and can become impacted into the frontal notch as a result. This often causes a blocked lacrimal duct on that side after birth. The frontal being driven back onto the sphenoid can create intraosseous distortion within the sphenoid: between the greater wing/pterygoid units and the body.

The temporal squama may be distorted in relation to the petrous part and the tympanic ring, particularly if the base has been subjected to sustained compression or there is significant vault base distortion.

The condylar parts and basiocciput are vulnerable to distortion as the head rotates against the resistance of the pelvic soft tissues under continuing strong uterine contractions. The long axis of the baby may be under compression from uterine contractions. The condylocervical junction is stabilized by ligaments such that in full flexion of the head relatively little rotation is possible between the occiput and atlas. With the passive resistance of the maternal soft tissues restricting the rotation of the head, strong rotatory forces are directed into the region of the condylar parts of the occiput. The condylar parts will distort under these forces. The direction of distortion will vary slightly in every birth. Often, due to the rotation of the occipital squama, one condyle is driven anteriorly and medially at the anterior pole of the condyle, and the other laterally at the posterior aspect of the condyle. For example if the occipital squama rotates anticlockwize the right posterior condyle will be taken laterally. Varying degrees of vertical distortion are also possible.

Towards the end of the second stage the head undergoes extension under the pubic arch of the mother. Normally the maternal sacrum and coccyx move backwards, and the innominates abduct to increase the diameter of the pelvic outlet. Now the shoulders have entered the pelvic bowl and, guided by the gutter of the pelvic floor, come to lie in an anteroposterior direction. They are rotated in relation to the head. At this stage the frontal bones are vulnerable to increased compression from the sacrum, particularly if the mother is reclining on her sacrum during labor. As the head extends under the pubic arch there may be further focal pressure on the condylar parts.

As the head is now born by extension under the pubic arch, with the face towards the sacrum, the extension transfers the emphasis of compression from the occipital condyles to C1 and the upper cervical spine.

The shoulders are now deep in the pelvis and are undergoing rotation under compression. This can be focused more on one shoulder than the other, and may also distort the diaphragm and crura. On osteopathic examination strong rotatory strains may be palpable in the thorax with the asymmetric distortion through the crura of the diaphragm. This is a common cause of difficulties in bringing up wind, colic, and reflux in infants (see Ch.11, Irritable infants and colic; Ch.12, Gastro-esophageal reflux).

When the head is born it is now free to rotate back into line with the shoulders. The shoulders may be delivered in two ways: either the anterior shoulder (the right shoulder in LOA) is delivered first, by a posterior and inferior movement of the head, if necessary aided by the midwife. This can place significant stretch on the lateral neck structures; in extreme cases it may cause brachial plexus injury (Erb's palsy). The posterior shoulder is born as the midwife lifts the baby's head anteriorly. The other possibility is the following: by lifting the baby's head towards the mother's abdomen the posterior shoulder is delivered first, and the anterior shoulder follows. This is often an easier delivery because the head continues to move in the direction it is travelling for the delivery; that is, anteriorly. Less strain is placed on cervical muscles and nerves.

Some babies are born with one hand up by the face. This not only increases the stretch on the maternal perineum, but also makes the vaginal wall more vulnerable to tearing as the elbow passes through. From the baby's point of view both clavicles are subject to enormous pressure, and the thorax undergoes greater distortion than normal.

Summary

After a normal labor, the commonly observed head shape is of flattened frontals and a high posterior vault, with the head elongated from front to back. Variable shape changes and stresses may be present through the whole basicranium. Commonly one or both condylar parts have undergone some distortion.

One can review the above sequence, thinking about the different parts of the body in turn and considering the forces imposed on each part as the infant descends and rotates down the birth canal. It is useful to use a doll and pelvis to practice the sequence, to get a visual impression of forces working on the cranial vault and base, shoulders and thorax, pelvis and spine.

Unusual presentations and their effects on the child

Occipitoposterior presentation (OP)

In an OP presentation the fetus is lying with the convexity of the spine approximated to the maternal spine, and the occiput adjacent to the maternal sacrum (back to back position; Fig. 5.12). Right occiput posterior (ROP) occurs in about 17% of all head presentations, and left occiput posterior (LOP) in about 3%. In late first stage, once the head is fully inside the bowl of the pelvis, the head can either rotate externally (long rotation) to come into the normal face posterior position. Or he can rotate internally (short rotation) to position himself with his face to the pubis of his mother. External or internal rotation is named in relation to the direction of movement of the occiput. The key to whether the child chooses the long rotation or the short rotation lies in whether the head flexes or extends on the neck as it enters the pelvis.

If the baby has spent some time with his head engaged in the bowl of the pelvis at the end of the pregnancy, a vault–base mismatch may develop. The base is primarily in flexion and compression of the sacral promontory causes flattening of the occiput so the squamous occiput is in extension. The vault is high as in an extension pattern.

Long rotation through 135°

If the child flexes the neck he will undergo a long rotation through 135° and end up facing the sacrum of the mother.

This happens because when the head flexes on the neck, the resistance of the occiput on the posterior pelvic structures slows the descent of the occiput, and the gutter of the levator ani guides the head into external rotation. This is the rotation of choice because the final delivery is easier on mother and child.

Common osteopathic findings

The rotation of the head is driven by strong uterine contractions; so compressive forces with rotation are felt down the long axis of the spine into the condylar region of the occiput. The vault meets the resistance of the birth canal in front, and this resistance may produce a contrarotation type of strain of the vault in relation to the base. On palpation this feels as though the vault is rotating in one direction (for example, clockwize) and the base and body in the other. The direction of rotation will depend on whether it is a LOP or a ROP presentation. It should be remembered that this rotation is occurring under great compression and can lead to vault-base distortion. There may be significant intrasphenoid and intraoccipital distortion and compression, including lateral strains of the sphenobasilar symphysis (SBS), which often produces a parallelogram shaped head (see Ch.15, Plagiocephaly). A lateral sheer may also be palpable between the upper and lower layers of the tentorium cerebelli, or between the layers of the falx cerebri.

Rotation under compression of the upper cervical complex and condylar parts can leave C1 impacted and rotated within the condyles on one side, and the baby finds it difficult to turn his or her head in one direction (see Ch.15, Torticollis). This commonly creates difficulties with breastfeeding on one side.

Considering what a large rotation thorax and shoulders have to make, it is not surprising that significant rotational stresses are often felt in the thorax. Distortions of the diaphragm and crura are also common. This is commonly associated with reflux or difficulty bringing up wind in the baby.

Short Rotation through 45°

If the head is not well flexed on the neck at the start of labor, as it approaches the pelvic brim the head is tipped into extension on the neck over the sacral promontory. As it continues to descend, the line of least resistance that it follows takes the head into internal rotation through 45º. It will then end up facing the pubis of the mother. This is initially easier for the baby than the long rotation; however, later on it is a much more difficult delivery.

Once in the face-to-pubis position, the head will usually continue its extension on the neck to become fully extended, and delivery is then by a face presentation in the face-to-pubis position. As this is a difficult delivery, it often leads to a caesarean section.

Common osteopathic findings

After such a birth the baby usually likes to hold his neck in full extension, with an extended occiput in relation to C1.

As the frontals come into contact with the pubic arch, this limits the extension of the head on the neck, and the head now moves into flexion. Full flexion enables the occiput to come clear of the maternal sacrum and coccyx. The occiput is delivered first, then the head extends again and the face is born. In this type of delivery there is severe compression back through the frontals as they come under the pubic arch. There is usually also severe compression of the face. Caused by the drag of the frontal area under the pubic arch, the sphenoid is often driven into extension while the occiput remains in a flexion position; so inferior vertical strain may be felt.

The angulation of the pubic arch means that the head has to pass under in a relatively more posterior position, making the perineum more vulnerable to tear due to the increased stretch required.

Deep transverse arrest

A deep transverse arrest occurs in 20% of cases. When descending, the long axis of the head often gets caught between the ischial spines of the mother and the child is then unable to complete the long rotation. Changes of position of the mother at this point may help the baby to turn past the ischial spines. Commonly, however, forceps or ventouse are used to assist complete the delivery.

Common osteopathic findings

Osteopathic findings are similar to those in long rotation, but are usually more marked. Additionally, there may be increased focal areas of compression from the application of forceps or ventouse.

Face presentation

In face presentation the head extends fully on the neck as it enters the pelvis (Fig. 5.13). As it descends, the mandible comes into contact with the gutter of the pelvic floor; this causes the head to rotate into a mentoanterior position. The head can be delivered by flexion under the pubic arch. This way of being born puts extreme stretch onto the skin on the anterior of the neck, and often there is much contusion around the face.

Common osteopathic findings

Individual cases will vary, but these are common features: severe extension strain through the upper cervical spine, and atlanto-occipital junction. The baby often holds the head in extension. The arch of the atlas and condylar parts of the occiput are very impacted, with a decrease in angulation between the squamous occiput and condyles. Intraosseous strain within the occipital squama condylar parts and upper cervical complex is common.

There is marked compression in the face and a lot of compression directed back through the mandible towards the temporals. Extreme shearing forces drive the frontal posteriorly onto the sphenoid, and vault-base stresses are common. The falx cerebri and tentorium cerebelli are also exposed to considerable forces.

Brow presentation

Here the maximum diameter of the head (mentovertical) meets the cervix (see Fig. 5.13). It is virtually impossible for the head to be born vaginally in this position. If it does not resolve into either a face presentation by further extension, or a vertex delivery by flexion, a caesarean section is performed.

Common osteopathic findings

Individual cases will vary, but common features are intraosseous distortion between the pre and post sphenoid, as well as between the body and greater wing/pterygoid units. The frontal also suffers intraosseous distortion; it is driven back into the sphenoid, carrying the greater wings posteriorly. The petrous temporals may be compressed and 'sandwiched' between the greater wing of the sphenoid and occiput. The remainder of the finding depends on how delivery takes place: in flexion, extension or by caesarean section.

Breech Presentation

Many breech babies are born by caesarean section these days, but you may see children who were born vaginally. In a vaginal delivery the baby's pelvis as the leading body part opening the cervix is exposed to a strong compression. After delivery of the body the head needs to delivered quickly because the stimulation of the baby's skin by physical handling and temperature can trigger the baby to try to take a first breath. When the head enters the birth canal it easily extends on the neck and presents the large anteroposterior diameter of the head. Delivery is eased by encouraging the head into a flexed position on the neck either by the midwife placing her finger in the baby's mouth to flex the head or by the use of forceps.

Common osteopathic findings

Fluid is forced upwards into the cranium from below, giving it an 'overinflated' feel on palpation. TMJ may be present due to the rapid delivery of the fluid filled head.

A ring of pressure may be palpable around the head, from the occiput to the zygomatic arches.

Intraosseous strains within the sacrum and pelvis are common, as these parts are not designed to withstand the pressures imparted by the cervix in labor.

The sacrum may be pulled superiorly by the dural membranes and the ischial tuberosities are held medially. Wales (1995) describes how such babies may have difficulty in learning to sit because they do not have a stable base plane. Treatment to allow the sacrum to assume its normal position within the pelvis will rectify this situation.

Developmental dysplasia of the hip (DDH), formerly known as congenital displacement of the hip, (CDH, see Ch.15) is more common in babies who have been in a breech position during all or part of the pregnancy. With the leg in full flexion, the head of femur is not situated in the optimum place in relation to the acetabulum. In children with DDH there is always distortion between the three parts of the innominates, and this generally responds well to osteopathic treatment.

Bibliography

Amiel-Tyson C, Sureau C, Schnider S: Cerebral handicap in full term neonates related to the mechanical forces of labor. Baillières clinical obstetrics and gynaecology 2(1) 1988

Arbuckle B: The selected writings of Beryl Arbuckle D.O. American Academy of Osteopathy, Indianapolis 1994

Llewellyn-Jones D: Fundamentals of obstetrics. 2nd edn. Faber and Faber, London 1977 (reprinted 1979)

Maternity Center Association: A baby is born. George Allen and Unwin, London 1966

Wales A: personal message 1995

PREMATURITY AND ASSOCIATED COMPLICATIONS

Eva Moeckel

A baby that is born before the end of the 37th week of pregnancy is called premature. A very immature preterm is a baby that is born before the 32nd week of pregnancy. Almost 6% of all babies in Germany are born too soon, and similar numbers apply to UK and most European countries. Because premature delivery often leads to developmental delay or other more or less serious long-term consequences, the proportion of premature children that we see in our osteopathic practice is undoubtedly relatively high.

Thanks to modern neonatal care, more children survive today. In 1981, the mortality rate of babies born in Bavaria weighing less than 1000 g was 53%; by 1991 it had dropped to 25%. This tremendous improvement in the chance of survival is the main reason why the overall rate of mortality at birth has dropped so dramatically in recent years.

Possible risk factors

Possible risk factors for premature delivery include:

- infection or malformation of the baby
- pathology of the mother, such as diabetes mellitus, kidney, heart or respiratory disease, hypo- or hyperthyrosis
- maternal infections
- EPH gestosis, HELLP syndrome
- anomalies or myoma of the uterus
- cervical insufficiency
- multiple pregnancy
- uterine bleeding during the pregnancy
- previous deliveries of ≤ 2500 g, previous stillbirth
- underweight mother (body mass index ≤ 18)
- polyhydramnios
- early contractions
- positional anomalies
- premature rupture of the membranes
- nicotine, alcohol, drug abuse
- psychosocial problems

Often the best therapy is reducing stress in the life of the pregnant woman (see Ch. 3). Relier (1999) quotes a study by Richard that compares the effects of stressors in pregnancy. In the group of women who had a pregnancy with no psychological stress, the rate of premature delivery was 4%. In the group of women who suffered a disturbance of psychological balance, perhaps because they rejected the baby, were deserted by a partner or experienced the death of a close relative, the rate increased to 17%.

Case history taking

In case history taking, the following questions are important:

- What was the gestation of the baby?
- How heavy was the child at birth?
- Was it a spontaneous delivery or a planned caesarean section? According to one investigation, in Bavaria in 1995 60% of all premature babies weighing less than 1500 g were born by C-section (Marcovich 2001).
- How did the bonding process between the baby and parents proceed?
- Was any further medical treatment necessary and if so, what? (In particular: methods of respiratory assistance.) Were other interventions such as suction, venepuncture, sedation or intubation carried out?
- Were there any complications such as infection?

- Was the baby in intensive care or an incubator and if so, for how long?

It is important not to make any judgmental remarks even if the circumstances were not ideal. Feelings of guilt should, if possible, be reduced during consultation and treatment, not added to.

Effects on the parents

A sudden, premature delivery may overwhelm the parents. It may be experienced as a shock, especially if it involves an emergency caesarean section. The mother may wake up afterwards and find her baby has been taken somewhere else for medical care, and all she has is a photograph. It may have been easier to deal with the shock if the mother has been able to hold the baby after giving birth, even if just for a short while.

If the child needs to be in intensive care, the role of the father is especially important after a C-section, as he will often be able to go to the intensive care unit, report back to the mother who may be unable to get up in the first few days and comfort her. This important early involvement of the father may have long term consequences. One study has shown that the fathers of prematurely born babies are more active in the care of their child at home than the fathers of term babies (Marcovich 2001).

Separation from the baby, fears for his survival and worrying about his future development affect the whole family.

Kangarooing, a method whereby the preterm baby is placed directly on the skin of the mother's or father's abdomen, may be used to encourage bonding and alleviate symptoms of stress in the child; the method was originally devised in Central America as an emergency measure to help deal with a lack of conventional facilities. Marcovich investigated it in her neonatal intensive care unit in Vienna and it is now common practice in many clinics throughout Europe. 'For mothers, the close physical contact is something like a home-coming. Almost all agree that the first time they feel their baby's skin against their own is when they truly feel like a mother' (Marcovich 2001). Not only is the bond between parents and child strengthened considerably, but the physical proximity also helps to deal with symptoms of stress. Children who are cared for by this method suffered, for example, far fewer respiratory problems. This may be because when we are stressed we need more oxygen, but when we are relaxed we use less.

Effects on the child

After a normal term delivery the baby can and should rest on the mother's abdomen; it is time to greet each other.

This is a very important stage in bonding. But it is often not possible after a premature delivery, whether vaginal or caesarean section, if the baby needs medical attention and observation. Instead of being close to the mother, the newborn has to get used to being in a high-tech environment.

Moderately premature babies can often stay with their mother. They probably feed more slowly than babies that have gone to term, and are also more likely to develop jaundice.

Premature babies weighing less than 1500 g at birth almost always require intensive care. There are usually many interventions such as suction, artificial respiration, infusions of fluid, nutrients and drugs to stimulate the circulation, either initially or long-term. It may be necessary to suction mucus from the bronchi and lungs; however, this is not a pleasant experience for the child, and causes fear and feelings of suffocation. In my opinion both artificial respiration and suction can hinder the physiological transition from placental breathing to lung breathing. The osteopath may notice this in the lung field (treatment see Ch.14, The first breath).

Lungs

Surfactant, a surface-active substance, reduces surface tension at the liquid/gas interface of the pulmonary alveoli. An adequate layer of surfactant prevents the lungs from collapsing. The unborn baby starts to produce surfactant around the 24th week of pregnancy, and in a sufficient quantity from the 35th week. The reason why premature babies born before the 35th week often suffer from respiratory problems is believed to be a lack of surfactant. Glucosteroids may be given to the pregnant woman 48 hours before delivery, if possible, to help the lungs mature. Directly after delivery, or as early as possible in the treatment for respiratory distress syndrome, the preterm baby is given surfactant by intratracheal application.

Other causes for respiratory distress are poor respiratory control from the brain, infections, adjustment difficulties due to stress or circulatory problems.

Neonates in need of artificial respiration are usually given a sedative to prevent them from extubating themselves. However, sedated preterm babies will not be able to indicate pain when they feel it because the medication impairs their muscle functions.

Consequences of artificial respiration

A long term effect of artificial respiration may be bronchopulmonary dysplasia.

After artificial respiration, especially if it continues for long, the osteopathic examination with the aid of the involuntary motion will often reveal restrictions in the bronchial and lung area and also in the area of the pharynx and larynx. If you know that a child has received artificial respiration then you need to assess the mobility of the ribcage and motility of the lungs, and treat if necessary.

Central nervous system

The more immature the preterm baby, the more likely there is to be cerebral hemorrhage (rare after the 32nd week). The brain is still immature; the supporting tissue and blood vessels are not as strong as in a mature baby. The tissue at the floor of the brain ventricles is particularly delicate. The lack of autoregulation of the cerebral circulation easily leads to subependymal bleeding and bleeding into the ventricles, which in turn may cause ventricular tamponade and circulatory disturbance of the periventricular region with hemorrhagic periventricular infarction.

Even if there is no bleeding, cerebral hypoperfusion (hypotonia, hypocapnia) may cause ischemic periventricular infarction (periventricular leukomalacia).

If the pressure of artificial respiration is too high, small blood vessels in the brain may rupture. A vascular lesion is not the only danger; any disturbance of the blood circulation often results in a reduction in oxygen saturation. A change in position can easily change the pressure in the delicate vessels.

Ultrasound checks are performed regularly so that cerebral hemorrhage can be identified early on. However, cerebral hemorrhage does not necessarily imply long-term consequences; often the child compensates well.

Just under 30% of preterm babies born before 28 weeks will develop cerebral palsy, as opposed to only 2% of those born between weeks 32 and 36 (De Jong 2003). Fits and epilepsy are also consequences of cerebral hemorrhage. In order to prevent cerebral hemorrhage, preterm babies are usually treated according to the principle of minimal handling, which means they are moved and irritated as little as possible; overstimulation, for example by noise, is avoided if at all possible, and interventions that are not strictly necessary are also avoided. One study showed that 83% of all hypoxemias, 93% of all brachycardia and 38% of all apnea in preterm babies occur during or after some form of nursing intervention (De Jong 2003). Fear and stress increase the metabolic rate, and thus the requirement for energy and oxygen. Stressful measures include frequent interruptions of sleep and rest, painful examinations such as the heel prick, inserting drips or suction.

Movement and motor function

Until the end of the 36th week the unborn baby changes his position frequently and quickly. The premature delivery puts an end to these activities. Immature preterm babies are exposed to the laws of gravity too soon, and are often weak; their spontaneous motor activity is slow to get going. This development is undoubtedly further hindered by the use of sedatives. Everything that helps the child's general well-being supports the development of the motor system.

Bones

In the last 10 weeks before the due date the bones increase in resistance and hardness many times over. A baby born early has very soft bones, depending on the extent of the prematurity, which means there is even greater exposure to the mechanical stress factors at birth. The child may be unable to adequately correct birth-related asymmetrical strain patterns without outside help. Amongst the reasons for this often reduced ability to self-correct may be the processing of drugs, shock, or an inadequate 'first breath.' It could also be that the baby's body is so busy establishing the vital functions that resolving intraosseous restrictions after delivery is not a priority.

Often, the lack of change of position in the incubator may cause further asymmetries, or restrictions of intraosseous motion. If the baby spends more than a few days in the incubator not only are intraosseous dysfunctions of the cranium common, but also of the pelvis and even the spine. If left untreated they may remain evident for years. The health of the neonate permitting, his position in the incubator should be changed regularly. Tiny preterm babies are unable to lift their head or turn it to the other side, and they are unable to hold it central while lying on their back. They stay in the position they are put in, which is why the sides of their head, which are very soft anyway, may flatten. Careful positioning of the head using small supports or a half-filled water cushion can help reduce this deformity.

Feeding

Healthy preterm babies weighing 1500 g or more are often happy to breastfeed a few hours after delivery. 'Pre term babies born between weeks 34 and 36 will be able to meet their requirement for their mother's milk by breastfeeding. If they are unable to feed very well, they may be given a bottle to help' (Conrath-Pelotte 2004). Very early preterm, small or poorly babies are usually fed through a tube, ideally on expressed breast milk. Both expressing and breastfeeding usually require the intensive support of a midwife, clinic staff or a specially trained breastfeeding advisor. Marcovich (2001) is of the opinion that even very small preterm neonates can suck and breastfeed well if they have not been on artificial respiration and therefore not been sedated.

The combination of sucking, breathing and swallowing is very difficult for a preterm baby to master since it requires the coordination of the swallowing, sucking, gag and search reflexes. A mature newborn also needs usually up to 5 days to establish an effective sucking pattern. According to Conrath-Pelotte (2003), preterm babies need a lot longer. A baby born between weeks 33 and 36 needs between 1 and 4 weeks, and a baby born between weeks 24 and 32 needs 6–8 weeks.

Breastfeeding is also calming: 'Pre term babies have a more stable heart rate and saturation values while breastfeeding than if they bottle-feed' (Conrath Pelotte). Preterm babies also digest their mother's milk better than formula.

Tiny preterms weighing less than 1500 g and sick or weak babies are fed through a duodenal or stomach tube, especially those born before weeks 30–32. Additionally, they may be fed by bottle. As soon as that works tube feeding may be reduced. Babies born between weeks 32 and 33 can usually breastfeed, even though they may need a long time and will probably also have to be fed by bottle or tube.

If a baby has been tube fed for some time, the osteopathic examination will often find a restriction of motion in the mediastinum. The soft tissue surrounding the area where the tube was positioned will have adapted to it. This area can be treated using point-of-balanced-fascial-tension techniques.

The mouth is a complex organ of perception that is exercised by sucking. Being tube fed for a long time may lead to delayed language development later on. Language development not only requires efficient mouth and neck muscles, but a correct physiological breathing rhythm as well.

If the stomach tube goes through the nose rather than the mouth, this will obstruct the baby's breathing, which often leads to arrhythmic breathing patterns.

Being tube fed for too long can also lead to eating disorders. According to Müller-Rieckmann (2000), almost every preterm baby needs help to develop mouth functions. If it is possible for a premature baby to receive osteopathic treatment whilst still in hospital, treatment will be, amongst other goals, aimed at helping the ability of the neonate to suck properly. Especially important is to ensure that the breathing pattern works well. Locally, it is important to establish good intraosseous mobility of the occipital bone in order to facilitate good function of the hypoglossal nerve.

Heart and circulation

At birth the baby's circulation functions virtually like it has since the early fetal period; however, the ductus arteriosus, the physiological bypass of the fetal lung, which usually closes in response to the stimulation of delivery, will often only close if the baby was at least 34 weeks old. A persistent ductus arteriosus may therefore be more common in a preterm baby and is closed surgically.

Also the opening in the cardiac septum, which is physiological in the fetal circulation, may persist as ventricular or atrial septal defect; this often closes by itself during the first year. If not, surgery will be performed. Resultant scars need to be treated frequently in order to ensure the symmetry of the growing body. It may be necessary therefore to continue treating the child once or twice a year while he is still growing.

Eyes

At birth, the eyes and their neurological connections are the least well developed of all the sensory organs. The eyelids are still very thin and transparent. Nor is the pupil function in children born before the 31st week fully developed. So the eyes of a preterm baby are exposed to daylight or artificial light at a time when they are not intended to be able to cope with this stimulation. That is why incubators are often – but unfortunately not always – covered.

Artificial respiration can cause retinopathy of prematurity. The blood vessels in the retina contract if they receive too much oxygen. The resultant lack of oxygen in the tissue causes a neovascularization of retinal vessels followed by scarring.

Preterm babies are more likely to squint than those that have gone to term. This may be connected with the commonly occurring cranial asymmetries. Symmetrical alignment of the eye sockets will support a balanced function of the eye musculature. Even if the child does not seem to have suffered any damage, the health of the eyes can be supported by treating osteopathically and dissolving any restrictions that might hinder the arterial and neurological supply to the eyes.

Senses of hearing and smell

Unlike the eyes, a preterm baby's hearing and sense of smell are ahead of the general development. Preterm babies are very sensitive to acoustic and olfactory stimuli. The use of perfume should therefore be avoided, nor should any scented burners be used in the practice.

Other after effects

One-third of babies born before the 32nd week will have problems processing information especially if several stimuli occur at the same time. There are often also problems with gross motor skills, especially in very early preterm children. Behavioral disturbance and concentration problems are 3 to 4 times more common than in term babies.

Children with delayed development often respond remarkably well to osteopathic treatment. Physiotherapy should be given as well; these treatment approaches complement each other. Areas of increased connective tissue tension that are diagnosed on osteopathic palpation as restricted or asymmetrical motion probably pass increased proprioceptive feedback back to the CNS. This more chaotic proprioceptive information may disturb the ability of the CNS to function normally in the motor, language and other areas. When explaining this to the parents, I often use a radio as an analogy: if the radio is set just off the station (symmetry disturbance and chaotic information) and you try to talk above the hissing, it is far more difficult – disproportionately so – than if the radio is set correctly and you are listening to the radio clearly (symmetry and balanced information).

Drugs
Drug-based treatment of the child

Antibiotics have often been given and can have a long-term negative effect on intestinal flora. Osteopathic treatment of the gut may be of benefit, and later the intestinal flora may be restored by microbiological products.

Blood pressure regulating drugs and sedatives have also often been given. Preterm babies, and neonates in general, take a long time to process any drugs they are given.

Treatment of the mother with drugs during pregnancy

Ask whether the mother was given any labor-inhibiting drugs before her premature delivery. Betamimetics stimulate the labor-inhibiting betareceptors, but the side effects include tachycardia, which in turn is treated with calcium-channel blockers. Opinions differ on the postnatal side effects for the child. There is some talk of cardiotoxic symptoms and disturbances in lung maturity. There is also a more frequent occurence of hyperbilirubinemia.

Sometimes nervous pregnant women will be given a psychopharmacologic drug or sedative such as diazepam. These drugs may impair the baby's ability to process and self-correct birth patterns without additional support.

The corrected age

Preterm babies need more time to mature physically. Use the calculated due date, not the actual date of birth, to determine the preterm baby's level of development. The difference between the planned due date and actual date of birth is calculated (e.g. 8 weeks if the baby was born in the 32nd week) and then subtracted from the actual age for the corrected age. Use this corrected age to estimate the child's development. It is important to know the corrected age when vaccinating a child, as otherwise vaccination may be too early.

Touch heals

Preterm infants and their parents may well have experienced a lot by the time the babies are a few months old and presented in the osteopathic practice for the first time. If the infants had to go through a lot of pain and many fearful situations, they may not have much trust in a therapeutic touch. Patience and a slow approach are the key. Preterm babies with developmental problems in particular often make surprisingly good progress with the help of osteopathic treatment.

The parents have also been through a lot, which is why I usually offer them a few treatments as well. Then they are not only able to experience for themselves how osteopathy works, but it also helps the whole family to process this difficult time together.

Bibliography

Conrath-Pelotte A: Ein besonderer Weg: Stillen von Frühgeborenen. Hebammenforum 5, 2004

De Jong T, Kemmler G: Kaiserschnitt. Wie Narben an Bauch und Seele heilen können. Kösel, Munich 2003

Marcovich M, De Jong T: Frühgeborene – zu klein zum Leben? 3rd edn. Fischer, Frankfurt 2001

Müller-Rieckmann E: Das frühgeborene Kind in seiner Entwicklung. 3rd edn. Ernst-Reinhardt, Munich 2000

Relier J: Liebe und Stress im pränatalen Leben. Lecture, 3rd European Osteopathy Symposium, Fraueninsel Chiemsee, February 1999

Schäper A, Gehrer B: Pflegeleitfaden Intensivpflege Pädiatrie. Urban & Fischer, Munich/Jena 1999

Weiss P: Sectio caesarea und assoziierte Fragen. Springer, Vienna 1994

Willard F: Development of the CNS and the Neurocranium. Audiotape, Sutherland Society UK 1993

6 Developmental physiology

William Goussel, Dina Guerassimiouk, Jens-Peter Markhoff

CONDITIONS FOR PHYSIOLOGICAL DEVELOPMENT

The creation and development of life depends on the existence of an appropriate environment. In this respect, the physiological conditions of the mother and father play a key role in ensuring that the egg can be fertilized and become implanted in the uterus.

The maturing processes that lead to the formation of the female and male gametes are dependent on functions of the central nervous system (CNS), the autonomic nervous system, the hormonal regulatory mechanisms and the functional condition of the testicles, ovaries and uterus.

Good health in the parents-to-be is obviously a decisive factor in enabling the child to develop her full potential. A prophylatic examination of the future parents from both an allopathic and osteopathic medical viewpoint may be useful in establishing functional disturbances and treating them if necessary. Osteopathy, and other treatments, may improve the vitality of the future parents. Osteopathic treatment is aimed at helping people achieve their optimum level of health. Other aspects in this optimization are, of course, a balanced diet, emotional well-being and a beneficial psychosocial environment.

In order to provide the right support for the physiological conditions in the future parents it may be a good idea to treat osteopathically any dysfunctions that restrict the function of the reciprocal tension membrane (dura mater) and the mobility of the cranial bones, especially at the base of the skull. Such dysfunctions may have a negative effect on the function of the CNS and the hypothalamo-hypophyseal regulation of hormone levels. Also of importance are mobility of the spine and the vertebrocostal relations, especially in regard to the anatomic position of the autonomic ganglia of the sympathetic nerve trunk in front of the rib heads. Treating the psoas muscle is no less important, as abnormal tension here can irritate the sympathetic ganglia at T12-L4. Free motion of the iliac bones, the sacrum, coccyx and pelvic floor and all the ligamentous relations must be checked and treated as appropriate (Benninghoff 1994, Netter 1994). Visceral dysfunctions of abdominal and pelvic organs can be relevant, as can hemodynamic aspects that may impair the

homeostasis of the sexual organs. Certain anatomical peculiarities such as drainage of the left ovarian or testicular vein to the left renal vein and possible vascular restrictions and backflow phenomena in this area may need to be considered. By adopting an appropriate prophylactic concept that includes examination and treatment of the parents it is possible to prepare the body physiology for a regular pregnancy. Especially if conception is difficult, interdisciplinary cooperation between gynecologists, fertility centers, urologists and osteopaths may be of benefit to the prospective parents.

PRENATAL DEVELOPMENT

Human embryological development is divided into five stages, most of which overlap or occur simultaneously. Rather than being a chronological sequence, this division is more a didactic classification.

Fertilization, cleavage, implantation

The development of a new human life begins with amalgamation of the female and male gametes. Before that, the ovary will have released an ovum. Actual fertilization occurs in the ampulla of the uterine tube, with usually one of the 300–500 million male gametes in the ejaculate fusing with the ovum. The fusion of these two gametes, each with one haploid set of chromosomes, creates the zygote, which in turn has a diploid set of chromosomes. Thus the new life that has now been created contains the hereditary information of both parents: 46 chromosomes, as is typical of every cell in the human body apart from the mature gametes, which have 23. Now several cleavages occur in the ampulla and the uterine tube through a series of mitotic cell divisions that produce the morula which consists of 16 newly formed cells, the blastomeres (Moore 1990, 1996; Drews 1993). At this stage, ciliary activity and contractions of the uterine tube transport the morula to the uterus by about the 4th day after fertilization.

There is undoubtedly more than just a 'genetic programme' to explain the initial activation and driving force behind the cleavages, divisions and continued differentiation of the blastomeres. Blechschmidt (1982, 2002) regards growth itself as the elementary factor in differentiation. Growth consists, among other things, of more molecular particles penetrating the still tiny ovum than, conversely, particles departing from the growing ovum as metabolic waste products. Thus metabolism is an essential part of organic growth. In that respect, the development process not only has a direction from the inside out, in the sense of implementing a genetic programme, but also from the outside in since it is necessary to provide nutrition.

The growing organism can be described as a metabolic field in which spatially organized metabolic conditions generate the process of differentiation. The main design forces are material movements that occur as the result of decreasing concentrations of molecules, and thereby overcoming membrane resistance. They follow the dominant hydrostatic or osmotic pressure. Creative powers are already in action at the first division of the ovum into two daughter cells. The cell limiting membrane absorbs substances, thereby increasing the size of its surface, which leads to cleavage. Surface growth occurs against the resistance of the cell plasma. So it needs energy, which is generated by metabolic processes.

This observation has significance for one particular aspect of osteopathic treatment. Very often our aim is to encourage the unrestricted interchange of body fluids – blood, lymph, cerebrospinal fluid (CSF), intra- and intercellular fluid – and the particles dissolved in them. With this in mind, these embryological findings are not only useful to the osteopath in understanding organ development, tissue derivatives and fascial associations; Blechschmidt's interpretation of embryology shows us that the same fundamental principle is at work there as the osteopath uses to support the patient's body in its striving for homeostasis.

To return to the further development, the fluid produced by the uterine membrane fills the intercellular spaces between the blastomeres, which results in the formation of a blastocystic cavity. Once this cavity has appeared, the embryo is known as a blastocyst and the outer cells as trophoblasts.

The next stage to follow, after dissolution of the zona pellucida that had been protecting the ovum, is implantation of the blastocyst in the endometrium of the uterus, which occurs on around the 6th day. As the invasively growing trophoblast embeds in the endometrium, a lacunary system becomes identifiable as early as the 11th–13th day, which is filled with cell debris, gland secretions and maternal blood. This is already the precursor of a primitive uteroplacental circulation. Following further cell divisions and growth processes during the first embryonic stage (fertilization and implantation), the 2nd week after fertilization sees the creation of the two-leafed germinal disk containing ectoderm and endoderm.

With regard to this initial stage of development, certain anatomic-functional associations in the mother's body may be of relevance in osteopathic treatment. The physiological processes explained above may be disturbed by restrictions in the fascial balance; for example:

- dysfunctions of the tubacolic ligaments, i.e the uterine tube in relation to the sigmoid colon or caecum.

- dysfunctions of the ligaments of Richard which connect the ovary with the fimbria of the uterine tube.

- mobility or motility disturbances of the entire gastrointestinal tract that may disrupt the physiology of the ovum and uterine tube.

- dysfunctions in the area of the iliac bones, the lumbar spine and the sacrum, especially in relation to the sacro-uterine ligaments.

Gastrulation

Next, in a flowing transition with the first stage of embryogenesis described above, follows the gastrulation stage, which ends with the creation of the three-layered germinal disk (Fig. 6.1): At the beginning of the 3rd week the primitive streak can be seen as a median, band-like cell aggregation of

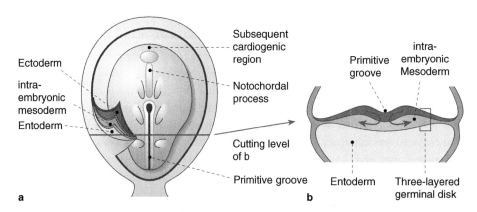

Figure 6.1 Formation of the three-layered germinal disk (15th–16th day). **a:** Dorsal view of the germinal disk; **b:** cross section of the germinal disk at the height given under a.
With permission, Henriette Rintelen, Velbert

the ectoderm at the dorsocaudal end of the germinal disk. Cells proliferate from this primitive streak and push themselves between the ectoderm and the endoderm. This results in a layer of loose mesenchyme cells that now form the intraembryonic mesoderm.

At the cranial end of the primitive streak, the ectoderm cells increase to create a raised primitive node. From here, cells migrate cranially under the ectoderm and form the notochordal process. The cranial limitation of the same is defined by the prechordal plate, which consists of endoderm and is firmly connected to the ectoderm. These two, here adhering, layers form the buccopharyngeal membrane and indicate the future position of the mouth. Transformation of the notochordal process results in the notochord, a cellular band that gives the embryo solidity and provides the axis for further growth processes. The notochord controls growth by inducing differentiation and the development of the nervous system. The spine develops around the structure of the notochord. The notochord degenerates almost entirely during the fetal stage; the only cells to remain are in the nucleus pulposus of the intervertebral discs.

At the same time, on the 16th day, the mesoderm cells around the prechordial plate shift further cranially to form the cardiogenic zone. So the result of gastrulation is a three-layered germinal disk that is the basis for all tissue types that will develop:

• The **ectoderm** is the origin of the CNS, peripheral nerves, skin and the epithelial construction of the sensory organs.

• From the **endoderm** develop the epithelial coverings for the gastrointestinal tract, the bronchi and lungs, the liver, pancreas and thyroid.

• From the **mesoderm** develop the bones, skeletal musculature, smooth muscle cells, connective tissue, heart, vascular system, kidneys and spleen.

Closer observation of gastrulation reveals that the mesoderm descends from the ectoderm, which could explain why osteopathic treatment of mesodermal derivatives can have such a major effect on the structures of the nervous system.

Neurulation

Under the influence of the notochord, around days 18 and 19 there is a thickening of the ectodermic cell layer above the notochord, which is called the neural plate and forms the anlage or primordium of the CNS. Growth inhibition by the notochord and fast growth of the neural plate results in a medial neural groove that continues to fold inwards before differentiating into the neural tube and the paired neural crests (Fig. 6.2). The latter go on to develop the spinal ganglia, the ganglia of the autonomic nervous system, the sensory

ganglia of the brain nerves V, VII, IX and X, pia mater and arachnoidea, and the Schwann cells which form the myelin sheath around the peripheral nerves. From the neural crests also develop the pigment cells, the cells of the adrenal medulla, the cranial bones and the muscles of the head.

From the cranial part of the neural tube emerge the cerebral vesicles, while the caudal part goes on to become the spinal cord. This differentiation is also a result of growth processes: there is a great increase in the numbers of the cells in the wall of the early brain. It consumes a tremendous amount of energy, and there is the corresponding gradient in metabolism. The consequence is a flow of fluid intercellular substance with nutrients from the body stalk along both sides of umbilical margin towards the brain. This transportation of nutrients occurs between intercellular tissue gaps that will

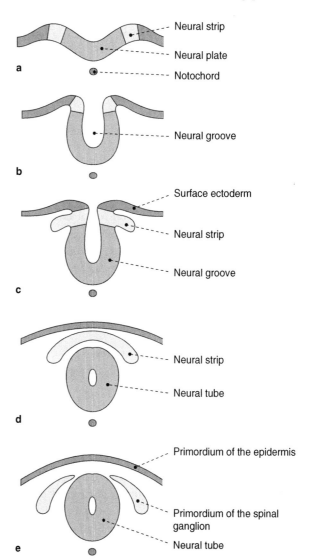

Figure 6.2 Stages in the development of neural groove, neural tube and neural crest.
With permission, Henriette Rintelen, Velbert

Table 6.1 Stages in prenatal development of various CNS structures and the associated malformations

Stage	CNS structure	Malformation
Day 17–21	Formation of the neural plate	Araphia (not viable)
Day 19–26	Formation of the neural tube	Anencephaly (not viable)
Day 26	Closure of the upper neuropore	Encephalocele
Day 27–28	Closure of the lower neuropore	Myelocele
Day 29–30	Formation of the cerebrum	Holoprosencephaly
Day 33–34	Formation of the cerebellar vesicle	Cerebellar aplasia
Day 47	Three-layer formation of the cerebral cortex	Agyria, pachygyria
Month 2–3	1st migration wave	Micropolygyria
Month 2–5	Cerebellar development	Cerebellar dysplasias (e.g. Dandy walker syndrome)
Month 2–6	Formation of the commissural plate	Agenesis of the corpus callosum
Month 3–4	2nd migration wave	Micropolygyria
End of 7th month	Formation of the six-layer cortex	Heterotopia

differentiate into vessels in just a few days. The supplying vessel anlagen converge in a collecting duct in the upper umbilical margin and directly beneath the brain: the heart anlage. Seen like this, the anlage of the heart directly serves the development of the brain during this stage of embryogenesis.

The pronounced growth of the brain is accompanied by the growth of the heart anlage, the walls of which are expanded by the stream of fluid. This expansion is that creative force that allows the wall cells to dilate into muscle cells. Thus the heart is already capable of rhythmic activity in the 4th week.

Three, and later on five fluid-filled cerebral vesicles develop in this metabolic field:

- the **telencephalon**; i.e. the two hemispheres with the lateral ventricles
- the **diencephalon** with the 3rd ventricle
- the **mesencephalon** with the aqueduct of Sylvius
- the **pons** and the **cerebellum** with the upper part of the 4th ventricle
- the **extended spinal cord** with the lower part of the 4th ventricle.

The spinal cord with its central canal develops from the caudal part of the neural tube. The ventricles and the central canal are all interconnected and filled with CSF, which also surrounds the brain and spinal cord in the subarachnoid spaces. At the 4th ventricle, the inner and outer fluid-filled spaces communicate by means of the foramina of Luschka and the foramen of Magendii. Furthermore, communication not only takes place between these described fluid-filled spaces, but there is also an exchange between CSF and the intercellular fluid of the nervous tissue.

Together with the blood, CSF is the medium that maintains the homeostasis of the nervous system, which is why its physiological fluctuation is of the utmost importance for the human organism. Sutherland describes this fluctuation in CSF as an important expression of the primary respiratory mechanism, and as containing a potency with an intelligence (Sutherland 1990). Accordingly, osteopathic treatments that affect this fluid are important as they can help to promote self-regulation of the entire body.

The stage of neurulation ends with the closing of the lower neuropore, about 26 days after fertilization. Then the neuroblasts develop into nerve cells, differentiating according to their particular metabolic field. The first synapses can already be seen in a 7-week-old embryo, facilitating a metabolic exchange, and thus also of information, between the nerve cells by means of their processes, the axons and dendrites. The continuing growth of the brain, especially the two cerebral hemispheres, leads to the formation of the sulci and gyri.

As far as malformations are concerned, neurulation is of the utmost importance (Table 6.1). Malformations may be limited to the nervous system, but they can also affect organs, bones, muscles or skin. Causes may be genetic, metabolic problems, environmental factors, infectious diseases in the mother or medication taken by the mother during pregnancy (see p.35). Such influences can cause such serious malformations as spina bifida. In about 85% of all congenital malformations of the CNS, the neural tube will not have closed properly. However, anencephalus or development disturbances

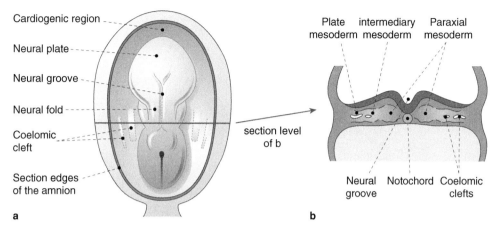

Figure 6.3 Representation of the intraembryonic mesoderm (approx. 20th day). **a:** Dorsal view of the embryo. **b:** Cross section of the germinal disk at the height given under a.
With permission, Henriette Rintelen, Velbert

of the ventricular system and the CSF function may also occur. There is a difference between an internal hydrocephalus due to a disturbance in CSF circulation in the actual ventricles, and an external hydrocephalus, which is the result of a blockage in the circulation of the subarachnoid space.

Other factors that can also play a part in causing malformation include various toxins, such as alcohol, nicotine, other drugs or poisons, and some medication. In the event of lower-grade damage with no anatomical change of the CNS, the above influences may still lead to behavioral disturbances and developmental delay of cognition and language.

Metamerization

During metamerization, which takes place between about the 20th and 30th day after fertilization, the embryo gains its segmental character. This process is based on the intraembryonic mesoderm which develops from the primitive streak and differentiates in three parts (Fig. 6.3):

- The **paraxial mesoderm** develops along both sides of the notochord as a longitudinal column that soon develops into cuboid structures, the **somites,** This results in 42–44 pairs of somites, further development of which produces the vertebral bodies, ribs, the muscles of the axial skeleton, the fibrous ring of the intervertebral discs and finally the dura mater.

- The more lateral **intermediary mesoderm** is the origin of the 42–44 primordial kidneys that develop into the **urogenital system.**

- The **plate mesoderm**, which appears to be the furthest lateral, forms spaces that are called the **intraembryonic coelom**. This divides the plate mesoderm into a parietal plate (somatopleura) and a visceral plate (splanchnopleura). Together with the overlying ectoderm, the former creates the embryonic body wall while the visceral plate and the endoderm form the wall of the primitive intestinal tube. Over the course of the 2nd month the intraembryonic coelom divides into three body cavities: the pericardial, pleural and peritoneal.

Delimitation

In this stage of embryogenesis, which also begins in the 3rd week, at the same time as the two previously described stages of neurulation and metamerization (see preceding sections), the embryo gains its definitive body shape. As the result of massive growth of the neuroectoblastic material, the embryo rotates or folds around two axes:

- **Folding around a transversal axis** (Fig. 6.4), brings the pericardial coelom, heart and septum transversum as the origin of the diaphragm into the final thoracic position in the area of the head-fold and shapes part of the yolk sac into the ventral intestine. In the area of the tail-fold, these growth processes shift the cloacal membrane ventrally, part of the yolk sac is shaped into the rectum and the actual caudal body stalk also moves to the ventral side.

- The **folding around a longitudinal axis** (Fig. 6.5) draws part of the yolk sac into the embryo as its midgut.

Summary

The embryonic period, which covers the first 8 weeks of the intrauterine life of a human being, is the time when the embryo develops most extensively. Most differentiations will have taken place by the 9th week, and the following fetal

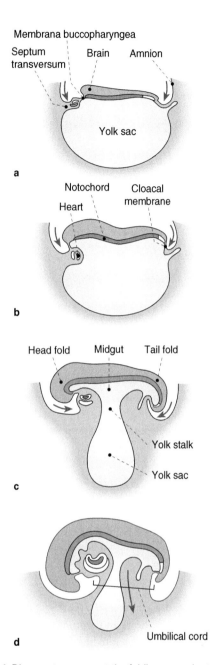

Figure 6.4 Diagram to represent the folding around a transversal axis of a 4-week embryo. **a:** around day 22. **b:** 24. day. **c:** 26. day. **d:** 28. day.
With permission, Henriette Rintelen, Velbert

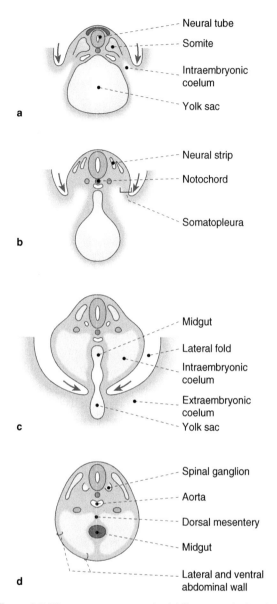

Figure 6.5 Diagram to represent the folding around a longitudinal axis of a 4-week embryo. **a:** around day 22. **b:** 24. day. **c:** 26. day. **d:** 28. day.
With permission, Henriette Rintelen, Velbert

period serves mainly for further growth and specialization of the organs.

A knowledge of the embryonic development of a human being can provide important information in the practice of osteopathy. For instance, because they share an origin, it is possible to identify the various relationships between the derivatives of the three germinal layers (Fig. 6.6). The extremities and the serous skins of the body cavities share an origin. The buds for the limbs develop from the visceral plate of

the plate mesoderm, the splanchnopleura, from which the pleura, pericardium and peritoneum are developed. This explains the influences on the parietal structures of the osteopathic treatment of the visceral structures.

In neurophysiology this is called the viscerosomatic reflex. For instance, a disturbance in the function of the gall bladder can cause a musculoskeletal dysfunction in the form of pain and impaired mobility in the lower left thoracic region. This can even be perceived as a subjective skin symptom, although the real cause is the chronic problem with the gall bladder. Conversely, a chronic segmental facilitation of the

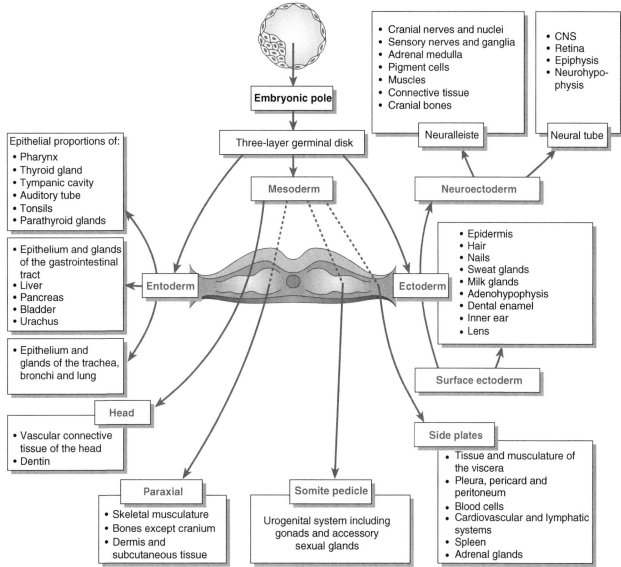

Figure 6.6 Origin and derivatives of the three germinal layers endoderm, mesoderm and ectoderm.
With permission, Henriette Rintelen, Velbert

opposing path can also be taken: in this somatovisceral reflex a somatic or musculoskeletal problem will sensitize the corresponding segment of the spine, which may in turn irritate the visceral organs that are connected to it, which can lead to a functional disturbance. Thus for instance, a chronic bad posture or an old trauma can cause a disturbance in the function of the gall bladder (Korr 1979).

Another example is the shift of the heart anlage during the delimitation stage (see see above) from the cranial pole of the germinal layer to the area of the fourth somite. This will result in a relationship between the pericardium and neck segment C3/C4. One further result of embryological folding is the innervation of the diaphragm and the peritoneal covering of

the organs of the upper abdomen by the phrenic nerve C3/C4, C4/C5. Corresponding reflectory influences emanating from the upper abdomen to the shoulder-neck region are a consequence of these embryonic associations.

To summarize, we should again emphasize the important role of the perspective represented by Blechschmidt (1982, 2002) with regard to the role of embryology in the practice of osteopathy. In his opinion, it is these metabolic exchanges and growth processes that condition the cell and organ differentiations in the embryo, and which form it and create it. The function characterizes the structure.

And are they not the same forces that we find again in the osteopathic palpation of the involuntary movement expression of primary respiration in tissue and fluids? Blechschmidt (1982, 2002) speaks of a biodynamic that accompanies development and growth. And are not the fundamental osteopathic principles of the reciprocal influence of function and structure reflected inasmuch as these biodynamic processes correspond to the function that creates the structure?

Thus the first months of a newborn's life in particular seem to be destined for the corresponding approach in osteopathy, since the tissue with its high content of fluid is still extremely adaptable and dynamic, unlike in later years when the skeletal and structural circumstances are more developed. Before dysfunctions of fluid possibly manifest themselves structurally, the osteopath will have the opportunity to diagnose and treat them, and thereby support the body in its full expansion and development.

POSTNATAL DEVELOPMENT

The cognitive, motor, linguistic and social development of a child within and outside the mother's body is dependent on the maturing processes of the CNS. Stimuli from the outside world and bodily functions in the form of a feedback effect are key factors in the quality of maturity of the brain.

Physiological development

It is important, for daily work in an osteopathy practice, to have a knowledge of the age-appropriate physiological abilities of children in order to be able to assess presenting children according to their level of development. This chapter is therefore intended to provide a broad outline of the harmonious development of a child. This is followed by information on the possibilities of developmental diagnosis (Ayres 1984, Pikler 1988, Flehmig 1996, Largo and v. Siebental 1997, Michaelis and Niemann 2001, Aksu 2002).

Month 1

In the 1st month of life, the newborn is still very much influenced by her position in the mother's body and will therefore largely still be flexed. When supine, the head will usually be turned to the side, and the baby is unable to hold it on the midline. The hands are often clenched with the thumbs adducted; the arms are angled beside the body. The knees are bent, the hips rotated to the outside and the feet dorsally flexed (Fig. 6.7). The newborn makes uncoordinated limb movements. When prone, the baby will turn her head to the side and lift it briefly.

The newborn will respond by reflex to certain stimuli. If a cheek is brushed, she will turn her head in that direction – a

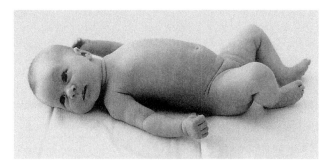

Figure 6.7 Position patterns of a newborn, supine, at 1 month. With permission, Ambühl-Stamm: Früherkennung von Bewegungsstörungen beim Säugling – Neuromotorische Untersuchung und Diagnostik. Urban & Fischer, Munich/ Jena 1999

reflex that is intended to help her find her food. Also during the 1st month, the newborn will automatically reach out towards an object that touches the palm of her hand.

Newborn babies are already able to recognize a face and their sense of smell is highly developed at birth. They can recognize the mother by her smell and taste. This sense is probably very important during the first few months of life while the other senses are still underdeveloped. Baby responds to noises; for example, by starting. This response to noise can be considered the first piece of the mosaic of linguistic development. Slight muscular contractions in the throat can also be observed, and tiny throaty sounds are produced.

Months 2–3

Because the motor development of a child occurs in a craniocaudal direction, the first parts of the body that a baby learns to control are the eye and neck muscles. They are important when orientating the head to the body or within a room.

In the 2nd and 3rd months the baby will stretch more and more and also will turn her head from side to side (Fig. 6.8). When on her front the flexion tone still dominates (Fig. 6.9), but gradually the baby learns to lift her head for longer.

The hands are now often unclenched. The child reaches out to objects and people, but the hand/eye control that is needed in order to reach the desired object is still lacking. Reaching out is still generally a 'palmar grasping'; this is because the baby is unable to differentiate the use of the thumb and forefinger.

The baby's eyes now fix on a face, vocal sounds become more varied, and social contact is increasingly made by smiling.

Months 4–6

By this age the babies are able to lie on their back symmetrically. They can bring their hands together on the midline

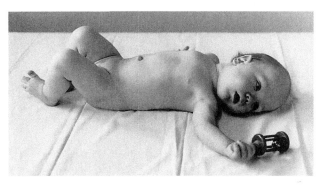

Figure 6.8 Supine position at 3 months: because the baby is able to stretch her neck fully, the head can be turned freely to either side by up to approx. 70°.
With permission, Ambühl-Stamm: Früherkennung von Bewegungsstörungen beim Säugling – Neuromotorische Untersuchung und Diagnostik. Urban & Fischer, Munich/ Jena 1999

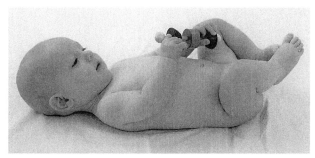

Figure 6.10 Grasping with both hands and hand-eye coordination at 6 months.
With permission, Ambühl-Stamm: Früherkennung von Bewegungsstörungen beim Säugling – Neuromotorische Untersuchung und Diagnostik. Urban & Fischer, Munich/ Jena 1999

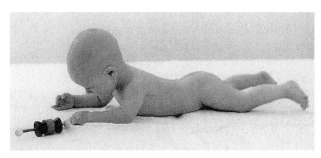

Figure 6.9 Prone position at 3 months: the upper arms are 90° in anteversion and 90° abduction from the trunk; the elbows are flexed by 90°.
With permission, Ambühl-Stamm: Früherkennung von Bewegungsstörungen beim Säugling – Neuromotorische Untersuchung und Diagnostik. Urban & Fischer, Munich/ Jena 1999

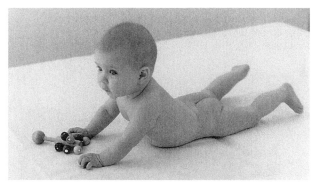

Figure 6.11 Prone position at 6 months.
With permission, Ambühl-Stamm: Früherkennung von Bewegungsstörungen beim Säugling – Neuromotorische Untersuchung und Diagnostik. Urban & Fischer, Munich/ Jena 1999

of the body, which is a major step in development. Babies play with their hands, and are able to hold an object and take it to their mouth (Fig. 6.10). They begin to use their thumbs and forefingers, although their grasp still lacks precision. Towards the end of this period the wrists become more mobile so babies are able to observe an object in their hand from all sides and maneuver it better.

From supine, the baby can now turn onto either side, occasionally ending up on her front. When lying on her stomach she has better head control, can lift her head by up to 90° and support herself well on her lower arms (Fig. 6.11).

The baby experiments more and more with her voice, combining a wide range of gurgling noises.

Months 7–9

The baby becomes increasingly active during these months. She turns herself around her longitudinal axis from her stomach onto her back and vice versa; she crawls, backwards at first,

but will later learn to crawl forwards on all fours (Fig. 6.12). One of the most important aspects of development in these months is moving forward, which enables the child to experience her environment and the distance between herself and the objects in it.

The baby also learns to sit up by herself, which helps to exercise her sense of balance (Fig. 6.13). Grasping is more deliberate, and thumb and forefinger are now used together in a pincer movement.

The baby is able to vocalize some syllables and imitate various sounds. The child is pleased to recognize her mother or another familiar person, and is more reserved with strangers.

Months 10–12

The child's ever-increasing radius of movement stimulates her nervous system by the perceptions of muscles, bones and gravity. These influences stimulate the nervous association of the two halves of her body and facilitate the first approaches

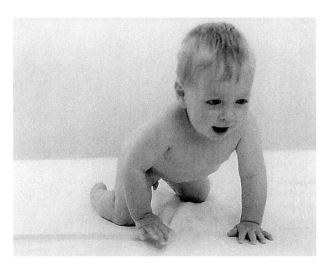

Figure 6.12 Crawling at 8 months.
With permission, Ambühl-Stamm: Früherkennung von Bewegungsstörungen beim Säugling – Neuromotorische Untersuchung und Diagnostik. Urban & Fischer, Munich/ Jena 1999

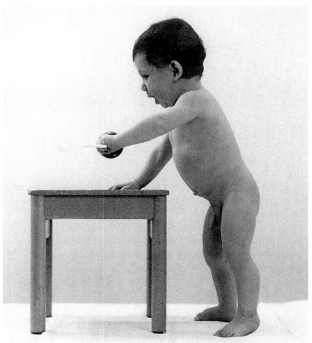

Figure 6.14 Standing at 10 months with lots of weight on the feet.
With permission, Ambühl-Stamm: Früherkennung von Bewegungsstörungen beim Säugling – Neuromotorische Untersuchung und Diagnostik. Urban & Fischer, Munich/ Jena 1999

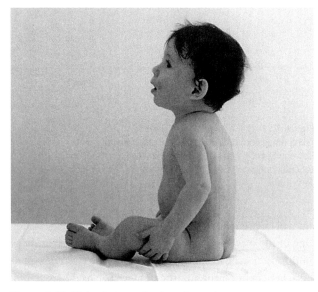

Figure 6.13 Sitting independently at 9 months.
With permission, Ambühl-Stamm: Früherkennung von Bewegungsstörungen beim Säugling – Neuromotorische Untersuchung und Diagnostik. Urban & Fischer, Munich/ Jena 1999

to planned movement. Accordingly, the crawling becomes surer and free; the strength to sit with outstretched legs improves daily.

One of the major events in early childhood is without doubt standing unaided for the first time. Standing unaided (Fig. 6.14) is a product of the processing of all the information that the child has absorbed in the previous months regarding gravity, her own movements, and the perceptions of her muscles and joints.

The child uses objects to pull herself up by and walks along holding on to them, taking her first active sideways steps. She is able to walk forwards if holding someone's hand, and then learns to walk unaided.

This extended movement also develops her visual perception. The child loves looking at things and exploring them. When playing she crosses over the midline more and more often, which aids general integration.

By now the infant also knows her own name and will respond to simple commands and restrictions. She learns to mimic gestures such as waving, and is able to repeat simple words such as 'mama' and 'dada'.

Year 2

As she becomes more able to process stimuli, the child learns to walk more safely. Now she really wants to explore her environment and improve her ability for spatial orientation. She starts to climb onto furniture and jump down again with someone's help, and to play with a ball.

By processing tactile and proprioceptive stimuli, the child is able to perceive her own body better and to plan and carry out complex activities. This makes her fine motor control more specific, and she is now able to do simple puzzles or take objects apart and put them back together again. The child has her first attempts at drawing by holding a crayon in a clenched fist and scribbling around on some paper. She is also able to play simple hide-and-seek and role-play games. Her awareness of her body is now so well developed that she is able to point to parts of her body when asked to do so.

At the end of the 2nd year the child will have a vocabulary of about 20 words.

Years 3–5

The 3-year-old toddler is able to jump from a step on both feet and run swinging both arms. Her fine motor skills are much more precise so she is able to point three fingers to manipulate small objects. This position is also extremely useful when drawing or scribbling with crayons.

In the 3rd year the child becomes more independent with regard to eating and dressing herself. She is usually toilet trained by the age of 3 or 3½.

The child's linguistic skills consist of three-word sentences. She might play with dolls, cars, Duplo, Lego, building blocks and Playmobil. She is able to play social games and exchange objects while observing some simple rules. In role play she will mimic the adults' activities.

Between the ages of 2 and 4 many children enter a stage of defiance. This stage is an important step on the way to self-discovery.

The gross motor skills become more complex between the ages of 3 and 5. At 3 years of age, a child will be able to ride a tricycle safely, and at 4–5 may progress to a bicycle. She can skip on both legs with stable balance control. The child learns to climb stairs alternating between legs, to stand on one leg and to hop, and to catch a ball thrown from a distance of 2 m. Seesawing, swinging and climbing frames become increasingly interesting and help to further develop the nervous system.

When drawing, the 4-year-old will hold a pencil with the tips of her thumb, index and middle fingers. She can draw figures and cut out shapes using special children's scissors. At about 5 years of age she is able to write her name in large letters, as well as various other letters and numbers. She draws objects differently, and is now able to reproduce a car, a house or the sun on paper.

The child becomes increasingly better at playing with peers; learning to show consideration to others, to observe certain game rules and to give and take.

A 4-year-old child can undo buttons and laces, and will be able to tie the latter when aged about 6. From 5 years the child is able to understand quantity, and can count up to five objects on a picture. But many children are already able to count to 10 and beyond by the age of 4 years. Temporal orientation regarding the day, month and year develops slowly but is usually complete by the age of 8 or 9 years.

Linguistically, sentences are becoming increasingly complex, with subordinate clauses also being included now. Articulation is faultless by 5 years old. The child's favourite words, which she uses frequently, are 'why' and 'how,' used to establish the reasoning behind everyday events. Events are retold in temporal and logical sequence, although individual segments are usually connected with '… and then … and then …'.

Summary

The postnatal physiological development of a child is a highly individual process that depends on many complex and usually interacting factors. They include the child's genetic background, psychosocial environment and the cultural and economic circumstances under which the child is growing up, and also personality and temperament. The possibilities offered by the child's direct environment are extremely important in the development of motor skills and cognitive abilities.

Thus, for instance, it is hardly surprising if a 3-year-old whose mother is an artist and whose father is a graphic designer should draw a brightly coloured Christmas tree with lots of prettily wrapped gifts beneath it. Children who live in single-storey houses and do not experience the vestibular challenge in their ground-level nursery school only learn to climb stairs when the opportunity presents itself. Likewise, there are children who are naturally shy and take a long time to feel bold enough to try something new. However, they are still well developed in their coordination and vestibular regulation, and in the sphere of motor skills development they reach all the important levels, albeit possibly a little later than their peers.

There is also a tremendous range in the sphere of linguistic development. Some children are already able to speak clearly and in complete sentences by the age of 2 years, whereas others are still only just able to form 3-word sentences at 4 years and then often 'swallow' bits of the words or get their letters mixed up, with the result that their parents end up acting as interpreters. It is not unusual for children of the latter category to turn out to have recurrent middle ear infections or a middle ear effusion in anamnesis; that is, they might have been unable to hear properly for a long period of time, and this will undoubtedly have impaired their linguistic development quite severely. If we now consider that both hearing and the vestibular regulation are closely related to the function of the inner ear, then it is easy to understand why these children not only have a poor knowledge of language but also appear to be somewhat clumsy.

Developmental diagnosis

Developmental diagnosis at an early age concerns a child's development-based abilities and skills, with various aspects being analyzed. Thus, for instance, when checking the motor skills look out for the quality of the child's movements with regard to coordination, balance and tone regulation. Assess head control, midline orientation, hand-hand, hand-mouth and hand-foot coordination, trunk symmetry and the occurrence of bilateral reflexes. When assessing linguistic development the crying of the newborn, the babbling of a baby and the word or sentence formation of the toddler are relevant. Observing the child's behavior is also extremely important: how does she enter into contact with other people; how interested is she in her environment, and how does she handle toys?

The child's sleeping and waking pattern is also extremely important; that is, the child's ability to go to sleep and sleep through the night without difficulty. One other aspect of diagnosis is the assessment of awareness and the ability to concentrate, which should increase steadily with age.

Milestones in development

Motor skills development

- End of 1st month: raises her head for at least 3 seconds while lying on her stomach, turns her head to the side when lying on her back
- 3rd month: confident at lifting her head while lying on her stomach, trunk straight
- 6th month: confident head control, targeted grasping with her whole hand, turns from back to front
- 7th–9th month: moves while lying on her front, turns around on her own axis, stands on all fours, crawls, scissor or pincer movement, sits unaided
- 9th–11th month: coordinated crawling on hands and feet, able to stand while holding on for support, walks with assistance, grasps with thumb and index finger
- 10th–14th month: moves from standing, while holding on, to sitting down
- 11th–16th month: walks unaided, bends down to pick up items
- 24th month: runs, walks backwards, able to climb stairs
- 3 years: rides a tricycle, able to stand on one leg for 1 second
- 4 years: able to stand on one leg for longer than 3 seconds, able to close a press stud
- 4–5 years: walks on tiptoes, can jump five times on one leg, able to draw a circle and square

Playing

- 3rd month: plays with her own fingers, follows a rattle from the corner of one eye to the other
- 6th month: looks for a toy, reaches out for objects, moves objects from hand to hand
- 9th month: investigates objects with her hands, eyes and mouth
- 12th month: shakes and bangs objects, pulls toys along on a string, throws blocks into box
- 18th month: sorts objects, able to stack 2–4 blocks
- 24th month: imitates the actions of adults, stacks different sized beakers inside each other
- 3 years: participates in role play, knows colours
- 4 years: plays simple, constructive games
- 5 years: plays games with rules

Linguistic development

- 1st week: cries lustily
- end of 1st month: makes short guttural sounds
- 3rd month: vocalizes spontaneously (babbling)
- 6th month: vocalizes when spoken to
- 9th month: chains of syllables with 'a' sound (e.g. ba-ba-ba-ba)
- 12th month: double syllables with 'a' sound (e.g. mama, dada)
- 15th month: imitates sounds
- 18th month: appropriate use of single words, two-word sentences
- 24th month: three-word sentences, active vocabulary of 100–300 words
- 3 years: able to use singular and plural
- 4 years: able to recount experiences independently
- 5 years: eight-word sentences, correct pronunciation

Social development

- end of 1st month: is soothed when picked up and spoken to
- 3rd month: smiles at a face
- 6th month: displays pleasure when acknowledged, spoken to
- 9th month: able to differentiate between familiar people and strangers
- 12th month: close emotional bonds with attachment figures

Table 6.2 Physiological reflexes and reactions in the 1st year

Reflex	Cause and reaction	Pathology
Sucking reflex (see fig. 6.15)	Rhythmic sucking and tongue movements when an index finger is inserted between the lips	None: e.g. vigilance disturbance, damage to brain stem
Oral search reflex (rooting)	When the corner of the mouth is brushed baby moves mouth and turns head to the side of the stimulus	Asymmetry: facial nerve or trigeminal paresis
Glabella reflex	Squeezes eyes shut on tapping against the glabella	• Extrapyramidal lesion, central facial nerve paresis: increased • Peripheral facial nerve paresis: weakened
Protective reaction	Turns head to side when lying on front to keep airways free	
Doll's eye sign	When head moved slowly in one direction eyes move in opposite direction	• None: abducens paresis, gaze paresis • Persistence: developmental delay
Stepping reaction (see Fig. 6.15)	Makes stepping movements when held under the arms with feet on a surface	• None: e.g. vigilance disturbance muscular hypotonus
Babkin reflex	Opens mouth when pressing on both palms together	Persistence e.g. with CP
Crossed extensor reflex	When bending hip and knee on one side, bends and then stretches other side while pointing toe	Stretching only: diplegia of lower limbs
Symmetrical tonic neck reflex (STNR) (see Fig. 6.15)	Bending the head causes arms to bend and legs to stretch, stretching head back causes arms to stretch and legs to bend	Persistence e.g. with CP, affects postural control
Tonic labyrinthine reflex	Observing spontaneous posture: lying on front flexion hypertonus, on back opisthotonus posture	Persistence e.g. with CP, affects postural control
Asymmetrical tonic neck reflex (ATNR) (see Fig. 6.15)	When turning head to side, extension of extremities on facial side and flexion of opposite side (fighter stance)	Intensified and/or persistent: e.g. spastic movement disorder
Moro reflex (see Fig. 6.15)	Holding child on back with one hand, supporting the head with the other; sudden backward movement of the head by 4–5 cm in the 1st stage: shoulder abduction, arms stretched, opening of the hands, spreading of the fingers, stretching of the legs 2nd stage: arm adduction, flexion	• none or asymmetry: central or peripheral paresis • intensified: hyperexcitability, hypoglycaemia, hypocalcaemia
Galant reflex (Fig. 6.15)	when the back is stroked 2–3 cm to the side of the spinous process from cranial to caudal ipsilateral flexion of the spine	• some failure: disorder of spinal cord segment • persistence: e.g. CP
Willingness to stand	when supported under the arms (feet touching a surface) active positioning of the feet on the surface and some supporting of weight	• none: e.g. muscular hypotonus • with increase in tonus, plantarflexion, inner rotation: e.g. in diplegia of lower limbs

(*Continued*)

Table 6.2 (Continued)

Reflex	Cause and reaction	Pathology
Palmar reflex (see Fig. 6.15)	Grabs finger and holds on when placed in palm of hand	• asymmetry: central or peripheral paresis • persistence, exaggerated: brain damage
Plantar reflex	Plantar flexion of toes when pressure on balls of feet	• asymmetry: central or peripheral paresis • persistence, exaggerated: brain damage
Babinski reflex	Dorsal extension of big toe when brushing against lateral foot sole	Persistence: e.g. CP
Labyrinthine righting reflex	When on front adjusts head to see room, lifts head	None: muscular hypotonus, lack of central coordination
Bauer reflex	Alternating crawling on pressing against sole of foot while on front	
Parachute reaction (Parachute reflex)	When face quickly brought towards a surface, arms stretched forward with opening out of hands	Asymmetry: central or peripheral paresis

- 15th month: imitates gestures
- 18th month: understands instructions and prohibitions
- 24th month: plays hide-and-seek, plays with a ball, defends her 'property'
- 3 years: shares with others
- 4 years: appropriate interaction with adults and peers, friendships with peers, follows rules, recognizes associations between behavior and consequences
- 5 years: able to count to 10, draws the first figures, feeling of belonging to a group

In all these criteria it must be emphasized that there is a tremendous variability in the development of children until they reach adulthood. Accordingly, care is to be taken to avoid making a hasty diagnosis (Largo and v. Siebenthal 1997, Michaelis and Niemann 2001). And finally, it must also be pointed out that the behavior and social competence of children is determined by their individual upbringing and temperament.

Physiological reflexes in the 1st year

Early diagnosis of any deviations in development during the 1st year are of particular practical relevance. The earlier any deficits in this area are identified, the more efficiently conventional and osteopathic treatment approaches can help.

Thus, for instance, in recent years Prechtl and his school have developed a method for diagnosing infantile cerebral palsy (ICP) in the first months of life. Deviations from the physiological pattern are established in video analysis of the fetus's spontaneous motor skills in the 8th and 9th months of pregnancy, and afterwards of the baby. By this means, the suspicion of future development of ICP can be addressed with the extraordinarily high rate of probability of approximately 95%. This is a highly differentiated procedure that is only to be carried out by experienced, specially trained neuropediatricians.

Another aspect of neurological diagnosis that can also be used in osteopathic practice is the provocation of certain reflexes and reactions and the assessment of their occurrence or level of development in respect of the child's age. The main point to be checked is the development of psychomotor skills, which are a mirror image of the successive brain development in the child.

Thus the reflexes and reactions in the 1st year are a good indicator of the structure and development of the brain. The newborn or baby will display many characteristic reactions that are under the dominance of subcortical cores as they mature before the cerebral cortex. As the brain matures further, these primary behavior patterns are inhibited and disappear from the child's motor response repertoire.

These reflexes and reactions are characteristic for the 1st year (Table 6.2, Fig. 6.15) and the time they appear and disappear

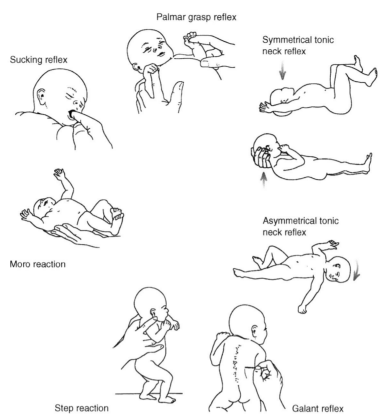

Figure 6.15 Physiological reflexes in the 1st year.
With permission, Stange, Borrosch: Pädiatrie in Frage und Antwort. 3rd edn. Urban & Fischer, Munich/Jena 2003

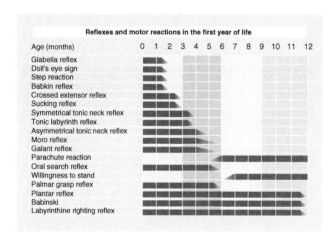

Figure 6.16 Time of occurrence of primitive reflexes in 1st year.
With permission, S. Adler, Lübeck

palate, dental anomalies, abnormally shaped ears, changes in the palmar creases, syndactylia, and changes to the genitalia (Aksu 2002). In the event of any of the above it is advised to contact the appropriate specialists. Nevertheless, osteopathy can be extremely beneficial in treating symptoms; any support for the mobility or motility of the bodily structures is a prerequisite for improvement of the function of the organ systems. With this in mind, even if there are existing genetic defects much can still be done to encourage the development of the child.

Bibliography

Aksu F: Neuropädiatrie, Diagnostik und Therapie neurologischer Erkrankungen im Kindes- und Jugendalter. Uni-Med, Bremen/London/Boston 2002

Ayres J: Bausteine der kindlichen Entwicklung. Springer, Berlin/Heidelberg/New York/Tokyo 1984

Badaljan L: Kinderneurologie. Medizin, Moscow 1975

Benninghoff A: Anatomie Band 1 und 2. Urban & Schwarzenberg, Munich/Vienna/Baltimore 1994

Blechschmidt E: Sein und Werden – Die menschliche Frühentwicklung. Urachhaus, Stuttgart 1982

Blechschmidt E: Wie beginnt das menschliche Leben – Vom Ei zum Embryo. Christiana, Stein am Rhein 2002

(Fig. 6.16) can be included in the individual assessment of development (Badaljan 1975, Flehmig 1996).

Children with persistent reflexes in particular and/or combined developmental delays may have a genetic syndrome or metabolic disease. Other indications of this may be morphological anomalies such as an unusually shaped skull, unusual hair growth, epicanthus, Brushfield spots of the iris, a high

Drews U: Taschenatlas der Embryologie. Thieme, Stuttgart/New York 1993

Einspieler C, Prechtl H: Der Vorhersagewert von 'general movements' beim jungen Säugling. In: Heinen F, Bartens W (publ.): Das Kind und die Spastik. Hans Huber, Bern/Göttingen 2001

Ernst B, Ernst W: Münchner Funktionelle Entwicklungsdiagnostik für das 2. und 3. Lebensjahr – Rationelle Testdurchführung. Der Kinderarzt 21, 1990: 1265–1268

Ferrari A, Cioni G, Prechtl H: Zusammenhänge zwischen Spontanmotorik und Hirnschädigung in den ersten Lebenswochen. In: (publ.): Ferrari A, Cioni G: Infantile Zerebralparese. Springer, Berlin/Heidelberg/New York 1998

Flehmig I: Die Denver Entwicklungsskalen (DES). In: Frühe Hilfen - wirksame Hilfen. published by the Bundesvereinigung Lebenshilfe für geistig Behinderte e.V., Bundeszentrale, Marburg 1975

Flehmig I: Normale Entwicklung des Säuglings und ihre Abweichungen. 5th edition, Thieme, Stuttgart/New York 1996

Korr I: The collected Papers of Irvin M. Korr. 5th edition, American Academy of Osteopathy, Indianapolis 1979

Largo R, v. Siebental K: Prognostische Aussagekraft von Entwicklungsuntersuchungen im ersten Lebensjahr. Kinderärztliche Praxis 67, 1997: 201–207

Michaelis R, Niemann G: Entwicklungsneurologie und Neuropädiatrie – Grundlagen und diagnostische Strategien. Thieme, Stuttgart 2001

Moore K: Embryologie – Lehrbuch und Atlas der Entwicklungsgeschichte des Menschen. Schattauer, Stuttgart/New York 1990

Moore K: Grundlagen der medizinischen Embryologie. Enke, Stuttgart 1996

Netter F: Atlas der Anatomie des Menschen. Ciba-Geigy AG, Basel 1994

Pikler E: Laβt mir Zeit – Die selbständige Bewegungsentwicklung des Kindes bis zum freien Gehen. Pflaum, Munich 1988

Sutherland W: Teachings in the Science of Osteopathy. Edited by Anne L. Wales, Sutherland Cranial Teaching Foundation, Texas 1990

7

Osteopathic diagnosis

Liz Hayden, Dion Kulak, Maxwell Fraval, Stefan Wentzke

CASE HISTORY

Liz Hayden

General considerations

Regardless of age, children presenting for treatment have a story to tell about their life so far. This begins during their pregnancy. Sometimes relevant events happened even before conception, such as a mother with a history of repeated miscarriage or infertility problems, who is likely to have a higher anxiety level about the pregnancy.

The importance of taking a thorough case history cannot be understated. This is a unique opportunity for you to get to know both the child and family, a chance that may not be repeated because during follow up treatments there is often only time for a brief discussion with the parent or carer bringing the child to update on progress.

You are interested in a factual account of the health history of the child. But at the same time there is a lot of useful information that can be gleaned on a subliminal level, such as the emotional state of the parents, the family environment, the relationship between the parents, or the parents' expectations regarding their child.

Some children find it very difficult to be brought in for treatment and to have to sit and listen while their parents talk about them to you. It is important to greet children when you meet them, even young babies respond to a greeting and eye contact. I provide toys and books to entertain the child during the case history and treatment. A younger child might find the time of case history taking a good chance to settle in and relax, when he can observe you without any contact, and hear you talk to his parent or carer in a relaxed way. If the child is old enough I try to involve him in the conversation as much as possible, so that he feels the center of attention and not ignored and talked about. You need to try to let him know that you are on his side.

In taking a case history, it is a good idea to adopt a systematic approach. This is where a good case card design can help give you invaluable prompts in your questioning.

The following is a summary of the main areas that you should be thinking about during the case history, but it is only a guide, and in reality you may need to explore other relevant events in this child's life.

Your first question is usually: why has the child been brought in for treatment? This includes presenting symptoms, but it may also be that he has been brought for a routine check up.

Conception and pregnancy

In questioning about the pregnancy, you are trying to get an idea of the health state of the baby before birth. This will have an effect on how that baby deals with the birth experience, and can help to explain why some babies with an apparently easy birth can be unable to recover from it, and others who have a very difficult birth recover very well.

It is advisable to begin asking questions about the pregnancy first because the conception issue can be a very sensitive topic and need to be broached gently. But it is useful to know about previous pregnancies or miscarriages, how long they took to conceive, or whether any fertility treatment, like IVF, was used. At the very least it helps your understanding of a 'precious baby'.

Physical health of the mother

- Raised blood pressure
- Pre-eclampsia, eclampsia
- Gestational diabetes
- Prolonged sickness
- Frequency of ultrasound scans
- Other prenatal diagnosis
- Any illnesses, especially febrile, at any stage of the pregnancy: recent evidence suggests that hyperthermia at any stage of pregnancy can have a detrimental effect on the baby. Depending on the stage of pregnancy it may be associated with neural tube defects, miscarriage, or growth retardation (Gardella and Hill 2000).
- Any health concerns related to the pregnancy, e.g. a threatened miscarriage or a history of previous miscarriage, can make the mother overanxious about the welfare of the baby.

Stress factors

- Anxieties about the pregnancy and the baby
- unrest in the home environment, e.g. by moving house, as the arrival of a new baby is a common time to move house.
- difficulties in the parents' relationship. This may be something that you draw out gradually. It is vitally important to know because the developing baby will respond to the stress in the mother, pregnancy being a time of 'nesting', when the mother craves the security of a stable home environment and a stable understanding relationship. If she does not have this and feels insecure, the baby may also feel insecure.
- Financial worries: this again is best not phrased as a direct question, but it may come out in general conversation.
- Death or severe illness in the family
- Other stress factors, e.g. in the work environment, seem to have less effect on the emotional state of the baby.

Family environment

You are also using the case history to assess the type of family environment that a child lives in. Babies and young children are acutely intuitive to their emotional environment, in particular to the mother, and will be taking in everything around them – even though parents may think that the child is unaffected by a situation, and the child may not be able to communicate it at this stage. You can often feel the physical and emotional tension in a child when they live in a stressful situation (see Ch.9, Diagnosing and treating emotional factors). Although your treatment may help them to cope with this, it can be more important at times to treat the mother to relieve some of her tension and anxiety. This can have a direct effect on the child. Many is the time in practice, when a baby is responding slowly to treatment, that once the mother is treated, the baby responds immediately. whether or not he has been treated on the day.

Last month of pregnancy

- How active was the baby at the end of pregnancy? A very active child in utero is often also a very active baby.
- Was the child really cramped for space, was there too little or too much amniotic fluid?
- How long was the baby engaged at the end of the pregnancy or was he not engaged at all? This gives an indication of the likelihood of in utero molding having occurred. A baby who was deeply engaged and unable to move much during the last month of pregnancy may well

have begun the molding process. This in utero molding can be more difficult to remodel with treatment after birth, because it has developed slowly in a non-traumatic way. Often the involuntary mechanism is actually working well and in balance in spite of an asymmetrical head. Also breech babies often have very molded heads because the head gets stuck under the mother's ribs.

Birth

It is helpful to get as much information as possible about labor and delivery. Parents of young babies are often very keen and happy to tell you every detail of the birth. But the intensity of the experience of birth soon fades, and with older children, especially when a mother has more than one child, it can be difficult to ascertain exact details.

Questions regarding birth

- Length of gestation
- Birth weight, length, head circumference
- Presentation
- Spontaneous onset or induced
- Pain relief (medication or epidural)
- Were there any of the following:
  - fetal acidosis, pH monitoring of umbilical cord
  - heart monitoring, changes in heart rate
  - fetal distress, fetal hypoxia
  - meconium in the amniotic fluid
- Length of first stage
- Length of second stage
- Delivery position
- Assisted delivery
- Elective or emergency caesarean
- Nuchal cord: was the cord round the neck, looped over the baby's head before delivery, or did it have to be cut before delivery of the shoulders? Was it cut immediately after birth, or after a few minutes, allowing time for breathing to establish itself?

Questions regarding the immediate postnatal time

- Apgar scores
- Was breathing established immediately?
- Did the baby cry excessively immediately after birth or was he calm?
- Was the baby given straight to the mother?

- When was he first breastfed?
- Did the baby spend any time in Intensive Care?
- Visible bruising/molding (photos can be helpful in this respect).

Development of the child

First 2 weeks

- Feeding: Were there any difficulties getting feeding established? Is the baby breast or bottle fed? If bottle fed, what was the reason: is it the mother's preference, difficulties of suckling or inadequate milk supply that may be caused by a poor suckling action? Can the baby feed equally easily on both breasts? Frequency of feeds, length of feeds.
- Colic: Colic is rare in the first 3 weeks. If it appears that if the baby has colic before this time, the likelihood is that the baby is suffering discomfort from the birth.
- Sleep patterns: At this stage the baby should sleep most of the time between feeds.
- Crying: Most babies do not cry excessively in the first 2 weeks. If they do it is usually an indication that they are in discomfort from birth. A high pitched cry can be an indicator of raised intracranial pressure, meningeal irritation or cerebral edema.
- Startle response: A baby that startles very easily may have an irritable nervous system, often caused by retained birth molding.

2 weeks to 6 months

- Disposition: How contented and happy is the child? Does the baby need constant attention and to be carried around, or can he be put down to play or to sleep?
- Establishment of feed patterns: Weight gain, breast feeding, bottle feeding, weaning, bowel motions, colic.
- Sleep: Is the baby developing a rhythm?
- Illnesses: How has the child recovered after an illness? Which, if any, medication has been given?
- Teething: Does the child suffer with teething? Some children become ill, or may show disturbed behavior or sleep.
- Vaccinations: Which ones, if any, did the child get? Were there any reactions? Was there a change in behavior, sleep or feed patterns afterwards, or did the child become ill?
- Physical development: Eye contact, smiling, holding toys, rolling
- Accidents and trauma.

6 months to 18 months

- Feeding: Feeding is not usually a problem at this age; babies will usually eat almost anything. However, food sensitivities or intolerances can start to show.
- Sleep: Sleep is often a problem. This may be due to the effects of retained birth molding that maintains a level of alertness in the central nervous system (CNS), preventing the child falling into a deep sleep. The style of parenting may also have an influence on the establishment of good sleep patterns. Do the parents respond instantly when the baby cries? Has the baby got a regular routine? Does the baby sleep in a cot or with the parents?
- Accidents: As the baby learns to move around, he is more vulnerable to accidents and falls. Even the most vigilant parents cannot prevent all falls. You do not want to make parents overanxious about falls, but do urge them to be observant for changes in behavior afterwards – often a child will succumb to an illness immediately after a fall, as the immune system is temporarily disabled due to the shock.
- Illnesses: Ask about acute episodes, medication or hospitalizations. Recurrent infections can begin to show a weakness in one system, e.g. ears or chest. Often children who are put into day-care nurseries suffer severe immune challenges and can suffer from recurrent infections as a result.
- Vaccinations: Which ones did the child get? Was there any reaction? Was there a change in behavior, sleep or feeding patterns afterwards, or did the child become ill?
- Establishment of locomotion: Age of onset of sitting, crawling and walking. Are these stages unduly early? A child who learns to be mobile very early may be one who is driven by physical discomfort, so it is not always a sign of healthy development. A child who is late with locomotion may be completely normal, or it may be an indication of a more global delay.
- Does the child have an appropriate activity level, or does he seem overactive or underactive? This is something that parents may be unable to assess, particularly if this is their first child.
- Speech: Is the child developing a range of sounds and first few words?
- Ability to entertain himself.
- Head banging: A child can head bang with frustration, but will usually choose a soft surface for this. A child who persistently head bangs, especially on a hard surface, may be trying to relieve discomfort or pressure in the head and

in doing so is obviously creating more problems for himself than he solves.

18 months to 3 years

- Speech development: The child should be developing a range of words and by 18 months old be connecting short phrases (see p.442; Ch.19, Language development). Delayed or unclear speech may indicate difficulties in controlling the tongue. Check on the child's feeding history as a young baby. Poor breast feeders may have found breastfeeding difficult because of difficulties in tongue control, and this shows later as articulation difficulties with speech.

- Development of the individual: The child begins to develop a sense of self, of being a separate individual from his mother. He will enjoy beginning to control his environment by asserting his own will, often more than his carers will! Shyness may begin, which is acceptable, but does the child seem basically confident in himself? If not, why? Is he picking up on other stresses around him?

- Concentration span: Watching the child play can give early indications of the concentration span developing. Some children are more physical, and others are more naturally sedentary and 'thinkers'.

- Illnesses and accidents: For illnesses and accidents the same can be said as above. Be aware of a child who seems unusually accident-prone. It may be that he has some degree of poor coordination or dyspraxia.

3–12 years

- Behavioral problems: Behavioral problems can continue, and are usually simply a continuation of behavior patterns that were present when the child was younger.

- Academic development: Academic development can only take place easily if child is balanced physically, mentally and emotionally. The early precursors to difficulties at school (poor concentration, inability to sit still for prolonged periods, poor fine or gross motor skills, poor short-term memory, etc.) have usually been present in the younger child, but it is only when expectations are increased that the problems show.

- Growth and maturation: Growth and maturation of the physical body continues rapidly through these years. Poor development of fine or gross motor skills can be an indicator of dyspraxia. Useful questions are: at what age the child learned to ride a bike, catch a ball, or swim unaided. The sutures are fully formed by 8 years old, and this is a common time for headaches to present. If a child complains of headaches before the age of 8, this is a sure sign

that the cranium is in severe difficulties either from birth trauma or acquired accident trauma.

- Accidents and acquired trauma: These may be common.

Teenagers

An important issue with teenagers is whether a parent is present during the consultation. In the UK it is advised that all children under the age of 18 should be accompanied by an adult, for the protection of the osteopath from allegations of inappropriate questions or physical contact. In the case of teenagers this can be difficult because they often have issues that they would like to discuss with you that they would not discuss in the presence of another adult. However, the teenager may not be able to supply all the information you require about their early history, and of course they are not always the most articulate communicators. I always ask a parent to be present at the initial consultation and treatment, but once I have got to know the family, for follow up treatments I may see the child alone if I feel it is appropriate.

Teenagers may present with physical symptoms, such as back pain or headaches, but it is also a time when you must consider the emotional and social pressures on them. They are often very stressed, and can be depressed. Chronic fatigue illness is not uncommon and is usually related to stress.

All the points from case history taking in a younger child are still relevant here, but particular issues also need to be taken into account.

Physical development

- Rapid growth: Physical problems often arise as a consequence, such as osteochondritic problems, or ligament and muscular strains because the soft tissue structures take time to catch up with the tone and strength needed to support the larger frame.

- Hormonal changes: The age of puberty should be established: the onset of periods in girls, the age of the voice breaking in boys. Undue delay in these changes may indicate poor pituitary function, as can delayed growth.

- Orthodontic appliances add enormous forces and pressure to a system that may already be struggling to cope with existing strain patterns. Secondary symptoms such as headache, backache, knee problems, depression, hormonal imbalances, lack of energy and digestion problems are all common.

Social challenges

- Educational/academic pressures
- Peer pressure

- First sexual relationships
- Smoking, drugs and alcohol
- Family problems
- A teenager is part child, part adult. It can be difficult for parents to retain a close relationship. It may be important to ascertain whether they still try to control the child or are they allowing him to develop into his own person?

Bibliography

Gardella J R, Hill J A: Environmental toxins associated with recurrent pregnancy loss. Seminars in Reproductive Medicine 18(4), 2000: 407–424

THE PEDIATRIC OSTEOPATHIC EXAMINATION

Dion Kulak

When looking at the scope of osteopathic practice, it becomes apparent that the osteopathic physical examination will need to include more than just a musculoskeletal assessment. Ideally the osteopathic pediatric assessment should be an integration of osteopathic as well as orthopedic, orthodontic, optometric and medical screening procedures.

Osteopathic sources describe how 'somatic dysfunction' may be an influencing factor in relation to a number of different areas of disease. Jane Carreiro (2003) summarized the possible relationship between somatic dysfunction and the neuroendocrine system. She described the influence of altered nociceptive input on the neuro-endocrine-immune system as it affects the general health of the child. Other authors (Ward 1997, Barral and Mercier 1998, Stone 2001) have described the role of somatic dysfunction in relation to visceral disease. Both, Magoun (1976) and Fryman (1976) mentioned the potential effects of cranial articular dysfunction on the subsequent growth and development of the cranium and the face. They also talked about the potential effects that such dysfunction might have on occlusion and extraocculomotor function. Clinical research by Fryman (1992) showed that osteopathic treatment may have a positive influence on the developmental progress of children with developmental delay. Consequently the use of palpation in the search for biomechanical impairments related to somatic dysfunction is an important part of the osteopathic physical assessment of the child.

Diagnosing somatic dysfunction

The subtle skill of palpation is an important tool in the diagnosis of somatic dysfunction. It enables us, as osteopaths, to become aware of the different connective tissue stresses and the ways in which they may be affecting the body. The clinical findings commonly associated with somatic dysfunction have been described by the mnemonic TART, which stands for: Tissue texture changes, Asymmetry, Restriction of motion and Tissue tenderness.

DiGiovanna and Schiowitz (1997) explained how 'in somatic dysfunction a joint is restricted or meets a barrier and is usually found to be restricted in one or more planes of motion. Motion in the opposite direction is normal or free.' Keppler (1997) mentioned how the perception of motion by way of palpation could be described as '… a sensation transmitted through the fingers … which estimates the weight of objects, the amount of pressure needed to move them, and the resistance of force exerted against your pressure …'.

Different means by which to assess any restrictions of motion

- An assessment of active range of motion (AROM): This is a movement which is being initiated by muscular activity and consciously acted out by the patient.
- The evaluation of passive range of motion (PROM): In this case the motion is induced and performed by you, the practitioner. The 'end feel' of the induced motion (of the motion barrier) gives you important diagnostic clues as to the type of tissue dysfunction present. Please note that the musculoskeletal system as well as the visceral structures can be assessed in this way.
- An assessment of inherent motion (IM): The palpation of inherent motion is the sensation of a motion which is being 'generated unconsciously' within the body (Goodridge 1986). IM is said to occur at cellular or subcellular level and to be of biochemical origin. It could be caused by the occurrence of multiple electrical patterns of activity or it may be the combined result of circulatory and electrical activities in the body. Involuntary motion has been described as exhibiting different cyclical patterns, which occur in the body simultaneously but are measured at different rates per minute. This 'phenomenon' has been measured but its origin is still very little understood. Sutherland (1990) described this involuntary activity in the body as the action of a 'primary respiratory mechanism', which occurs independently of respiration and of the heart beat. The clinical assessment of IM includes palpatory findings such as an alteration of the quality, the amplitude and direction of inherent motion. IM can be palpated in relation to all tissues of the body. This includes structures of the body, such as the vault, the cranium, the face, the viscera and the rest of the body including the spine, trunk and extremities.

- Barral and Mercier (1988) described how, in addition to the assessment of visceral mobility, an inherent motility of the different organs (inherent motion) can be palpated. He detailed different hand placements for the IM assessment of the different organs.

The clinical value of observation

The clinical observation of the child forms an important part of the youngster's physical examination. The way in which he interacts with people in the waiting room as well as with his care givers will provide invaluable information in relation to the child's psychosocial and speech development, as well as the general state of health. A lot of clinically relevant information can be gained regarding the child's musculoskeletal function. Gross motor skills are easily observed while the child moves around the room. Fine motor skills can be assessed by watching how the child manipulates and plays with the toys. Is the child unsteady when walking? Does he use both sides of the body equally well? Is there any difficulty with coordination? Can you observe any behavioral difficulties when observing the child's interaction with his parents? Does he make good eye contact? Are there any clinical signs suggestive of a visual or hearing impairment? (An abnormal response to noise or visual stimulation may be indicative of just that.) What is the child's general state of health?

Many children are too shy to speak to strangers but will readily speak to someone they already trust. I personally find it useful to watch the child, inconspicuously, as he is moving towards the toy box, whilst I am talking to the parents. A good opportunity for us to observe the child's levels of skill arises when the child is laying down on the table for treatment. Whilst treating the child, give the youngster an opportunity to play with different toys, or ask the parent to read a book to him. With an older child, allow him to read a book for himself, or play with a hand-held puzzle. Treat the toddler in the sitting position whilst initiating spontaneous play.

Conditions of cerebral palsy, muscular dystrophy, or mental disability may become apparent during the observational stage of the clinical examination. Valuable information can be gained about a child's disability by simply observing the youngster as he moves towards the toy box. This may shed some light on the extent of the child's disability. Cerebral palsy or a myopathy is best observed when the child is unawares. Also note that many physical abnormalities are associated with different syndromes or chromosomal abnormalities. A close observation of the physical appearance of the child may give important clues towards the clinical diagnosis.

The child who does not cooperate

The child's full and active cooperation is needed in order to gain clinically useful information. The clinician must take note of the basic temperament of the child and adjust the examination accordingly. One child may be extremely shy or inattentive whereas another one seems to be extremely anxious. In other instances the parents of the child may interfere with the examination, or have poor authoritative control of their youngster.

The following are some suggestions on how to deal with the difficult child:

- The hyperactive or inattentive child: In this case you will need to be flexible in the approach to examination and treatment. Try not to restrain the child's movements too much and allow him to move freely around the room. Engage in activities with the child and offer toys to play with. Try to positively reinforce any cooperative behavior, and quickly change the tasks in order to keep his attention.

- The anxious child: Try to use a gentle and non-threatening approach. Remove all objects from the examination area which the child may consider to be threatening. This also includes wearing a white coat. Keep any medical instruments out of sight. Once you have gained the confidence of the child, introduce the youngster to the examination by initiating a play situation with the equipment (e.g. let the child play doctor with the stethoscope). Do not stare at an anxious child or rush any procedures. Sit and chat with the parents first until he has gained some confidence and makes eye contact with you. It is also helpful to offer toys to the child whilst talking to the parents and allow the child to stay close to the parent in order to encourage a non-threatening environment. Leave the developmental assessment to the next appointment if cooperation cannot be achieved during the initial consultation. With an autistic child, observe the child's spontaneous play, the way in which he makes eye contact as well as the social interaction of the youngster with the environment. Watch the child as he moves around the room. This may give you sufficient clinical information regarding the child's condition so that treatment can be commenced safely.

- The non-cooperative child: In this instance you need to stay calm and patient. Try to develop ways in which you and the parent will be able to work together in a joint attempt to gain the child's cooperation. In some cases the parent is the reason as to why the child behaves in an obstructive way, especially as some care givers seem to have very little control of their youngster. Coping strategies need to be developed and discussed with the parents. In some instances the child may be more cooperative when the parent is not present. A reward system such as stickers, balloons or other little presents may provide a helpful incentive for gaining the child's cooperation.

- Inappropriate parent behavior: Parents may interfere during the examination and treatment process. In some cases inappropriate and discouraging comments in front of the off-spring are being made, or anxiety about their youngster's condition is being expressed in front of the child. Try to discourage such situations by offering to talk to the parents in the absence of their child. Alternatively you could suggest that they may ring you later in order to discuss any issues concerning their child. Questionnaires filled out as part of the case history give the parents an opportunity to express some of their concerns prior to the consultation. Stresses about childcare arrangements and divorce situations are clinically relevant. These are topics frequently dealt with by the practitioner. It may also be important for the mother to discuss any trauma, emotional or physical, as well as any sickness that she or her immediate family have suffered, as these maybe affecting her child's well-being.

The signs of physical, emotional and sexual abuse

Although the majority of your time spent in the clinic is about managing children who are being loved and well looked after, we need to be aware. The maltreatment of children does exist, and at times, whether consciously or unconsciously, we will come into contact with youngsters who have been physically or emotionally abused. This is the reason why, as primary health care providers, we have to be prepared and need to know our legal responsibilities. In some localities it is mandatory for the osteopath to report any cases of child abuse or maltreatment.

Find out which local facilities exist and what services are being offered to the victims of abuse and their families. Be prepared for the time when a child under your care discloses the fact that he has been abused to you. Remember that it is rare for a child to lie about their mistreatment. Always believe the child unless proven otherwise and proceed to look at ways in which to initiate intervention without upsetting or frightening the youngster any further. Also keep in mind that most situations of abuse are of a repetitive nature. It is rare to find that you are dealing with a singular event only.

The mistreatment of children may take on different forms. It can be physical, sexual, deprivational or may involve physical neglect. Ebrall and Davies (1998) summarized some of the physical, behavioral and non-specific indicators as they relate to the different types of abuse.

Physical abuse

This is where a non-accidental injury has been inflicted to the child. These may include bruises, burns, scalds, hematomas, fractures, or retinal hemorrhages. Become suspicious when you are detecting bruises on areas of the child's body that usually are not affected by ordinary trauma. Such areas include the thigh, the back and the torso. A fracture of the shaft of the femur, for example, which occurs under the age of 1 year, is highly suspicious. Be aware if an older child presents with fractured ribs; this is usually caused by severe trauma. Consider abuse when a burn resembles a pattern. Reports of seizures and associated unconsciousness in a child under 1 year of age will need to be differentiated from ordinary trauma. Be aware that a retinal hemorrhage in a youngster under 4 years of age may be related to the shaking of the child (shaken-impact or whiplash-shake syndrome; Coody et al 1994).

Physical neglect

This is when the caregiver of the child fails to provide proper nutrition, medical care, clothing, shelter or supervision, and consequently is putting the child's health at risk. Contemplate neglect when the child suffers from 'failure to thrive' or malnutrition (i.e. vitamin B deficiency). Also look at the family background and signs of poor hygiene and physical neglect to support your suspicion.

Emotional abuse

Garbarino (1993) describes emotional abuse as psychological maltreatment where the caregiver fails to meet the needs of the child. Some of the commonly accepted forms of emotional abuse include situations where:

- a parent ignores the child or is emotionally unavailable
- the youngster is being isolated by the care giver or being removed from his usual social environment.
- the child is being encouraged into self-destructive or antisocial behavior.
- or the youngster is continually being rejected or blamed for things for which he should not be held responsible.

The behavioral indicators of emotional abuse were summarized by Ebrall and Davies (1998). They include low self-esteem, depression, extreme anxiety, poor social and psychosocial skills, self-destructive behavior, unexplained poor learning, developmental delay, and habit disorders including rocking, biting, head banging, or sucking.

Sexual abuse

A situation of sexual abuse exists if someone older uses his or her power to engage with a child in sexual activities. Please note that this does not only relate to the penetration of the vagina or anus with a finger or the penis, but also includes other sexual activities such as touching of the genitals, oral sex or exhibitionism.

Please remember that it is not an abusive situation when sexual games are occurring between children of similar ages. No force or suffering is usually caused by these games. Most of the time the sexual explorations are innocent, as the child is searching for his own identity.

A youngster who is suffering abuse is not always easy to detect unless the child volunteers information to you personally. Contemplate the possibility of sexual abuse if the child seems to be suffering from persistent vaginal infections, unexplained injuries of the genital or anal areas, or suffers from recurrent urinary infections. Be aware if you detect unexplained bruises, scratches, burns or bite marks. In the younger child, become suspicious if the child displays sexual behaviors and knowledge inappropriate for their age. Children who fear to have their nappies changed or are anxious about being bathed need to be assessed with the possibility of sexual abuse in mind. Also consider mistreatment when a teenager displays aggressive or delinquent behavior, suffers from depression, has a tendency to self-mutilate, or is unusually sexually promiscuous.

The osteopathic physical examination
Examination setup

In many instances, the clinical examination of the infant differs from that of a toddler, the preschooler, or the school age child. Not all clinical areas have to be examined in the same detail with every child. The presenting signs and symptoms, as well as the age of the child at the time of examination, will be the deciding factors regarding the detail and sequence of the assessment for each individual case.

In most instances the physical examination is performed in a 'Head to toe' fashion, which on some occasions may need to be altered (see p.110). This is often the case with a toddler, or with an autistic or uncooperative child. However, try to adhere to a set sequence of the examination as much as possible as this helps you not to forget certain important screening procedures.

Try to disturb the child as little as possible in the clinical set up; the examination should provide a secure environment for the child (e.g. sitting on mum's lap for the toddler). The assessment should be integrated in a way which will cause minimal disturbance to the youngster. Where possible, change the positioning of the child as little as you can, and examine everything that relates to one area of the body at once.

Earlier in this chapter (see pp.100, 101)I described ways in which to get maximum cooperation from a child. We should consider that our main aim is not just to assess the child, but also to focus on how to get maximum compliance during the actual treatment session. If the child is getting too distressed by the examination procedures, he is not going to cooperate well with the actual treatment. This is why we should use our time spent during the physical assessment to establish a trusting relationship with the child rather than unnecessarily upsetting him by too many tests, which would serve only to put a distance between you and the young patient.

First impressions

Record your first impressions when meeting the youngster, asking yourself whether the child seems 'well' or 'not well'.

- Does the child seem to be feverish, showing signs of lethargy, or not responding in the way you would expect? We need to be aware that infection does not necessarily cause a fever in the young infant. The only clinical signs may be that we are dealing with a sleepy baby who does not want to feed.

- Is the child dehydrated? Clinical signs include sunken eyes. The infant may present with a sunken anterior fontanelle.

- Look for obvious signs of respiratory distress such as nasal flaring in the infant. Intercostal and subcostal retractions may be apparent in the infant and in the older child.

- Does the child show signs of central cyanosis such as blue lips indicating cardiac or respiratory disease?

- Are you observing any pallor in the child's complexion indicating anemia?

- Does the skin have a yellowish appearance? Jaundice may be present pointing to liver or gallbladder disease. In the infant you may be looking at hyperbilirubinaemia.

- Inspect the skin for rashes, bleeding or purpura (bruising). In the case of unexplained bruising always contemplate child abuse until proven otherwise.

- Does the child exhibit any dysmorphic features? Where a child has inner epicanthal folds and the eyes seem to be slanting in an upwards direction, you may be dealing with Down syndrome.

Physical growth

Pathological disturbances of growth are not always obvious at first sight. This is because the majority of children with growth abnormalities present at the extremes of normal. The accuracy of your measurements will be important.

Also take into account familiar traits, and be aware that the normal growth values of children from other ethnic backgrounds may differ from the set norms of the growth charts available. Adjusted growth charts should be used in children of different ethnic backgrounds, or in the case of Down syndrome.

The measurements of body length, head circumference and weight are plotted on the appropriate growth charts and compared with the recorded values of any past measurements. Be aware that from 2 to 18 years the stature by age is being measured rather than the recumbent length by age. Make sure not to compare the measurements taken in the recumbent position with any measurements of stature, because the values are distinctly different.

The growth charts used in practice commonly show the 5th–95th percentiles. This enables the clinician to diagnose the children whose measurements lie outside the normal limits. Any child who's weight or height is below the 5th percentile is considered to be underweight or of short stature, respectively, whilst any child above the 95th percentile is considered to be overweight or of large stature. To decide whether the child's clinical measurements are within the normal range or not, you will need to include the youngster's genetic background. Ask the parents for their height and weight measurements when they were the same age as their child.

Indications for referral

A referral for further investigation may be indicated:

- If there is a sudden increase or decrease of a previously steady growth pattern, especially if the recorded drop or rise comprizes more than two levels in the percentile chart. Please note that a drop of more than two levels in weight suggests that the child is suffering from 'failure to thrive', which urgently needs to be investigated.

- If the recorded height and weight percentiles are measuring far apart (e.g. height in the 10th percentile, and weight in the 90th percentile).

- If the child fails to achieve the expected growth rates in height and weight, especially during the times of rapid growth such as in infancy and during puberty.

Compare your growth measurements over a longer period of time in order to make a diagnosis. Tables indicating normal growth and weight values may be useful in practice when trying to analyse your data. Take into account the high velocity of growth and weight increase during the first 6 months of life. Also consider that between 3 and 7 years of age, the body weight increases by 2 kg per year, but between 8 and 12 years the increase is 3 kg per year.

Micro- and macrocephaly

Microcephaly may be benign and familiar in origin. Compare the size of the mother's and father's head with the child's measurements where head circumference is recording two standard deviations below normal. A small head may be associated with poor brain growth or developmental delay warranting referral to the neurologist for further investigation. A premature fusion of a suture (see Ch.15, Craniosynostosis) may be present when the head circumference measures below normal. An X-ray in this instance may show an exaggerated view of the bony impressions of the cerebral gyri on the inner table of the cranium. This X-ray feature is due to the prolonged increased intracranial pressure caused by the craniosynostosis. Papilledema is one of the diagnostic features of this condition. Palpating the affected suture may reveal a bony ridge.

If the head measures too large (macrocephaly), look for signs of hydrocephalus. Clinical findings include a bulging fontanelle, a dilation of the veins of the scalp, or an appearance of the eyes as if depressed in their socket. The affected child may be irritable and present with neurological signs.

Proportional and disproportional growth

When the child seems unusually short, assess the growth retardation in relation to the rest of the body. Are the growth measurements of the head, trunk and extremities in proportion, or are they not? When the child is suffering from dwarfism (see Ch.17, Achondroplasia), the trunk usually is longer relative to the length of the limbs.

Vital signs

Assess the vital functions of the child by measuring the quality of the pulse and its rate, respiratory rate, heart rate and body temperature. As the readings differ with age you will need to compare your measurements against the age-adjusted normal values. It is easy to get a false reading in the young child. This is because the different states of alertness of the baby will significantly alter your measurements. In the infant it matters whether the child is asleep, awake or is crying. In order not to upset the infant too much, count the respiratory rate first, take the pulse next, and measure the temperature last.

Respiratory rate

In the older child you can assess the respiratory rate like in the adult. In the under 5-year-old, however, respiration will primarily be abdominal. This is why you observe the abdominal movements of the younger child when counting the respiratory rate. It is only when the child reaches school age that respiration becomes thoracic. In the baby, count the respiratory rate for no less than 1 minute, as respiratory movements at that age tends to occur in an irregular pattern.

The ranges of respiration per minute may vary greatly depending on the age of the child (Table 7.1). In the newborn it is said to range between 30 and 80/minute and between 20 and 40 in early childhood (Hoekelman 1987). Be aware that respiratory rates exceeding a rate of 100/minute are symptomatic of lower respiratory tract obstruction, bronchiolitis, or bronchial asthma and warrant referral for medical management.

Heart rate (Table 7.2)

In the young infant, count the heart rate (pulse) by observing or palpating the pulsations of the anterior fontanelle or by palpating the brachial artery on the upper arm, Assess the pulse rate of the older infant and the toddler by listening to the apical beat of the heart. In this case use a stethoscope, placing it over the apex of the heart or palpate the radial artery with

your index and middle finger proximal of the child's wrist. Because of common irregularities in the rhythm of the heart at that age, the pulse needs to be counted for as long as 1 minute in order to assure accuracy of the measurement. In children over 2 years of age it is sufficient to palpate the pulse of the radial artery at the wrist.

Temperature

Different ways exist to measure the child's temperature, the most common method being the digital thermometer. Take the temperature rectally, orally, or in the axilla.

When measured orally the normal body temperature in the adult reads approximately 37°C. The temperature in infants and young children, however, is not as constant as in the adult. Fever is defined as an increase in temperature above 38°C measured rectally. The temperature can be physiologically elevated above 38°C in infants and toddlers through bodily activities, a meal containing large amounts of protein, high levels of anxiety or strong thirst ('thirst fever').

I personally like to use the tympanic membrane sensor in my clinic. This is because this is a less intrusive way of taking the temperature. The sensor of the instrument records the temperature of the tympanic membrane and thereby the hypothalamus, the center of temperature regulation (Fig. 7.1).Tug upwards on the child's ear in order to straighten the ear canal to insert the instrument. This enables the sensor to measure the heat of the tympanic membrane. Take three measurements and record the highest reading. Be aware that the measurements may be affected in their accuracy when you find it difficult to correctly place the sensor into the ear canal.

Also observe the young child for any clinical signs of fever such as flushed skin, increased respiratory and heart rate, malaise, or a 'glassy look' of the eyes. Please remember that the temperature of the young infant suffering from an infection may read normal or even subnormal.

Table 7.1 Normal range of respiratory rate

Age	Child awake	Child sleeping
Newborn	50–60	40–50
6–12 months	58–75	22–31
1–2 years old	30–40	17–23
2–4 years old	23–42	16–25
4–6 years old	19–36	14–23
6–8 years old	15–30	13–23
8–10 years old	15–31	14–23
10–12 years old	15–28	13–19
1–14 years old	18–26	15–18

From: Illing S, Klassen M: Klinikleitfaden Pädiatrie. 6th edn. Elsevier/Urban & Fischer, Munich/Jena 2003

Table 7.2 Normal range of heart rate

Age	Child awake	Child sleeping	With exertion, fever
Newborn	100–180	80–160	≤220
1 week–3 months	100–220	80–200	≤220
3 months–2 years of age	80–150	70–120	≤200
2–10 years old	70–110	60–90	≤200
>10 years old	55–90	50–90	≤200

From: Illing S, Klassen M: Klinikleitfaden Pädiatrie. 6th edn. Elsevier/Urban & Fischer, Munich/Jena 2003

Blood pressure

It is difficult to accurately measure the blood pressure in the infant. However, children over the age of 3 years are usually fascinated by the blood pressure instrument and may cooperate well with the procedure. Medical sources (American Academy of Pediatrics 1987) suggest that the blood pressure should be taken at least once a year in children with symptoms of hypertension.

It is best to use a sphygmomanometer. To ensure an accurate reading, it is important to choose the right cuff size (Table 7.3). If it is too small, the sphygmomanometer reading may be too high. If the cuff covers almost the full length of the arm with the forearm bent, you have chosen the right cuff size (Roy 1992). Where the child is obese try to cover the entire upper arm. Before inflating the cuff, supinate the hand in order to make the radial artery more accessible. Hold the arm in an extended position when taking the blood pressure as this ensures accuracy of the reading.

The bloodpressure measurements depend on the age of the child (Fig. 7.2).

The musculoskeletal assessment

When looking to assess the musculoskeletal system, you need to differentiate whether the youngster's symptoms are caused by a neurological, pathological, orthopedic, or musculoskeletal condition, or whether they are benign in origin. Common causes of musculoskeletal pain and movement dysfunction are:

- inflammation (local or systemic)
- growing pains
- somatic
- trauma

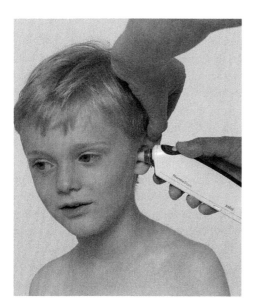

Figure 7.1 Taking a child's temperature with an ear thermometer. The auditory canal is pulled upwards by pulling on the ear. With permission, Karsten Franke, Hamburg

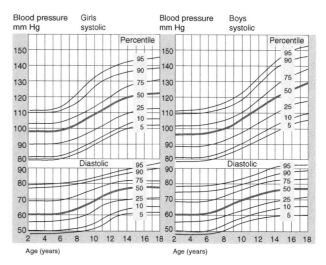

Figure 7.2 Normal blood pressure. With permission, S. Adler, Lübeck

Table 7.3 Appropriate cuff sizes for taking blood pressure

Alter (Age)	Length of extremity	Diameter of extremity	Breadth of cuff
Infants	5–7 cm	1.5–2 cm	2.5 cm
Toddlers	7.5–10 cm	2–3 cm	3–4 cm
<8 years old	12.5–15 cm	4–5 cm	5–6 cm
8–10 years old	15–20 cm	5–6.5 cm	7–10 cm
>10 years old	≥22.5 cm	≥7.5 cm	12 cm

From: Illing S, Klassen M: Klinikleitfaden Pädiatrie. 6th edn. Elsevier/Urban & Fischer, Munich/Jena 2003

- joint pathology (Perthes, slipped capital epiphyses, inflammatory or infectious disease)
- referred pain (nerve root, joint pathology, visceral)
- infection (osteomyelitis, pyogenic arthritis)
- tumor, cyst (benign, malignant or metastatic)
- hematological disorders (hemophilia)
- immunodeficiencies
- cystic fibrosis
- psychological (family stress, abuse, abnormally symbiotic parent-child relationship)
- neuropathy (cerebral palsy, hypotonia)
- myopathy (myasthenia gravis)

If the youngster displays aberrant patterns of movement, try to determine whether you are looking at a protective reaction to the pain, or whether there is evidence of any neurological dysfunction. In the latter case we need to differentiate between a myopathy such as myasthenia gravis, or a neuropathy such as cerebral palsy.

Spasticity usually presents with restricted mobility, muscle weakness and wasting. The continued increased muscle tone associated with spasticity often causes abnormal connective tissue stresses which are progressively acting on the developing bone. This is why, in the child with cerebral palsy, you may find a relative shortening of the affected limb, as well as developmental bony deformities affecting the hip joint or the ankle. Other clinical findings may include a dislocated hip or a scoliosis.

A child suffering from an upper limb peripheral nerve injury, such as Erb's palsy, may present with muscle wasting and an anteriorly displaced radial head of the affected limb. This is due to the unopposed flexor tone acting on the elbow joint.

Assessing pain and injury

If the child is suffering from pain, deal with this first. Simply observe the child and the way in which the youngster moves. This will give you clues as to the severity of the pain and the extent of the problem.

Assess the type and the severity of an injury by asking the child to show you where the pain is. Also encourage the youngster by asking him to point to the affected area with his finger. Involve the parents by asking their opinion on where they think the location of the pain is and when they became aware of the child's discomfort, as well as what type of activities seem to relieve the symptoms. In the case of a recent injury or concussion, the youngster should be left for at least 48 hours before commencing any osteopathic treatment.

Find ways in which to gain the child's trust by using an extremely gentle approach to the examination of any painful area. Ask the care giver to comfort the child during the examination when assessing the area for bruising or swelling. If the child lets you touch the injury, palpate the area for signs of edema, or increased temperature. Compare your local palpatory findings with other areas of the body. Are other joints also swollen or hot, indicating a systemic involvement? Is there any past history of respiratory infection or have antibiotics been used recently? In the latter case consider the possibility of osteomyelitis or pyogenic arthritis. Can you palpate any bony abnormalities or masses indicating a tumor or a cyst? Test the range of motion as well as determining the end feel of the joint motion.

The pediatric musculoskeletal examination

The musculoskeletal examination of the child includes an orthopedic assessment as well as an osteopathic evaluation of the biomechanical function of the body. Diagnose any structural asymmetry, as well as assessing the youngster for any restrictions of motion. Start by observing the child's active movements and postural habits. Continue your examination by evaluating the local regions of the body, including the range of motion and restrictions of individual joints.

Note the qualitative differences in the end feel of a joint; use your osteopathic palpatory skill in addition to performing the standard orthopedic procedures. Note any changes in the muscular and connective tissue make up as it is affecting the biomechanical function of the body. Especially, be aware of the tissue changes occurring as a result of somatic dysfunction. The qualitative difference perceived by palpation of any metabolic and biochemical connective tissue changes may add valuable information towards the clinical diagnosis of the child's condition.

The routine examination of the musculoskeletal system of the child includes

- assessment of gait and mobility
- static examination of anatomical landmarks for symmetry and position.
- dynamic assessment of individual segmental mobility
- assessment of somatic dysfunction as a contributing factor
- evaluation of pain and discomfort suffered by the child
- orthopedic tests
- referral for further investigation including blood tests and imaging such as X-ray, MRI and ultrasound or specialist referral.

Even though the pediatric musculoskeletal examination is described here as a separate sequence of examination, it should be performed as an integrated part of the medical and neurodevelopmental assessment of the child. When the child is suffering from chronic respiratory problems, for instance, you may choose to assess the respiratory and cardiac functions as well as performing a musculoskeletal examination of the thorax.

The neurodevelopmental examination

Clinical assessment of the child with developmental delay

When developmental delay in a child is being suspected, the examiner must consider a neurological cause as well as look for signs of visual, auditory or mental impairment. These are well-known factors which may negatively be influencing the developmental progress of the youngster.

Also look for dysmorphic features, some of which are frequently found in children presenting with developmental delay. Congenital abnormalities such as heart disease, a cleft palate or syndactyly may be present in children diagnosed with chromosomal abnormalities or a specific syndrome. Keep in mind that many of these children also suffer from an intellectual impairment associated with developmental delay.

The potential negative influence of systemic disease on the child's development will need to be considered in your assessment, as well as any genetic influences. Neurological disease, whether it be progressive or due to an injury will, no doubt, be affecting the child's developmental progress.

It has been found (Spreen et al 1995) that a child's developmental progress is not only dependent on the maturation of the CNS, but that a multitude of sensory, nutritional, psychosocial and many other environmental influences stimulate and determine the eventual architecture of the nervous system as the different functional systems develop. Environmental influences are thought to influence the 'fine wiring' of the nervous system, especially in relation to the development of higher cortical tasks such as cognition. The need for an early diagnosis and treatment of all potentially negative influences on the child's development becomes apparent.

As osteopaths, we need to consider how somatic dysfunction may be one of the influencing factors affecting the child's developmental progress. A clinical study conducted by Viola Fryman (1992) found that the neurological performance of children diagnosed with developmental delay significantly improved in the group of children who received osteopathic treatment, when compared with a control group which had not been treated. Osteopathic intervention at an early stage of the child's development may therefore be important. This

is why, as a pediatric osteopath, it is crucial to have a good working knowledge of normal development so that an early diagnosis of abnormal trends will result in early intervention. A chart listing the important milestones of normal development against which to compare the clinical findings is a useful tool in clinical practice (see p.90).

In most instances the developmental progress of the child is being assessed in the following areas:

- Gross motor skills (use of large muscles of the body).

- Fine motor skills and vision (small muscle use in relation to hand-eye coordination and visuospacial skills).

- Cognition (higher cortical function in relation to mental processes such as memory, learning and thinking).

- Language, hearing and psychosocial interaction (receptive and expressive language in relation to understanding, and the expression of meaningful communication by using symbols as well as emotional interaction).

In your assessment of the youngster you will be looking for strengths and weaknesses. Any discordance of achievement between the different areas is significant and may be an early indicator of potential problems later on. For example, if a child scores average in the area of gross motor development but seems to be delayed in the psychosocial and language areas, consider the possibility of a hearing deficit.

We also must keep in mind that there are great variations of what is considered to be normal. Whereas one child will crawl at 8 months, it may be normal for another one to achieve the same task at 18 months of age. The family history may be a helpful guide, enabling us to decide whether the relative late development in one area can be seen as normal or may need further investigation.

Important clinical information can be derived from the case history. It is useful to compare other clinical assessments of the child with your own findings. If the youngster has performed unusually badly on the day of the examination, the parent's feedback about their child's progress may be able to verify your clinical findings. Also ask whether any other members of the family have a hearing impairment and whether the child has been suffering from recurrent episodes of middle ear infection or 'glue ear'. This is because a hearing loss may be one of the factors negatively affecting speech development as well as the youngster's psychosocial adjustment.

A referral for further investigation may be indicated if a significant delay in the gross motor development of a child is also associated with:

- delayed speech

- slow development in the psychosocial area

- an asymmetric use of a limb
- the loss of a previously achieved developmental milestone.

Infantile primitive reflexes – their role in the development of antigravity responses and locomotion

It is important to be familiar with the infantile reflexes (see p.91–3), especially as they relate to early motor development. Most motor activity in the newborn is being initiated by involuntary reflex activity, which is stimulating an integrated function of multiple muscle groups. With time these primitive reactions will be replaced by other more sophisticated ones that eventually lead to the development of voluntary muscle control.

In the case of the 2- to 6-month-old, for example, the asymmetric tonic reflex (ATNR) is active. This reflex is being elicited by the turning of the infant's head to one side. In response, the upper and lower limbs of the child will assume a 'fencer position'. From 6 months onwards, however, this reflex will be replaced by a neck righting action, where the whole body will follow when the neck is being rotated to one side. Be aware that you may be looking at a spastic response when the whole body follows the head in an infant younger than 3 months old.

As the infant is starting to develop voluntary control of the body, the primitive reflexes will be suppressed by voluntary postural mechanisms. In the case where a primitive reflex persists beyond its normal time of disappearance, gross motor development may become compromised. In order for the child to crawl, for instance, he will need to be able to release the upper extremities independently from the lower ones. For this to be possible the primitive reflexes will need to be replaced by postural mechanisms under voluntary control. In order to achieve this, the youngster will need to develop vestibular as well as proprioceptive reactions for the successful development of the appropriate antigravity responses. If these reactions are dysfunctional, the fine and gross motor skills of a child may be compromised.

Developmental screening tests

A number of standardized intelligence and neurodevelopmental screening tests have been developed in order to help differentiate between normal and abnormal development. Remember that these tests often have very little predictive value as to what the future may bring for the child.

I personally do not use any standardized screening tests in the under 5-year-old. I usually manage to derive enough information regarding the child's development by observation and the initiation of spontaneous play. In the case where a developmental screening assessment seems relevant for the clinical management of the child, I usually refer the youngster to a practitioner specializing in this field.

Intelligence tests

When developmental delay is being suspected, we must also consider the possibility of mental impairment. In this case it may be appropriate to refer for an assessment of the child's cognitive abilities.

A diagnosis of mental impairment is made if the IQ of a child is 70–75 or below. A child with an IQ of between 50–55 and 70 often appears normal and is able to develop social and communication skills. In the case of an IQ between 35–40 and 50–55, the preschooler usually presents with poor social skills, can communicate but is in need of supervision. When the IQ is below 20–25 the youngster is usually dependent on care and the sensorimotor development may be poor.

General considerations regarding the neurodevelopmental assessment of the infant, toddler and preschool child

When performing a neurodevelopmental examination the clinician should consider the following factors which may be affecting the child's developmental progress. Check the child's growth parameters and physical appearance for evidence of:

- failure to thrive
- syndromal and chromosomal abnormalities
- malnutrition or chronic illness (e.g. cardiac or respiratory disease)
- small or large head size (microcephaly/hydrocephalus)

Assess the child's cognitive development. According to Illingworth (1983) the following clinical findings may be indicative of mental subnormality in a child:

- The child with mental impairment will be delayed in all areas of development. Such children show little interest for their environment, lack alertness, and are less responsive than would normally be expected. The mentally impaired child is often easily distracted, and not able to concentrate on any one task for too long. In the older child delayed speech is often associated with intellectual impairment.
- The mentally impaired newborn is more likely to present with sucking and swallowing problems. Difficulties with feeding are more common.
- The affected baby may sleep more than one would normally expect. Parents often comment that their child seems to be 'so good and hardly ever cries'.
- The infant may be late to smile.

Check the child's vision and hearing. Any problems in these areas may have a negative influence on the child's development.

Observe the youngster's behavior for signs of autism. Note whether there is any evidence that the child is lacking eye contact with you, or you are observing any age-inappropriate emotional responses, or behavioral tics. Watch for signs of psychosocial neglect and child abuse. This includes any evidence of unexplained bruising or unusual psychoemotional behavior. Check for signs of neurological disease. The clinical findings below may be indicative of CNS disease (Hoekelmann 1987):

- abnormal localized neurological findings
- failure to elicit expected neurological responses
- late persistence of normal reflex responses
- re-emergence of vanished reflex responses
- signs of developmental delay associated with developmental arrest or regression of already achieved developmental milestones.

In the infant the following signs and symptoms may warrant a full neurological screen:

- abnormal or asymmetric posturing, such as scissoring of the legs or a C-shaped body when in the supine position
- evidence of hypotonia, hypertonia, muscle weakness or wasting
- persistent primitive reflexes
- asymmetrical body or limb movements
- one-sided preference in the use of the limbs
- sudden twitching or jumps of the body indicative of infantile spasms
- sleepiness/floppiness
- lack of response to auditory or visual stimulation
- lack of eye contact/absence of smiling.

The neurodevelopmental assessment needs to have a different emphasis depending on the age of the child (Egan 1990).

- In the 6-week to 6-month-old, the examination needs to focus on the communication of the child with the parent, the visual function, and the infant's response to sound as well as the development of gross motor skills.

- If the child is between 7 and 19 months old, it will be essential to examine the child's visual behavior, gross motor skills, fine motor and visuomotor abilities and the development of expressive and perceptive language.

- The 20 months to 4½-year-old is able to cooperate better with more sophisticated clinical tests for hearing.

- From 33 months old onwards visual acuity can be tested. A substantial difference between expressive and receptive language skills, as well as an overall low score in the language area, is a reason for concern at this age and may indicate a developmental problem.

Bibliography

American Academy of Pediatrics: Report of the second taskforce on blood pressure control in children. Pediatrics 79 (1), 1987: 1–25

Barral J P, Mercier P: Visceral Manipulation. Eastland Press, Seattle 1988

Carreiro J E: Pädiatrie aus osteopathischer Sicht. Elsevier, Munich/Jena 2003

Coody D, Brown M, Montgomery D, Flynn A, Yetman R: Shaken baby syndrome: identification and prevention for the nurse practitioner. Journal of Pediatric Health Care 8, 1994: 50–56

DiGiovanna E L, Schiowitz S: An osteopathic approach to diagnosis and treatment. 2nd edn. Lippincott-Raven, Philadelphia 1997

Ebrall P S, Davies N J: Non-accidental injury and child maltreatment. In: Anrig C, Plaugher (eds): Pediatric Chiropractic. Williams and Wilkins, Baltimore 1998

Egan D F: Developmental examination of infants and preschool children. Clinics in Developmental Medicine, No. 112, Mac Keith, Blackwell Scientific Pub, Oxford 1990

Fryman V M: Learning difficulties of children viewed in the light of the osteopathic concept. JAOA 1976: 46–61

Fryman V M: Effect of osteopathic medical management on neurological development in children. JAOA 1992: 729–744

Garbarino J: Psychological child maltreatment, a developmental view. Primary Care 20, 1993: 307–315

Goodridge J: Biomechanics syllabus. Michigan State University College of Osteopathic Medicine, 1986, quoted by Keppler RE: Palpatory Skills. In Ward RC (Ed.): Foundations for Osteopathic Medicine. Williams and Wilkins, Baltimore 1997

Hoeckelman R A: Pediatric examination. In Bates B: A guide to physical examination and history taking. 4th edn. Lippincott, Philadelphia 1987

Illingworth R S: The development of the infant and young child: normal and abnormal. 8th edn. Churchill Livingstone, Edinburgh 1983

Keppler R E: Palpatory skills. In Ward R C (ed.): Foundations for osteopathic medicine. Williams and Wilkins, Baltimore 1997

Magoun H I: Osteopathy in the cranial field. 3rd edn. Journal Printing, Kirksville, Mo. 1976

Riley D (ed.): Sexual abuse of children: understanding, intervention and prevention. Radcliffe Medical, Oxford 1991

Roy D L: in Goldbloom R B (ed.): Pediatric clinical skills. Churchill Livingstone, New York 1992, pp. 171–193

Spreen O, Rissers A T, Edgell D: Developmental neuropsychology. Oxford University, New York 1995

Stone C: Visceral interactions within osteopathy. Australian Osteopathic Association Handout, September 2001

Sutherland W G: Teachings in the science of osteopathy. Anne Wales (ed). Sutherland Cranial Teaching Foundation, Fort Worth, Tex. 1990

Ward R C (ed.): Foundations for osteopathic medicine. Williams and Wilkins 1997

Zitelli B J, Davies H J (ed.): Atlas of pediatric physical diagnosis. 2nd edn. Gower Medical, New York 1992

THE 'HEAD TO TOE' SEQUENCE OF THE PHYSICAL EXAMINATION

Dion Kulak

The 'head to toe' sequence of the physical examination helps the practitioner examine the different systems in an ordered sequence. This form of assessment is least disturbing to the child and makes sure that all the necessary procedures have been included in the assessment.

Even though the musculoskeletal examination (see p.102), the neurodevelopmental assessment (see pp.126, 134, 136), and the examination of the ears and the eyes (see Ch.7, Examination of the visual and auditory system, Osteopathic considerations of sensory development) have been described separately here, wherever possible try to integrate these examinations with the head to toe sequence. For example, the child's hearing and vision tests can easily be integrated with the head and neck examination, and the musculoskeletal examination of the thorax can be put together with the assessment of the cardiac and respiratory systems.

Inspection of the hair, nails, hands and arms

The child sits on the treatment table facing the examiner.

Inspect the hair for strength and elasticity. In a child of poor nutritional status, the hair may be stringy, brittle and dry. Also check the head for any bald patches of hair. In the infant note any cradle cap.

Look at the child's hands counting the fingers. Check the shape and condition of the fingernails. The color of the nails is usually pink, the shape convex, and the nails should appear hard and smooth, but not brittle. Changes in shape are of clinical significance. A concave shape (spoon nails) may be associated with anemia; a clubbing of the nails indicates chronic cyanosis. This is where the base of the nail is springy on palpation and visibly swollen. Check the capillary refill time by pressing down on the nail and assessing the time it takes for the color of the nail to normalize. A yellow discolouration of the nail maybe associated with jaundice; a bluish-black color may have been caused by a hemorrhage following trauma. In fungal infections the entire nail is white and has a pitted surface.

Look at the palm of the child's hands to inspect the palmar creases for abnormalities such as a single horizontal crease as is the case in Down syndrome (Simian crease). Also look for clinodactyly as may be present in Russel-Silver, Down or Seckel syndrome. Ask the child to make a fist to detect a short fourth metacarpal which may be present in Turner syndrome, fetal alcohol syndrome (FAS), or pseudo-hypoparathyroidism.

Hold the arms of the child straight with the palms up in order to assess the carrying angle at the elbow. Note any cubitus varus. The presence of valgus maybe associated with Turner or Noonan syndromes.

Bend the child's elbow to touch the shoulders with their thumbs. This procedure detects a proximal or distal segmental shortening of the upper limb as seen in achrondroplasia.

Inspection of the head and the neck

Stand behind the child to observe the position of the head, neck and the shoulders. Try to detect any postural asymmetries and structural abnormalities such as:

- a short neck as in Klippel-Feil or Noonan syndrome
- a webbing of the neck (pterygium colli) as in Turner or Noonan syndrome.
- a low hairline, e.g. in Turner, Noonan, or Klippel-Feil syndrome.

Palpate the paraspinal muscles of the neck for any tenderness and pain as well as assessing the range of motion. In the case of torticollis you find cervical motion to be limited and the head held to one side with the chin pointing in the opposite direction. When the child is holding the head in hyperextension (opisthonos) and pain can be elicited during neck flexion, you may be dealing with a meningeal irritation (Brudzinski sign), which needs to be referred immediately for medical management.

Inspection of the head and the face

With the child sitting, check the head and the face for any swelling. Note any unusual sites of edema which could be related to conditions such as Cushing syndrome, kidney disease, or steroid therapy. A bilateral swelling in front of the earlobe may be associated with mumps as you are palpating an enlargement of the parotid gland.

Assess the head for general shape and symmetry. Is one cranial bone unusually flat? Observe the head for any obvious asymmetry of shape, which may be associated with craniosynostosis (see Ch.15). This is where the sagittal suture has fused, the lateral growth of the cranium is being prevented (dolichocephaly). The shape of the skull will therefore become long and narrow. When the coronal suture is fused the cranial growth in an anteroposterior direction is being restricted.

Note any asymmetries affecting the skull. Plagiocephaly (see Ch.15) may be associated with a lateral molding strain of the cranial base. Magoun (1976) suggested that a left lateral strain of the cranial base could be associated with clinical findings where the left eye and the left inferior-lateral angle of the occiput are in a relative anterior position when compared with the right eye and occiput. In this situation the mandible frequently appears to be in a position to the right, off the midline. Where the child is presenting with a molding strain related to a right torsion of the cranial base, the right ear is flared and the right eye may seem bigger than the left one.

Recent clinical studies (Yu et al 2004) investigating torticollis and plagiocephaly have found that cranial and facial asymmetries related to infantile torticollis may become permanent when the associated sternocleidomastoid contracture is being left untreated. This finding underlines the need for an osteopathic treatment of conditions where biomechanical stresses are thought to be a contributing factor to the developing asymmetries affecting the head. This is why it is important to assess the infant for restricted cranial articular motion as well as for spinal somatic dysfunction associated with the observed musculoskeletal asymmetries.

Palpate the skull, the sutures and the fontanelles for patency and, if applicable, measure the length and width of the anterior fontanelle. Note any fractures or swellings. Normally the anterior fontanelle fuses between 12 and 18 months of age whereas the posterior has already closed at 2 months of age.

Inspect the face for unusual proportions. Do the eyes of the child seem widely or closely spaced, or are you observing a small or a receding chin? Ask the child to make a face, or watch the baby smile in order to assess the movement of the face. In the case of Bell's Palsy, the mandible will deviate to the unaffected side when the baby is smiling, and the corner of the mouth will stay depressed on the affected side (see facial nerve (CN VII), p.137).

Observe the level of the ears. If they are set low you maybe dealing with mental retardation or a kidney abnormality. Normally the top of the pinna of the earlobe should meet an imaginary line which is being drawn from the outer orbit to the occiput. Also assess whether one pinna is pointing outwards more than the other, indicating a temporal bone dysfunction or a positional change due to intraosseous molding. If the temporal bone is being held in a position of relative external rotation, the ear will be flared, whilst the opposite temporal bone may be held in relative internal rotation where the earlobe seems closer to the head (Magoun 1976). Palpate the inferior-lateral angles of the occiput in order to assess the relative position of the temporal and occipital complex.

Examine the child's hearing (see vestibulocochlear nerve, p.136) and test his visual abilities and the movement of the eyes (see optical, occulumotor, trochlear and abducent nerves p.136).

Examination of the nose

Normally the nose is located along a vertical line running from the midpoint between the eyes to the notch of the upper lip. Inspect the nose for any deviation that could be due to childhood trauma or birth. Note the size and shape of the nostrils and whether there is any nasal flaring as may be the case in respiratory distress of the infant. Examine the patency of the nasal passages by alternately covering one nostril and then the other.

Inspect the internal structures of the nose with the otoscope using a short and wide speculum. Push the tip of the nose up whilst tilting the child's head backwards, illuminating the nasal cavity (see Fig. 7.3). The otoscope needs to inserted away from the nasal septum and be tilted upwards in order to straighten the nasal passageway. This position will help with the viewing of the posterior wall of the nasal cavity. It is important to explain this process so the child will not become upset by this procedure.

Observe the color of the nasal mucosal lining, noting any swelling, discharge, dryness or bleeding. In the common cold the lining usually appears to be red and swollen. But if the nasal membrane looks pale, greyish pink and swollen, we are dealing with a nasal allergy. Another differentiating feature is the type of nasal discharge. If the exudate is thin and clear, an allergic situation may be causing the postnasal drip. A purulent, green discharge, however, will indicate the presence of an infection. If you smell a foul odour, suspect a foreign body or a chronic infection. When looking deeper into the nose, inspect the concha. Do they seem enlarged, or has the mucosal lining a boggy, pale or greyish appearance? Check the nasal septum for any deviation.

Inspection of the mouth and the throat

Examine the mouth and the throat by inspecting the lips, tongue, teeth, bite, gums, palate, uvula, tonsils, mucosal lining

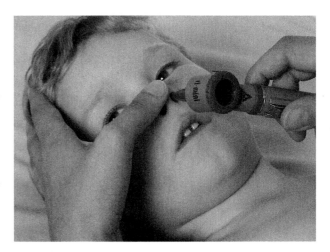

Figure 7.3 Inspection of the nose.
With permission, Karsten Franke, Hamburg

of the oral cavity and the posterior pharynx. Start the examination with an inspection of the lips, looking for ulcerations such as herpes simplex, as well as any cracking or fissures at the corners of the lips. The latter may be related to deficiencies of niacin, riboflavin, Vitamin C or iron.

The inspection of the internal structures of the mouth will be difficult in infants and toddlers and may be upsetting for the child. In the infant it is best performed during episodes of crying when the child spontaneously opens his mouth. A tongue blade usually elicits a strong reflex elevation of the base of the tongue, which tends to occlude the view of the pharynx. When inspecting the tongue and mucosal lining of the oral cavity of the infant, check it for thrush (candidiasis), which presents as a lacy, white lining of the tongue with an erythematous base. Try to remove this lining from the tongue. If you are successful at removing it, you are dealing with milk curd residues rather than thrush.

In the preschooler you can use a tongue blade. But all children who are able to stick out their tongue at you can usually be examined without it. Ask the child to open his mouth wide and to say 'ahh', in order to encourage a full view of the oral and posterior pharyngeal cavities. If you are using a spatula to depress the tongue, always try to place it away from the midline of the tongue, which is less likely to cause any gagging. This also encourages a view of the lateral gums and the posterior pharyngeal cavity. A flash light may be used to transilluminate the pharyngeal cavity. Children resist this examination by pursing their lips and clamping their teeth. This can be overcome by gently inserting the tongue blade along the buccal mucosa between the alveolar ridges and behind the molars. This initiates a gagging by the child and therefore opens the mouth so that the pharynx can be fully inspected.

Observe the color of the mucosal lining of the oral cavity. Look for any Koplik spots in the case of measles (rubeola). They usually appear on the oral mucosa opposite the first and second molar and look like grains of salt sitting on individual erythematous bases. In the case where the Koplik spots are associated with fever and coryza, the diagnosis of a prodromal stage of measles is likely.

Look at the size of the tonsils, assessing the position and shape of the uvula. If the tonsils are enlarged and red, and there are white patches on them and the surrounding areas, the child may be suffering from tonsillitis or a throat infection. A white exudate over the surface of the tonsils is suggestive of streptococcal tonsillitis requiring medical management with antibiotics. An exceptionally red and swollen tongue is a sign of systemic disease. The adenoids cannot be visualized other than when they are unusually enlarged.

In order to examine the gums and the teeth, ask the child to 'bite down hard' as this action encourages the child to part their lips. Inspect the health of the gums and the teeth. Is there any sign of crowding of the teeth? Also check the teeth for any discolouration and plaques as well as for cavities. Try to assess any obvious problems with occlusion. Observe how the upper and lower jaws meet in the vertical, transverse and anteroposterior planes. Also inspect the alignment of the teeth and watch how they interdigitate with each other. Is there evidence of any malocclusion such as a cross bite, a maxillary protrusion (overbite), a mandibular protrusion (underbite), or a receded mandible?

Check the position of the tongue. Is it protruding anteriorly or laterally between the teeth when the bite is closed? Is there any evidence of a 'tongue tie', where the tongue is restricted in its forward movement? A 'tongue tie' may be causing feeding problems in the infant, and speech difficulties in the older child. An anterior tongue thrust usually becomes apparent when the child is talking to you, as this often presents with a lisp. An open bite may be associated with a lisp as the tongue travels anteriorly when swallowing or speaking. Ask the child to stick out his tongue to test the function of the hypoglossal nerve.

In order to examine the structural integrity of the palate, ask the child to open his mouth. Use a finger cot to palpate the shape of the upper palate. If you feel a bony ridge along the cruciate suture you are dealing with a torus palatinus. Note whether the child's palate is unusually high. Is the child a mouth breather? Palpate the palate of the infant by inserting a cotted little or index finger into the mouth, stimulating the child to suck. This procedure also gives you the chance to evaluate the way in which the infant latches on to your finger and may give you clues in relation to any breast feeding problems experienced by the mother. Once the infant has latched on to the finger properly, it should be drawn backward and up by the sucking motion and come to rest on the upper palate. When feeding problems are affecting the infant you may find that the baby fails to draw the finger backwards but instead is clamping down on your fingers with the anterior palate. This is frequently the case when the mother complains of cracked nipples and mastitis.

Examination of the anterior structures of the neck

Inspect the neck for any swelling and unusual masses. Marked edema may be indicative of an infection involving the mouth or the throat.

Palpate the lymph glands of the neck looking for any abnormalities. Check the supraclavicular nodes situated just posteriorly to the clavicle. Tilt the child's head upwards in order to palpate the cervical lymph nodes which lie anterior and posterior to the sternocleidomastoid muscle. Also check the submental, submaxillary and suboccipital nodes. Lymph nodes tender, warm and enlarged may be associated with a local infection or inflammation. Cervical adenopathy is often seen with an infection of the throat or the mouth. In many children, the existence of small, easily delineated and moveable lymph nodes are commonly found. They involve calcified lymph glands and are frequently found in children who have suffered a lot of upper respiratory tract infections. Differentiate such findings from lymph node enlargement associated with malignancies, where the glandular tissue seems immobile and irregular in shape.

Palpate the isthmus of the thyroid gland, which is the band of glandular tissue connecting the two lobes of the thyroid situated at the base of the neck. The thyroid gland cannot easily be palpated in the infant.

Place the thumb and index finger on either side of the trachea in order to assess its position. Any shift away from the midline may be associated with lung disease, a tumor, or a foreign body.

Check the function of the accessory nerve (see p.138).

Examination of the thorax

The chest of the infant is almost circular and a barrel shaped chest is normal in the very young child. At that age the anteroposterior diameter of the chest equals the lateral diameter from side to side. The ratio between the two diameters (the thoracic index) is 1 in the infant, 1.25 at 1 year and 1.35 at 6 years of age. However, if you observe a barrel shaped chest in the older child, you are looking at chronic obstructive airway disease such as asthma or cystic fibrosis. A larger than normal inferior costal angle is characteristic of lung disease and is often associated with a barrel-shaped chest. A smaller angle than usual may be a sign of malnutrition. The normal costal angle measures between 45 and 50º.

Make a note of any chest asymmetry. A bulging left chest may be associated with the presence of serious cardiac or pulmonary disease. Look for spinal scoliosis affecting the shape of the chest. Inspect the ribs at their costochondral junctions and the sternum. The junction is normally smooth. The presence of any swelling or knobs at the side of the sternum may indicate a vitamin D deficiency as found in rickets. Associated with this deficiency you may also find a Harrison's groove. A severe impression of the lower part of the sternum as is the case in a funnel chest (pectus excavatum) may impair cardiorespiratory function and may be associated with Marfan syndrome. In a pigeon chest (pectus carinatum) the sternum is protruding outwardly, a variation of the normal without any implications of pathology.

Examination of the respiratory system
Searching for symptoms

Look at the child's presenting clinical signs and symptoms for diagnostic clues. They include: cough (especially a barking cough), fever, nasal discharge, stridor, wheeze, cyanosis and whoop. The time of onset of the symptoms as well as their duration will be of diagnostic value. The case history may help you differentiate between acute (less than 3 weeks duration), long-standing (lasting longer than 3 months), or recurrent symptoms (the presence of symptom-free periods of at least 2 week's duration between sickness).

Where a stridor started overnight and is associated with a barking cough, croup is most likely. However, when you observe a chronic stridor in an infant without a cough, a problem with the larynx may be causing the child's symptoms, as is often the case in hypotonia affecting the throat. When a cough presents with a wheeze, the child may be suffering from asthma. This diagnosis is likely, especially when environmental stimuli such as exposure to cold, dust, smoke, or exercise seem to be triggering the respiratory symptoms.

In the child who is suffering from a wheeze, a recurrent and persisting cough, and shows symptoms of failure to thrive, a more serious respiratory disease such as cystic fibrosis may be the cause. The case history may help with your diagnosis of the child.

Begin the physical examination by looking for any obvious signs of respiratory disease such as central cyanosis. Assess clubbing of the fingers by inspecting the lateral side of the fingers and looking at the angle formed at the junction between the nail bed and the skin. Finger clubbing is caused by increased tissue formation of the nail bed and is seen in cystic fibrosis and bronchiectasis.

Inspection

Observe the respiratory movements of the thorax and establish the respiratory rate per minute by observing the child (see p.102). Be aware that in the case of fever the respiratory rate will be increased. Note whether the child's breathing is regular or irregular. Also assess the child's respiratory efforts in relation to its quality and depth, as well as the character of the breath sounds. Does the child find it difficult to breathe? Is the respiration shallow or deep? What type of breath sounds can you hear? Are they noisy, grunting, snoring or heavy? Is there any stridor indicating an extrathoracic problem involving the larynx or trachea?

Does the child show any signs of respiratory distress or are you observing any soft tissue retractions associated with labored breathing? Look for nasal flaring and abnormal patterns of breathing in the infant. Watch for symmetry of movement as the chest and abdomen rise and fall together during respiration. During expiration the chest falls and decreases in size as the thoracic diaphragm rises and the infer-ior costal angle narrows. In inspiration the reverse occurs. A decreased chest movement on one side may indicate a pneumothorax, pneumonia, or an airway obstruction caused by a foreign body or by a musculoskeletal problem affecting the excursion of the ribs.

As the infant predominantly uses abdominal breathing, a paradoxical breathing effect is being produced where the lower thorax is being drawn in and the abdomen is protruded during inspiration and the reverse occurs in expiration. When this type of breathing changes into predominantly thoracic breathing in the infant, intra-abdominal or intrathoracic pathology needs to be considered as this tends to limit the diaphragmatic excursion during respiration.

Also consider that infants often exhibit irregular breathing patterns that are even more obvious in the premature baby. It is characterized by 'periodic breathing' which alternates with breathing at a normal rate. During the time of periodic breathing the rate of respiration may be reduced or even stop for more than 3 seconds. Where episodes of apnea are lasting longer than 20 seconds and are accompanied by bradycardia, you need to investigate the child for cardiopulmonary or CNS disease. When such episodes of apnea are experienced by the infant, the child may be at risk of SIDS (sudden infant death syndrome).

Where the child extends the head or the neck during inspiration and uses the accessory muscles, severe respiratory disease is likely. Look for any soft tissue retractions associated with the child's respiratory effort, such as suprasternal, supraclavicular, lower sternal, or intercostal retraction. Subcostal or lower costal retractions are associated with a flattened diaphragm caused by a hyperinflation of the lungs or by trapped air. This is when the flattened thoracic diaphragm contracts whilst pulling at its attachments on the chest wall. This situation frequently creates a horizontal groove along the diaphragmatic attachments called a Harrison's groove. This happens because in younger children and infants, soft tissue retractions associated with labored breathing are usually due to large changes in intrathoracic pressure, or an existing airway obstruction.

Palpation

With the child sitting, palpate the respiratory movements of the thorax and the individual movements of the ribs. Stand behind the child, placing your hands along the lateral chest walls with your thumbs meeting in the midline. Start at the lower costal margin to test the lower ribs and their bucket handle motion. Then place the hands more superiorly in order to assess the pump handle movement of the upper part of the ribcage. Then place each hand on either side of the shoulder with the fingertips contacting the first rib in the supraclavicular fossa. Ask the child to take in a few deep breaths when testing the rib movement .The different hand positions can also be used to assess the position and the range of motion of the individual ribs, including their involuntary motion. When palpating the movement of the thorax during respiration, note the presence of any decreased, asymmetrical movements.

Altered vocal fremitus always warrants further investigation. This is a vibration associated with the conduction of voice sounds. Ask the child to repeat words such as 'one, two or three' or 'ninety-nine.' Normally vocal fremitus is most intense at the apex of the lungs. If it is decreased or not able to be heard then the ribs' ability to vibrate may be compromized as, for example, in pleural effusion. It could also indicate an interruption of the conduction of the vibration from the lungs to the chest wall, as is the case with an obstruction of a major bronchus caused by a foreign body.

The vocal fremitus is increased when the lung tissue consolidates and the conduction of the vibration is easier. This is the case in infections. In the infant, fremitus is best palpated when the baby is crying.

A pleural friction rub may also be palpated. This is a grating sensation caused by the inflammation and rubbing together of the pleural linings of the lungs. A crepitation is a coarse and crackling sensation that is felt when air is escaping the lungs into the subcutaneous tissues, as can be the case in injury. Both crepitations and pleural friction rubs can be palpated as well as auscultated.

Percussion of the lungs

Percussion is used in order to demarcate the parameters of the lungs and the liver, the position and size of the heart, and also the movement of the lungs during respiration and their expansion. With the child in the sitting position, assess the child's chest in relation to the different densities of the viscera. Percuss and compare the sounds of one side with the other side of the lungs. Start with the anterior aspect at the apex of the lungs then progressively work your way towards the base of the lungs. Please note that findings of tympany on the left side and dullness on the right side of the lungs are normal and relate to the positions of the stomach and the liver, respectively. When percussing further in a downward direction, the dull sound changes into a flat sound when the lower border of the liver is reached. The percussion of the heart is perceived as a dullness over the left side of the sternum reaching from the second to the fifth intercostal spaces. Below the fifth intercostal space on the left side, however, the presence of tympany usually indicates an air-filled stomach. A resonance is heard over the lobes of the lungs whereas a dullness is heard at the fifth intercostal space on the right, at the midclavicular line, due to the position of the liver. When percussing the posterior thorax a resonance is usually heard down to the level of the 8th to the 10th ribs, after which the sound becomes more dull towards the base of the lungs when the thoracic diaphragm is being percussed.

Pathological findings are:

- hypersonoric percussion, indicating pulmonary emphysema or stress pneumothorax.
- muted percussion that occurs in atelectasis, inflammation of the lung tissue, pleural effusion or pleural fibrosis.
- tympanitic percussion heard via a pneumothorax or large caverns in the lung tissue.

Note the anatomical dimensions of the respiratory system: The trachea bifurcates below the sternal angle; the apex of the lungs are situated about 2–4 cm above the inner third of the clavicles. The boundaries of the lungs are as follows:

- parasternal line.
- posteriorly the base of the lungs is situated at the level of the 11th rib.
- in the midaxillary line it is found at the level of the 8th rib, whilst in the
- midclavicular line the lungs extend to the level of the 6th rib.
- parasternal line at the level of the 4th rib on the left and the 6th rib on the right.
- midclavicular line at the level of the 6th rib, and on deep inspiration approx. 3 cm further to caudal; on deep expiration approx. 2 cm further to cranial.
- anterior axillary line at the level of the 7th rib.
- midaxillary line at the level of the 8th rib, on deep inspiration approx. 6–8 cm further to caudal; on deep expiration approx. 4 cm further to cranial.
- scapular line at the level of the 9th–10th rib, on deep inspiration approx. 5 cm further to caudal; on deep expiration approx. 3 cm further to cranial.
- paravertebral line at the level of the spinous processes from T10–T11, on deep inspiration approx. 3 cm further to caudal; on deep expiration approx. 2 cm further to cranial.

Keep in mind that any areas of consolidation will sound more dull, whilst an area of perfusion will have a flat quality to it. A hyperinflated area of the lungs will seem to be hyper-resonant. Please note that it is normal to find a hyperresonant percussion sound throughout in the young infant and that any decrease in the hyperresonance of the thorax in the infant may have the same relevance as a percussed dullness in

the adult. The force of your percussion will need to be much lighter than in the older child and adult.

Auscultation of the lungs

Use a pediatric stethoscope for infants, as the adult size of the bell and the membrane are usually too large for you to be able to localize any clinical findings in a small child. The stethoscope assesses the breath and the voice sounds. Although the open bell of the stethoscope will be more sensitive to any low-pitched sounds, the diaphragm side of the stethoscope is better for the perception of high-pitched sounds as it filters out any low ones.

The breath sounds are louder and harsher in the infant and during childhood than in the adult. Take into account that infantile breathing can be intermittently slow and shallow, and then rapid and deep. Also consider that the infant's breath sounds maybe reduced on the side to which the head is turned. Crying in the infant will enhance the breath sounds. In the older child where cooperation can be gained, ask the child to take a deep breath. Remember that any absent or diminished breath sounds are always abnormal findings indicating the presence of fluid, air or a solid mass interfering with the conduction of sound.

Normal breath sounds include:

- Tracheal breath sounds: high pitched and usually heard during inspiration and expiration.
- Vesicular breath sounds: can be heard everywhere in the lungs except in the upper intrascapular space and beneath the manubrium. The sound is often described as a soft, swishing sound. These are mainly heard on inspiration.
- Bronchovesicular breath sounds: can be auscultated over the manubrium and the intrascapular area, where the trachea and bronchi divide into two branches. These sounds are higher in pitch than vesicular sounds.
- Bronchial sounds: short breath sounds over the bronchi with a tubular quality which are short during inspiration and long during expiration.

Pathologic findings are:

- Decreased breath sounds: occur during infiltration, decreased expansion, emphysema, asthma, atelectasis.
- Missing breath sounds: pneumothorax, pleural effusion.
- Increased breath sounds (loud and hissing): beginning infiltration.
- Bronchial breathing (hissing): physiologic over the bronchial tree, over other parts of the lung if infiltration present, in cystic fibrosis.
- Wheeze (continuous hissing sound with a high pitch): associated with a partial airway obstruction caused by

asthma, a tumor or a foreign body. An inspiratory wheeze indicates a narrowed upper airway whilst an expiratory wheeze is associated with narrowed lower airways. Keep in mind that wheezes will be heard more readily in the young child as the small lumen easily narrows in response to a small amount of mucous or a swelling of the mucous lining of the airways.

- The auscultation of a coarse crackle (sounds like a discontinuous, interrupted, and loud sound with a low pitch): occurs when air passes through large airways containing fluid.
- A fine crackle (quieter and higher in pitch): usually caused by air passing through smaller airways containing fluid.
- A rhonchus (continuous, low pitched snoring sound): caused by thick mucous secretions which are partially obstructing the large upper airway.
- Moist rale (on inspiration): constant, deep 'snoring' sounds due to thick mucous discharge.
- coarse bubble (low frequency) with fluid in the bronchial tubes and acute pulmonary edema, bronchiectasis.
- fine bubble (high frequency) with fluid in the bronchioles and alveoli with chronic left ventricular insufficiency and pulmonary congestion.
- sonorous = close to ear on infiltration.
- non-sonorous = away from ear with blockage, pulmonary edema.

Examination of the cardiovascular system

The etiology of coronary disease is unknown. Possible causes are:

- if the mother has been in contact with rubella during her pregnancy
- if there been exposure to drugs during the pregnancy such as lithium, dilantin, thalidomide
- excessive intake of alcohol
- exposure to radiation
- maternal diabetes (increases the risk of congenital heart defects)
- if the child suffers from a chromosomal abnormality such as Down or Marfan syndrome.

Searching for symptoms

Remember that the physical signs and symptoms of heart disease are not limited to the cardiovascular system alone. Cyanosis, fatigue, poor weight gain, liver enlargement and

respiratory difficulties may be important symptoms when trying to evaluate a heart murmur and its clinical significance. For instance, a child with primary cardiac disease may present with a pulmonary infection as the only obvious clinical presentation.

Heart disease associated with respiratory distress may present in different ways depending on the condition that causes the symptoms. The signs of heart disease maybe dyspnea. In the case of low cardiac output the child may be suffering from tachypnea.

Heart disease associated with cyanosis, or heart conditions causing low cardiac output, are associated with a rapid respiratory rate, which becomes more obvious on exertion. Fatigue may also be associated with such a condition. In young infants with low cardiac output the infant may be exhausted whilst feeding. This is because this is a time of high metabolic demand. However, an older child may need to squat as he tires after exertion. This is a typical presentation in tetralogy of Fallot, where squatting decreases the amount of right to left shunting thereby increasing the systemic oxygen saturation.

Children with cyanotic congenital heart disease may suffer hypoxic spells. If the spell is severe there maybe a loss of consciousness. A typical hypoxic spell is associated with a sudden increase of cyanosis. This is because the infundibular muscle contraction further restricts the right ventricular cardiac output whilst increasing the right to left shunt of the blood.

Symptoms of angina are rare in infants and children, and peripheral edema related to heart failure presents quite differently than in the adult. The infant suffering from heart failure has periorbital edema. However, this is usually being preceded by tachypnea, dyspnea and hepatomegaly. We seldom see angina pectoris symptoms in infants and children.

The clinical manifestations of congestive heartfailure

- Impaired myocardial function: tachycardia, inappropriate sweating, decreased urine output, fatigue, weakness and restlessness, anorexia, pale and cool extremities, weak peripheral pulse, decreased blood pressure, gallop rhythm, cardiomegaly.
- Pulmonary congestion: tachypnea, dyspnea, costal retractions and nasal flaring in infants, exercise intolerance, orthopnea, cough, hoarseness, cyanosis, wheezing and grunting.
- Systemic venous congestion: weight gain, hepatomegaly, peripheral edema especially in the periorbital region, ascites, distension of the veins in the neck.

If congestive heart failure develops (Roy 1992) before 3 months of age the probability is high of it being caused by congenital heart disease. If heart failure develops after 3 months then myocarditis, cardiomyopathy or paroxysmal tachycardia are the more likely causes. By the time a child is 3–5 years old, most pathologies causing cyanosis or congestive heart failure have already been revealed. Cardiac lesions which may have gone undiagnosed include atrial septal defect (ASD), a small ventricular septal defect (VSD), a bicuspid aortic valve, and acquired cardiac disorders such as pericarditis, myocarditis, and cardiac symptoms associated with hereditary muscular or neuromuscular diseases. Also consider that congenital heart disease is associated with many syndromes such as Down and Marfan.

Inspection

- Look for any chest deformities because an enlarged heart can lead to a bulging left side of the chest.
- Look at the anterior chest of the child whilst comparing both sides; in some cases pulsations of the chest wall may be visible.
- Observe the movement of the chest wall during respiration for tachypnea and dyspnea.
- Look for any obvious flaring of the lower ribs or a horizontal depression in the lower part of the rib cage known as a Harrison's groove.
- Check whether there is any clubbing of the fingers.
- Look for evidence of cyanosis, pallor or inappropriate sweating.

Central cyanosis is difficult to detect in the infant. Carefully look in the baby's mouth or watch the cyanosis become more obvious when the baby is crying. In aortic coarctation, a persistent pulmonary hypertension or a right to left shunt in patent ductus arteriosus, the lower body of the child maybe cyanosed whilst the upper part is maintaining its pink color. Differentiate central cyanosis from peripheral cyanosis. In the latter case the mouth and tongue are usually pink.

Examine the hands and fingers. Assess the palmar creases (Down syndrome) and the nail bed looking for clubbing of the fingers. This can best be assessed when looking at the fingertips from the side. Assess the capillary refill time to test the peripheral circulation. Use a sustained pressure over the nail bed for a few seconds and then release it. In the healthy child the induced blanching of the nail bed disappears in less than 2 seconds.

Palpation

Pulse

The quality of the pulse relates to cardiac function in that it gives you feedback regarding the peripheral resistance the blood meets when exiting the heart. When trying to assess the quality of the pulse start with the brachial pulse not the radial. This is because the closer the pulse is felt to the heart the more accurate will be the reading. Use the first and second digits of your right hand when palpating the brachial artery. In the older child you may want to support the right arm of the child with your left arm whilst using the right thumb to palpate the pulse.

Compare the radial and femoral pulses. A weak femoral pulse or a delay between the two pulses may indicate a circulatory impairment, as is the case in coarctation of the aorta. In some instances this may be the only presenting sign of the condition.

Assess the volume of the pulse in relation to heart disease (Roy 1992). If the pulse volume is increased you should check for a 'water hammer' pulse. This is when the pulse is still present when the arm is being elevated and encircled with one of your hands. A normal pulse volume should not be palpable in such a situation, whilst a positive finding indicates an aortic insufficiency, a hyperkinetic circulation, or a patent ductus.

Check for pulsus paradoxus, which appears when a decrease greater than 10mmHg during normal inspiration is being observed. The presence of a pulsus paradoxus greater than 8mmHg may indicate cardiac tamponade.

Measure the blood pressure and heart rate (detailed description see p.105).

Heart

In the infant palpate the right ventricle by laying your right hand on his chest. Use the tips of your first and second fingers and position them just left of the xyphoid process whilst lightly depressing the thorax. In the normal situation a faint impulse may be palpated, but if a forceful movement is being felt under your fingers an enlarged heart is likely.

Palpate the apical impulse (AI) by using your index and middle fingers in order to depress the thorax. In the normal infant the AI can be palpated at the beginning of a systole at the level of the fourth intercostal space left to the midclavicular line. This is where it will be situated at up to 4 years of age. From 4 to 6 years of age the AI is usually positioned on the midclavicular line. From 7 years onwards it is situated at the level of the fifth intercostal space to the right of the midclavicular line (Hoeckelmann 1987).

Your aim is to feel:

- additional pulsation: in arrythmia
- strong pulsations: in aortic insufficiency
- a thrill (a palpable vibration produced by blood flowing through an abnormal or narrowed opening): possible stenosis of a heart valve, or a septal defect which can best be palpated during expiration.

- left laterocaudal displacement: left ventricular hypertrophy.

In the normal infant a strong pulse originating from the pulmonary artery can be palpated by contacting the second intercostal space just left of the sternum. Use your index and middle fingers. In the older child, however, a palpable impulse here may indicate pulmonary artery pathology.

In order to palpate any abnormal pulsations such as thrills or any heart murmurs, place the index finger of your right hand in the suprasternal notch. Where the older child presents with a palpable impulse in the suprasternal notch, suspect an increased flow through the aortic arch, a patent ductus arteriosus, or an aortic insufficiency.

Liver

Sit on the right side of the child in order to palpate the inferior margin of the liver. In the infant use the tip of your right thumb. Start by placing the thumb in the inferior end of the lower right quadrant of the abdomen. Palpate the liver by moving the thumb inward and in a cephalad direction. If in the infant you find an enlarged liver as well as an increased action of the heart, the diagnosis of heart failure is almost certain.

Percuss the liver by contacting the abdomen with the second and third digits of your left hand whilst tapping it with the third digit of your right hand. Begin low in the lower quadrant of the abdomen whilst placing the digits of your left hand right along the edge of the liver, which, in the infant, is usually found approximately 1 cm below the right costal margin. The older child is less likely to suffer from heart failure, and clinical findings where the liver is found to be 2 cm or more below the costal margin are more likely to be caused by pulmonary disease. This is why for a differential diagnosis the upper margin of the liver will need to be percussed as well.

Auscultation

During the auscultation the surroundings should be as quiet as possible. The child can be examined lying or sitting.

Listen to the child's cardiac auscultation points (Fig. 7.4):

- aortic valve : second intercostal space (ICS) right on edge of sternum.
- pulmonary valve : second ICS left approx. one transverse finger from edge of sternum.
- tricuspid valve : fourth ICS right above the base of the 5th rib on the sternum.
- mitral valve: fifth ICS left approx. three transverse fingers from edge of sternum on the midclavicular line.

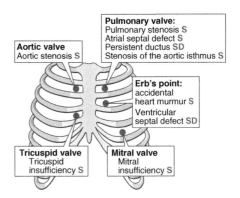

Figure 7.4 Cardiac auscultation points and causes of systolic (S) and systolic-diastolic (SD) murmurs.
With permission, Henriette Rintelen, Velbert, in association with the series Klinik- und Praxisleitfaden, Urban & Fischer Verlag

- Erb's point : third ICS left approx. two transverse fingers away from edge of sternum.

In the normal child two heart sounds (S1 and S2) can be auscultated producing a familiar 'lub-dub' sound. If you have any difficulties in distinguishing between S1 and S2, simultaneously palpate the carotid pulse.

The first heart sound (1st HS, myocardial tension sound) is initiated at the beginning of systole by the closing of the mitral and tricuspid valves. It is longer and muted; the punctum maximum is above the Erb's point. It is muted with reduced contractility in, for example, myocarditis, and loud when there is an increase in the stroke volume and contractility, such as in the event of fever, anemia or after exertion.

The second heart sound (second semilunar valve, closing sound) is initiated by the closing of the semilunar valves. It is longer and light; the punctum maximum is above the Erb's point. It consists of two components: the aortic valve closes first, then the pulmonary valve. This can lead to a physiological, respiratory-dependent division of the second HS. It is muted in aortic or pulmonary stenosis, and loud in arterial or pulmonary hypertension. A fixed, respiratory-independent division occurs when the right ventricle is under stress; for example when there is ventricular septal defect, pulmonary stenosis or pulmonary hypertonia. As the aortic valve is late closing in stenosis, sometimes only a single sound is heard. A thrill can be palpated in the incisura jugularis sterni.

A third heart sound is heard as a ventricular filling tone in the early diastole. In children, a fourth heart sound as an atrial contraction sound in late diastole may be physiological or indicate cardiac insufficiency or that the atrium is working extra hard.

Evaluate the heart sounds for their clarity and intensity as well as in relation to the site of their auscultation. Also assess the heart rate and the regularity of the heart sounds.

Normally S1 is louder when auscultated at the apex of the heart whilst S2 is louder at the pulmonary and aortic sites of auscultation. In the case of anemia, fever or after exercise, the first heart sound appears to be loud. The second heart sound maybe unusually soft in pulmonary or aortic stenosis, and appears to be widely split in atrial septal defect (ASD). In the latter the splitting will not vary with respir-ation. Because of the late closure of the aortic valve in the case of stenosis, you may only hear one single heart sound. In this situation you may also be able to palpate a thrill in the suprasternal notch.

A heart rate that increases with inspiration but decreases during expiration may be due to a sinus arrhythmia. Differentiate this from a normal situation by reassessing the rhythm of the heart when the child is holding the breath.

A murmur is an extra noise heard on auscultation of the heart. It can occur in systole or in diastole. A murmur may be innocent or indicative of cardiac disease. Pathological murmurs may be associated with cyanosis or they may be acyanotic. However, not all heart pathology presents with a murmur.

Heart murmurs need to be classified according to location, duration, volume, when they occur in the heart cycle, the type of tone and punctum maximum. They may occur during sys-tole or diastole, may be harmless or indicate heart disease. A heart murmur may be detected during the examination of a neonatal if the transition from fetal to neonatal circulation fol-lowing birth is not entirely concluded. This is often seen in premature babies. We differentiate between:

- accidental sounds – occurring during systole, these are short, more obvious when sitting than lying down or dis-appear when sitting, are auscultated in the 2nd–3rd ICR left parasternal, and frequently occur physiologically in healthy children.

- functional sounds – occur frequently during systole, less so during diastole, with increased cardiac output resulting from turbulence in the blood flow with no organic heart disease, e.g. in the event of fever, anemia, hyperthyrosis.

- organic sounds – occur systolically or diastolically with anomalies of the heart, heart valves or vessels.

A 'venous hum' is a constant sound that can be heard dur-ing systole and diastole, and is at its loudest when auscultated under the right clavicle. It is the result of turbulent blood flow in the major vessels and is harmless.

Murmurs need to be classified according to their location, their time of occurrence, their intensity and their loudness. As they need a lot of practice to be heard and distinguished, children with suspected heart murmurs should be referred to a cardiologist for further differential diagnosis.

The biomechanical dimension of cardiac and respiratory function

The functional integrity of the parietal pleura and the fibrous pericardium with the thoracic rib cage needs to be acknow-ledged when assessing respiratory and cardiac function. The parietal pleura is intimately attached to the internal aspects of the ribs, whilst the fibrous pericardium attaches to the sternum anteriorly and to the thoracic diaphragm inferiorly.

Stamenovic et al (1990) suggest that the movement of the ribcage does not only have an influence on the intrathoracic pressures but that it may also induce changes within the lung tissues themselves. The parietal pleura as well as the pericar-dium are separated from their respective external layers by a fluid space. This anatomical arrangement enables the heart and the lungs to move independently because the two layers of connective tissues allow for a gliding movement (Stone 2001). Where there are adhesions between the two layers, the biomechanical action of the thorax may be compromised, which, in turn may have an effect on heart and lung func-tion. It is for this reason that it is important to include a bio-mechanical assessment of the thorax with the examination of the cardiac and respiratory systems.

Liechtenstein et al (1992) explained how respiratory func-tion is affected by the combined influences of the lungs, the ribcage, the abdomen and the thoracic diaphragm.

When assessing the infant we should keep in mind that we are dealing with a soft and compliant chest wall. Papasta-melos et al (1995) described how, at that young age, the function of the lungs will be controlling the chest wall, whilst in the older child the opposite occurs, where the bio-mechanical integrity of the chest wall will be controlling lung function.

Biomechanical assessment of the thorax:

- Assess the biomechanical aspect of the thoracic rib cage by palpating the movement of the upper and lower ribs dur-ing respiration. Evaluate individual rib mobility as well as the involuntary motion of these structures. When palpat-ing the thorax, observe whether there are any torsional or shearing stresses of the connective tissues affecting pleural as well as pericardial function.

- Examine scapular mobility as well as any restrictive influences of associated myofascial structures on scapular mobility.

- Assess individual rib movement taking into account any connective tissue stresses originating from the pleura or pericardial sac, as well as any influence exerted by the thor-acic diaphragm on the individual ribs.

- Evaluate thoracic spinal mobility taking into account the effects of connective tissue stresses originating from the anterior longitudinal ligament and the crura of the thoracic diaphragm.

- Examine the function of the sternomanubrial joint as well as the mobility of ribs 1 to 3.

- Assess the sternoclavicular and acromioclavicular joints in relation to clavicular mobility.

- Evaluate the mobility of ribs 1 bilaterally during respiration. Stand behind the child whilst contacting the supraclavicular spaces on both sides with your index and middle fingers. Simultaneously palpate the clavicle and the scapulae by resting your hands on either side of his shoulders.

- The function of the upper portion of the pleura can be assessed by contacting rib 1. This is because the apex of the lungs is attached to this rib via the cervicopleural ligaments (Barral 1991). Caroline Stone (2001) mentioned how the parietal pleura of the apex of the lungs is connected to the fascia which envelops the apex of the lungs as well as connecting to the scalenes, the brachial plexus, the subclavius, the clavicle and the sternum. The same fascial sheath continues to form the suspensory ligament of the pleural dome.

- Palpate the apex of the lungs. With the child sitting and you standing at the side, contact rib 1 on either side of the spine using the thumb and the index finger of your left hand. The thumb and index finger of your right hand should be in contact with the first ribs anteriorly just beneath the clavicle and above the costal cartilages of ribs 2 on either side of the manubrium (Fig. 7.5).

- To palpate the pericardial sac as well as the aortic arch, take an anteroposterior contact with one hand contacting the posterior aspect of the thorax at the level of T2–T6, whilst the other hand is being placed over the area of the sternomanubrial joint. This hand placement allows you to assess the influence of the pleura as well as of the pericardium on the mediastinum. This also includes the aortic arch and the arteries supplying the head and neck.

- Move your anteroposterior hand contact inferior to contact T6–T12 posteriorly and the area of the xiphoid process anteriorly. This contact allows you to assess the pericardial sac with its inferior attachment to the thoracic diaphragm. With this handhold you may also become aware of any potential influences that pleural scarring on the lower lobes of the lungs might be having on diaphragmatic as well as pericardial function.

Examination of the abdomen and the genitourinary tract

The child is in a supine position on the treatment table.

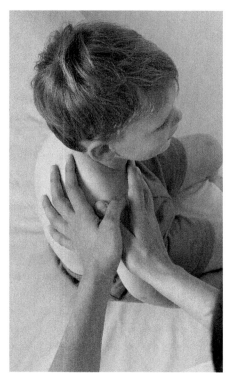

Figure 7.5 Palpation of the upper aspect of the lungs. With permission, Karsten Franke, Hamburg

Observation

It is important to assess the abdomen of the child looking at the shape of the abdomen and noting any asymmetry or abdominal distension. Check the umbilicus, the linea alba and the inguinal region for any hernias.

Find out about the history of any scars as surgery may have been performed early in the infant's life in order to correct any obstructive abnormalities affecting the gastrointestinal tract. These include duodenal or esophageal atresia, or Hirschsprung's disease, a distal obstruction of the digestive tract. In the latter case the child usually gets diagnosed because of the delayed passage of meconium and a progressively more distended abdomen (Gillis 1992).

Watch the movement of the child's abdomen during respiration. In the case where abdominal movement seems to be absent, you need to think of causes such as peritonitis, excessive gas, a paralytic ileus, or appendicitis. If the child is also suffering from rebound tenderness, abdominal distension and fever then a referral for medical management is indicated.

Auscultation

In order to auscultate the abdomen use the diaphragm of the stethoscope, placing it on each quadrant of the abdomen as well as on the umbilicus. You must listen for at least 2–3 minutes before you can be sure that the bowel sounds are absent (Gillis1992). Obstructive bowel sounds are higher pitched (tinkly) whereas hyperactive sounds are frequently associated with inflammatory bowel problems (Gillis1992).

Percussion

Percussion of the abdomen is important in order to identify any unusual areas of fluid or organ enlargements warranting urgent referral for specialist medical care. Gillis (1992) reasons that gentle percussion may overcome any diagnostic difficulties encountered by the practitioner due to voluntary muscle resistance. He suggests to gently percuss over the non-tender areas first before assessing any tender spots of the abdomen.

The presence of gas in the abdomen is often due to swallowed air or hypersensitivity reactions to cow's milk or lactose intolerance. Abdominal distension can be caused by benign clinical conditions such as obesity or air but may also be due to serious conditions such as organ enlargements, tumors, or the presence of fluid in the abdominal cavity.

Palpation

Palpation of the abdomen is important for the diagnosis of any serious medical conditions, but the subtle skills of osteopathic palpation may also be a helpful tool for the diagnosis of connective tissue stresses affecting the mobility of the organs within the abdominal cavity. Visceral mobility and involuntary motion are thought to be an important feature of healthy visceral function. Barral (1988) and Stone (1998) have described the biomechanical aspects of visceral function, as well as reminding us of the structural interdependence of the individual structures in relation to the abdominal cavity as a whole. Barral (1988) explained how the peritoneal membrane creates a continuous connective tissue structure by which the organs are suspended as well as allowed to glide in relation to each other without ever irritating a neighbouring viscera. This means that as osteopaths we will need to not only assess the position and shape of the individual organs for pathology but that we should also assess visceral mobility and inherent motility, noting whether any undue connective tissue stresses are interfering with normal peritoneal function, and test each individual organ for its ability to glide within its connective tissue suspension.

Standing to the right of the child, start with a superficial palpation of the four quadrants of the abdomen with the child lying in the supine position.

In the young child observe his face in order to assess whether you are eliciting any pain or tenderness with your touch. Continue your abdominal examination with the palpation of the individual organs.

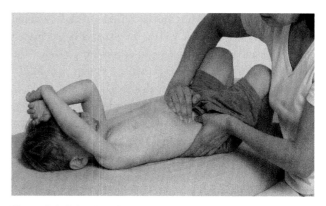

Figure 7.6 Palpation of the kidneys. With permission, Karsten Franke, Hamburg

The liver

See p.220

The spleen

With your left hand contact the posterior aspect of the child's thorax and lift the left side of the abdomen whilst your right hand is being placed anteriorly in order to palpate the inferior margin of the spleen. Note that the fingers of the superior hand should be pointing towards the left upper quadrant of the abdomen.

The kidneys

Davies (2000) described how to palpate the kidneys in the young child. With the child lying supine compress the lateral aspect of the abdomen just below the inferior costal margin by using your thumb above and your forefingers below. At the same time flex the infant's leg at the hip and the knee; this pushes the forefingers of the palpating hand deep into the soft tissues, thereby enabling a better palpation of the kidney. In the school-age child lift the kidney up with your forefingers which are contacting the posterior aspect of the abdomen and the kidney. A quick flick of the hand 'ballots' the kidney (ballottement maneuver), enabling the palpation of a rebound sensation of the hand placed superiorly on the abdomen (Fig. 7.6).

The bladder

Palpate the bladder with a cupped hand. Start by placing your hand at the umbilical level and then move closer towards the pubis.

The colon

Determine the presence of any fecal or other masses in the large bowel. In order to palpate the caecum locate the ascending colon by holding the lateral wall of the abdomen with the left hand whilst your right hand is being placed superiorly and applying lateral and downward pressure. The descending colon is being palpated in a similar manner. In this case you need to compress the abdominal wall laterally on the opposite side by using your right hand, whilst the left hand is being placed superiorly to palpate the descending colon and the sigmoid flexure. If the child has been suffering from constipation, fecal masses may be palpated.

The thoracic diaphragm and pelvic floor

The position of the viscera within the abdominal cavity is being maintained by the action of the thoracic diaphragm, the tone of the abdominal muscles and the ligamentous suspension of the individual organs, including the peritoneum, spinal column and the iliopsoas and erector spinae muscles. The muscles of the pelvic floor are providing a 'suspensory hammock' for the pelvic organs. It is therefore important to include an assessment of these musculoskeletal components of visceral function in your palpatory examination of the abdomen.

Assess the thoracic diaphragm and the associated viscera with the child lying supine and you sitting at the side of the child. Assume an anterior-posterior handhold with the posterior hand contacting the lower ribs and the thoracolumbar junction. Place the anterior hand over the lower costal angles and the xyphoid process.

The pelvic floor can be assessed by using an anterior-posterior handhold, contacting the sacrum and coccyx areas posteriorly and the pubic symphysis anteriorly.

Abdominal masses

Many normal structures can be palpated in the abdomen. These include the liver, spleen, abdominal aorta, colon, stool in the bowels, the kidneys and the bladder. The two most common abnormal masses found in children are intussusception and an appendix mass.

The highest incidence of intussusception is in the first 2 years of life. This is a situation where the bowel invaginates into the adjacent distal part of it. This is usually associated with pain, rectal bleeding and shock. A sausage shaped mass can usually be palpated which is associated with the clinical signs of bowel obstruction. Appendicitis usually presents with a palpable fixed mass in the right iliac fossa, which is associated with abdominal pain, fever and other signs of infection.

Pyloric stenosis (see Ch.12) occurs during the first few weeks of life. Boys are more often affected than girls. The child usually has a history of vomiting and dehydration. A hypertrophied pyloric sphincter can usually be palpated whilst the child is feeding.

Malign tumors occur in neonates as well as in older children. Leukemia and lymphoma are often associated with an enlargement of the spleen as well as with hepatomegaly. Weight loss, anemia and fever may be associated clinical symptoms.

Examination of the genitalia, rectum and anus

In a boy, check the genitalia for hypopspadius or an undescended testicle. Where an inguinal mass can be palpated, you need to differentiate between an inguinal hernia, a hydrocele, an undescended testicle, lymphadenopathy or a femoral hernia.

Inspect the sacrococcygeal region for any tufts of hair suggestive of spinal bifida occulta. A pilonidal sinus may also be found in this area. Examine the anus for any skin lesions such as rashes which may be apparent in a child suffering diarrhea irritating the skin around the anus. Where sexual abuse is being suspected, examine the genital area for any injury as well as assessing the vagina for any discharge related to infectious disease.

Bibliography

Barral J P and Mercier P: Visceral Manipulation. Eastland Press, Seattle 1988

Barral J P: The Thorax. Eastland Press, Seattle 1991

Davies J N: Chiropractic pediatrics – a clinical handbook. Churchill Livingstone, Edinburgh 2000, p. 26

Ebrall P S, Davies N J: Non-accidental injury and child maltreatment. In: Anrig C and Plaugher (eds) Pediatric chiropractic. Williams and Wilkins, Baltimore 1998

Field D, Stroobant J (eds): Pediatrics – an illustrated colour text. Churchill Livingstone, Edinburgh 1997

Gillis D A: Surgical assessment of the child's abdomen. In Goldbloom R B (ed.): Pediatric clinical skills. Churchill Livingstone, New York 1992

Goldbloom R B (ed.): Pediatric clinical skills. Churchill Livingstone, New York 1992

Hoeckelman R A: Pediatric examination. In Bates B (ed.) A guide to physical examination and history taking. 4th edn. Lippincott, Philadelphia 1987

Magoun H I: Osteopathy in the cranial field. 3rd edn. Journal Printing, Kirksville, Mo. 1976

Papastamelos C, Panitch H B, England S E, and Allen J L: Developmental changes in chest wall compliance in infancy and early childhood. Journal of Applied Physiology 78(1), 1995: 179–184

Roy D L: Cardiovascular assessments in infants and children. In Goldbloom R B (ed.): Pediatric clinical skills. Churchill Livingstone, New York 1992, pp. 171–193

Stamenovic D, Glass G M, Barnas G M, Fredberg J J: Viscoplasticity of respiratory tissues. Journal of Applied Physiology 69, 1990: 973–988

Stone C: Visceral interactions within osteopathy. Australian Osteopathic Association handout, September 2001

Wong D L (ed.): Whaley and Wong's nursing care of infants and children. 6th edn. Mosby, St.Louis 1999

Yu C C; Wong F H, Lo L J; Chen Y R: Craniofacial deformity in patients with uncorrected congenital muscular torticollis: an assessment from three-dimensional computed tomography imaging. Plastic and Reconstructive Surgery 113(1), 2004: 24–33

EXAMINATION OF THE INFANT AND TODDLER

Dion Kulak

Child sitting

Head

Start your examination by palpating the skull for any excess molding at the suture lines, as well as checking the anterior and posterior fontanelles for patency. The sutures close at the age of 2 years. If there is a premature fusing one should think of the possibility of a craniosynostosis (see Ch.15) a microcephaly or, if the sutures are too far apart, a chronic increased intracranial pressure might be present.

Check how far the fontanelles have already closed. The anterior fontanelle has a diameter of approximately 2–3 cm and closes between the 9th and 18th month. The posterior fontanelle has a diameter of about 0.5–1 cm and closes up to the 3rd month.

Check for signs of excess molding of the head during the birth process. Note any obvious skull asymmetries including relatively flat or bulging areas, as in the case of plagiocephaly (see Ch.15).

Also note any evidence of bruising, swelling or molding, especially in relation to apparent cranial base strains (as described by Magoun 1976), or unexplained bruising related to physical abuse.

Observe the face for asymmetry including the shape of the orbits, the nasal bridge and the relative position of the mandible. Also note the shape of the mandible as well as any evidence of mandibular retrusion, protrusion, or micrognathia. Note any dysmorphic features especially in relation to the position of the eyes, ears and the mandible. Assess the level of the ears, the spacing of the eyes and their sizes.

Measure the head circumference (check for hydrocephalus or microcephaly).

For more detail of the diagnosis of cranial somatic dysfunction please refer to the head and neck examination (see Ch.8, Intraosseous strains).

Thorax

Palpate the shape of the thorax. Also assess upper and lower rib mobility and motion by evaluating the movement of the ribs during respiration. Palpate the spinous processes of the

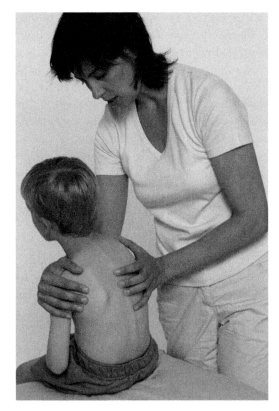

Figure 7.7 Palpation of the mobility of the spine. With permission, Karsten Franke, Hamburg

thoracic and lumbar spine for their alignment and assess their mobility. Note any evidence of thoracic and lumbar scoliosis, kyphosis or lordosis.

Test lumbar and thoracic spinal mobility (Fig. 7.7). Induce a side-bending movement of the child's trunk by contacting the opposite shoulder and encouraging a movement in an inferior direction with your hand resting on the shoulder, whilst the fingertips of the other hand are assessing the relative movement of the spinous processes of the thoracic and lumbar spines.

Child lying supine

Inspection and palpation

Observe the way in which the child is lying on the treatment table. Do you notice any side-bending of the trunk or asymmetry of head position? In torticollis (see Ch.15) palpate the sternocleidomastoid muscle for any lumps; these usually develop at the lower end of the muscle approximately 3 weeks after birth.

Check upper limb function by elevating the arm to 180° whilst palpating clavicular movement at the sternoclavicular junction and the acromioclavicular joints, respectively.

Assess the levels of the medial malleoli, the patellae, the anterior superior iliac spines and the iliac crests for symmetry. Is there any evidence of structural asymmetry such as excessive tibial torsion, metatarsus adductus (see p.341), or an abnormally short or long upper or lower limb? Observe the position of the lower limbs. In the young infant the legs are naturally held in a flexed position. This may differ in the premature neonate, when, in the case of cerebral palsy, a scissoring of the legs may be apparent. Check the feet for any deformities. These include metatarsus adductus varus, a club foot (talipes equinovarus), a calcaneovalgus, a pes cavus or a vertical talus.

Weight bearing and walking is only possible after the lower limbs have undergone changes in shape and position. This is when the acetabulum assumes a more anterior orientation and a straightening of the tibia occurs. This normal development may be disturbed by undue connective tissue stresses acting on the developing lower limbs. In this case femoral anteversion and persistent tibial torsion may lead to an abnormal foot positioning and intoeing of the child. The relationships between the upper body and the lower body segments are most rapidly changing in the toddler and preschool child, so that any dysfunctional growth patterns will be most obvious at that age. This is when the lower limbs will become relatively longer in relation to the upper body. Many parents will voice their concerns about the structural asymmetries they are observing in their 2- to 4-year-old. These include intoeing, the bow-legged or knock-kneed child, excessive ankle pronation and flat feet (pes planus).

The parents usually complain that their child seems to be clumsy, frequently falling over his own feet. An osteopathic assessment and treatment of the above-mentioned conditions is important as there is the potential to 'grow out' of the developing structural asymmetries once any undue connective tissue stresses have been treated, thus allowing the lower limbs to grow and assume the adult position and shape.

As osteopaths we should consider that any undue connective tissue stresses resulting from intrauterine compression forces acting on the limb will need to be addressed in order to encourage a normal growth pattern. Any tibial torsion (bow leggedness) should resolve by 2 years of age whilst a knock-kneed appearance of the limbs is thought to be part of the normal development from 2 to 7 years of age.

Spine

In the young infant, suspend the baby in the supine position by contacting the pelvis and the lower limbs with one hand whilst your other hand is supporting the head and the shoulder girdle (see Fig. 7.8). This way of holding the baby is useful for the assessment of any axial connective tissue stresses affecting the spinal alignment of the child. Such strains may

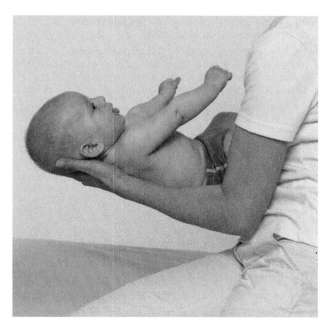

Figure 7.8 Assessment in suspended supine position.
With permission, Karsten Franke, Hamburg

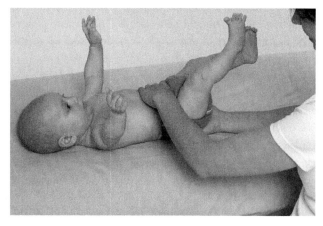

Figure 7.9 Assessing the involuntary motion of the pelvis in a supine position.
With permission, Karsten Franke, Hamburg

be related to the compression effects of a long or difficult labor on the spine.

Pelvis

Involuntary motion (IVM) of the pelvis

Sit at the side of the table, with the child lying supine.

Place one hand under the sacrum, with the elbow of your other arm contacting the ilium on the near side and the hand of that arm cradling the ilium on the far side of the infant. Assess sacroiliac joint involuntary motion by gently approximating the two ilia with each other (Fig. 7.9).

Contact the tip of the greater trochanter with your thumbs by placing them on top of each other. The fingers of the inferiorly placed hand will also be contacting the ischium, the sacroiliac joint and the posterior part of the ilium. The fingers of the superiorly placed hand are contacting the pubic arch as well as the anterior part of the ilium.

Hips

Examine the hips. The neonate should always be checked for hip pathology such as DDH (developmental dysplasia of the hip). An early screening should be able to disclose the presence of a frank dislocation. Special attention needs to be given to the infant with a family history of DDH or after a breech birth. All hips, however, should be re-examined at 6 months and definitely before the child is starting to weight bear. A number of infants diagnosed with hip instability recover spontaneously (1:80 hips at birth) and become stable in a few days after birth. Also consider that in the frankly dislocated hip (1:800 hips at birth), the Ortolani sign becomes negative at 2 months of age. Instead, tight adductors and a short leg will become evident as a diagnostic sign. It is less common these days for a child not to be diagnosed before weight bearing commences. This is because most developed countries have routine screening programs in place for DDH. Despite this promising situation, however, we should not forget to check the toddler and older child for any signs of DDH. A unilateral dislocation in the older child usually presents with a visible widening of the perineum due to the hip displacement. If the child has been walking with a dislocated hip you will also find a compensatory lumbar curve. The affected leg in this case may be of a slightly shorter appearance and in a position of relative external rotation. The gait will show an abnormal shoulder sway. Asymmetrical skin folds may also be present but are not a clinically reliable finding.

Ortolani test

Please note that the examination should be carried out on a firm surface and that the relaxation of the baby will be essential in order to satisfactorily perform this test (Fig. 7.10).

Flex the knees by cradling them in your hands, and with your thumbs resting along the medial sides of the thigh and your fingers over the greater trochanter, proceed to flex the hips to 90°. Gently abduct the hips whilst palpating with your fingers over the greater trochanters. If the hip is dislocated you feel the femoral head slip back into the acetabulum. An audible 'clunk' maybe heard. Where the dislocation is irreducible, a pathological restriction of abduction may then be perceived.

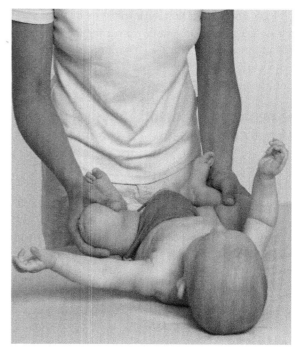

Figure 7.10 Ortolani's test. With permission, Karsten Franke, Hamburg

Faber test

Take the hip joint through a flexion, abduction and external rotation movement. In the normal newborn the knees should touch the table. A restriction of this movement may be indicative of hip disease. Perform this test again but, this time around, simultaneously palpate the tip of the greater tuberosity with the heel of your other hand. This gives you a chance to evaluate the connective tissue stresses acting on the ligaments of the hip joint in relation to somatic dysfunction.

Child lying prone

Observe the older infant and toddler for any developing scoliosis, or thoracic kyphosis. Palpate the spine for any restriction or asymmetry of function. Compare any clinical findings of gross spinal and thoracic mobility with your segmental findings.

Note whether the head control of the infant is age appropriate. Are you detecting any tilt of the head or a rotation of the cervical spine as the preferred position? In this case the child prefers to hold the head rotated to one side and side-bent to the other.

With the child lying prone on the treatment table or alternatively on your lap, stabilize the lumbar spine and sacrum with one hand whilst moving the lower limb to extend the hip with your other hand. This movement assesses sacroiliac function as well as the soft tissues of the joint.

Thoracic and lumbar segmental spinal motion can also be assessed in the prone position by contacting the relevant two spinal processes of the articulation with the fingertips of one hand whilst gently rocking the pelvis from side to side with the other hand.

The neurodevelopmental physical examination sequence for the infant child

Vertical suspension of the infant

Hold the infant in horizontal suspension. Make sure that you hold the infant under the axilla and you are not supporting the child at the chest. In this position the baby should be able to support his own weight, which is testing the proximal power of the arms.

Examination of the muscle tone

Watch for the positioning of the legs when the child is being held in vertical suspension. Note the child's legs. They should be flexed at the hip and the knees. Hypertonia of the hip adductors may be present if the legs are held in extension or are crossed (scissoring). If the child holds his feet in plantar flexion, spasticity is likely.

An increased tone in the arms will be most obvious in the hands, where fisting of the fingers will be apparent with the thumb being positioned beneath the fingers. Any muscle weakness, as is the case in neuromuscular disorders, usually presents as the 'floppy infant', who is lacking in proper antigravity control (see Ch.16, Hypotonia, Cerebral palsy).

The head-righting response

Whilst holding the child in vertical suspension, swing the child back and forth. At 4 months the infant should be able to keep his head in the midline in relation to the thorax. This head righting response is important in relation to posturing and the placement of the center of gravity for walking. It tests postural muscular control as well as the vestibular and proprioceptive systems.

Testing cranial nerve XI

Observe whether the infant is able to hold his head in the midline whilst being suspended in a vertical position. This tests Cranial Nerve XI (Accessory nerve supplying the sternocleidomastoid and trapezius muscles). The infant is usually able to hold his head steady at about 3 months of age.

Weight bearing

Check the lower limbs for any scissoring (as is the case in cerebral palsy) or the presence of lower limb hypotonia. Keep in mind that any age-inappropriate weight bearing may indicate cerebral palsy. It is normal for the 4-month-old child not to bear any weight because the placing reflex has usually disappeared by 6 weeks of age. If it can be elicited beyond this age further investigations may be warranted.

The placing and stepping reflexes (birth to 6 weeks)

Hold the child in a vertical position. When the infant's sole is being pressed to the ground, the legs of the child will reciprocally flex and extend. This reflex balances the flexor and extensor tone for future standing and walking as well as stimulating dorsiflexion of the foot and extension of the toes. The absence of this reflex is usually related to CNS damage.

Testing cranial nerves II, III, IV and VI

Keep the infant steady, whilst moving your own body from side to side. During this motion observe the child's ability to fix the eyes at a certain distance, which is testing Cranial Nerve II (Optic nerve). When the infant follows your movement with his eyes the extraoccular muscles are being assessed (Cranial Nerves III, IV and VI).

- At birth a full term infant should be able to track briefly with his eyes in a vertical and horizontal direction and focus on a face at a distance of 20–30 cm.
- The infant should be able to follow with his eyes from 5–6 weeks old.
- At 4 months old the normal baby should be able to fix with his eyes at a distance of 45 cm and actively turn his head as well as follow with his eyes.

Ventral suspension of the infant

Hold the infant in horizontal suspension.

Assessment of muscle tone

This position tests the baby's head control and ability to extend his trunk as well as muscle strength and tone. The hypotonic or floppy baby will hang in a U-shape, or form a C-shape if only one side of the body is being affected. The hypertonic child will have a tendency to hyperextend. Please note that from 3 to 24 months of age the Landau reaction will be active and enable the infant to extend his neck and pelvis. Between 6 and 9 months the 'parachute reflex' is developing, which involves a protective falling response involving the upper extremities.

The Landau reflex

Hold the infant with a flat hand under the tummy in horizontal suspension. Evaluate the position of the spine, head, arms, legs and feet.

- 1–6 weeks (first phase): the head, trunk and arms are slightly flexed, the hands are held in an open relaxed way.
- 7 weeks–3 months (second phase): the neck is held symmetrically straight; the trunk is slightly flexed from the middle thoracic spine downwards. The arms start to be held in a 90° angle in their neutral position, the legs are flexed.
- 4–7 months (third phase): the extension of the spine continues and is complete at 7 months of age. The arms are flexed and relaxed with a 90° angle at the elbow. The legs are gradually held at a 90° angle in all three joints.
- 8–12 months (fourth phase): the spine is completely extended; the knees are flexed and relaxed and not held at a 90° angle anymore. From the 9th month onwards at the earliest the legs are stretched at the knees in a relaxed way.

In the hypotonic infant the Landau reaction may be weak or absent and the child will have the spine flexed and the head and the limbs hanging down in a U-shaped position.

The parachute reflex

The parachute reflex appears between 6 and 12 months of age. It is commonly present at 9 months of age, and persists throughout adult life. Its absence is abnormal.

In order to test this reflex, hold the infant face down in the prone position, and move the child rapidly towards the floor. The normal child will respond by extending both upper limbs. The role of this reflex is to help break a possible fall by placing the arms in front, thus providing a protective response for the head.

This response may be asymmetric in hemiplegia, or in Erb's palsy. In my own clinical practice I have found that some cases of improper function of this protective response may be related to somatic dysfunction affecting the upper limbs or the shoulder girdle. In this case the inability of the child to extend the arms forward may be related to a pain response rather than a neurological deficit.

Examination with the infant in the supine position

Observation

Observe the infant's posture and the way in which the child moves:

- Does the child lie in C-shape?
- Is there an obvious head preference in position towards the left or the right side?
- Is there any abnormal limb positioning? In the newborn the lower limbs are usually held in a flexed position; in the spastic child, however, they may be extended.

- Does the child move all limbs equally well? Any difference in the movement of the upper limbs may be related to Erb's palsy (peripheral nerve injury).
- Is there any paucity of movement indicating the possibility of CNS injury?

Explore the interaction between yourself and the infant by making visual contact and starting to speak to him. This will test vision and hearing as well as giving you an opportunity to observe the baby's psychosocial interaction with you. Use the test for examining hearing and vision as described in sections from pages 139 and 141.

Sucking and gag reflexes

Examine the sucking and the gag reflexes. Insert your finger into the infant's mouth, which will encourage the child to latch and to suck. Evaluate the strength of the suck and the child's ability to close his mouth around your finger. In response, the normal infant will pull your finger inwards and upwards towards the upper palate. The gag reflex may also be elicited by this maneuver, indicating a sensitive or excessive gag reflex. Assess the child's ability to swallow by observing how the infant feeds.

Grasping

Fine-motor function of the infant and the child's visuospacial abilities are tested by observing the skill levels with which the baby is attempting to grasp and handle objects.

In the older infant watch the way in which the toys get manipulated and transferred from one hand to the other. In the neonate the fingers and the thumbs are tightly fisted when the palm is touched and only an involuntary grasp exists, which the infant is not able to release. This reflex disappears by 1 month old and the hands start to open at 2–3 months of age. This is when the voluntary grasp develops. The use of the upper extremities, the wrists, hands and fingers, as well as the child's visuospacial skills, are being progressively more fine tuned in relation to the child's ability to handle different objects.

Test the hand grasp in the 4- to 5-month-old by using one tongue depressor whilst in the 6- to 9-month-old offer two tongue depressors in order to test for independent hand control and the transfer of objects from one hand to the other. Also check the way in which the child is grasping the toy. At 9 to 12 months the baby is starting to use a pincer grasp. Up to the age of 18 months the child will use both hands equally well. If a hand preference develops before the age of 2 years, further investigation maybe indicated in order to find the cause for the neglect of the other hand.

Muscle tone and strength

Pull the infant from lying supine to the sitting position. Place your thumbs in the child's palms and pull her up slowly. Observe the degree of head control. Up to 6 weeks of age the infant usually presents with a complete head lag with arms and legs flexed. Up to the 3rd month the head is held in a straight line with the spine. From 4–6 months onwards the chin is held against the chest and arms and legs are completely flexed. At 7 months the arms are flexed and the legs are held straight in a relaxed way.

Muscle tone and strength is being tested here in relation to hand grasp and the neuromuscular function of the arms and the shoulder girdle. Watch for asymmetric head positioning when performing this procedure. In torticollis or in the presence of one-sided neurological symptoms the head may be positioned to one side, off the midline.

The asymmetric tonic neck reflex – ATNR (2–6 months)

Test this reflex with the child lying in the supine position. Rotate his head in one direction, which under normal conditions leads to a 'fencing posture'. The infant responds by extending his lower limb on the same side and flexing it on the opposite side. At the same time the upper limb on the same side extends and flexes on the other side. If this reflex can still be elicited after 6 months of age, an upper motor neuron problem may be present, as is the case in cerebral palsy. If the child maintains the 'fencing position' for as long as the head is being held in rotation, CNS disease may be present. The ATNR disappears when the infant is starting to roll over.

Testing the Moro reflex

With the child lying in the supine position, lift the infant's head up and let it fall backwards whilst guiding it. In response, all extremities of the child will symmetrically abduct and extend, which is then followed by a symmetrical adduction and flexion of all extremities.

This reflex is present at birth and usually persists until 4 months of age. It evaluates the integrity of the central as well as the peripheral nervous systems in relation to limb function. In cerebral palsy limb extension is being prevented by the existing excess flexor tone. An asymmetric response of the upper limbs may indicate Erb's palsy (brachial plexus injury) or a congenital disorder. If the Moro reflex persists beyond 4 months old, the clinician will need to check not only the infant's legs for symmetry but also the child's facial responses when eliciting this reflex.

Please note that the examination of the Moro reflex should be conducted towards the end of the physical assessment as it startles and may be upsetting to the child. This reflex also occurs spontaneously in response to a loud noise or can be inadvertently elicited by an abrupt change in the positioning of the child's head.

Examination of the infant in the sitting position

When supporting the infant in the sitting position, check the amount of head and trunk control as well as the developing lumbar curve.

At 1–2 months of age the head is being held up intermittently whilst at 4 months old the child should start to exhibit good head control. The 2- to 3-month-old infant will be able to raise his head and shoulders in the sitting position but still has no proper control in the thoracolumbar area. At 3 months old the baby should be able to sit when being supported, and at 4 months old he is starting to develop a lumbar curve below L3. The 7-month-old infant is starting to sit without any support, is holding the spine straight and the head erect.

The protective equilibrium response

A lateral propping reflex is present at 7 months of age. This infantile response is tested by pushing the baby laterally. The normal infant starts to flex his trunk against the applied force in an attempt to regain the center of gravity. At the same time the arm on the opposite side will extend in the direction towards which the examiner has pushed him. This reflex aims to protect against falling.

Examination of the infant in the prone position

The baby is placed in the prone position. The newborn will lie with his pelvis high and knees placed under the abdomen. At 6 weeks old the hips will be extended in this position.

Muscle tone and strength

We are looking to assess the muscle tone and strength of the infant in relation to the neurodevelopmental control of the upper body and the extremities. In the older infant put the child in the prone position, whilst at the same time ensuring that the baby's hands are being placed to either side of his shoulders with the palms facing towards the ground and his arms being flexed at the elbows. This will optimize the infant's ability to raise his head and trunk. The normal child will be able to lift his chin off to 45° at 6 weeks old, and to 90° at 3 months old. At that age the infant is usually able to support the weight on his forearms with his chest well off the ground, and at 6 months old the baby will bear the weight on his hands with the arms being extended forwards (Illingworth 1983). Watch out for any fisting of the hands. Look for symmetrical function of the head, neck and shoulders and assess the child's ability to control his arms.

Mobility of the spine

At this point of the examination it is also relevant to assess the baby's cervical, thoracic and lumbar spine mobility as well as the infant's pelvic mobility, including the sacroiliac joints and the psoas muscle. Somatic dysfunction, associated pain and discomfort as well as with restricted mobility, may potentially be a limiting factor to the child's neuromuscular abilities.

With the child lying prone on the treatment table, or alternatively on your lap, stabilize the lumbar spine and sacrum with one hand whilst moving the lower limb to extend the hip with your other hand. This movement assesses sacroiliac function as well as the soft tissues of the joint.

Thoracic and lumbar segmental spinal motion can also be assessed in the prone position by contacting the relevant two spinal processes of the articulation with the fingertips of one hand whilst gently rocking the pelvis from side to side with the other hand.

Sensory testing

Sensation can be assessed by initiating a stimulus on one limb whilst the infant is being distracted from this action by the care giver. Observe how the baby withdraws the limb in response to the applied pressure and/or a painful sensation.

Deep tendon reflexes

When eliciting the deep tendon reflexes, the test result may vary according to the relative maturity of the different reflexes. They are tested by applying the reflex hammer over the clinician's thumb or finger overlying the tendon. The biceps tendon reflex (C5–C6), radial periostal reflex (C5–C6), triceps reflex (C6–C8), patellar reflex (L2–L4) and Achilles reflex (L5–S2) are tested. Due to the predominance of the flexoral tone it is difficult to test the triceps reflex in babies under the age of 6 months.

Observe the strength and a lateral difference in reflex response. The reflex is:

- not activated: if there is damage to the second motoneuron or peripheral nerve (e.g. with spinal muscular atrophy, polyneuropathy), myopathy, erroneously if there is tension (attempts may be made to overcome this through facilitation, e.g. with Jendrassik's maneuver; interlace both hands in front of the chest and allow them to be pulled apart).

- exaggerated, i.e. there are cloni, or the actuation area is extensive: if there is damage to the first motoneuron (e.g. spasticity in infantile cerebral palsy).

Please remember that any clinically abnormal results should always be validated by further comprehensive neurological testing.

Pyramidal tract signs

A positive Babinski response is thought to be normal during the first year of life. When elicited, the big toe extends whilst the other toes are fanning out. Clonus may be present and is a normal occurrence in the first 2 to 4 months of an infant's life.

Gross motor skills

The evaluation of the infant's gross motor skills is best performed by putting the child on the floor and by encouraging spontaneous mobility such as asking him to crawl, cruise or walk, either towards you or in the direction of a toy or a parent. Compare the observed skills with the suggested ages at which the different gross motor skill are commonly achieved (described on p.90). Remember, however, that the average age listed below can only serve as a guideline. There may be great variations of what is considered normal. If a child seems to be late in achieving the different gross motor skills, discuss this with the parents; for example, ask whether there are any late walkers within the family. The child may be within normal limits in relation to his genetic background.

Cerebellar testing

It is difficult to examine cerebellar function in the infant.

Bibliography

Carreiro J E : An osteopathic approach to children; Churchill Livingstone, Edinburgh 2003

Habel A: Aids to pediatrics. 3rd edn. Churchill Livingstone, Edinburgh 1993

Illingworth R S: The development of the infant and young child: normal and abnormal. 8th edn. Churchill Livingstone, Edinburgh 1983

Magoun HI: Osteopathy in the cranial field. 3rd edn. Journal Printing, Kirksville, Mo. 1976

McRae R: Clinical orthopedic examination. 2nd edn. Churchill Livingstone, Edinburgh 1983

EXAMINATION OF THE PRESCHOOLER AND SCHOOLCHILD

Once the child is able to follow your instructions, the physical examination can be conducted in a similar fashion to the adult. Some of the examination procedures described have been adapted from Greenman (1996) whilst some of the orthopedic assessments originate from the Easter Seal Society (1982), from McRae (1983) and from Lang (1992).

The biomechanics of gait

Observe the gait as the child enters the treatment room. Note any limp associated with hip pathology or a short leg, as well as looking for any aberrant movement patterns suggestive of neurological disease or myopathy.

When looking at the child's foot placement, take note of any in- or out-toeing. Are both feet equally turned in or out? Or are you noticing excessively pronated or everted ankles, or does the child suffer from flat feet? Is the child knock-kneed (genu valgum) or bow-legged (genu varum), or are you observing toe walking indicating a shortened Achilles tendon?

The child first starts to walk between 9 and 15 months. In the early stages of walking there is no heel strike or toe-off. Instead the toddler will put his foot down flat onto the floor and lift it back up flat. In the early walker the foot will be naturally pronated, which is needed for the toddler to gain lateral stability when walking in a typically broad based walk.

In the 3- to 4-year-old a mature gait can be seen with a proper heel strike and lift-off phase as the postural equilibrium is being established. The normal 7- to 8-year-old has outgrown the foot pronation of the childhood gait and established a full adult function of the foot.

Ask the child to walk up and down, whilst looking for any aberrant or non-age appropriate gait patterns. Normally the feet at birth are held outwards in a valgus position or inwards in a varus position. As the child begins to walk his feet should be turning outwards no more than 30° and inwards no more than 10° (Wong 2001). Assess the gait angle of the child. Normally it measures 10° of out-toeing.

Observe the width of the child's gait, noting whether the child is walking inappropriately for his age. Does the child seem steady on his feet, or is he unstable and swaying from side to side, indicating the possibility of cerebellar or dorsal column involvement? Also observe how the child swings his arms during walking. Normally the arms should swing with the legs in a cross-crawling pattern.

Instruct the child to 'walk on your heels', then to 'walk on tiptoes'. This will assess distal muscle strength of the legs, balance and coordination. Any muscle weakness of the distal limbs also becomes apparent when asking the child to 'sit down and get up again'. Any difficulties may indicate Gowers' sign, which is diagnostic for myasthenia gravis.

Ask the child to 'hop on one leg and then on the other'. This assesses the vestibular system and the muscle strength of the lower extremities.

Assessment of the child standing

Posterior view

Check the following anatomical landmarks for symmetry:

- the tips of the acromion processes
- the inferior angles of the scapulae
- the iliac crests
- the tips of the greater trochanters
- the PSISs (posterior superior iliac spines)
- the lateral margins of the knee joints
- the medial malleoli.

Observe the weight distribution through the feet. In a short leg or a scoliosis the heel of the foot belonging to the shortened leg is not fully placed on the ground. In hip pathology the affected leg is externally rotated.

Are you observing any fidgeting of the child indicating the possibility of hyperactivity or attention deficit syndrome (ADS)? Any swaying from side to side or unsteadiness should be noted in relationship to neurological dysfunction or developmental delay.

Take a close look at the physical appearance of the child. Note the shape and size of his head, as well as the positioning of his eyes and ears. Are you detecting any dysmorphic features indicative of a syndrome or genetic abnormalities? Is there any evidence of microcephaly, hydrocephalus or plagiocephaly, or are you detecting any obvious postural asymmetries including torticollis, a spinal scoliosis, or an oblique pelvis?

Note any lateral head tilt as seen in torticollis. Check the length of the neck looking for any dysmorphic features such as a short neck in Klippel-Feil or Noonan syndrome, or a webbing of the neck in Turner or Noonan, as well as a low hairline in Turner, Noonan, or Klippel-Feil syndrome. Observe the carrying angle of the upper limbs, noting any varus or valgus deformities. A cubitus valgus exists if the carrying angle reads over 15° in girls, or more than 10° in boys. Can you see any deformity of the thoracic cage, such as a one-sided scapular prominence, and a thoracic or a lumbar scoliosis? A pelvic tilt may indicate hip pathology, a short leg, or a sacroiliac dysfunction. Are there any obvious spinal dimples or hairy patches suggesting the presence of spina bifida occulta?

Ask the child to take a deep breath in and then out to evaluate the movement of the ribcage. Palpate rib mobility by contacting the intercostal spaces with your the fingers on both sides of the thorax. Assess lower rib motion first, moving your hands superiorly towards the axilla to assess the upper ribs.

Sidebending test

Ask the child to run each hand in turn down his lateral thigh as far as possible for a lateral sidebending test. Make sure that the child is not bending forwards when doing this test. Check for symmetry of movement between left and right, as well as observing the spine as it is assuming a smooth C-shape during normal sidebending. Are you observing any spinal segments that stay in a straight position during sidebending, or is there any muscular fullness on one side of the paraspinals when compared with the other, suggesting a scoliosis? Take note whether the pelvis is shifting equally to the right and to the left when performing this test.

Standing flexion test

With the child standing, the feet slightly apart, use your thumbs to palpate inferior to the slope of the PSISs. Then ask the child to try touching his toes with his fingers, making sure that the legs are being kept straight for a standing flexion test. Observe whether one PSIS appears to be moving more cephalward and anteriorly when compared with the other, indicating restricted sacroiliac joint function.

At the same time also observe the segmental movement of the thoracic and lumbar spines during forward bending, as well as noting any sidebending of the curve. In the case of a scoliosis you may also find a stronger build up of the paraspinal muscles on one side of the spine. Measure the distance between the child's finger tips and the floor to assess the flexibility of the spine as well as the muscle tone of the hamstrings.

Stork test

Place your left thumb over the most posterior portion of the left PSIS with the right thumb overlying the midline of the sacrum at the same level. Ask the child to lift his left knee up for the stork test. Encourage a minimum of at least 90° of hip flexion. In the normal situation you would expect the PSIS to move in a superior direction in relation to your right thumb. Compare your findings with the other side.

Trendelenberg test

The Trendelenberg test assesses hip pathology. Ask the child to stand on one leg. In hip pathology, the buttock of the non-weight-bearing side fails to rise (the unaffected side) due to weak pelvic muscles (especially m. gluteus medius).

Lateral view

Observe the spinal curves for thoracic kyphosis, or a lumbar lordosis.

Check the child's posture in relation to the plumb line. This is an imaginary line, depicting the center of gravity, which runs from the external auditory meatus to the tip of the acromion process and continues through the greater trochanter to run just in front of the medial maleolus.

Check the arches of the feet for symmetry and flattening, a high arch or low arch. Ask the child to stand on tiptoes in order to assess the arch of the foot. In a 'true flat foot' the arch will not be reinstated when off weight bearing. If

the arch is being reinstated by this action we are dealing with ligamentous laxity instead (see Ch.15, Flat foot).

Assessment of the child sitting

The child is asked to sit on the treatment table.

Upper extremity screen

Ask the child to reach up towards the ceiling and make the heels of his hands meet above the his head. You may need to guide the child's action to ensure this movement is made correctly.

This maneuver assesses the function of the sternoclavicular, acromioclavicular, and glenohumeral, as well as the elbow and the wrist joints. Look for symmetry of function, noting the degrees at which the aberrant movement is occurring.

Trunk

Rotation

Stand behind the child contacting each of the shoulders. Ask the child to fold his arms then to turn and to look over his shoulder as far as possible, whilst guiding the trunk rotation. Assess the symmetry of this movement from side to side.

Sidebending

Grasp the child's shoulders. Press downwards on the right shoulder to induce a right sidebending of the trunk. Try to sense the range and quality, as well as the end-feel of the movement. Compare right sidebending with the left.

Cervical spine

Flexion and extension

With the child sitting at the end of the table, stand at the side and hold the child's head between your hands in an anteroposterior plane. Ask the child to move his head downwards and to look at his feet to test cervical flexion. Whilst guiding the neck through this flexion movement assess the range of motion by recording the distance between the chin and the child's chest. Introduce a backward bending motion by asking the child to look up at the ceiling; this tests cervical extension. In the normal situation the child will be able to directly look up at the ceiling. Make sure that you prevent the child from moving the chest anteriorly in order to assess pure cervical motion, rather than a combined movement of the body and the cervical spinal column.

Rotation

Introduce cervical rotation by asking the child to look over each shoulder in turn, whilst fixing the position of the shoulder girdle. Compare the two sides.

Side-bending

Position yourself behind the child. Whilst guiding his head with your hands placed over the temporal areas, introduce a side-bending motion to the neck. Assess the symmetry of motion between both sides.

Articular joints

Test for ligamentous laxity of the joints. In order to assess the child for joint laxity, see whether the child manages to touch his forearm with his thumb.

Examination with the child lying supine

Part of the examination can be done with the older child lying supine if the child is cooperative.

Observation

Observe the natural position of the upper and lower limbs, the head and the neck, as well as looking for any sidebending of the trunk, or structural deformities. Consider the congenital as well as the functional aspects of your clinical findings.

Are you detecting any loss in muscle bulk between the right and the left sides of the body? Measure the circumference of the affected limb in order to assess the severity of the condition. To rule out a neurological cause, you may at this point decide to test the deep tendon reflexes (see p.129) as well as assessing the child's muscle tone and strength. Palpate the affected joints for any swelling and bony or connective tissue masses, as well as for any differences in temperature.

Upper extremities

Look at the carrying angle of the child's arms. Check the acromio- and sternoclavicular joints by passively elevating the child's arm and at the same time palpating with your other hand the individual function of the joints. Test the passive elbow extension and flexion as well as pronation and supination. Assess wrist function in passive abduction and adduction as well as passive flexion and extension. Note any areas of increased bone density indicating a healed greenstick fracture.

Lower extremities

Observe the lower limbs for any structural asymmetry including tibial torsion or femoral anteversion. Does one limb seem more internally rotated than the other? Compare your findings with other asymmetries found in the upper extremities, neck, cranium or face.

To verify a case of genu valgum, measure the distance between the medial malleoli. In the case of genu varum, measure the distance between the medial joint margins of the knee.

Assess the following bilateral structures for symmetry:

- the iliac crests
- the ASISs (anterior superior iliac spines)
- the tips of the greater trochanters
- the inferior margins of the patellae
- the medial malleoli.

The hip

Circumduct the hip joint. Circumduction of the hip joint consists of a compound movement including flexion, extension, abduction and adduction as well as internal and external rotation.

The movement of the femoral head within the acetabulum is dependent on the smooth myofascial action of the rotator muscles of the hip. Carreiro (2003) pointed out, that, similar to the shoulder joint, these muscles are stabilizing and guiding the movement and the position of this joint. She underlined the importance of the functional integrity of this 'rotator cuff' arrangement in relation to the diagnosis of any joint dysfunction affecting the hip. Therefore try to also assess the myofascial and other connective tissue stresses affecting the hip joint.

Bend the knees of the child towards the chest whilst monitoring the lumbar spine for any fixed flexion deformity with the other hand contacting the lumbar spine. A fixed flexion deformity may be associated with an iliopsoas, rectus femoris or tensor fasciae latae contracture (Baxter 1998).

Check hip abduction with legs straight. Examine any difference in the range of motion between left and right limb abduction. Stabilize the ASIS when doing this test in order to prevent any compensatory lumbar lateral flexion.

Faber test

Ask the child to 'do the splits' in order to get the child's cooperation with this test. To test for hip pathology, take the hip joint through its full range of motion in the Faber test (flexion, abduction, external rotation).

Be aware of the quality of the passive movement at the hip as well as the joint end-feel. Differentiate between a bony end-feel (joint pathology), cogwheel rigidity (cerebellar involvement), any sudden twitching (possible epilepsy), myofascial stresses affecting the joint capsule, or any biomechanical stresses affecting the joint (somatic dysfunction).

Repeat the test with one hand on the child's knee and the palm of your other hand on the ischial tuberosity. This gives you information about the tissue tension, which may affect the ligaments of the hip, in comparison to the somatic dysfunction.

Examination of the knee

When assessing the range of motion of the knee you need to examine knee flexion, extension, and rotation. Jane Carreiro (2003) mentioned that knee flexion is associated with an internal rotation of the tibia, whilst during knee extension the tibia is rotating externally. This is caused by the asymmetric shape of the femoral condyles and the menisci. During knee flexion and extension, the medial meniscus is able to move in distance by up to 6 mm, whilst the lateral meniscus may be shifting its position by up to 12 mm. During knee extension the quadriceps muscle contracts, leading to an anterior glide of the tibia as the patella is being drawn upwards. The opposite occurs during flexion. Take these minor movements of the knee joint into account. Connective tissue stresses altering these minor movements of the knee may be a contributing factor to some knee conditions.

A normal flexion of the knee allows the child to touch his buttock with his foot.

Also look for any quadriceps muscle wasting or swelling around the knee. Check for any joint perfusion at the patellar articulation, as is the case with chondromalacia patella in the teenage girl. Also check the tibial tubercle, swelling of the joint and pain as these may be present in boys suffering from Osgood-Schlatter disease (see Ch.15).

With one hand contact the medial and lateral joint margins and the patella, whilst the other hand is holding the leg with the thumb contacting the tibial tubercle. The degree of tibial rotation should be noted by observing the tibial tubercle as it moves laterally during knee extension. A normal range of flexion at the knee exists when you can touch the child's buttocks with his foot.

With your right index finger contact the tibial tubercle whilst your left index finger is contacting the midpoint of the ankle mortis. Normally these two points should be in the midline, otherwise you may be looking at a persistent tibial torsion when assessing the preschool or school-age child. You can also use this handhold to assess the tibia for any intraosseous strains.

Assess the ligamentous stability of the knee by testing abduction, adduction and the medial, lateral, anterior and posterior glide of the tibia on the femur. Also monitor the superior and inferior motion of the patella during knee flexion and extension, as well as examining the transverse motion of the patella.

Contact the fibula by holding it at each end between your index fingers and thumbs. Test for ligamentous integrity of the tibiofibular joints as well as testing the interosseous membrane connecting the two bones.

The 'short leg'

Observe the lower limbs for unequal leg length by comparing the levels of the medial malleoli.

A 'true shortening of the leg' exists when the problem causing the short leg lies below the level of the greater trochanter. We need to differentiate such a situation from a 'false short leg' where a pelvic asymmetry is affecting the leg above the level of the greater trochanter. In order to diagnose a true short leg, use a tape measure to record the distance between the tip of the medial malleoli and the ASIS.

Verify your findings by assessing the pelvis because a pelvic deformity could lead to an error in your assessment. With the child in the supine position contact the ASIS on one side with your thumb whilst contacting the greater trochanter of that side with your other fingers (McRae 1983). If the distance between your thumbs and the greater trochanter is shorter on one side when compared with the other, we may be dealing with a pelvic deformity causing the short leg.

Compare the level of the two knees with the child lying supine, the knees flexed and the soles of the feet on the table. In the case where one knee seems to be more forward than the other, we are dealing with a femoral shortening. If, however, one knee seems higher than the other knee, we are dealing with a shortening of the tibia.

Measure the tibia by holding the knees in a flexed position. Then mark the medial joint line of the knee with a pen and measure the length between this mark and the tip of the medial malleolus. Compare both sides.

Measure the femoral shaft with the child lying supine with the knees flexed. Compare both sides by measuring the distance between the tip of the greater trochanter and the lateral joint margin of the knee.

The ankle and the foot

When testing the ankle we need to take into account the non-weight-bearing motions as they occur between the talus and the calcaneus. These are inversion, eversion, adduction, abduction, pronation and supination of the ankle mortis.

The four main motions of the foot during weight bearing include dorsiflexion, plantar flexion, inversion and eversion. Dorsi- and plantarflexion involve a motion at the talocalcaneal joint and some tarsal movement. Eversion involves the ankle mortis as well as the tarsals, with inversion mainly taking place in the tarsal joints.

When standing at the foot end of the treatment table, test the four main motions of the foot by cradling the heel of the child's foot with one hand and contacting the forefoot with the other hand. In order to examine the mid-tarsal joint, stand at the side of the table with the child lying supine. Test the movement of this joint by contacting the distal part of the foot with one hand whilst the other hand is contacting the proximal part.

Examination of the child lying prone

Ask the child to lie prone on the treatment table and assess the levels of the posterior iliac spines as well as the iliac crests. Continue by examining the spinal alignment by palpating the spinous processes and the paraspinal muscles of thoracic and the lumbar spines. Check for any dimples or tufts of hair indicating spina bifida. Contact the adjoining spinous processes with your fingers whilst rocking the pelvis from side to side in order to test the mobility of the individual spinal articulations.

Flex the child's knees in this prone position looking at the soles of the feet for any evidence of metatarsus adductus. This is a foot deformity in which the forefoot is adducted in relation to the hindfoot (see Ch.15, Intoeing). It is important to diagnose such a deformity as early as possible in the infant as osteopathy as well as casting and reversed boots may be used to normalize the foot. If it persists beyond 4 years of age, surgery will be the only way to correct it (Easter Seal 1982).

Look at the thigh-foot angle, which assesses the degree of internal tibial torsion. An external rotation of the foot in relation to the thigh is thought to be normal whereas any internal rotation of the thigh-foot angle indicates an internal tibial torsion. Please note that a metatarsus adductus also presents with an internal rotation of the thigh-foot angle; however, the heel of the foot will not be internally rotated in this case.

Test the passive range of motion (ROM) of internal and external rotation of the hip with the child prone and the knees flexed. The normal ROM is 45° of internal rotation in the hip, and 30° of external rotation. In the case of a femoral anteversion (internal femoral torsion) you are looking at a situation where you find an increased ROM of internal rotation of the hip (up to 90° in some cases), and a decreased ROM in external rotation (as low as 10° in some cases).

The neurodevelopmental physical examination

Gait and gross motor skills

Observe the gait (see p.129), the gross motor skills and the coordination of the child. This is best achieved by observing the way in which the child moves around the room. If old enough, ask the child to climb onto the treatment table, which gives you plenty of feedback regarding his motor skills, muscle strength and abilities to balance. The presence of an unsteady or wide based gait after the age of 2½ as well as an immature walk at 3–4 years may be warning signs of developmental delay (Field et al 1997).

In most instances preschoolers enjoy showing off their skills to the clinician. Encourage the child to jump, balance on one foot, to hop and to skip. Find out from the parent whether their offspring is able to ride a tricycle or a bicycle with support wheels.

Psychosocial interaction

It is important to observe the child's interaction with the parent. Do you detect any behavioral problems or difficulties with discipline? An ability to understand and follow instructions reflects the child's receptive and expressive language abilities.

Behavior while playing and speech

The psychosocial interaction of the child as well as the acquisition of speech will be at the center of the toddler's development. From 20 months onwards the child is starting to engage in symbolic play with toys. This is why the first part of the neurodevelopmental examination of the toddler and preschooler is best performed by observing how the child interacts with his environment.

Try to engage the child in spontaneous play and make a note on how he uses speech and is communicating. A playful interaction with the child may give you clues regarding ability to name shapes, colors, numbers, and letters as well as give you insight into his capacity to grasp abstract concepts. Depending on the willingness of the child, the second part of the assessment may also include some formal assessments.

Developmental delay needs to be considered if the child does not link two words together by 2 years old or if the parents are voicing concern about their child's ability to acquire new words. Also consider further investigation if a 3-year-old is not able to join three words together or does not form full sentences at the age of 4. Dysarthria can be related to problems with motor-sensory function of the mouth including cranial nerve lesions affecting VII, VIII, IX or XII, or a cleft-palate. Dysphasia is suggestive of a cortical problem in the dominant hemisphere.

Muscle tone and strength

Are you detecting any 'stiffness' in the child's limbs as the child moves around the room? This may indicate spasticity. The child with hemiplegia displays a specific body posture where the affected arm is being adducted and flexed at the elbow whilst the spastic leg is being circumducted at the hip when trying to walk or to run. Such a child also prefers to hold a pencil in the unaffected hand.

Muscle power can also be assessed by observing how the child is moving around the room. If a child has problems with getting up from sitting to standing, a weakness of the proximal limb muscles may be present. In this case the child may be presenting with Gowers' sign, where he is seen 'as if to climb up the legs with the arms' when trying to regain a standing position. This is diagnostic of muscular dystrophy. It is important to remember that a muscle weakness which is predominantly affecting the proximal parts of the limbs is associated with a myopathy whereas a distal muscle weakness frequently relates to a neuropathy in children, as is the case in cerebral palsy.

A good way to test the upper limbs in the toddler and in the preschool child is to establish a 'pretend wheelbarrow race'. In order to test the muscle strength of the upper extremities, put the child in a wheelbarrow position on the floor and encourage a race (Dooley 1992).

The muscle tone of the upper extremity can be tested by holding each forearm of the child and shaking it whilst at the same time observing the movement of the wrist. If the child is not willing to cooperate with this, simultaneously also pronate and supinate the forearm. This action will be difficult for the child to resist (Dooley 1992).

When testing the range of motion of the lower limbs, note whether you can detect any increased resistance indicating an increased muscle tone. Also make a note of any abnormal movements detected such as chorea. Athetotic movements usually present with a characteristic writhing action. Such clinical findings are suggestive of the likely diagnosis of cerebral palsy.

Coordination

Ask the child to lie down front-first on the floor and encourage him to creep on all fours, or to move like a soldier in combat. This assesses the preschooler's ability to cross-crawl. Note any asymmetrical use of the limbs, or any difficulty of the child to coordinate a cross-crawling action between the individual limbs.

Sense of balance

In the Romberg test ask the child to stand on one leg with the eyes closed. In unilateral vestibular dysfunction or cerebellar disease the child will tend to veer or fall to one side. In the case of a loss of posture sense the child will be perfectly stable with the eyes open but unstable with them shut.

This test can be used from 3 years onwards, at which age the child should be able to briefly stand on one foot. In the preschool child ask the parents to cover the child's eyes on your behalf. You may also want to do the exercise together with the child in order to get cooperation. Please note that Romberg's test is not a specific test of vestibular function.

Response to pain

Use the wheel and the pin prick test and observe the child's response to pain. Also move some tissue across the child's skin in order to assess his ability to perceive sensation. Be careful of how you introduce the child to these tests so as not to cause any upset. Ask the child to say 'now' whenever they become aware of the sensation.

Deep tendon reflexes

(see p.129)

Fine motor skills

Fine motor skills feature prominently in many daily activities of the child. The so called 'clumsy' child who lacks the dexterity to complete tasks such as using zips, closing buttons or cutting with a knife may develop a lack in self-confidence as a result. In the school-aged child the lack of fine motor-coordination may affect the speed at which he able to complete the set tasks in the school environment. It is therefore important to diagnose any problems in this area early, as therapeutic intervention may help improve the child's skills before going to school.

Toys provide the examiner with an opportunity to observe the fine motor coordination as well as the visuospacial skills. Children love to play with shapes that have to be fitted through holes. An easy way to test fine motor coordination in the smaller child is by asking the child to put a pen into a pen-top. The child affected by cerebral palsy will use the unaffected hand to manipulate the pen. Try to determine whether the child exhibits any difficulties with coordination or has more difficulties manipulating toys with one extremity when compared with the other. The latter may indicate a cerebellar lesion on the same side.

Drawing

Ask the child to draw on a magnetic drawing board (e.g. a Magna doodle), which gives you useful feedback on the manual dexterity of the child. Note the way in which the child is grasping the pen. Observe the child's visuospacial awareness and motor planning skills. Any signs of hyperactivity or attention deficit disorder may become apparent during this stage of the examination.

Assess the child's ability to draw. If a child can not do any circular scribbles by the age of 2½ years, is not able to draw a circle by 3½ years, or is not able to make a cross by 4 years, concern should be raised in relation to the child's development. An immature pincer grasp at 3 to 4 years of age should be reason for further investigation.

The child's cognitive abilities are being assessed with the 'draw a person test' (DAP), which can be used with children who are 3 years and older. Instruct the child to draw a person whilst encouraging the child to take as much time as needed and to try his best. Make sure that the child does not receive any cues or help from any other children or adults as this might influence the test results. Evaluate the drawing by counting how many details of the person are to be seen. The older the child is, the more 'natural' and detailed the person should be (see Ch.9, A child's world).

'Reading'

The osteopathic treatment session itself provides a good opportunity to further assess the child regarding the level of intellectual function. Encourage the child to choose a book and to be read to by the parent. The older child may be happy to read whilst lying down on the treatment table whereas the 20-month-old may not be willing to lie down, feeling more secure when sitting on his mother's lap.

Books with flaps are a useful tool of assessment. Most children like reading them. Such a situation allows you to engage in a verbal and instructional interaction with the child. Note how well the youngster is able to lift the flaps of a book and turn the pages. Watch how he points to different pictures on the page. This will give you a lot of information about the child's fine motor abilities as well as the receptive and perceptual language skills. Also evaluate the child's level of understanding of the story line; this will give you important feedback on cognitive ability.

From 18 to 21 months old a child is starting to turn the pages of a book and to point to objects. At 2 years of age the toddler should be able to turn the pages singly by using a pincer grasp. At this age the youngster should be able to identify the different parts of the body as well as recognize the finer details on pictures. Ask the child to point to different items in the book and to name them. Please note that frequent encouragement and praise by the clinician helps children become more confident and to show the best of their abilities.

Evidence of developmental delay

Field (1997) mentioned that if a 12- to 18-month-old does not recognize the use of certain objects and has not spoken any first words by 15 months, developmental delay should be suspected. If a 18- to 24-month-old does not link two words together or does not follow simple requests, and there is no symbolic play with toys, concern should be raised. This is also the case in a child where a pincer grasp is still absent after the age of 14 months. A series of good books are available that teach children about shapes, colors and numbers. Use these books in your practice to test the different skill levels. The 3½-year-old should be able to count to 10 and to match two or more primary colors.

Examination of the cranial nerves
Olfactory (I)
- **Function:** smell
- **Examination result after failure:** anosmia.

Examination

The sense of smell is present at age 5 to 7 months, but is very difficult to examine in a child. The examination is made individually on each side and with the eyes closed, using a number of aromatic substances (aniseed, coffee, cinnamon). The control is effected with trigeminus irritants (ammonia, vinegar), which should be recognized even with anosmia.

Optic (II)
- **Function:** sight
- **Examination result after failure:** optical hypoplasia or atrophy, edema of the optic disk.

Examination

The sight check is made separately for both eyes. The best way to check a small child's sight is by watching the infant play. Special boards can be used from 3 years of age.

With the child sitting, check the field of vision by distracting him with a toy and moving a red toy from the side into his peripheral field of vision. The child should respond to the red toy as soon as it appears at the height of an imaginary vertical line at the outside angle of his eyelid.

Shine a torch into the child's eye to effect miosis. This tests the integrity of cranial nerves II and III. This test also causes a 'blinking reflex' or grimacing by the child, and checks the integrity of cranial nerves VII and II.

The direct reflection of the ocular fundus should not be taken until the end of the examination when the child is more likely to cooperate, as the eyes must be kept still for this examination.

Oculomotor (III)

- **Function:** innervation of musculus (m.) rectus medialis, m. rectus superior, m. rectus inferior, m. obliquus inferior, m. levator palpebrae superior, m. ciliaris, m. sphincter pupillae.
- **Examination result after failure:** ptosis, pupil dilatation, downward and outward deviation of the eyeball.

Examination

The case history may show that the child sees double images.

Use an interesting toy, about 10 cm in diameter, that the child will like to look at, or else a torch. Hold it about 25 cm in front of the child's face and move it to lateral, medial, superior and inferior positions whilst observing the movements of the eyes. Look out for deviation in the eyeball, a nystagmus in adduction and strabismus.

Perform the Hirschberg test on children who can follow instructions. Assess the light reflex of the cornea. Hold a torch in front of the child's nose and ask him to follow the light. Observe the symmetry of the light reflex on the cornea.

Trochlear (IV)

- **Function:** innervation of the m. obliquus superior.
- **Examination result after failure:** upward and outward deviation of the eyeball.

Examination

See Oculomotor III above.

Trigeminal (V)

The three branches of the trigeminal nerve are the ophthalmic (V_1), maxillary (V_2) and mandibular (V_3).

- **Function:** innervation of the mastication muscles (m. masseter, m. temporalis) and m. tensor veli palatini, m. mylohyoideus, m. digastricus (venter anterior), sensitive facial nerve, parasympathetic innervation of the glandula lacrimalis, sensory innervation of the front two-thirds of the tongue.
- **Examination result after failure:** atrophy and loss of strength in mastication muscles (observable in babies by stimulation of the chin reflex), absence of corneal reflex.

Examination

The mastication muscles may be observed while watching the child eat. Watch for abnormal movements of the lower jaw to one side. Alternatively palpate m. masseter and m. temporalis with the jaw firmly closed. Ask the child to open the mouth slightly in order to stimulate the masseter reflex. A gentle tap of your finger, resting on the child's chin, will cause the mouth to close.

Test sensitivity by brushing the child's face gently with a cotton wool ball or your fingertip, following the expansion range of the three trigeminus branches.

Check the nerve exit points on the foramen supraorbitale (V_1), foramen infraorbitale (V_2) and foramen mentale (V_3) by pressing firmly and establishing the perception of pain.

To check the corneal reflex, lightly touch the edge of the cornea with a wisp of cotton wool, bringing the wool from the side of the eye.

Abducent (VI)

- **Function:** innervation of the m. rectus lateralis.
- **Examination result after failure:** horizontal inward deviation of the eyeball.

see Oculomotor III above.

Facial (VII)

- **Function:** motor innervation of the mimetic facial muscles, from m. digastricus (venter posterior), m. stylohyoideus, m. stapedius, sensory innervation of the front two-thirds of the tongue, parasympathetic innervation of the glandula lacrimalis and salivary glands.
- **Examination result after failure**
  - in **peripheral** paresis the ipsilateral muscles are weak to the perioral and periorbital areas, and around the forehead.
  - in **central** paresis only the perioral area is affected.

Examination

The case history of the child may indicate hyperacusis, problems with taste or a reduction in the secretion of saliva or tears.

Observe the face for facial asymmetry (drooping corners of the mouth are typical), differences in the eyelids and flattening of the brow or nasolabial folds. Observe the facial expression.

In order to test the facial muscles, ask the child to wrinkle his brow, squeeze his eyes closed, show his teeth (like a lion), to laugh and to whistle (or pucker his lips). Check for symmetry of the sides of the face; if one side is less able to respond, this is an indication of facial paresis.

Vestibulocochlear (VIII)

- **Function:** innervation of the organ of Corti and balance organ.
- **Examination result after failure:** hypacusis, dizziness.

Examination

The case history of the child may show complaints of tinnitus.

The orientation of the child's hearing may be tested using a rattle, bell or rustling paper whilst the child is being distracted by a parent. Test a preschool child by asking him to repeat a number or a word that you whisper quietly into his ear. Tuning fork tests (Weber and Rinne tests, see p.142) may also be carried out.

Check the function of the balance organ, by turning in circles with the child in your arms. Normal eye reaction would be a deviation in the direction of rotation, and a nystagmus in the opposite direction. Ask an older child to stand on both feet, then on one foot, first with his eyes open and then with them closed (see p.149).

Glossopharyngeal (IX)

- **Function:** innervation of the cranial part of the pharynx muscles, from m. levator veli palatini, m. uvulae, m. palatoglossus, m. palatopharyngeus, m. stylopharyngeus, sensitive innervation of the cranial section of the pharynx membrane and the tuba auditiva, sensory innervation of the back one-third of the tongue, parasympathetic innervation of the glandula parotidea.
- **Examination result after failure:** absence of, or asymmetrical, gag reflex.

Examination

Examining a small child's pharynx may be difficult. You will see it best if the child opens his mouth spontaneously or when he cries. Look for paresis of the soft palate, with the uvula moving to the healthy side. You can ask an older child to say 'aah' while you are examining the pharynx.

Ask the parents whether they have perhaps observed a dysfunction in the gag reflex. Children who tend to aspirate milk and food may have a less active gag reflex. Children with cerebral palsy often have an overactive reflex and gag more frequently. You can stimulate the gag reflex by touching the back of the pharynx, although it may well be absent in an otherwise healthy child.

Children with speech problems, especially with sounds such as 'b' 'd' and 'k' may indicate dysfunctional movements of the pharynx.

Vagus (X)

- **Function:** innervation of the soft palate, the causal section of the pharynx muscles, the larynx muscles, the vocal cords and from m. levator veli palatini, m. uvulae, sensory innervation of the root of the tongue, parasympathetic innervation of the throat, thorax and abdominal organs as far as Cannon's point.
- **Examination result after failure:** hoarse voice due to paralysis of the vocal cords, problems swallowing.

Examination

Listen to the child talking. A nasal or 'throaty' voice or hoarseness are indicators of paresis of the recurrent nerve. Bilateral vagal paralysis leads to aphonia and problems swallowing.

Accessory (XI)

- **Function:** innervation of the m. sternocleidomastoideus and m. trapezius.
- **Examination result after failure:** head turns to opposite side and weakening in the drawing up of the shoulders.

Examination

To test the strength of the m. trapezius ask the child to lift his shoulders while you press down gently on them. Test the m. sternocleidomastoideus by asking the child to turn his head first to one side, then to the other, whilst you prevent the movement. Watch for noticeable asymmetries and uneven muscle strength on the right and left sides.

Hypoglossal (XII)

- **Function:** innervation of the tongue muscles, from m. styloglossus, m. hyoglossus, m. genioglossus.
- **Examination result after failure:** weakness, atrophy, fasciculation of the tongue muscles, inability to extend the tongue if there is bilateral failure, dysphagia.

Examination

Observe whether the child tends to hold the tongue in a protruded position. Ask the youngster to 'stick your tongue out' and note any deviation from the midline. Test the strength of hypoglossal function by placing a tongue blade on one side of the tongue and asking the youngster to move it away.

Bibliography

Baxter R E: Pocket guide to musculo-skeletal assessment. W B Saunders, Philadelphia 1998

Carreiro J E: An osteopathic approach to children. Churchill Livingstone, Edinburgh 2003

Dooley J M: Pediatric neurological examination. In: Goldbloom R B (ed.) Pediatric clinical skills. Churchill Livingstone, New York 1992

The Easter Seal Society: The Easter Seal guide to children's orthopedics. The Easter Seal Society, Ontario 1982

Field D, Stroobant J (eds): Pediatrics – an illustrated colour text; Churchill Livingstone, Edinburgh 1997

Greenman P E: Principles of manual medicine. 2nd edn. Lippincott Williams and Wilkins, Philadelphia 1996

Lang B A: The pediatric musculoskeletal examination. In Goldbloom R B (ed.) Pediatric clinical skills. Churchill Livingstone, New York 1992

Mc Rae R: Clinical orthopedic examination. 2nd edn. Churchill Livingstone, Edinburgh 1983

Roy D L Cardiovascular assessment of infants and children. In Goldbloom R B (ed.): Pediatric clinical skills. Churchill Livingstone, New York 1992, pp. 171–193

Wong D L (ed.): Whaley and Wong's nursing care of infants and children. 6th edn. Mosby, St.Louis 1999

Wong D L, Hockenberry-Eaton M (eds): Wong's essentials of pediatric nursing. 6th edn. Mosby, St.Louis 2001

Zitelli B J,Davies H J (eds):Atlas of pediatric physical diagnosis. 2nd edn. Gower Medical Publishing, New York 1992

EXAMINATION OF THE VISUAL AND AUDITORY SYSTEM

Dion Kulak

The early detection of visual or auditory dysfunction is essential for the normal development of the youngster. Scientific research has documented the extent to which the developing brain is sensitive to the effects of environmental deprivation (Spreen et al 1995). Some researchers describe 'critical' or 'sensitive periods' for the acquisition of speech and the development of vision. For the child it is essential to be able to rely on the proper function of the visual and auditory systems. Any visual or hearing problem will have an effect on the process of learning as well as on the child's psychosocial development. Chronic glue ear in a child younger than 5 years old may have a significant influence on speech, whilst the development of binocular vision and proper tracking of the eye will be essential for reading and writing.

Examination of the visual system

Vision in the less than 3-year-old child is difficult to assess. In the young child you will need to rely more on your observational skills, but you can examine the older child in a similar way to an adult. Vision may be impaired if the youngster is frequently running into things, or is holding objects unnecessarily close to his eyes. Observe the way in which the child is able to fix onto an object and track with his eyes. Does the youngster seem to focus with both eyes or does one eye seem to wander?

The examination of the visual system includes:

- inspection of the eye including the eyelid, sclera, iris, pupils and cornea.

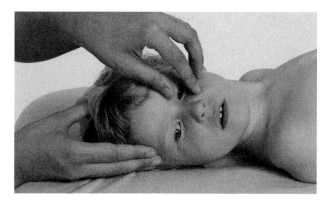

Figure 7.11 Palpation of the orbit.
With permission, Karsten Franke, Hamburg

- assessment of the shape, position and size of the orbits, as well as looking for any abnormal head positioning.
- palpation of the orbit and the eyeball in order to assess the biomechanical effects of any connective tissue stresses on eye function (Fig. 7.11).
- assessment of the child's ability to track with the eyes (examination of extraocular muscle function and nystagmus).
- testing for strabismus: corneal light reflex, cover-uncover test (Hirschberg test), cross-cover test.
- visual acuity.
- examination of the retina: ophthalmoscopic examination of the retina in the older child or test the pupillary red light reflex in the infant.

Inspection of the eye and the orbit

Check the eye for any redness, tearing, or discharge, as well as for eye pain or photophobia. Does the child present with ptosis of the eyelid? Consider causes such as occulomotor nerve palsy, Horner syndrome, a tumor, or a congenital cause. Look at the size, the shape and the position of the orbit. A protruded eyeball may warrant referral for further investigation to exclude a tumor. In the case of plagiocephaly examine the child for any biomechanical causes for the developing asymmetries of the shape and position of the orbits. Contemplate the potential effects of biomechanical dysfunction on the visual system; for example connective tissue stresses affecting the eyeball within the orbit, such as cranial base strains, torticollis and any spinal misalignment.

To assess the tension of the tissues of the orbit place the tips of your fingers evenly around the rim of the orbit and feel for the expression of primary respiration (see Fig. 7.11). At the same time it is possible to palpate the expression of primary respiration in the eyeball with one finger of the other hand.

Differentiate a biomechanical reason for the child's head tilt from a tilt caused by a trochlear nerve palsy. In this case the child tilts his head to avoid seeing double, the head is rotated to one side and side-bended to the other.

Extraocular motor function

In order to test cranial nerves II, III, IV, and VI, which supply the external eye muscles in the infant (see p.136), hold the baby in front of you whilst supporting him under the axillae. Keep the child steady, whilst at the same time moving your own body from side to side and observing the child's ability to fix and track with the eyes.

Test extraocculomotor function (occulomotor, trochlear and abducent nerve function) in the older child by evaluating the youngster's ability to track with the eyes. In the younger child use an interesting toy measuring about 10 cm for the child to happily focus on. Move it in lateral, medial, superior and inferior directions, whilst checking for any disconjugate eye movements. Also assess the eyes for nystagmus.

Testing for strabismus

Strabismus is often referred to as a 'lazy eye'. This is when the visual axes do not lie in a parallel direction, resulting in non-conjugate eye movement. A misalignment of the eyes can also be caused by two unequally clear images being sent to the cortex. In both cases the cortex attempts to suppress one image, so that one eye will eventually stop functioning, leading to a loss of bifocal vision. The 'lazy eye' usually assumes a position of ocular deviation either away from the midline axis (exotropia) or closer to the midline (esotropia).

The following tests are used to diagnose strabismus:

- **Hirschberg test:** Ask the child to keep looking at the light of your torch which is being held at a distance of about 30–35 cm away from the youngster. Look over the top of your light source and assess whether your light is being reflected in an equal position by both eyes (corneal light reflex). In a lateral deviation of the eye (exotropia), the light will be reflected more medial to the pupil on the affected eye. In the case of a medial deviation of the eye (esotropia), the light reflection will be more lateral to the pupil of the deviated eye than on the unaffected eye.

- The **cover-uncover test:** This test is used to diagnose a **manifested squint**. Cover one eye of the child whilst observing the same eye immediately after it has been uncovered. Do this test whilst the child is looking at an object held near to them at a distance of 33 cm. Then ask the child to focus at an object in the far distance, approximately 6 m away. A misalignment of the eye that has been left uncovered is present if it moves after the other eye has been uncovered.

The reason for this is that, when the stronger eye is temporarily covered, the weaker eye has to attempt to focus on the object. Once the stronger eye takes over again, the affected eye will reinstitute its deviated position.

- The **cross-cover test** (alternate cover test): This test is used to diagnose a dormant, concealed squint. Let the child focus on a point in front. Cover one eye and then the other, whilst observing the movement of the eye that has just been uncovered. Normally the eyes will not move when they are being uncovered. If a tropia is present, however, the eye will shift once the cover has been removed.

It is very important to discover a true squint since the suppression of the visual information of the eye with the squint may lead to amblyopia (weak-sightedness of one eye). An amblyopia can only be successfully treated in the first years of life as long as the visual system is pliable.

Assessing visual acuity

Visual acuity is difficult to assess in a child less than 3 years old. In the infant, shine a light into the eyes and observe the responses, such as blinking, a constriction of the pupils or following a light source. Also observe the child for any visual abnormalities. Does the child focus with the eyes properly? Does the youngster frequently run into things or put the toys unusually close to the eyes when playing with them?

In the older child the visual acuity can be assessed in a similar fashion to that of the adult. Instead of cards with letters, though, picture cards can be used.

Testing the visual fields

From 3 years of age the child is able to follow instructions so that the visual fields can be tested. Distract the child with one toy in front whilst moving a red toy from behind into the peripheral field of vision. The child will respond to the red toy as soon as it enters the field of vision. In the normal situation this point should be in line with an imaginary line perpendicular to the outer canthus of the eye.

The school age child will not need any distraction with a toy but the fields of vision may be tested in the same way as you would in the adult. Ask the child to look straight ahead whilst introducing an object to the peripheral field of vision. In order to delineate the expanse of the field of vision, ask the child to tell you when he is able to see the object, then move it further outwards, asking the youngster to tell when the object disappears again from his field of vision. Each eye should be tested separately.

Examination of the retina

It is difficult to perform an opthalmoscopic examination in the infant. Test the 'red light reflex' instead by shining a light into his eyes and observing its red reflection. In the case where the reflection is white rather than red, urgent referral is indicated as you may be dealing with cataract or retinal disease warranting further investigation and medical management.

Also assess the pupillary reaction of the child to the light. Shine a light in to the infant's eyes to test the pupillary light reflex and observe whether the pupils constrict equally in both eyes in response to the light source.

Examine the pupils and the retina in the older child as you would in the adult. Start with the assessment of the direct and the consensual pupillary light reflexes. The direct reflex is being elicited by observing an equal constriction of the pupils in response to a bright light which is being flashed across the outer surface of the child's eye. Test the consensual pupillary light reflex by observing one eye whilst the light is being flashed across both eyes simultaneously.

The pupillary light reflex is testing the integrity of cranial nerve II and III function. Note whether both pupils react and constrict equally in response to the light source. An unequal pupil size may be caused by cranial nerve III palsy, or Horner syndrome.

Test the pupillary near and far accommodation by asking the youngster to focus on a light source in front of them. Start at 30 cm, then move the light source closer towards the tip of the child's nose and further away again. Observe the distance at which the binocular focusing on the light source by the child is being broken by one eye.

The examination of the fundus of the eye with the ophthalmoscope is best left to the end of the examination. Full cooperation is needed to perform this test, as the youngster needs to keep the eyes still to allow for the examination. Hold the child's head firmly in the midline when positioning the ophthalmoscope at a fixed distance from the eyes. Start with the highest dioptre in order to view the outer surface of the eyeball. Then proceed to reduce the dioptre settings in order to view the back of the eye at the level of the retina. Watch for papilledema related to increased intracranial pressure. This examination may also detect a dislocated lens as seen in Marfan syndrome, where it is dislocated upwards.

The biomechanical dimension of visual dysfunction

Jane Carreiro (2003) described the impact a torticollis may have on the vestibular system and hence the visual system. She explained how the eyes are involved in balance and that vestibulo postural reflexes exist which help with the horizontal orientation of our visual axes. This means that the examination of the visual system will also need to consider any biomechanical factors affecting visual function. These include torticollis and other postural asymmetries.

Carreiro (2003) and Magoun (1976) proposed a mechanism by which connective tissue stresses affect the ligamentous suspension of the eye within the orbit. They imply that such stresses can potentially affect the vertical and horizontal tracking of the eyes. Cranial base strains affecting the tracking mechanism of the eyes have been described by Magoun. He explained how inferior and superior strains of the cranial base may have an effect on the vertical tracking of the eyes, and that lateral strains of the cranial base may influence the horizontal tracking.

Also consider the effects of cranial molding on the shape of the orbit. The frontal bone, the sphenoid as well as the maxilla provide for the attachment of the extraorbital muscles. A cranial articular dysfunction of these bones may be one of the many etiological factors involved in strabismus. Strains of the cranial base, the zygoma, as well as the maxilla may play a role in visual dysfunction, as they provide for the attachment of the suspensory ligaments of the eyeball.

Magoun (1988) described how the effect of connective tissue stresses on the tentorium cerebellum might influence the neurotrophic function of the cranial nerves involved in strabismus. A detailed description of these mechanisms is beyond the scope of this text.

When assessing the biomechanical stresses affecting the orbit and influencing visual function, we need to assess the cranial bones making up the orbit for cranial dysfunction. These include the frontal bone, the zygoma, the lacrimal bone, the ethmoid, the sphenoid, the palatine bone and the maxilla. The following anatomical structures may have a biomechanical influence on visual function and should be examined:

- the cranial base
- the tentorium cerebellum
- the vault
- the orbit
- the suspensory ligaments of the eyeball
- postural asymmetries affecting the head and neck
- the spinal vertebral alignment of the body
- intraosseous strains between the greater and lesser wings of the sphenoid.
- connective tissue stresses affecting the common tendinous ring, which provides for the attachment of the extraocular motor muscles.

Assessing auditory function
Observation and palpation

Inspect the shape and position of the ear for any abnormalities. Are the ears set low? In the infant check for skin tags, pits or fistula. These may be located just anterior to the tragus of the ear. Gently take hold of the pinna of the ear to check for any pain or tenderness. If pain can be elicited then otitis externa may be a likely diagnosis. Pain elicted by pressing the tragus is a sign that an otits media may be present. Inspect the mastoid area as well as posterior to the ear for any swelling. Also examine the lymph nodes of the head and the neck.

Tests with technical devices

Several types of hearing test are available which measure the degree of hearing loss in a child. Referral for specialist assessment is needed for an audiometric evaluation. It provides information regarding the severity of the hearing loss. The electrical audiometer evaluates the threshold of hearing for loudness and pure tone frequencies. The procedure involves the transmission of a sound to the child's ear. The youngster is then asked to indicate the point at which the sound disappears.

Bone conduction can be tested by audiometry. This examination passes different sounds through a plaque placed over the mastoid bone. Air conduction is being assessed by audiometry by passing the sounds to the child through an ear phone.

Tympanometry assesses tympanic membrane mobility by measuring the pressure in the middle ear. It detects middle ear disease such as middle ear effusion involved in conductive hearing loss but it does not evaluate the degree of the condition. It is difficult to perform this test in young children who are not always able to sit still for very long.

Examination of the infant and toddler for hearing loss

It is not easy to properly assess a hearing loss in the toddler. Much of your information here may need to come from the parents, who may have become aware that their toddler is not always responding to their voice or other sounds as they would expect. Check the hearing of a toddler by making sounds when the child is turning away from you playing. Also observe the child's interaction with the parents and siblings for any clues regarding the youngster's hearing.

The baby quietens when being spoken to and usually starts to smile at 4 to 6 weeks old. In order to test the infant's hearing, ask the parent to distract the child so he looks away from the examiner. Clap your hands next to the infant's ear and observe the response. When a rattle is being held at ear level, a newborn infant's reaction will be to blink, whereas at 4 months old the child will turn towards the sound. Be aware that the sudden noise may startle the child, initiating the Moro reflex.

An OAE or evoked otoacoustic emissions analyser can be used in the infant in order to test objectively for any sensorineural hearing loss. The OAEs being measured by this test are thought to be sound energy generated by the movement of the outer hairs of the organ of Corti. The results, however, do not give any clue as to the severity of the hearing loss. The integrity of the auditory system in the infant can also be assessed by measuring brainstem-auditory evoked responses (BAER). This measures the waveforms transmitted by the brain after repetitive, short acoustic stimulation. The acoustic signal changes the electric activity of the vestibulocochlear nerve (CN VIII) and the brain for a short period of time. This change in voltage can be measured by electrodes placed on the scalp similar to an EEG.

Assessing the hearing of the school-age child

Assess the hearing of the school-age child by using the Rinne and the Weber tests, both of which measure the conduction of sound.

The Weber test assesses the air conduction of sound. Hold the stem of the tuning fork (440 Hz) in the midline of the head. In the normal situation the child will be able to hear the sound of the tuning fork equally well in both ears (positive test result). With loss of air conduction (e.g. after an episode of otitis media) the child will hear the sound better in the unaffected ear (Weber negative).

The Rinne test examines whether any interference exists in the middle and external ear chambers to the bone's conduction of sound. Place the stem of the tuning fork (440 Hz) against the mastoid process until the child ceases to hear the sound. Then move the prong near the auditory meatus making sure that it is not touching it. When bone conduction is compromised the sound will not reappear (Rinne negative) and we have a middle-ear hearing loss. If the air conduction is more sensitive and persistent than the bone conduction, then the child will hear the sound again when the tuning fork is held in front of the ear. In this case the test is positive and we are dealing with a perceptive hearing loss.

The otoscopic examination

Please note that this procedure may upset the child, especially when the youngster is suffering from pain with an existing ear condition, which is why it is better to leave it until the end of the examination.

It is best to restrain the youngster from moving, so as not to be hurt by the placement of the otoscope in the external auditory meatus. In the infant and toddler the otoscopic examination is best performed where the youngster's head is being steadied by the mother with the child sitting on her lap. Due to the different position of the ear canal in the infant, pull downwards and back on the pinna of the

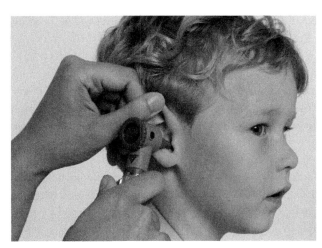

Figure 7.12 Otoscopic examination.
With permission, Karsten Franke, Hamburg

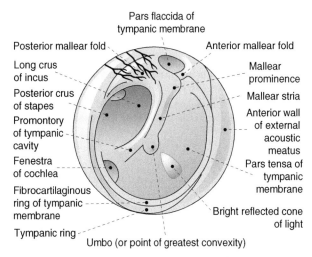

Pars flaccida of tympanic membrane
Posterior mallear fold
Anterior mallear fold
Long crus of incus
Mallear prominence
Posterior crus of stapes
Mallear stria
Promontory of tympanic cavity
Anterior wall of external acoustic meatus
Fenestra of cochlea
Pars tensa of tympanic membrane
Fibrocartilaginous ring of tympanic membrane
Bright reflected cone of light
Tympanic ring
Umbo (or point of greatest convexity)

Figure 7.13 Orientation points and quadrants of the ear drum. With permission, Sobotta: Atlas der Anatomie des Menschen. Publisher: R. Putz and R. Pabst, 21st edn. Elsevier/Urban & Fischer, Munich/Jena 2000

ear in order to straighten the ear canal for better visibility of the tympanic membrane. To insert the speculum hold the otoscope upside down between your thumb and index finger, whilst steading the instrument with your other fingers against the child's skull (Fig. 7.12). Please remember that in the older child the pinna has to be pulled up and backwards instead in order to allow for a good viewing of the internal structures of the ear.

The cooperative or older child can be examined in the supine position. In this case tilt the head slightly towards the child's opposite shoulder to achieve a better viewing of the tympanic membrane.

Start with examining the external ear canal for cerumen (wax), abrasions, discharge or a foreign body. Continue with checking the color and the integrity of the tympanic membrane (Fig 7.13). A healthy membrane appears to be translucent, a light pink, or a grey color. Is there any evidence of scarring of the tympanic membrane or holes indicative of past middle ear disease? The presence of a black area in the membrane suggests a perforation, whilst a healed perforation or a scar in the tympanic membrane usually appears to be ashen grey in color. If the child has grommets, check their positioning. Is there any discharge and, if so, of what color? Middle-ear infection usually shows as a reddening of the membrane. In middle-ear effusion a degree of fluid may be detected and sometimes an air bubble sitting above the fluid may also be seen.

An absent light reflex is commonly due to a bulging tympanic membrane, suggesting the presence of fluid in the middle ear. A retracted tympanic membrane may be associated with chronic 'glue ear'. A pneumatic otoscope may be used to assess the mobility of the tympanic membrane.

The biomechanical dimension of auditory dysfunction

Spreen et al (1995) reported studies describing long term otitis media as a contributing factor of long term language delay. This underlines the importance of normal middle-ear function for the development of the child. A carefully controlled study found a significant association between middle-ear effusion during the first 3 years of life with poorer language skills and IQ performance scores in maths and reading.

Carreiro (2003) discussed the potential vulnerability of the eustachian tube to congestion in the newborn and the infant, describing how the osseous part of the tube is still cartilaginous at that age and that it runs more horizontally than in the adult. This may be one of the reasons why the drainage of fluid from the eustachian tube maybe more vulnerable to congestion in the children younger that 5 years old than in the adult (see p.279).

Degenhard and Kuchera (1994) found that an association exists between middle-ear infection and cranial strain patterns. When considering the potential long term effects of otitis media on the development of the child, an assessment of cranial articular dysfunction (with special reference to the connective tissue structures attaching to the temporal and sphenoid bones) will be essential when looking at the biomechanical integrity of the auditory system.

Bibliography

Carreiro J E: An osteopathic approach to children. Churchill Livingstone, Edinburgh 2003

Degenhard B F, Kuchera M L: The prevalence of cranial dysfunction in children with a history of otitis media from kindergarden to

3rd grade. Journal of the American Osteopathic Association 94, 1994: 754

Goldbloom R B (ed.): Pediatric clinical skills, Churchill Livingstone, New York 1992

Magoun H I: Osteopathy in the cranial field. 3rd edn. The Journal Printing Co, Kirksville, Mo. 1976

Magoun H I: Entrapment neuropathy, part 1, 2 and 3. In Feely R A (ed.): Clinical cranial osteopathy. The Cranial Academy, Meridian, Idaho 1988, pp. 184–203

Spreen O, Rissers A T, Edgell D: Developmental neuropsychology. Oxford University Press, New York 1995

Ward R C (ed.): Foundations for osteopathic medicine. Williams and Wilkins, Baltimore 1997

Wong D L (ed.): Whaley and Wong's nursing care of infants and children. 6th edn. Mosby, St.Louis 1999

Wong D L, Hockenberry-Eaton M (eds): Wong's essentials of pediatric nursing. 6th edn. Mosby, St.Louis 2001

Yu C C; Wong F H, Lo L J; Chen Y R: Craniofacial deformity in patients with uncorrected congenital muscular torticollis: an assessment from three-dimensional computed tomography imaging. Plastic and Reconstructive Surgery 113(1), 2004: 24–33

OSTEOPATHIC CONSIDERATIONS OF SENSORY DEVELOPMENT

Maxwell Fraval

The neurodevelopmental examination of the school-aged child between the ages of 5 and 12 years requires a consideration of both his function of coordination and balance, and visual and auditory processing abilities, because of their complex influence on the development of the child.

The visual system

Improved visual function will of course lead to improvements in the ability to learn; osteopathy has much to offer those children who have mechanical strains as an underlying etiology of this dysfunction.

Symptoms of impaired vision

When learning difficulties arise, vision is often checked at an early stage. Distance vision is only one component in the complex sense of sight. It was only in 1990 that the work of Lovegrove (1990) and later Galaburda (Livingstone et al 1991) demonstrated that there was a twin cell system, the parvocellular and magnocellular system, operating within the visual pathway. The parvocellular system monitors the ambient, background or ongoing visual input, whereas the magnocellular system monitors rapid changes within the visual field. Lovegrove (1990) found that in children with a learning problem, the processing speed of the magnocellular system was much slower, and therefore any child attempting to read from the blackboard or from a book would much more

rapidly become overloaded. Because of this rapid overloading of the system, the eyes will tend to move to and fro rather than in an orderly sequential manner.

As a result of his resulting perceptual problems, the child may misread words or repeat words or lines, may read very slowly, become easily fatigued, or may even read with one eye covered or sit sideways when reading so as to make sense of the images.

In order for a child to be able to read he must be able to successfully achieve convergence, accommodation, and tracking. In order for the eyes to scan along a line of letters and send a clear single image to the brain the eyes and must be able to achieve convergence. For a child to be able to follow words on a page from one line to another, he must be able to track smoothly along the line of print. Accommodation allows a sharp image to be seen when moving from a far to a near point. A child also needs to have the spatial and directional ability to distinguish similar but directionally different symbols such as 'p' and 'q', 'b' and 'd', 'on' and 'no', and so on (Goddard 1996).

Osteopathic considerations on vision

As osteopaths we assess the body for the presence of somatic dysfunction to see whether it has influenced physiological function; we look at the interface between structure (anatomy) and function (physiology).

Sutherland (1990) noted that, at birth, the sphenoid bone is in three parts (see p.175), a central one consisting of the body and lesser wings and two lateral ones, each comprising a greater wing and pterygoid process. Fusion of these three parts occurs by the time the child is 1 year old. Prior to that time an intraosseous strain (with some warping, however small) may occur – either prior to, during or after birth. If that occurs, a distortion of the shape of the superior orbital fissure between the greater and the lesser wing may occur. This may affect the function of the tendinous ring of Zinn which forms the origin of the four rectus muscles of the eye and is attached to the roots of the lesser wing and the margin of the greater wing. All the nerves to the extraocular muscles (the occulomotor, trochlear, and abducens) pass through the superior orbital fissure and so may also be affected. Finally, the autonomic supply also follows this pathway, as does the venous drainage so that circulation to the area may be affected by sphenoid lesioning.

For instance, in a child a lateral strain of the basisphenoid bone (which includes the lesser wing) relative to the base of the occiput, apart from causing a shearing strain at the sphenobasilar synchondrosis (SBS), may cause a concomitant intraosseous lesion at the cartilaginous joint between the basisphenoid and the greater wing pterygoid unit (and distortion of the superior orbital fissure) such that there is a displacement of the axis of the orbit due to rotation of the sphenoid around an anteroposterior axis between nasion and basion. Distortion in the shape of the orbit due to medial pressure on the greater wing may also occur.

A lateral strain can also distort the relation of the base of the occiput between the petrous portions. The squama of the temporal bone moves with the greater wing of the sphenoid. This results in production of an intraosseous lesion of the temporal bone in which the squama is carried anteromedially, and there is increased angulation of the petrous axis within the base. The intraosseous lesions of the temporal and the sphenoid bones are liable to disturb the third, fourth, and sixth cranial nerves and the ophthalmic division of the fifth, as well as to disturb the cavernous sinus and superior and inferior petrosal sinuses, which provide venous drainage from the orbit.

Pressure on or stretching of the nerves controlling the muscles of the eyeball can occur as they pass in relation to the forward reaches of the free and attached borders of the tentorium cerebelli. The petrosphenoid ligament coming off the apex of the petrous portion of the temporal bone and attaching to the posterior clinoid process of the sphenoid is of particular importance insofar as the sixth cranial nerve (abducens) is concerned. The abducent controls the lateral rectus – flaccidity of this muscle results in an esotropia (where the eye turns inwards) whereas spasticity results in an exotropia (where the eye turns outwards).

Additionally, as a result of the somatic dysfunction described, a phoria (defined as a transient tendency to misalignment; Behrman 1992), or other difficulties which involve dysfunctions of convergence, accommodation or tracking may occur. The child may say that the letters he sees are blurred or that he has difficulty seeing them. Sometimes the child does not attempt to describe the difficulty he has in seeing letters or numbers, assuming that everyone experiences the same difficulty. The difficulty may have been there since birth.

Osteopathic treatment can remove somatic dysfunction, neutralizing intraosseous strains of the sphenoid and thereby normalizing the annular tendon of Zinn and restoring normal venous drainage of the orbit. It also restores the balanced membranous tension to the reciprocal tension membrane (RTM) removing irritation to one or more of the nerves controlling the external ocular muscles.

The auditory system

Development of the ability to hear

Myelination of auditory fibres occurs very early, between the 24th and 28th week in utero. Sound perception develops slowly from this time onward. At this stage, the ear is tuned specifically to the sounds heard in utero, and bone conduction is the only means by which sound is transduced. The fetus does respond to some external auditory stimuli as well (see p.30).

The newborn infant's ears become exposed to a vast range of sound frequencies, something in the region of 0–20,000 Hz and beyond. Postnatally the child must learn to respond to air conduction rather than the bone conduction that was relied upon in utero. The baby begins to use his ears to focus on and distinguish the specific frequencies of his own language. It is at this time that the child has the potential to learn any language if exposed to the sounds of that language continuously over a period of time, no matter what language the mother speaks. After the age of 3 years, when these fine-tuning adjustments should have been made, it becomes far more difficult to assimilate a new language.

In order for sounds to be processed successfully, a child must be able to discriminate between the same and different sound, to make an association between environmental sounds and words, to fill in missing parts of verbally presented information and to correctly identify the source of the sound and identify its sequence. The child also needs to be able to isolate relevant sounds that need to be attended to and screen out background noise.

In processing sound that has been registered both at the tympanic membrane and in the surrounding bone, impulses pass from the cochlea to both superior olivary nuclei and other nuclei in the brain stem; so there is a cross over at this early stage. This is important for sound localization in space. It takes only 30 ms of difference between right and left ears to pinpoint a sound. From there impulses are relayed to the inferior colliculus and medial geniculate nuclei in the thalamus where integration with other sensory modalities takes place. Impulses then travel to the auditory cortex in the temporal lobes, particularly to the left hemisphere.

In the auditory cortex, there are specific areas connected with processing of simple sounds, tones, words, phrases, melodies, auditory attention and auditory/motor speech and singing. Research (Tallal et al 1995, Tallal et al 1993) has shown that individual neurons are responsive to specific frequencies and represented spatially in the cortex, just as they are in the cochlea.

Otitis media is one of the most common diagnoses made by the practicing pediatrician (Williams 1992) (see p.283). Frequent ear, nose and throat infections in early childhood resulting in intermittent hearing loss over a period of time can prevent the development of such auditory discrimination skills. Lack of auditory stimulation, or a hypersensitivity to background noise in early life, can discourage early 'listening' and the child may learn to shut out and ignore sound from an early age.

When sound arrives at the superior olivary nucleus, feedback is relayed back to the muscles of the eardrum. This is called the attenuation reflex. It allows the brain to control the tension in the eardrum and the motion of the stapes at the oval window, thus deadening a sound that is too loud or amplifying a soft sound as needed. Hearing too much or 'auditory hypersensitivity' can be just as much of a problem as hearing deficit. The autistic child utilizes the attenuation reflex to turn off to sound when certain frequencies are too distorted and disturbing.

A second feedback loop, known as the olivocochlear bundle appears to be important in the detection of sound background noise, and in attention mechanisms. The inability to filter or occlude miscellaneous sound suggests poorly developed listening skills and can have a profound effect upon later learning, language, communication and behavior.

Symptoms of impaired auditory function

The common signs are that are reported in relation to a child who is experiencing difficulties with auditory processing are that he processes too slowly and can only manage to understand short blocks of words, often only half a sentence. The child seems to get overloaded quickly and his attention wanders; memory and output is often scrambled. He is assessed as having late/poor language skills in receptive and expressive areas and is poor at phonics; that is, in deciphering packets of sound, decoding new words, reading, spelling and comprehension.

So a child with auditory processing problems may be easily distracted or misinterpret questions because it is so hard to hear what is being said. As a result, instructions are ignored or there is an inability to follow sequential instructions. He may show confusion of similar sounding words and often need to have a word repeated. Such children are often unable to sing in tune or demonstrate confusion or reversal of letters.

Keith (1986) described 11 central auditory abilities which are measured by tests of central auditory function. Tomatis discovered the link between ear and voice early in his career (1991). Initially, he applied his discoveries to help musicians, especially singers, regain audio-vocal control. It was not long, however, before his work extended to children whose parents wanted to improve their musicality in order to enrol them in top music programs in Europe. Tomatis was surprized to discover reports that both the adults and children were coincidentally experiencing improved memory, focus, attention span and a diminution of their learning difficulties (Campbell 1997). Determined to get to the root of these findings, Tomatis embarked on a lifelong pursuit of understanding the relationship between the ear and its role in communication, learning and brain function.

Tomatis' pioneering discoveries explains why the way we listen has a profound impact on almost all aspects of our being, including reading, writing, singing, speaking, and even control of our bodies (Madaule 1994). Tomatis also discovered that listening problems are the root of many learning disabilities and his ideas have changed the way we think of education, learning difficulties, listening and communication. He defined the physiological and cognitive differences between hearing and listening. Tomatis' method of sound stimulation to improve listening is called the Tomatis method.

Tomatis (1991) emphasized that hearing is not the same as listening. Hearing is the ability of the ears to take in sound. The ear's mechanics or structure is capable of responding to sound. Listening is the result of our auditory processing or how our brain processes and makes sense of the sounds received from the ear; in other words, our understanding. Auditory processing is the ability to make sense of the sound that comes into the ear and to process or interpret what is heard.

Tomatis (1991) has shown that there is a difference in the way that sounds are transmitted to the language processing center in the brain, depending on which ear is used as the dominant listening ear. Pinkerton and associates (1989) compared 18 'good readers' with 14 'poor readers' in an ordinary classroom of 8- and 9-year-old children. Brain-stem auditory evoked potentials in the right ear were significantly different from those in the left in the good readers, but such asymmetry was not found in the poor readers.

To lay down the sounds of the English language, the infant and young child needs to hear up to 8000 Hz at −10 decibels. The French child needs a slightly different range, so the curves for the two languages differ. Tomatis discovered that all language is spoken between certain ranges, each being specific to the language concerned.

Tomatis also found that we are born with ears able to hear all sounds at −10 decibels. Our hearing will never be as acute as it is once the birth waters have drained out of our outer ear, at about 10 days post delivery. Over the next few years, as we listen to the sounds of our own language our ears gradually close to those frequencies and loudness that are not needed for our language. By the age of 7 years this process is complete. This explains why younger children speak a new language better than their older siblings – their ears are not yet closed, so they hear more accurately, and can therefore match their attempts to their teachers more nearly. After the age of 7 it is very hard for the French to hear the 'th' sound of the English language; they need to be hearing at −5 to −10 decibels at 6 to 8 kHz, and most are not.

It has been shown by Gallaburda et al (Livingstone et al 1991) that within the auditory pathway, as in the visual pathway, there are two cell systems: the magnocellular and parvocellular systems. The magnocellular or transient pathway relays onset/offset (i.e. fast changing stimuli), so it is concerned with fast changes in the sounds of speech and music, changes in localization and changes in figure ground perception. The parvocellular cells monitor ambient sound and relay slow/non changing stimuli; that is, long tones and stable background noise, and emotional content. Gallaburda et al (Livingstone et al 1991) showed that children with an auditory processing problem have minor but significant anatomical deficits in the magnocellular system. By sending sudden bursts of high harmonic sound, therapy is able to stimulate the on/off attentional switch which recognizes fast changing stimuli.

It has been established that the speed of processing in the left hemisphere where Broca's area is located needs to be less than 100 ms for adequate sequential decoding of speech. Tallal et al (1995) showed that the speed of processing is often slower than it should be in the child with attention deficit. Children with hyperactivity are usually normal or very fast. Take the words 'ticket' or 'ticked.' If your sequential processing is slower than 100 ms, you will not be able to distinguish 'it' from 't' so you cannot sort out which sound came first, and spelling will be very hard. If your processing is slower than 200 ms, you will add to the confusion with the 'ck' sound, and if it is slower than 400 ms it will be difficult to make any sense of it at all, because there will be no order of sounds whatsoever. Children have been found with processing times as slow as 700 ms. These children have severe language delay and speech problems. Sound therapy can help to improve the speed of processing in these children. The Listening Program is a home-based set of eight CDs that has been produced by Advanced Brain Technologies that is based on the work of Tomatis. A more sophisticated, clinic-based system, the Dynamic Listening System uses state of the art technology and provides the ability to design programs that respond to be exact needs of a particular patient (see internet addresses at the end of the references).

Osteopathic considerations in hearing

Sutherland (1990) noted a general situation, which makes anatomical function of certain apertures more vulnerable to mechanical embarrassment, with consequent effects upon fluid systems.

The petrotympanic fissure opens just above and in front of the tympanic ring. It is a small slit, and the anterior process and ligament of the malleus attach here. The anterior tympanic branch of the internal maxillary artery, which supplies the tympanic membrane, passes through it. This supply can be affected by compressions of the petrous portion of the temporal bone, thereby affecting the ability of the tympanic

membrane to respond to, and accurately transmit, sound to the oval window.

The veins terminate in the pterygoid plexus which drains into the cavernous sinus and the superior petrosal sinus. The cavernous sinus drains into the jugular vein via the superior petrosal sinus. The jugular vein leaves the cranium via the jugular foramen. The superior petrosal sinus can be affected by dural strains, being formed by the splitting of the tentorium as it attaches along the petrous ridge. Drainage via the inferior petrosal sinus may be compromised by somatic dysfunction of the petrobasilar suture. Sutherland also noted a general situation, which makes certain openings or foramena more vulnerable to mechanical embarrassment than others. These are places where two bones meet to form the opening as at the jugular foramen or the petrotympanic fissure as mentioned above. The case of the cartilaginous portion of the auditory tubes is similarly vulnerable. It lies in a groove formed by the junction of the petrous portions of the temporal bones and the greater wings of the sphenoid.

Sutherland noted a regular physiological action that opens and closes the auditory tubes. Swallowing, yawning and sneezing have a similar effect. The characteristic involuntary movement of the bones of the cranial base with primary respiration is flexion and extension of the midline structure with coincident external rotation of paired lateral structures; internal rotation of paired lateral structures is coincident with extension. The auditory tube is positioned where the petrous portion of the temporal bones meet the posterior borders of the greater wings of the sphenoid. These structures are paired lateral structures not far from the midline.

As the sphenoid moves into its flexion position the posterior border of the greater wings rises and the medial pterygoid plates move down and back. At the same time, the petrous portions of the temporal bones are moving into the position of external rotation. The effect of this action changes the tension in the auditory tubes and siphons fluid from the middle ear whilst permitting the movement of air.

As the sphenoid moves in extension the posterior border of the greater wings lowers, the medial pterygoid plates move forwards and up, and the petrous portions of the temporal bones turn into internal rotation coincident with the circumduction of the occiput. Dr. Sutherland noted that as the petrous portions of the temporal bones move into external rotation they also undulate laterally; as they move into internal rotation they also undulate medially. The effect of these changes in relationship is to relax and close the cartilaginous portions of the auditory tubes.

Once the anatomical-physiological mechanism is understood it is possible to see varieties of circumstances in the area that modify or handicap the function of opening and closing the auditory tubes. Besides aerating the middle ear and mastoid air cells this physiological opening and closing of the tubes is clinically important. A detailed description of the anatomy and physiology of the auditory tubes can be found in Ch.13, p.279.

With catarrhal conditions and inflammation of the mucosa, the drainage of excess secretions is of great importance. These air spaces that are part of the air sinus system cannot function properly when filled with liquid. Osteopathic management of problems of this sort has much to offer in diagnosis and treatment when drainage through the auditory tubes as outlets is desired. A recent study (Mulls et al 2003) has shown that osteopathic treatment can assist children with recurrent otitis media.

Once mechanical function has been restored, the child may still require assistance in order to restore normal patterns of processing. Researchers have shown that some cells at all levels of the auditory pathways respond to onset and offset of tone, and to increase or decrease in frequency.

The vestibular system

The vestibular system and its impairments

In order to undertake the early activities associated with learning the child must have adequate balance and coordination. Whether he is stacking bricks, fitting cups of various diameters one into the other or attempting to hold a crayon or paintbrush, the child in the early stages of schooling is very dependent upon vestibular function.

Ayres (1972) drew attention to the importance of the vestibular system to the developing child's ability to gauge distance, depth, space and velocity. The vestibular system is one of the first to be fully developed and myelinated and it operates closely with the reflexes to facilitate balance.

Blythe (1979) considers that the primitive reflexes, which should be abolished during the first year after birth, may persist and thereby confound the normal developmental process. When, therefore, the tonic labyrinthine reflex has not been inhibited as it should have been by the end of the 6th month, then the child fails to acquire a sense of gravitational security (Blythe 1979). This is because the ampulla, a component of the vestibular apparatus, is constantly reporting on gravity throughout life. On the other hand the semicircular canals are reporting the speed and direction of movement of the head. If head control is lacking then eye coordination may be affected, since the vestibular system has a powerful influence on the movement of the eyes during activity (Patten 1977).

Vestibular function is important in the establishment of a normal gravitational response. It is also important for coordination and balance and for ensuring that the appropriate alignment of the eyes in relation to the direction and velocity of movement can be achieved. Some children may be sufficiently supported by virtue of all other systems being well integrated to enable them to cope with the confusion generated from the vestibular system; others will be subject to constant confusion. Interactions between the vestibular apparatus and the eyes and the proprioceptive reflex response to incoming stimuli will adversely affect the rapid exchange of information between the systems, thereby affecting the smooth operation of the whole.

Symptoms of impaired vestibular function

The child may struggle with activities that involve coordination of both sides of the body, and may find it difficult to maintain a normal body posture whilst carrying out a task which involves fine motor controls such as writing (Pyfer 1981).

The parents may report that if their child is lifted suddenly off the ground he will express fear and cling to the parent. The vestibular system may be facilitated, thereby producing a barrage of afference to the brain stem. Sometimes the opposite may occur and the child may seek to stimulate the vestibular system at any and every opportunity. The child may have spatial and organizational difficulties and may find it easier to relate to physical objects rather than abstract concepts. The parent may report that when the child is in the car, a recurring and negative response to acceleration and deceleration occurs.

Assessment of vestibular function

Goddard (1996) described the primitive reflexes and the effects that are observed when a child has retained any of those primitive reflexes beyond the point at which they should persist. Ways in which the child's vestibular function can be assessed are:

- Ask the child to stand with his eyes closed and arms held at 90° abduction to the body. Then move the child's head, rotating it first to left and right and then carrying it from easy-normal to full extension and then to full flexion. If the child has a retained **tonic labyrinthine reflex** then there will be a progressive resistance to the rotation, extension or flexion.

- Seat the child on a stool that is able to rotate through 360° and then spin first clockwise and then counter clockwise. Observe whether post-rotary nystagmus occurs and, if so, for how long the eye movements persist. If there is no post-rotary nystagmus or if the nystagmus persists, then there is either an inhibition or a facilitation of the labyrinth.

- Ask the child to walk along an imagined line, placing his feet one directly in front of the other (first with the eyes open, then with them closed). If there is an impairment of the vestibular system the child will waver off the line.

- To perform the **Romberg test** ask the child to stand with the feet close together and with closed eyes. If the child sways from one side to the other or falls (positive Romberg sign) you can assume a spinal impairment or a loss of depth perception. If the child sways or falls with open eyes it is a sign of a problem of the cerebellum or the vestibular system.

- Ask the child to skip and jump. If there is a loss of function of the vestibular system soft neurological signs may be seen; for example curling or stretching of fingers with an extended or flexed wrist. This occurs especially when the child walks on the heels, tiptoes or on the medial or lateral border of the foot.

- To test via the **Finger-nose test** ask the child to stretch both arms straight ahead and touch first his nose and then your index finger with one index finger and then with the other one. The child's other arm is held extended. Change the position of your index finger each time.

If you see any difficulties while the child performs these tests a clinical examination is necessary. Beside an osteopathic treatment, occupational therapy (ergotherapy) may be necessary.

Osteopathic considerations on the vestibular system

Learning is a process of layering, with a progression towards a greater sophistication where abstract concepts frequently form the basis of activities that are performed. If the early layers of learning are not soundly laid down then more complex forms of thought and consequent action become increasingly difficult to achieve. Speed of processing can also be compromised where this layering process has not occurred.

Where there is a strain of the cranial base with consequent counter rotation of the temporal bones, one being in relative internal rotation and the other in relative external rotation, the child will evince no post-rotary nystagmus on one side and an exaggerated response on the other side.

An asymmetry between the two temporals is often seen after primary cranial trauma or as an adaptation to other asymmetrical problems of the body. This kind of lesion can lead to a confusion of the vestibular system. Treatments resolving primary or secondary lesions of the temporals can improve this situation, especially if it is done in the early years of age when the dynamic interaction between all sensory systems is crucial for the further development of the child.

In relation to vestibular nerve function Magoun (1976) also drew attention to the fact that the vestibular nerve '... passes in close relation to the jugular tubercle, which should not be forgotten in understanding and treating pathology. Lesions of the sphenoid, occiput or temporals, leading to dural tension around the internal auditory meatus, associated tension in the adjacent cervical fascia, approximation of the common parts crowding the nerve centers in the ponds, or other pertinent pathology, must be considered. Pressure may result in affecting the endolymphatic mechanism. Pressure may be the result in lymphadenitis in the facial canal.'

Primary lesions of the reciprocal tension membrane as is the case in inertia of the membranes caused by trauma (see p.67) may also be important in this context and should be treated.

As described above, children with sensory problems are able to compensate with the help of other systems in the body. That means that even if osteopathic treatment may not always help to improve the vestibular function directly, it can enhance the ability of the body to compensate.

All senses and their coordinated functioning are important. Information from our environment is usually not perceived by one sense only. Perception is nearly always a combination of the function of several sensory organs. The sum of sensory processing is called sensory integration and is described in detail in Ch.16, Sensory integration disorders.

Bibliography

Ayres A J: Sensory integration and learning disorders. Western Psychological Services, Los Angeles 1972

Behrman R (ed.): Nelson textbook of pediatrics. 14th edn. W B Saunders, Philadelphia 1992, p. 1569

Blythe P, McGlown D J: An organic basis for neuroses and educational difficulties. Insight Publications, Chester, UK 1979

Campbell D: The Mozart effect. Avon Books, New York, 1997

Côtè L, Crutchen M D: The basal ganglia. In: Kandel E R, Scwartz J H, Jessel T M (eds) Principles of neural science. 3rd edn. Appleton and Langer, Norwalk, Conn. 1991, pp. 649–653

Goddard S: A teacher's window into the child's mind. Fern Ridge Press, Eugene, Ore. 1996

Keith J L W: SCAN: a screening test for auditory processing disorders. Psychological Corp., San Antonio, Tex. 1986

Kupferman I: Learning and memory. In: Kandel E R, Scwartz J H, Jessel T M (eds) Principles of neural science. 3rd edn. Appleton and Langer, Norwalk, Conn. 1991, pp. 1005–1006

Livingstone M S, Roseim G, Drislane F W and Galaburda A M Physiological and anatomical evidence for a magnocellular deficit in developmental dyslexia. Proceedings of the National Academy of Sciences of the USA 88, 1991: 7943-7947

Lovegrove W J. et al: Experimental evidence of a transient system deficit in specific reading disability. Journal of the American Optometric Association 61, 1990: 137–146

Madaule P: When listening comes alive: a guide to effective learning and communication. Moulin Publishing, Ontario, 1994

Magoun H G: Osteopathy in the cranial field. 3rd edn. Journal Printin, Kirksville, Mo. 1976, p. 150

Mulls M V et al: The use of osteopathic treatment as adjuvant therapy on children with recurrent otitis media. Archives of Pediatric Adolescent Medicine 15, 2003

Patten J: Neurological differential diagnosis. Harold Starke, London 1977, p. 60

Pinkerton F, Watson D R., McClelland R J: A neurophysiological study of children with reading, writing and spelling difficulties. Developmental Medicine and Child Neurology 31, 1989: 569–580

Pyfer J, Johnson R: Factors affecting motor delays. In: Adapted physical activity. Human Kinetics, Champaign, Ill. 1981

Sutherland W G: Teachings in the science of osteopathy. Anne Wales (ed.) Sutherland Cranial Teaching Foundation, Fort Worth, Tex. 1990

Sutherland W G: Contributions of thought. 2nd edn. Ada Strand, Anne Wales (eds) Sutherland Cranial Teaching Foundation, Fort Worth, Tex. 1998

Tallal PM, Ffier S, Fitch J: Neurobiological basis of speech: a case for the pre-eminence of temporal processing. Annals of the New York Academy of Sciences 14(682) 1993: 27–47

Tallal P M, Wer S, Delaney G: Speech and other central processing insights from cognitive neuroscience. Current Opinion in Neurobiology 1995

Tomatis A: The conscious ear, Station Hill Press. NY, 1991

Willard F: Medical neuroanatomy. JB Lippincott, Philadelphia. 1993, p. 216

Williams R L: Otitis media and otitis externa. In: Hoekelman A (ed.) Primary pediatric care. 2nd edn. 1992, pp. 1417–1420

See the website at www.advancedbrain.com

See the website at www.dynamiclisteningsystems.com

WARNING SIGNS AND DIFFERENTIAL DIAGNOSES: THE LIMITS OF OSTEOPATHIC TREATMENT

Stefan Wentzke

The purpose of osteopathic treatment is to escort the pediatric patient to his or her inner balance. The experienced osteopath is skilled in harnessing the great potential of self-healing forces, even in problematic situations, whereas to influence these forces is beyond the scope of a less experienced practitioner.

Increased attentiveness is mandatory in disorders that show no change or are of uncertain etiology, especially in all acute complaints. Children possess less reserves of strength than adults and their immune system is not yet fully developed. Life-threatening situations may emerge over an extremely short period.

The knowledge and in particular the experience of the osteopathic practitioner will determine at what point secondary measures are to be recommended or even when emergency measures are to be set in motion. As well as recognizing what can potentially be achieved, good osteopaths are also aware of their limitations. Regular training courses and critical self-assessment are therefore established elements in pediatric osteopathy. The following sections summarize the most important warning signs and differential diagnoses to be considered in everyday practice.

Neurological diseases

Febrile seizure

A febrile seizure is not epilepsy. A simple occasional febrile seizure generally lasts for between 3 and 15 minutes and in most cases occurs during a sudden fever spike. Its tonic-clonic, generalized character is alarming and resembles a grand mal seizure. Febrile seizures are encountered most commonly in children between the ages of 6 months and 6 years, and their onset peaks during the 2nd year of life. A complex febrile seizure lasts for longer than 15 minutes and is characterized by focal onset, post-paroxysmal paresis, multiple seizures within a 24-hour period, previous cerebral injury, or occurrence outside the usual age range.

What do to

It is important to stay calm and to protect the child from injury.

Repetitive febrile seizures can be interrupted by prophylactic prescription of medication. First-line therapy consists of administration of a diazepam rectal tube (5 mg in children weighing up to 15 kg, 10 mg in children weighing more than 15 kg), which may be repeated after 5 minutes if necessary, and fever reduction with paracetamol suppositories. Alternatively, treatment may be given by an experienced homeopath using belladonna before seizure onset, copper (cuprum metallicum) during the febrile seizure, and black hellebore during the post-ictal drowsy phase.

However, because the differential diagnosis should also consider meningitis or encephalitis as possible causes, at the first occurrence of a febrile seizure the emergency medical services should be contacted immediately and specialist pediatric assistance should be enlisted.

Hydrocephalus

Excessive accumulation of cerebrospinal fluid (CSF) in the CSF spaces due to an imbalance between CSF production and reabsorption may be of genetic, infectious, tumor-related or traumatic origin.

In infants, because the cranial sutures and fontanelles are still open, hydrocephalus is characterized initially only by an accelerated rate of growth of the head. Prominent scalp vein dilation, raised fontanelles, widened sutures, bulging forehead, shrill crying or the 'setting sun' phenomenon (downward deviation of the eyes) appear later. As a rule the development of hydrocephalus in infancy is noticed by the parents or during routine health checks.

In preschool and older children, because the cranial sutures have closed, the development of hydrocephalus produces autonomic symptoms of increased cranial pressure, such as dull headaches, vomiting on an empty stomach, bradycardia and arterial hypertension. Ophthalmoscopy reveals papilledema.

What to do

If hydrocephalus is suspected during a course of osteopathic treatment, immediate contact with a pediatrician is essential because of the necessity for CSF drainage.

Infantile cerebral palsy

(See Ch.16 Cerebral palsy).

Intrauterine, peripartum or postnatal brain damage which is non-progressive but which leads to permanent motor deficits is termed infantile cerebral palsy. The condition may be characterized additionally by intellectual disturbances and seizures. Causal factors may include central vascular occlusion, infection, genetic disorders, cerebral hemorrhage or hypoxic-ischemic encephalopathy.

The child with infantile cerebral palsy presents with unusual body posture and movement patterns. The classification of infantile cerebral palsy is made on the basis of the clinical picture in each case. One typical feature is spasticity, which is characterized by raised muscle tone, increased deep tendon reflexes or positive pyramidal tract signs. Dyskinesia is a movement disorder typified by continuous changes in muscle tone and by involuntary movements that cease or subside during sleep. While the dominant features of dystonia are slow, worm-like movements, chorea is distinguished by rapid, irregular and jerky movements. Depending on location and severity, further forms are differentiated: spastic hemiparesis, spastic tetraparesis, spastic diplegia and ataxia.

In particular, spastic hemiparesis affecting just one side of the body often only becomes apparent after the end of the first year of life; it is recognized because the child displays asymmetric movements, delayed motor development, and shortening or atrophy of one extremity.

What to do

If infantile cerebral palsy is suspected, a pediatrician must immediately be contacted so that a comprehensive treatment strategy can be set in motion; this should be complemented by a course of osteopathic treatment.

Headache

(See Ch.16 Headache).

Now and then children react to stress with a headache. In such cases simple home remedies such as fresh air, rest or a cold compress will be sufficient to drive away the 'headache'. Headache may also be the first symptom of incipient infection.

Chronic headaches are not uncommonly the result of previously unrecognized defective vision. Sometimes the pain is referred from the paranasal sinuses or middle ear. Crooked or carious teeth and dental malocclusion may also give rise to headache. Tumors or hydrocephalus may be responsible for childhood headaches in rare cases.

Childhood migraine is often accompanied by nausea and vomiting.

What to do

As a prelude to osteopathic treatment it is important to establish which specialist medical investigations have already been carried out. Sudden unaccustomed headaches may point to meningitis, arterial hypertension or a fractured skull. These require immediate hospital treatment.

Craniocerebral trauma

Depending on severity, craniocerebral injuries include the following types:

- **Cranial contusion:** head injury with or without lacerations, hematoma, abrasions, nausea or vomiting, but never with loss of consciousness or amnesia.
- **Concussion:** head injury without damage to the brain with short-term loss of consciousness and amnesia that resolves completely.
- **Cerebral contusion:** trauma-related brain damage with neurological deficits.
- **Cerebral compression:** a marked rise in intracranial pressure due to bleeding, cerebral edema, meningeal rupture or fractures. Cerebral regions, vessels and nerves may be compressed and irreversibly damaged.

What to do

There have been instances where a child with a recent head injury attends for osteopathic treatment. It is advisable to defer such treatment. As a precaution the child must first undergo examination in A&E and receive treatment as appropriate.

In children with cranial injuries the possibility of abuse must also be considered.

Cerebral seizures

(See Ch.16, Epilepsy).

Seizures may occur at any age. The pattern of their appearance in children is very varied. A distinction is made between partial seizures (focal seizures) and generalized seizures. In comparison to complex seizures, simple seizures do not entail any loss of consciousness.

Partial seizures (focal seizures)

Partial seizures are usually a symptom of an underlying brain disorder. Inflammation, injury, vascular lesions or tumors involving a region of the brain produce a focus from which the seizure emanates. Partial seizures are limited to one cerebral hemisphere and may become generalized as a secondary phenomenon.

Motor Jacksonian seizures (involving one side of the body) are rare in children. They begin with jerking movements of one hand or one side of the face, and these may spread to involve an entire body region. Reversible paralysis of one side of the body may be seen in the aftermath of the seizure.

Adversive seizures are defined as focal events that manifest themselves only in turning movements of the eyes or head. In addition, a focal seizure may have sensory symptoms. The child complains of unpleasant sensations such as tingling-paresthesia or abnormal temperature sensations in *one* half of the face, *one* hand or *one* foot, lasting from a few seconds to several minutes. A sensory seizure rarely occurs in isolation. If accompanied by autonomic symptoms it may appear as an 'aura' and involve all the senses.

An aura is a prodromal feature of the particularly common psychomotor seizure (temporal lobe seizure, complex focal seizure). During the seizure itself, consciousness is clouded or lost, and this may be accompanied by a wide range of symptoms: motor automatisms such as lip smacking, chewing, fumbling with the hands, plucking and pawing movements are just as typical as confused speech and singing, through to dramatic and disorderly behavior.

Generalized seizures

An absence (or petit mal seizure) is a disturbance of consciousness that starts and ends abruptly and lasts for 5 to 30 seconds, and is followed by amnesia. In most cases unwittingly misinterpreted as day-dreaming or inability to concentrate, simple absence is often not recognized until a late stage. However, notable features include recurrent interruptions to the continuity of conversation, writing or other activities. The course of myoclonic absence is so discrete that the fine rhythmic jerking movements can only be perceived on careful observation. In comparison, complex absence manifests itself very impressively in upward turning of the eyes or backward tilting of the head. Absence seizures generally occur without an aura.

An abrupt onset is specific for generalized tonic-clonic seizures, or grand mal seizures. There is no aura, and the child suddenly loses consciousness and falls to the ground. The tonic seizure phase involving all skeletal muscles begins with hyperextension of the body, possibly with an initial cry and brief apnea, followed by the rhythmic jerking movements typical of the clonic seizure phase. For those unaccustomed to it, a tonic-clonic seizure is most alarming. Other typical symptoms of grand mal seizures include involuntary urination, open eyes with fixed pupils, and foaming salivation, and patients will occasionally bite their own tongue.

Many infants with brain damage due to malformation or degenerative diseases suffer from infantile spasms (BNS seizures). This seizure type is characterized by sudden flexion spasms of the trunk lasting for fractions of a second, while the head, arms and legs are simultaneously flung forwards or upwards.

What to do

The first steps to be taken in the event of a cerebral seizure are straightforward; it is sufficient to remain with the child, to maintain calm and not to attempt any repositioning. Sit on the floor and place your thighs under the child's head to prevent injury, allow free flow of saliva so as to guarantee unhampered respiration. The seizure will usually end spontaneously. However, if it lasts for longer than 30 minutes, medical assistance is essential. After the seizure has passed, the child will feel extremely tired and frequently falls asleep.

At first occurrence or if there is uncertainty regarding a possible cerebral seizure, immediate referral to a pediatrician is imperative because possible differential diagnoses also include syncope, poisoning (due to medication, alcohol), brain injury, vascular disease, heat stroke, infection, hypoglycemia and tumors. Epilepsy is said to be present after two or more non-febrile seizures.

Respiratory tract diseases

Respiratory distress (dyspnea)

Acute respiratory distress

Chest indrawing is indicative of respiratory distress in neonates and infants; additional symptoms include nasal flaring as well as jugular and epigastric retractions. Older children also use their accessory respiratory muscles when breathing.

Common causes of acute respiratory distress are predominantly febrile pneumonia with asymmetrical lung sounds, also obstructive bronchitis and bronchial asthma with symmetrical rhonchi and wheezing. Absent respiratory sounds on one side may be indicative of foreign body aspiration or pneumothorax.

What to do

Acute respiratory distress requires immediate investigation by the emergency medical team.

Chronic respiratory distress

A child with chronic respiratory distress will generally have previously undergone thorough examination. Nevertheless, it is important to understand that the cause of respiratory distress need not necessarily be located in the territory of the respiratory organs. The following possible etiologies should be considered:

- **Lungs:** The commonest cause is bronchial asthma. Malformations or cystic fibrosis are very much rarer.
- **Thorax:** Mediastinal lymph nodes and tumors, cardiac malformations, extremely severe scoliosis or other advanced skeletal deformities may result in respiratory distress.
- **Abdomen:** Ascites, growing tumours and increasing hernia volume may cause massive impairment of diaphragmatic function.
- **Other causes:** Swollen tonsils and adenoids, extreme obesity, anemia and allergies may lead to respiratory distress, especially at night.

Hyperventilation

Rapid shallow breathing, in many cases caused by anxiety and, in rare instances, by fever. If intensified to panic levels, muscle spasms may develop, with the typical 'obstetrician's hand' deformity.

What to do

First provide calming reassurance to the parents and child, and then encourage the child to re-breathe into a paper or plastic bag.

Gastrointestinal diseases

Acute abdomen and stomach pain

(See Ch.12, Nervous (functional) stomach ache).

Children frequently report stomach pain, even in the context of other diseases that are not localized to the stomach. A full physical examination should therefore always be performed. Even unspectacular ailments may be indicative of life-threatening diseases, such as appendicitis or ileus.

Acute abdomen is the clinical term used to describe a cluster of abdominal symptoms, usually of acute onset. Hallmark symptoms are acute-onset pain, changes in peristalsis and bowel sounds, evacuation disturbances, abdominal wall 'guarding', deterioration in general health, possibly fever, circulatory disorders and shock.

What to do

Strict fasting and rapid diagnostic clarification in a pediatric unit are essential in all cases.

Appendicitis

Appendicitis is the commonest inflammatory disease of the abdominal cavity in children. The danger with appendicitis is associated with perforation and peritonitis. Alongside all the symptoms of acute abdomen, which do not always occur routinely or as a complete set, two forms of appendicitis are distinguished:

- **Acute appendicitis:** Within hours, up to a maximum of 1–2 days, the symptoms begin with pain in the epigastric region, which migrates to the right lower abdomen and which may be relieved by slightly flexing the right leg. The child has no appetite, complains of nausea, sometimes with vomiting, and may have fever and diarrhea.
- **Subacute or chronic appendicitis:** The history may cover a period of months. Right-sided abdominal pain is episodic and the child often suffers from constipation.

What to do

If appendicitis is suspected, the child should be admitted at once to a pediatric surgery unit. Therapy takes the form of appendectomy.

Vomiting

Parents use the terms 'vomiting' or 'being sick' in very different ways and therefore it is essential to obtain a history with precise details of the volume and frequency involved. In all age groups, the commonest cause of vomiting is gastroenteritis.

Other causes of vomiting, depending on age, include:

- **Neonates:** Gastrointestinal obstruction, e.g. pyloric stenosis, intestinal malrotation, raised intracranial pressure, cerebral edema, hydrocephalus.
- **Infants:** Intussusception, hereditary metabolic disorders, copious vomiting (with the accompanying symptoms of acute abdomen, may be indicative of a strangulated inguinal hernia).

- **Any age:** Hiatus hernia, gastro-esophageal reflux, intolerance to cows' milk protein, intracranial space-occupying lesion, respiratory tract infections, otitis media, urinary tract infection, meningitis, encephalitis, hypertensive crisis, sunstroke, incipient appendicitis, and in rare cases diabetes mellitus. Vomiting with pallor, loss of consciousness through to shock should prompt possible consideration of poisoning (medication, alcohol), sepsis, meningitis and raised intracranial pressure.

What to do

Depending on the child's medical history and condition, careful observation may be sufficient or the emergency medical services will need to be called immediately.

Dehydration

Inadequate fluid intake coupled with increased fluid output leads to a combined disturbance of fluid and electrolyte balance. The commonest cause of dehydration in infants and preschool children is gastroenteritis with diarrhea, vomiting and refusal to eat. Diabetes mellitus, diabetes insipidus or renal failure are discovered much more rarely in association with dehydration.

The child's general state of health will vary depending on the degree of dehydration. In mild cases the symptoms first encountered are mottled skin, decreased skin turgor and dried oral mucosa. Moderate dehydration is presumed to be present if the fontanelles are already depressed, the eyes are sunken, blood pressure is low and pulse rate is accelerated. Deepened, rapid breathing, shrill crying, disturbed consciousness and seizures should alert to the presence of severe dehydration.

What to do

Only the mild form of dehydration can be compensated for easily by oral fluid and electrolyte intake (lemonade and salt sticks). Even moderate dehydration requires treatment with infusions because the ratio of fluid to electrolyte loss needs to be corrected.

Nutritional problems

In worldwide terms, being underweight in children is due primarily to malnutrition. In the industrialized world it is more commonly the result of chronic illness. An underweight child is seriously at risk in terms of his health and overall capacity for development. It carries an increased risk of infection. Children become underweight due to reduced food intake (malnutrition), nutrient losses resulting from impaired absorption (malabsorption) or increased energy consumption (infections, endocrine diseases, tumours).

Lifestyle factors in the developed nations combine to make obesity the commonest nutritional disorder in children, with immense long-term implications for the musculoskeletal and vascular systems, metabolism, hormone balance and psychosocial equilibrium. Endocrine or genetic disorders are present in a very small proportion of obese children.

Psychological eating disorders, such as anorexia nervosa and bulimia, need to be distinguished from genuinely nutritional problems.

What to do

The patient should be referred to a pediatrician to eliminate any possible underlying disease.

Ileocolic intussusception

In contrast to harmless ileocolic dysfunction in adults, ileocolic intussusception in children carries an inherent risk of intestinal obstruction. The symptoms are mostly of sudden onset and take the form of violent, colicky abdominal pain. Unlike the situation in acute abdomen, the abdomen is usually soft, concave and the intestinal invagination can be readily palpated. The child is pale and lethargic and in the advanced stage of the condition exhibits signs of shock.

What to do

Repositioning is performed in hospital under ultrasound or X-ray control. Surgery is required in the event of ileus, perforation or peritonitis.

Inguinal hernia

In most cases indirect inguinal hernia occurs as a result of adhesion failure of the processus vaginalis of the peritoneum. It is more than twice as common on the right side as on the left. An inguinal hernia may contain fluid, intestinal and omental elements as well as gonadal structures. Protrusion of the hernia is palpable on coughing, straining or crying.

Strangulation of the contents of the hernia sac occurs spontaneously in most cases and is often the first symptom of an inguinal hernia. The inguinal region and the scrotum or labia majora are massively swollen. The child experiences pain, cries, refuses food and vomits.

What to do

Attempts to reduce an inguinal hernia should never be undertaken in the absence of ultrasound control because the contents of the hernia sac may become strangulated, resulting subsequently in necrosis. An appointment with a pediatrician is always necessary to assess whether surgery is indicated.

Meckel diverticulum

The rudiment of the embryonic yolk sac only becomes symptomatic if complications occur. Essentially, the symptoms include inflammation, ulceration, perforation, intussusception and intestinal obstruction. The symptoms are the same as those described for appendicitis.

Vitamin deficiency and excess

Vitamins need to be taken regularly and in sufficient quantities because they are not synthesized in the body's own metabolic processes. Unfortunately, poor food quality, unbalanced diet or malnutrition commonly lead to vitamin deficiency, as does impaired uptake from the digestive tract (malabsorption). In cases where the mother is suffering from vitamin deficiency without clinical symptoms, severe signs of vitamin deficiency may be seen in the breastfed infant after just a few months. Vitamin deficiency may also be caused by vitamin-antagonistic medication or by increased urinary excretion.

The specific implications of a deficiency syndrome depend on the particular vitamin that is lacking. The following symptoms may generally point to a vitamin deficiency: inflammatory changes involving the skin and mucous membranes, persistent diarrhea, disorders of hematopoiesis and blood clotting, as well as bone structure deformities. Failure to thrive, developmental and visual disturbances, paresthesias, ataxia, seizures or increased muscle tone are also possible manifestations of a vitamin deficiency.

In the event of vitamin excess water-soluble vitamins are excreted via the kidneys, whereas fat-soluble vitamins are stored and may produce pathological symptoms if taken in extreme doses.

What to do

If vitamin deficiency or excess is suspected, diagnosis and treatment by a pediatrician is essential.

Urological diseases

Urinary retention and hematuria

A child with acute urinary retention generally has stomach pain and palpable distension of the bladder. In neonatal boys this is sometimes caused by urethral valves, and in infants and preschool children by urethral polyps, phimosis and inflammation of the bladder. In preschool and school-age children tumours, extreme constipation or occult spina bifida may lead to urinary retention or to blood in the urine.

What to do

Diagnostic clarification by an urologist or pediatric surgeon is required in such cases.

Testicular torsion

A testis may undergo torsion about its longitudinal axis spontaneously or as a result of trauma (during sporting activity). Testicular infarction may threaten within a short time due to strangulation of the spermatic cord vessels. The sudden violent pain is referred to the testes and groin. Nausea and vomiting frequently ensue due to irritation of the peritoneum. The scrotum is swollen and the affected testis is higher than its partner.

What to do

Even a suspicion of testicular torsion – i.e. any swelling of the scrotal contents of uncertain etiology – constitutes an immediate absolute indication for surgery.

Hydrocele

A hydrocele is an inguinal hernia filled with peritoneal fluid and communicating with the abdominal cavity. In most cases there is painless scrotal swelling.

What to do

While hydroceles regress spontaneously by about the age of 3 years in one third of children, they should nevertheless be examined by an urologist.

Paraphimosis

Although it fits relatively tightly, the penile foreskin is in principle retractable. Following retraction behind the coronal sulcus, however, the phimotic prepuce may trap the glans, causing it to swell to such an extent that spontaneous reduction becomes impossible. The first-line response is to gently compress the swollen glans and reposition it under the foreskin.

What to do

Because of the risk of necrosis, further treatment by a urologist is required promptly.

Diseases of the musculoskeletal system

Epiphysis of the femoral head

(See Ch.15, Slipped capital femoral epiphysis).

Acute or chronic slippage of the upper femoral epiphysis out of the neck of the femur may be encountered primarily during the prepubertal growth spurt. Swift diagnosis is required particularly in the event of sports-related sprain injury to the legs, sudden severe hip pain, and load-bearing incapacity. However, an insidious form also exists, characterized initially merely by dragging pains in the hip, thigh and knee and possibly taking the form of an abnormal gait pattern. When the patient is supine, there is a noticeable internal rotation and adduction deficit in the affected hip. Once flexion is completed, the hip 'escapes' into external rotation and abduction (Drehmann sign).

What to do

Depending on the degree of dislocation, epiphyseal slippage usually requires surgery for bilateral repositioning and fixation.

Craniosynostosis and microcephaly

(See Ch.15, Craniosynostosis).

A functional disturbance of the cranium in neonates and infants may result in bizarre cranial asymmetry without any adverse repercussions for health. A structural disorder, such as premature closure of a fontanelle or cranial suture (craniosynostosis), also leads to cranial asymmetry or microcephaly but this may be associated with mental retardation.

What to do

Whereas functional cranial asymmetry can be very readily corrected using osteopathic treatment alone, surgery is required to release premature closure of a fontanelle or cranial suture. The child may subsequently undergo further osteopathic treatment.

Perthes disease

(See p.329).

If a child complains of exercise-related hip pain, sometimes limps slightly, and easily tires when walking or running, or if the parents suspect 'growing pains', this situation may conceal early signs of ischemic necrosis of the femoral head. In particular, younger children with Perthes disease report knee and stomach pain. The picture is further obscured because these symptoms already exist before bony transformation becomes visible on X-ray. When the child is examined in the supine position, limitation of internal rotation and abduction ('sign of four') is already present in the early stages. Structural leg shortening may occur in the later stages and in older children, necessitating prompt corrective osteotomy or hip joint replacement in adulthood.

What to do

Perthes disease is not a contraindication for osteopathic treatment. Quite the contrary: for preschool children osteopathy is probably a highly suitable treatment modality in order to successfully restore the physiological shape of the femoral head.

However, because the symptoms present may also be suggestive of inflammation and tumors, the treatment delivered should be agreed in consultation with an orthopedic surgeon.

Spina bifida

This is the commonest congenital malformation of the spinal column and it occurs in various degrees of severity. All segments of the spine may be affected but the lumbar region is most commonly involved. The neurological deficits are determined by the highest spinal segment involved.

The rare severe form of spina bifida with detectable external manifestations is an inhibitory malformation of the spinal column and spinal cord and is detected immediately after birth. The following types are distinguished:

- **Dermal sinus** (dermal fistula): a communicating tract between the skin and spinal canal.
- **Meningocele:** protrusion of the meninges (dura mater and pia mater).
- **Meningomyelocele:** protrusion of the meninges and spinal cord.
- **Open myelocele:** meningomyelocele with cutaneous defect.

Far more common is the mild form, known as occult spina bifida, which is a defect of the vertebral arch, usually without involvement of the nerve structures. Generally asymptomatic, it tends to be detected opportunistically during X-ray examination. In quite rare cases fusion may cause damage to the sacral region of the spinal cord.

What to do

If spina bifida is suspected, the child must be referred for an appointment with a pediatrician.

Eye diseases

Orbital phlegmon

Whereas disturbed lacrimation via the tear duct constitutes a classic indication for osteopathic treatment, a swollen eyelid may conceal an orbital phlegmon due to sinusitis.

What to do

Particularly in cases where the eye secretions are purulent, rapid specialist pediatric assistance must be sought because of the imminent threat of complications such as blindness and intracranial abscesses.

Strabismus (squint)

Aside from the multifactorial, genetic and central causes of strabismus (concomitant strabismus), there are numerous forms that are attributable to ocular muscle or ocular nerve disorders (paralytic strabismus). Mild internal strabismus during accommodation is often associated with long-sightedness and is therefore easy to correct. However, strabismus may also be a symptom of retrobulbar tumors or infections and should not therefore be trivialized.

What to do

An ophthalmological examination is an absolutely essential prelude to osteopathic treatment for strabismus.

Infections

Infections in childhood often run their course with few symptoms and improve spontaneously after a few days. They are commonly associated with fever, and once this has subsided the child is kept under observation for a while. In osteopathic practice, too, body temperature should be checked, along with a complete assessment of lymph node status. Liver, spleen and joints should be examined for enlargement or swelling, the patient's throat and eardrums inspected and a special watch kept for skin rashes. It is always worthwhile to enquire about other family members who are also ill so as to gain a clearer picture of the infection.

What to do

In acute infections and immunization reactions osteopathic treatment sessions are only conditionally recommended as an accompaniment to mainstream medical care. Very high-grade fever, uncertain etiologies and fever in infants must always be investigated by a physician.

Lyme borreliosis (Lyme disease)

Pain and inflammation of the joints may both already be present in the early stage of Lyme borreliosis. Because typical symptoms such as erythema chronicum migrans or lymphocytoma may be absent, the condition can be confused with mechanically induced or traumatic capsulitis. The complications are particularly feared: facial nerve palsy, carditis and meningitis.

What to do

Antibiotic therapy is indispensable.

Meningitis, encephalitis

Whenever a child presents with fever, headache, nausea, vomiting, photosensitivity, listlessness and any neurological symptoms of uncertain etiology, a check should be made for the presence of meningism: nuchal rigidity and pain on passive elevation of the legs. Patients are unable to 'kiss their knees'. The child adopts a position on its side as a relief posture. These symptoms are not routinely present in young children. In infants the symptoms include respiratory disturbances and skin discoloration, refusal to feed, lethargy or irritability, increased muscle tone and vomiting.

Petechial hemorrhaging into the skin is indicative of meningococcal meningitis.

What to do

Because of the high mortality and possible sequelae, no time should be lost if meningitis or encephalitis are suspected – immediate admission to hospital is absolutely imperative.

Otitis media

Acute otitis media

Because of the good results achieved, treatment for ventilatory disturbances of the middle ear is an established element in the osteopathic repertoire. Performance of the routine procedures associated with this treatment should nevertheless be coupled with constant alertness for possible complications. Ear pain and general signs of infection, such as fever or lymph node swelling, may be absent in the infant who may then attract attention merely because of a refusal to feed or restlessness.

What to do

Mastoiditis with redness and swelling behind the ear is an unequivocal alarm sign in this context, necessitating mainstream medical treatment. Because of the high risk of meningitis, otitis media is an acutely life-threatening condition for infants, especially up to the age of 6 months.

Chronic otitis media

In chronic, non-suppurative otitis media there are also certain limitations on the indications for osteopathy: latent infections present over a period of weeks and months constitute a drain on the child in terms of overall well-being. The not inconsiderable auditory disturbances inhibit the child's general, linguistic and social development. Thus, inexplicably aggressive behavior may be the only symptom of previously unrecognized hearing problems.

What to do

Where conservative efforts have remained unsuccessful, the parents' decision to opt for a surgical procedure should generally be respected.

Paronychia, whitlow

What to do

Infections of the nail margin, nail bed or subcutaneous tissue with painful swelling and redness must be treated surgically in the event of massive suppuration; in neonates or infants these conditions are always treated in a hospital setting because of the major risk of sepsis and meningitis.

Pilonidal sinus, coccygeal fistula

A pilonidal sinus of embryonic origin may be the underlying cause of a fluctuant soft-tissue swelling over the sacrum or coccyx. The highly acute phase is characterized by severe pain, redness and often by purulent secretions from a fistula track.

What to do

Pilonidal sinus occurs primarily in young adults and requires surgery. Children are rarely affected.

Abuse and maltreatment

In most cases this will remain only at the level of suspicion because a child almost never makes an open accusation of abuse or maltreatment. The suspicion may arise in situations where the details of an alleged accident keep changing or are unclear, absent or obviously untrue. Multiple bruising, hematomas, burns or fractures of differing age, point to the application of force. Failure to thrive and malnutrition may also be indicative of maltreatment. An abused or maltreated child has major difficulty in establishing social contacts. On examination the child will sometimes display a peculiar mixture of mistrust, lack of reserve and indifference. It is unusual if a child submits to an unpleasant therapy without any comment.

An abused or maltreated child is commonly presented for medical attention after some delay, repeatedly at untypical times and to different therapists. It is important to obtain a full history from the child and parents and to conduct and document a full physical examination. A circumspect approach is absolutely necessary because parents who feel pressurized will withdraw themselves and the child from treatment.

What to do

The help of further therapists and institutions should be enlisted immediately. Children are also exposed to subtle forms of violence apart from that of a physical nature. This is not always exerted by the parents or by other persons close to them. Violence or bullying ('mobbing') practised in school or en route to school may go so far as to cause children to react against others or themselves with extreme aggression or even suicide.

Bibliography

Breusch S, Mau H, Sabo D: Klinikleitfaden Orthopädie. 4th edn. Urban & Fischer, Munich/Jena 2002

Doose H: Epilepsien im Kindes- und Jugendalter. 11th edn. Desitin Arzneimittel, Hamburg 1998

Hasse F-M, Nürnberger H-R: Klinikleitfaden Chirurgie. 3rd edn. Urban & Fischer, Munich/Jena, 2002

Illing S, Claßen M: Klinikleitfaden Pädiatrie. 6th edn. Urban & Fischer, Munich/Jena 2003

Iro H et al: HNO 52, 2004: 395–408

Koletzko B: Kinderheilkunde und Jugendmedizin. 12th edn. Springer, Berlin 2004

Lentze M-J, Schaub J, Schulte F-J: Pädiatrie, Grundlagen und Praxis. 2nd edn. Springer, Berlin 2003

Riedel F: Kinder- und Jugendarzt 35, 2004: 187–188

Siebenand R, Siebenand S: Leitfaden Interdisziplinäre Notfälle. 2nd edn. Urban & Fischer, Munich/Jena 1999

8

Principles of osteopathic treatment

Alison Brown, Sibyl Grundberg, Susan Turner, Noori Mitha

DIAGNOSIS AND TREATMENT WITH THE PRIMARY RESPIRATORY MECHANISM

This chapter is a personal view of principles for the perception, diagnosis and treatment with the primary respiratory mechanism (PRM) with reference to the teachings of Still, Sutherland, Rollin Becker and other osteopaths. It is based upon lectures given as part of the Sutherland Cranial College's Module 2/3 in Germany and experiences of working with infants and children in practice.

We feel the effects or expression of the PRM as a whole body shape change. This is an expression of the inherent health and healing of our patients. I propose that the whole body shape change, or involuntary motion, is the 'Language of the Primary Respiratory Mechanism'. It is a means of communication: it allows us to perceive, understand and influence the health and healing of our patients. In this chapter, I would like to pursue the analogy of involuntary motion as a language to review the principles of perception, diagnosis and treatment with the PRM.

The language of the primary respiratory mechanism

How do you learn a language? We will have experienced two different approaches: immersion and phrases. As a child you were immersed or surrounded by your native language: its sounds, rhythms, alphabet and culture. Day by day, you practised the pronunciation, vocabulary, and grammar. Gradually you developed your unique voice in that language and there are no limits to the potential communication. As adults, most of us learn second languages from key phrases so we understand and can speak basic elements of the language. This is a starting point for communication and we can 'get by' in a wide range of situations with a few well chosen phrases. As we use these phrases, we gradually learn more and become better at understanding and, subsequently, speaking the language.

When learning the language of the PRM, we use both approaches. We learn to 'tune-in', listen and perceive its sounds and rhythms. With practice, we learn to recognize and understand what the PRM is saying and 'answer' promptly and appropriately. We also learn key phrases which provide a starting point for understanding and responding. As you become more aware and fluent in the language, you are able to perceive the unique 'voice' of each patient and find your own unique ways of treating them. There are no limits to the potential of healing.

Communication skills

In simple terms, language is composed of words and silences, and the language of the PRM is composed of motion and stillness. How do we learn to 'tune-in' and listen to its language? We begin with the osteopathic communication skills of centring, contact, fulcrum, divided awareness and resonance.

Centering

Centering describes the shift in perception as we acknowledge the noise around and within us and, gradually, find a sense of comfort and peace from which to observe our patients. We continue to develop and refine our ability to center as we understand more about our patients and ourselves. We encourage students to start by getting physically comfortable and relaxed: feet on floor, ischial tuberosities on chair, back supported, and taking a moment to allow posture to settle so that breathing and body are at ease. Sometimes it helps to acknowledge the quality and organization within our own body or mechanism. Then to explore our awareness: beginning by focusing entirely on our body and then, gradually, expanding our awareness and noticing sensations and qualities nearby, within the room, outside the building and up to the sky. Then, bringing our awareness back towards the body, noting and remembering where we feel most comfortable and peaceful.

Contact

Contact of the whole hand on the patient can help shift perception from the touch sense (e.g. finger tips) towards proprioception (e.g. motion and three-dimensional sense) as we enlist the help of proprioceptors in all the small joints of the hands.

If osteopaths have strong and stiff hands because muscles are hypertrophied it may be necessary to:

- stretch and relax the hands like a pianist before a performance, or
- take a moment to visualize hands as harmonizing and moving freely with the patient. Susan Turner (a fellow osteopath and teacher) talked about the way seaweed moves in the ocean and encouraged students to imagine that they had 'seaweed hands'.

Fulcrum

A fulcrum is normally formed by the forearms resting on the table. Being aware of the support under your forearms is important for determining the lightness and comfort of the contact. Engaging the forearm fulcrum, by modest contractions of the forearm flexors, seems to influence the responsiveness of the fulcrum and open awareness to different depths and qualities of tissue. This acts as an automatically shifting suspension fulcrum. We can adapt this fulcrum from moment to moment and respond to the patient as they are telling their story.

When working with children, it is not always possible to have a fixed support for your arms. However, you can establish a fulcrum by settling elbows against your body, or in space, if you are centered, relaxed, and aware of the changes around you. This is analogous to photography: using a tripod may not always be feasible, yet you can still get great photographs when just holding a digital camera. In treating toddlers, or older children with behavioral difficulties, it is sometimes necessary to move around the room with them in order to treat. This is not easy but it is possible. You function as a whole body 'automatic shifting suspension fulcrum' and can spontaneously respond to them, as in a dance. There is a point when you can 'let go' and 'go with it' and this seems to be when the treatment happens.

Divided awareness

Divided awareness is a natural human ability which we can develop and refine so that we choose where and how we direct our awareness. This is important when we are monitoring shape change with the PRM. We need to be aware of our patients but also aware of ourselves, so we can check that we remain centerd and refine our centering as necessary. This is like having a conversation with someone: you listen and respond to them but, at the same time, think about what they are saying and what you need to say (or not say). You also notice how the conversation is going, and anything you need to change to help it develop.

Resonance

This was a concept which I learnt from Rachel Brooks and involves finding the point of optimum communication or interchange between practitioner and patient; I have called this 'resonance'. It is analogous to perceiving the appropriate physical separation between you and a person in conversation. This will vary for person to person and from day to day. If you get too close then they will move away a little, become less at ease or distressed. Have you had the experience of treating infants or children who start crying as soon as you touch them? Do you ever feel exhausted after treating a particular patient? If so, then the concept of resonance may well help. I have found this invaluable when treating infants and children.

The practitioner starts by focusing their awareness on themselves; and then gradually expanding awareness, little by little, out towards the patient until they feel the point of meeting, resonance or rapport. If the practitioner expands too far, the patient may feel slightly imposed or intruded upon. Infants and children seem particularly sensitive in this way. I suspect that it feels like suddenly hearing a radio which is too loud and this can be distressing for them. If the practitioner does not expand enough, the patient may feel unsupported or abandoned, and the practitioner has to strain their perception to feel the involuntary motion. Some infants and children are so 'compressed' that you have to reach out to them in order to support their mechanisms: otherwise it is like straining to hear a radio which is too quiet, and this can be tiring for the practitioner. The point of resonance may change during the treatment. When I work from here, I can feel my patient's mechanisms more easily and clearly and I rarely feel tired afterwards.

Principles of perception

Rollin Becker discusses palpatory skills in his book *Life in motion*, and I would recommend that you read this. There seem to be stages in developing our palpation and perception of the PRM and I would like to explore these in terms of learning a language. At each stage, we do not 'forget' what we have learnt before in order to move onto something different and better. Instead, we harmonize and integrate our new insights with existing awareness so that we gradually develop our unique voice and perception in that language.

Our earliest perception and consciousness of language is its sounds and rhythms. Babies will respond to their mothers by copying their mother's speech; small children learn the sounds and rhythms of phrases, nursery rhymes or Christmas carols (even though they may use their own words). At the same time, we begin to learn the communication skills of body language and eye contact.

Our first perception and consciousness of the language of the PRM is the motion and rhythm of the whole body shape change. We learn to perceive the rhythm, symmetry and synchrony of the whole body shape change and variations within the body.

We then shift from sounds to words in spoken language, which enables us to identify and communicate with more consciousness and precision. At the same time, we begin to learn the communication skills of volume, pace and emphasis.

Once we have an impression of the whole body shape change (its rhythm, symmetry and synchrony) then we become more aware of the motion present. We experience the characteristics and variations in the quality and vitality of involuntary motion, and how that is expressed through different areas of the body and different tissues. We develop and refine our contact, our fulcrum, and keep in resonance whilst the patients are telling their story. We begin to build a 'sensory vocabulary' or 'library' so that we can recognize sensations again and again. The characteristics of healthy tissues, or exhaustion, shock, membranous inertia, post-meningitis, even hormonal changes such as hypothyroidism or diabetes – the list is endless.

Once we understand the words then we can hear the meaning: the emotions, intentions and ideas behind the words. We shift awareness from the words to the silence between the words. As adults, we know that we don't need speech to communicate and recognize the value and need for silence. A shared silence can be restoring, inspiring and transforming.

The same is true in the language of the PRM as we turn our awareness from the motion present towards the stillness. Where motion is the effect, the stillness is the cause: 'Life resides as stillness and manifests as motion' (Brooks 2002). We become more conscious of the stillness between the motion and behind the motion and open to the possible changes and healing which occur in stillness.

'The stillness is that which centers every molecule of being of that living body. The body physiology is the outward expression of that stillness' (Becker 1997).

This is only possible when we have a sense of stillness in ourselves; we are continually unfolding and developing our personal sense of stillness. I never feel that I am still enough, yet I can normally sense stillness somewhere within myself or the universe around me. I would like to quote one of Rollin Becker's writings which greatly helped my relationship with stillness when palpating my patients: 'To do this, the physician must feel from the heart of his stillness into the heart of the stillness within the patient' (Becker 1997).

This opens our perception further so we can experience something of the living physiology or the inherent healing processes or potency at work: the 'causes' behind the 'effects'. 'The unerring potency of the body to heal itself has more power than anything you can safely bring to bear from any force from without' (Sutherland 2004). Sutherland used the word 'potency' and it is important that you read the osteopathic literature; ponder this and develop your own understanding of this word and the idea. In the meantime, I find the following definitions or descriptions particularly useful: 'Potency is the potential for change' (Grundberg 2003). 'Potency is that force or forces which tend to move the body towards homeostasis, a process honed by millions of years of evolution and common to all organisms. The task of the osteopath is to harness that potency and facilitate the move to homeostatic balance'(Dove 2003).

Conversations in the language of the PRM

The principles of diagnosis and treatment are described in osteopathic texts (Magoun 1976). As a student of 'osteopathy in the cranial field', I initially found it difficult to learn these ideas; therefore I would like to pursue the 'language' analogy and present them differently.

Diagnosis and treatment are on-going and interdependent conversations in the language of the PRM. The diagnosis is a 'working hypothesis' to guide and inform your osteopathic treatment. It will be developed and refined as you treat and learn more about your patients and their unique health and healing.

You could learn to diagnose and treat by listening to many patients and learning from your experiences, which is how Sutherland learnt. However, previous osteopaths have identified diagnostic and treatment 'phrases' which often occur. This is a starting point for communication and we can 'get by' in a wide range of situations with a few well-chosen phrases. As we practise these phrases, we learn more and gradually become better at understanding and speaking the language of the PRM.

Like any conversation, the amount we 'say' will vary and, for me, this is particularly evident when treating infants and children. Sometimes, as practitioners, we don't 'do' very much and the body does all the work. Sometimes, it feels like we need to 'do' a lot in order to perceive the potential for health and how it is trying to be expressed.

For this chapter, I shall consider diagnostic and treatment 'phrases' separately. I hope that this will help you to understand, identify and apply the phrases with your patients.

Principles of diagnosis

In the following text the diagnostic phrases and those concerning treatment will be described separately. I hope that will help you to understand and identify and use them while treating your patients.

Models for diagnosis

'There are always three factors to consider every time a patient enters your office: the patient's ideas and beliefs of what he considers his problem to be; the physician's concepts of what he considers the patient's problem to be; and finally, what the anatomical-physiological wholeness of the patient's body knows the problem to be' (Becker 1997).

I heard this quote when I began to study osteopathy in the cranial field and struggled to reconcile these three aspects. It seemed a matter of luck rather than judgement whether I could perceive and sustain these diverse, and potentially contradictory, viewpoints in any kind of relationship.

I now consider that these three elements can be reconciled but this calls for a shift in our model of diagnosis. As undergraduate osteopaths, we are taught a medical model: we learn what is 'normal' and 'abnormal' so that we can identify what is wrong and put it right. This model has its place, especially when we are learning, but I believe that it can limit our perception and communication with our patients as osteopaths in the cranial field. In its place, we need an osteopathic model of diagnosis. We must focus on health, and try to understand the way the body is functioning at that moment. Remember that, at any moment, the body is expressing the best health possible. 'Life is always trying to express health' (Becker 1997). We acknowledge the relationship between present health and potential health and the capacity to change: in other words, how the body is trying to heal itself. Our treatment supports and facilitates the inherent healing processes and enables the body to realize its potential health more fully.

With vigilance and practice, the osteopathic model can be applied throughout the consultation so that we are respectful, accepting and positive in attitude and language. It can be difficult to focus on health when children have major medical conditions or have needed complex interventions, and parents may be judging themselves (or the child), but it is worth the effort. I believe that infants and children (and their parents) are highly sensitive to non-verbal and verbal communication. When I avoid being judgmental or negative, it is easier to find resonance or rapport for palpation, establish communication in the language of the PRM and begin to perceive their unique 'voice': 'This is what I want to be: that pattern individually designed for that one soul, that one individual'. (Becker 1997).

The process of diagnosis with the help of the PRM

During a consultation, we listen and ask questions, observe and examine and gather lots of information. These findings are not your diagnosis but the beginning of the diagnostic process. This will involve acknowledging, analyzing, and evaluating each of these findings and then integrating them in order to make a diagnosis. As we are trained to think like osteopaths, we may not be aware of the separate stages in making a diagnosis because we do this automatically. Not all findings will be equally relevant.

The diagnosis is a statement of your understanding of the patient at that time: their present health, their potential health and their capacity to heal. These elements may not be equally clear but are all necessary in order to guide treatment and form a prognosis.

I would like to explore the process of diagnosis of the involuntary mechanism in more detail as this may not be quite so familiar.

As we begin to monitor our patient, we get a general sense of their shape change with the PRM. Theoretically, this is rhythmic, synchronous and symmetrical. In health, it is rhythmic and synchronous but rarely symmetrical. We can acknowledge the rhythm, symmetry or asymmetry and synchrony of the whole-body shape change and variations within the body.

We know: 'The forces of embryogenesis become the forces of healing in the adult' (Jealous 2001). It therefore can be useful to acknowledge our experience of the shape change with the PRM in relation to embryological principles. For example, we know from Blechschmidt that the body is a fluid system; it is organized around a central, segmented and longitudinal axis. Questions one might like to ask:

- Can I feel fluid in the patient's body?
- Is the quality, depth and vitality of fluid the same throughout the body? If it varies, how does it vary?
- Is the shape change organized around a midline?
- Do the neighbouring segments show similar intensity and energy?

We become more aware of the motion present: the qualities, amplitude and health expressed through different areas of the body and different tissues. We notice whether the motion present is consistent with the theoretical axes and fulcra or any of Sutherland's cranial base patterns.

It is often useful to consider the five principles of Sutherland's hypothesis of the PRM separately:

- **fluctuation of the cerebrospinal fluid:** how is the fluctuation? Imagine it as a mountain stream – how does it flow? Does it bend or disappear? How deep and vital is the water?
- **function of the reciprocal tension membrane** (RTM): what is the quality of the membrane? Where is the automatic shifting suspension fulcrum (e.g. is it in the region

of the straight sinus?) Can it accommodate changes in any direction? Imagine the RTM as a spider's web – what does the web look like? Is it symmetrical or not?

- **motility of the neural tube:** is the central nervous system (CNS) moving? Is it moving around the lamina terminalis? Imagine the CNS as the weather affecting the whole body.

- **articular mobility of the cranial bones** is like a dance involving all the bones of the body. They express their own 'style' (i.e. organized around their own ossification centers and moving around their own axes) but remain an integral part of the dance as there is harmony within and between all bones. Living bones are like sponges and it is helpful to identify variations in the density of the sponge and intraosseous 'breathing'. When it is not expressing involuntary motion, or breathing, with the PRM it can feel more like a brick wall.

- **involuntary mobility of the sacrum** between the ilia: is the sacrum rocking around S2? Lifting and lowering with the RTM? Expressing intraosseous breathing? The sacrum is composed of five bony segments or 'sponges', floating in a membranous bag. Are all five segments floating? Are they organized around the same fulcrum? Are they moving together? And are they synchronous with the occiput?

This is like a dialogue between your 'feeling' and 'thinking' brain as you analyze and express your experiences in objective or subjective language. If you are trying to understand an unfamiliar or unexpected experience then, like a child learning to speak, make up your own words and analogies. Later, take time to talk with colleagues and read osteopathic literature to help develop your vocabulary and find out whether anyone else has had a similar experience.

Gradually, we weigh up all the findings to complete our diagnosis. This is like finding the meaning behind the words; so that you understand how the patient is trying to heal and where to begin treatment.

At any moment, there may be several areas that are not expressing their potential health, but this does not mean that you treat them all straightaway. How do we evaluate which areas are capable of changing today and receptive to treatment? Where are the healing processes most dynamic? Where is the greatest potential for change? I think that the quality of the 'diagnostic conversation' helps you decide. As you palpate, you are listening to the body and 'how it is feeling' and this will be easier to perceive in some areas than others. This indicates where the mechanism is more dynamic and active and where to begin treatment. After all, your treatment is to reinforce and facilitate the natural healing of the body – the unerring potency of the body to heal itself. This is analogous

to having conversations with lots of different people at a party. You soon know which conversations flow and feel dynamic and when it is worth waiting to hear what unfolds.

Sometimes, we can perceive the meaning behind the words more clearly. We may feel the potential health 'trying to get through' and can sense how the patient 'wants to be'. We may glimpse the precise cause of their present state and understand its effects throughout the living physiology, and the change needed to reveal the potential health. For me, these moments are a precious reminder of the inherent order and healing within my patients, but I don't always have this clarity. Most of the time, it feels like their mechanisms are telling a story. This unfolds over a few treatments, so I can gradually begin to understand what has happened and why.

Principles of treatment

The first principle of treatment is listening: 'something happens' when you are centered and listen to the language of the PRM. As osteopaths in the cranial field, there are times when we don't know what is happening, yet we may feel changes and our patients get better. The best description of the dynamics of listening I have found is from a book about education, written by a psychotherapist and teacher (Rogers 1979):

- '**I like to hear.** When I can really hear someone it puts me in touch with him. It enriches my life … So there is both the satisfaction of hearing this particular person and also the satisfaction of feeling oneself in some sort of touch with what is universally true.

- **I like to be heard.** I can testify that when you are in psychological distress and someone really hears you without passing judgement on you, without trying to take responsibility for you, without trying to mold you, it feels damn good. When I have been listened to and when I have been heard, I am able to re-perceive my world in a new way and to go on.'

We have discussed the language of the PRM and there are certain phrases which occur again and again during treatment. I would like to consider these in terms of fluid conversations and balanced tension conversations – but do remember that they normally occur together.

Principles of treatment with fluid

Sutherland considered that cerebrospinal fluid had a vital role in sustaining the health of the central nervous system and the whole body, and seems to have anticipated research on neuroendocrine–immune system integration. In the foreword to *Teachings in the science of osteopathy* Becker describes the five principles of the cranial concept including 'the fluctuation of the cerebrospinal fluid, or the potency of the Tide.' This is an important reminder that Sutherland's understanding of cerebrospinal fluid was more than just the physical fluid around the brain and spinal cord.

Our understanding comes from experience with patients and observations as the body treats itself. Sutherland described longitudinal fluctuation, stillness, directional fluctuation and lateral fluctuation.

Longitudinal fluctuation

This is like seeing waves in a bay but perceiving the tidal rhythms of the ocean behind it. It may take a while to establish resonance and perceive the longitudinal fluctuation. Sometimes I am aware of it appearing like a tide, but not disappearing, which is when I start to wonder what I am feeling! In health, it is expressed throughout the whole body.

Some osteopaths relate the longitudinal fluctuation to the longitudinal organization of the embryo around the notochordal axis. They describe longitudinal fluctuation as a 'tide' appearing from the coccyx, ascending through center of each segment of the spine and body and then disappearing. Variations in the presence, position and quality of the longitudinal fluctuation may indicate areas of altered function which need treatment.

The treatment conversation may involve 'hearing' how the body is self-correcting: the way distortions correct themselves, compressed segments begin to find more space, or areas of restricted fluctuation draw in fluid from somewhere else. Listening to and facilitating fluid self-corrections is an important aspect of treatment. Alternatively, the treatment conversation may involve you gently asking what the PRM would like to do:

- 'Is this how you want to be?' is often sufficient to initiate realignment, which you can support if you are centered.

- 'Would you like more space between these segments?' can help you to identify which, if any, segments are trying to make changes.

- 'Would you like more fluid in this area?' will show whether fluid is trying to get into an area and needs a little help.

Improvement in the quality and continuity of the longitudinal fluctuation indicates that a significant change has occurred and can signal the end of a treatment.

Stillness

During treatment, you will experience stillpoints; these are moments of no involuntary movement and a normal feature of the healing process as the physiology pauses to allow reorganization. This has been described as a 'pause for the breath of life'. In a stillpoint, all the tissues are receptive to the stillness and health within. You can learn about the PRM by noticing when stillpoints happen spontaneously and their effects; and we can initiate stillpoints with certain treatment approaches such as the CV4 or balanced tension. With experience of stillpoints, we become more familiar with stillness, the 'pauses between words' in the language of the PRM. As we treat our patients, we may become more aware of stillness than motion. It is not always possible to perceive what is happening during stillness so we have to watch and wait, and trust the 'physician within'.

Directional fluctuation

During treatment, you may notice 'directional fluctuations' or waves within the body which ebb and flow. These may be experienced as 'directional waves', which seem to appear from nowhere, cause turbulence then stillness, and then disappear, leaving a change in the amplitude or quality of motion. The body seems to use directional waves to remove obstacles or restrictions to motion.

We can initiate directional fluctuations as 'fluid drives', from the opposite longest diagonal, when we identify an obstacle to motion or disturbance in the quality of motion.

Lateral fluctuation

Just as longitudinal fluctuation has been related to the midline longitudinal organization of the embryo, lateral fluctuation relates to the lateral segmental organization and has been described as lateral expansion or external rotation from the center of each segment outwards throughout all the structures supplied by that segment. As with the longitudinal fluctuation, I am aware of it appearing like a tide, but not disappearing, and there may be variations in the symmetry, synchrony and quality of expansion between segments. In health, the longitudinal and lateral fluctuations are integrated so that there is an expansion along the midline and also outwards through each segment. Sometimes the lateral fluctuation can dominate and it is important to check that there is also longitudinal fluctuation as well.

Sometimes we perceive a paradoxical movement as one side feels to externally rotate and, at the same time, the other side feels to internally rotate: then it seems as if there is a lateral fluctuation from one side to the other across the limb, sacrum, body or head of the patient. This may occur:

- spontaneously during treatment, if we lose balanced tension between practitioner and patient (particularly if we impose upon the patient's mechanism) or as a part of the self-correcting and self-healing process.

- as a presenting feature when there is a history of shock, fever, or major trauma.

- as a treatment reaction; either when the patient did not fully re-establish their longitudinal fluctuation at the end of treatment or has not been able to assimilate the changes initiated during treatment (e.g. if over-treated).

We may learn to initiate lateral fluctuations as an alternative to the CV4 to restore vitality in the body or calm them as part of the management of treatment reactions.

Principles of treatment with balanced tension

The body uses the same 'phrases' or principles of treatment to find balance within bone, ligaments, membranes, the CNS, fluids or energy. The optimal balance may be represented by blocks arranged around a midline axis; these blocks could be neighbouring bones, membranes, viscera or areas of brain or fluid. When 'something happens' (like a trauma), then the blocks shift in relation to the midline axis (Figs 8.1, 8.2).

We may perceive the motion as organized around a different fulcrum; we can support the motion to establish 'a neutral point' when all the forces are balanced equally in all directions. At this point, the kinetic energy trapped within the strain can begin to release so there is no motion but a state of poise or stillness or potency for change. We experience this in different ways: an absence of motion, a change in fluid dynamics, a sense of heat, or, maybe, an awareness

of stillness. During this phase, 'something happens' and it is followed by motion in a different pattern (about a different fulcrum) which is closer to the physiological optimum.

By observing and monitoring the 'motion present', we can facilitate these self-corrections. This is considered the safest way to treat and is particularly recommended in the care of infants and children. Sometimes, it is difficult to feel 'motion present' and it helps to gently ask what the PRM would like to do. This does not involve any gross physical movement but the momentary 'thought' or 'intention' of the shape of a movement then pausing to gently observe and monitor the mechanism's response. Is it a 'yes' as the movement is readily taken up by the tissues or 'no' as the body subtly but definitely resists that movement? This requires care and skill as it is all too easy to 'ask too much' and to 'impose' rather than to simply, and precisely, 'facilitate' self-correction.

There are five principles of treatment, or 'phrases' which the body uses naturally to establish balanced tension.

Direct action

Direct action is by far the most common way to establish balanced tension in infants and children (or adults with acute or recent strains) (Fig. 8.3). We feel the body trying to

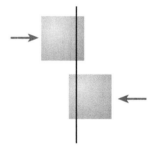

Figure 8.3 Direct action as treatment principle. Two blocks, *midline* and *arrows* to show balanced tension with direct action. With permission, Henriette Rintelen, Velbert

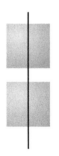

Figure 8.1 Balanced tension as two blocks aligned around a midline.
With permission, Henriette Rintelen, Velbert

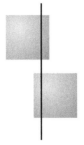

Figure 8.2 Something happens, so blocks no longer aligned around a midline.
With permission, Henriette Rintelen, Velbert

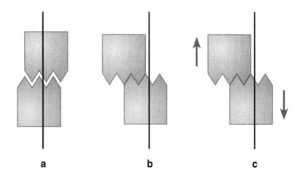

a   b   c

Figure 8.4 Disengagement as treatment principle **a:** balanced tension irregular blocks aligned around a midline; **b:** something happens, so irregular blocks are not aligned around midline; **c:** in order to regain balance the blocks have to be disengaged from one another before they can be shifted.
With permission, Henriette Rintelen, Velbert

move out of the strain pattern back towards the position of neutrality or health. This is most common in very acute or recent strains. If you attempt to guide it back, allowing physiological function to help you do it, the patient feels more comfortable and you feel tissues release and balance themselves. This treatment approach is treatment of choice with babies and children under 7 years old.

Molding

This is a form of direct action and particularly evident with intraosseous strains when you feel the bone structure trying to 'breathe' and reorganize itself around its ossification center. It is usually necessary to facilitate release of any interosseous restrictions first before the intraosseous strains can resolve.

Exaggeration

Somebody is in distress about something, and needs to tell you about their experience. You are listening and sympathizing and, after some time, they get to the point when it does not seem so bad and they do not need to talk about it anymore.

Exaggeration as a treatment principle is contraindicated in acute trauma and inflammation of the head or other structures, as reinforcing the pattern could exacerbate the condition and damage that has already occurred. It is also generally avoided in children under 7 years because they have insufficient sutural development. However, exaggeration can occur spontaneously in children and infants (and, occasionally, it is needed) but it is very precise and only exaggerated to the point of balance (see p.183).

Disengagement

Disengagement is the treatment principle which is characteristic of irregular sutures when there is compression trauma and impaction, but it can occur in fluid and energy when there is trauma or emotional shock. The body has to disengage tissues *before* they can begin to shift and find balance (Fig. 8.4).

Opposite physiological motion

Opposite physiological motion is characteristic of severe trauma between midline and paired structures or severe emotional shock. It is most common at sacroiliac or occipitomastoid joints, which cannot sustain their normal complex motion when strained.

On palpation, we experience paradoxical motion between neighbouring structures, which may be represented as the treatment phrase of 'yes, but': 'yes I would like to go to the theatre but I have to finish writing a lecture' and the two

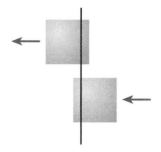

Figure 8.5 Opposite physiological motion as treatment principle. To balance the blocks one motion is exaggerated and the other lessened.
With permission, Henriette Rintelen, Velbert

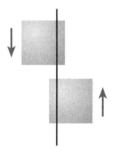

Figure 8.6 Compression as the treatment principle to achieve balanced tension.
With permission, Henriette Rintelen, Velbert

contradictory messages can be brought into balance by supporting one and lessening the other (Fig. 8.5). For example, if the occipitomastoid has been strained so that the occiput is held in relative flexion and the temporal in relative internal rotation, we can support the body's attempts at resolution by subtly exaggerating flexion of the occiput and applying direct action to guide temporals towards external rotation. Thus, we are supporting one component and lessening the other component to resolve the paradox.

Opposite physiological motion may occur within bones; for example the basisphenoid may be moving into flexion whilst the greater wing is moving into internal rotation. Or between viscera (e.g. the mediastinum and the lungs) where there has been trauma or surgery. It is important to be aware of this treatment 'phrase', especially when working with infants and children who experience birth trauma and shock.

Compression

Compression may be considered as a type of exaggeration rather than a treatment phrase in its own right. But Rollin Becker (1997) and Rachel Brooks (2002) highlighted the importance of compression in establishing diagnostic and treatment dialogue with patients. In treating infants and children, I am often surprized at the degree of compression within their tissues and the changes that happen once I am able to acknowledge and support this quality (Fig. 8.6).

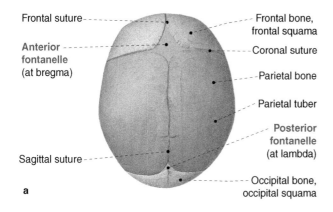

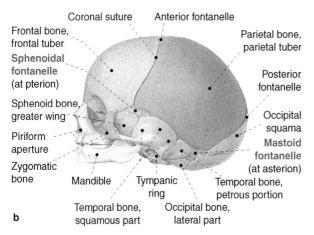

Figure 8.7 Skull of a newborn with the membranes (fontanels) on the skullcap. **a:** from above. **b:** from lateral.
With permission, Sobotta: Atlas der Anatomie des Menschen. Publisher: R. Putz and R. Pabst, 21st edn. Elsevier/Urban & Fischer, Munich/Jena 2000

Conclusion

- Accept the 'living mechanism' in you and in the patient. Life is always trying to express health.

- Surrender comes after acceptance. Accept the fact that what the mechanism is telling you is true.

- Develop palpatory skills. The body is smarter than you are, so learn from it (Becker 1997).

- Trust the body's ability to tell its story and your ability to understand.

References

Becker R E: Life in motion. Brooks Rudra, Portland, Ore. 1997

Becker R E: Stillness of life. Brooks Stillness, Portland, Ore. 2000

Blechschmidt E, Gasser R F: Biokinetics and biodynamics of human differentiation. Thomas, Springfield, Ill. 1978

Brooks R: SCC Rollin Becker Memorial Lecture 2002

Grundberg S: SCC Module 2/3, Lecture April 2003

Jealous J: Lecture notes 2001

Magoun HG: Osteopathy in the cranial field. 3rd edn. Sutherland Cranial Teaching Foundation, Kirksville, Mo. 1976

Rogers C: Freedom to learn. Merrill Publishing Company 1979

Sutherland W G: Teachings in the science of osteopathy. edited by Anne Wales. Sutherland Cranial Teaching Foundation 1990

Sutherland W G: Contributions of thought. 2nd edn. Ada Strand, Anne Wales (eds) Sutherland Cranial Teaching Foundation 1998

INTRAOSSEOUS STRAINS

Sibyl Grundberg

There are many things that distinguish the child from the adult, but none is more dynamic than the process of development that each child is undergoing. Dr Anne Wales tells us, 'Growth is slow motion.' A child is literally growing under our hands, and this makes treatment of children a roller-coaster ride.

Those parts of the developing skeletal structure that protect the central nervous system (CNS) are of particular importance. The spine and cranium must grow synchronously with the developing CNS in order to make room for its adaptation to the sensory, motor, emotional and intellectual stimulation that drives the growth process. In this chapter I will focus on the bones of the cranium and pelvic girdle, but the infant body as a whole is a cartilaginous/membranous entity which is as tough and flexible as it is delicate. This is the context in which intraosseous strains (strains *within* bone) occur – in infancy, in childhood, and beyond.

Intraosseous motion

All bones, in health, express intraosseous motion. If this were not so, it would not be possible for the cranium as a whole to broaden into external rotation in the inhalation phase. The sphenoid is a bone with the ability to express inhalation and exhalation within itself that allows widening of the orbits when the midline bones go into flexion. On palpation a healthy occiput is felt not just to flex and extend, but also to express widening and narrowing (external and internal rotation) within itself.

When we palpate any bone in the body, whether we realize it or not, we are assessing the health of that bone to ascertain whether it expresses a breathing function or whether it feels hard and dead. Because each bone moves and breathes, it follows that it is capable of absorbing intraosseous strains, such as compression, torsion or shearing patterns. When we set out to address strains in joints – or sutures – we will find that that articulation will only be as good as the integrity and vitality of the two bones that compose it.

Living bone is a fluid tissue. In mature bone the matrix surrounding the cells contains 10–20% water, as well as 60–70% of mineral salts and 30–45% organic materials including collagen. In early, developing bone, the proportion of mineral salts is much smaller, and that of water (much of it in the gel-like state characteristic of connective tissue ground substance), greater. This confers flexibility and tensile strength.

In this chapter, we will concentrate on strains that occur because of the unossified unions within the cranial bones at birth. These are particularly prone to strain, especially in the growing years, but also throughout life. These unossified areas exist because all bones develop *within* more primitive tissue, growing outward from two or more, sometimes many, centers of ossification.

The origins of bone in the embryo

The early embryo is a bag of fluid-filled cells in a gel-like state, organized into three distinct layers of tissue: ectoderm, mesoderm and endoderm. These primitive cells are 'plenipotent' and thus can develop into many kinds of more specialized tissue. The future forms of endoderm are easy to remember, as endoderm is the forerunner of all the viscera. Ectoderm doubles as the precursor both of neural tissue and of the skin. Mesoderm originally lies between these other two. Although it starts out as the 'meat in the sandwich', it eventually surrounds, protects, supports and separates these developing structures. It differentiates to provide a backing fabric for the skin, a tough covering for the central nervous system (dura mater), and as the tunica adventitia, it keeps blood vessels patent. Fibres with a contractile potential appear and form muscles. Membrane which is called fascia in this context remains around these muscular tissues, giving muscles their separate shapes and identities. Early on the heart starts to take form as a muscle of intricate design, which exists within its own bag of tough, protective membrane, the pericardium. All these tissues earn the name 'connective tissue' by being continuous and communicative throughout the body.

Embryonic connective tissue is called mesenchyme, signifying its origins in mesoderm. Under the influence of stretching, it forms membrane; when compressed, it develops into cartilage. Either of these may ossify to bone. The cranial base forms from mesenchyme that has condensed around the notochord in response to compression to become the median axial stem. This mesenchymal structure, upon being compressed between the growing brain and the developing heart, becomes cartilaginous before it is ossified (endochondral ossification). The cranial vault, on the other hand, ossifies directly within the membrane that is formed when mesenchyme is stretched (endomembranous ossification).

In the cranium, by the end of the 2nd month of life in the womb, small condensations of bone matrix are forming within both cartilage and membrane. Ossification proceeds rapidly but is not complete at the time of birth.

Bone develops within connective tissue

After birth there are thin islands of bone visible and palpable within their membrane (now renamed periosteum), and separated by more flexible areas either of cartilage or, in the vault, of membrane alone. We are accustomed to 'seeing', in the infant skull, areas of cartilage and membrane. The most obvious spaces between the bones of the vault are the fontanelles (Fig. 8.7).

Less obviously, certain bones, which are forming from two or more separate ossification centers, may incur strain between these centers. The two halves of the frontal bone for example are not yet joined at the metopic suture. Compression, overlap, distortion and even distraction are possibilities.

In the cranial base, there is a tough framework of cartilage surrounding the islands of bone, but this is still subject to strain during the birth process and afterwards. As these islands of bone meet and unite to form the bone whose form we recognize, we can see a certain symmetry of the paired bones.

The various cranial bones fuse at different times (Table 8.1). The bones protecting the foramen magnum (the atlas and the occiput) unite synchronously, as do the bones of the middle cranial fossa (sphenoid and temporals). The cranial base and sacrum relinquish their cartilaginous flexibility at approximately the same mature age. As the diagrams will show, both the occipital parts and those of the atlas unite first posteriorly, then anteriorly.

Ossification

The complex pattern of skeletal ossification from mesenchyme can be lost in a welter of detail. The important principles to remember are that:

- bones form within membrane, or within cartilage formed from mesenchyme
- they ossify outward from centers that appear during the fetal period, or sometimes after birth
- this process is a gradual one, the final events occurring usually around the age of 25
- certain bones unite synchronously, and this may have implications for function

Table 8.1 Time of fusion of the bones of the skull

Bones	Number of parts at birth	Fusion of the parts
Occipital bone	4	Up to 6–7 years of age
Atlas	2 (lateral), one 3rd center appears later	By 6–8 years
Sphenoid bone	3	During the 1st year
Temporal bone	2	During the 1st year
Solitary segment of the Sacrum	5	Completed by 8th year
All segments of the Sacrum	5	In 25 years or later, 1st and 2nd segment do not unite in some cases
Occiput and Sphenoid		Up to 25 years
Coccyx	3	Up to 18 years, ossification continues up to 25 years of age

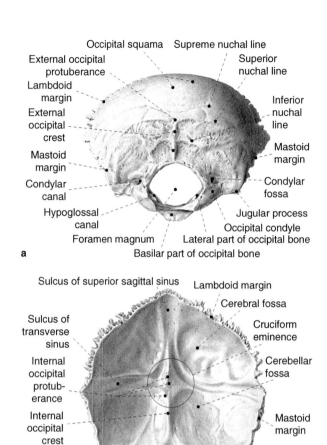

a

b

Figure 8.8 Os occipitale (occipital bone). **a:** from below. **b:** from front.
With permission, Sobotta: Atlas der Anatomie des Menschen. Publisher: R. Putz and R. Pabst, 21st edn. Elsevier/Urban & Fischer, Munich/Jena 2000

- in synchrony, the posterior parts of the occiput and atlas unite first, the more anterior parts later; the sphenobasilar synchondrosis (SBS) is last of all, in early adulthood, and about the same time as the sacral segments complete unification with each other
- owing to all these factors, the head of an infant or very young child is like a 'soft-shelled egg' and, while allowing accommodation to the challenges of birth and other trauma, it is also extremely vulnerable to distortion.

Let us look at these bones in detail.

The occiput

The occiput (Fig. 8.8) provides a classic illustration of the importance of this type of strain. Its four parts surround the foramen magnum, and serious distortion may result in injury to the brainstem causing disability or death. No wonder that, as Dr Anne Wales tells us, Dr Sutherland *started* his teaching programme with a close study of the occiput as it is at birth. The child's future motor and sensory coordination, intelligence, shape and structure will all be influenced by the ease or stress with which the central nervous system is housed in this area. Apart from the most obvious potential for catastrophic events occurring at birth, or pre- and post-natally, the effects of intraosseous distortion and compression may be chronic and subtle. Clinical effects may be absent until later in childhood, when scoliosis, dental occlusal problems, or some accidental injury brings the underlying problems to notice. In the adult, one sees that many chronic problems apparently originating in hormonal or infectious events may have their true origins in the unresolved intraosseous distortions of early life.

Warning: Because of the slow ossification of the parts of the occiput and the delicate structures it protects it is not advisable to use the CV4 (compression of the fourth ventricle) until a child is at least 8 years old.

Intraosseous strain of the occiput

Three factors predispose to intraosseous strains of the occiput. These are:

1. the uterine forces of labor on the spine

2. the resistance of the cervix against the presenting part (normally the vault)

3. the responses of the partly ossified atlas and occiput to these combined, opposing forces.

At birth, the occiput is in four parts (Fig. 8.9): the squama, the two condylar parts (also called the lateral parts) and the basiocciput. The squama is in two parts up until shortly before or after birth when the interparietal occiput unites with the supraocciput. The flexibility of this aspect of the occiput – and its capacity for compression and distortion – are important factors in treatment. The junctions between the condylar parts and the squama will unite between 2 and 5 years; the condylobasilar junctions before 8 years.

It follows that the window of best opportunity for the osteopath to treat a pattern originating in the occiput is in the first 2 years. Wales says that the pattern is difficult to change after 3 months, and particularly after the infant has started to sit up; in other words, when she uses her muscles to hold her head up. What we must remember is that the process of ossification and union of the parts is *continuous* into early adult life. During this time bone is constantly remodelling. The body's capacity for homeostasis uses this 'living' quality of bone to move ever towards normal *function*, even if the actual degree of structural change is small.

Although the atlas (Fig. 8.10) is often described as having threes at birth, the anterior arch of the atlas is fibrocartilaginous and its center of ossification does not appear until the end of the first year. The two lateral centers, which are present at birth, join with each other posteriorly at around years 3–4 and unite with the anterior center in years 6–8. Ossification of the atlas mirrors ossification of the occiput.

The surfaces of the occipital condyles are very slightly convex in the infant, while the pits of the atlas are concave. The flexible articulatory surfaces of both occiput and atlas converge anteriorly and diverge posteriorly. Those of the occiput face slightly laterally whereas those of the atlas face slightly medially. In ordinary circumstances this allows rocking in the anterior-posterior plane, with a very limited degree of sidebending. When uterine forces act on the infant vault, the occipital condyles may become trapped in a 'headlock' by the anterior convergence and posterior divergence of the atlas, either unilaterally or bilaterally (Fig. 8.11).

Because the articular condyles of the occiput are formed from parts of both the basiocciput and the condylar parts (note the confusing distinction between 'condyles' and 'condylar parts' (see Fig. 8.8), compression into the pits of the atlas can involve three of the four parts of the newborn occipital bone. If the forces operating in this way are asymmetrical, all four parts rotate in a compensatory pat-

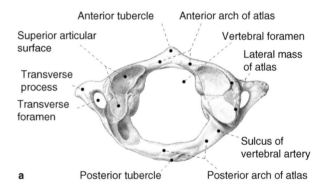

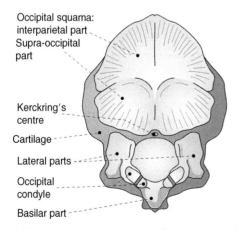

Figure 8.9 The occipital bone consists of four parts at birth: squama occipitalis, condylar parts and pars basilaris. With permission, Henriette Rintelen, Velbert

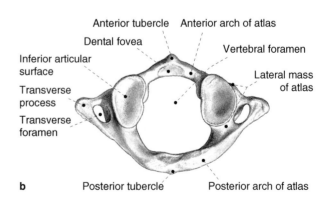

Figure 8.10 Atlas. **a:** from cranial; **b:** from caudal. With permission, Sobotta: Atlas der Anatomie des Menschen. Publisher: R. Putz and R. Pabst, 21st edn. Elsevier/Urban & Fischer, Munich/Jena 2000

tern; essentially, the PRM does its best to balance tensions between the parts. Each part may turn on an anterior/posterior axis, a transverse axis, rotate around the foramen magnum on a vertical axis or more likely, a combination of these. However, their directions of movement will be determined by the restraining influence of the cartilage in which they are embedded, as well as the adjoining bones.

One would expect that the atlas could be more vulnerable, owing to the broad areas of cartilage present posteriorly and especially anteriorly. However, the transverse ligament of the atlas holds the two lateral parts securely so distortion is minimized. As the occiput is driven forward, the mobility of the two ossifying bones will absorb strain and then shift according to the resilience and 'give' in the cartilage around them. Too much compression or distortion will result in some functional compromize in the occipitoatlantal area.

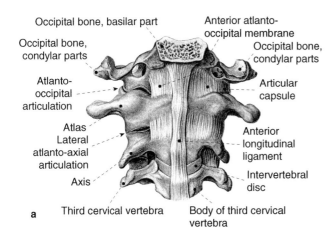

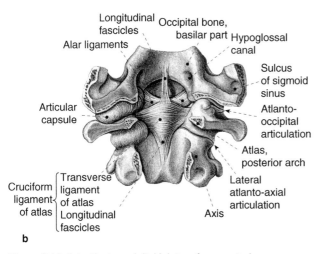

Figure 8.11 Art. atlantooccipital joint: **a:** from ventral; **b:** from dorsal.
With permission, Sobotta: Atlas der Anatomie des Menschen. Publisher: R. Putz and R. Pabst, 21st edn. Elsevier/Urban & Fischer, Munich/Jena 2000

Assessing the infant occiput

There are many possible patterns of strain or compression. When assessing a newborn, it is necessary to keep an open mind. It is counterproductive to 'hunt' for lesion patterns. The field of operation is tiny, and recognizing 'structure' is extremely difficult. It may be more helpful merely to think of the tiny head as the sum of many influences – from the different textures of its emerging tissues to the dynamic interaction of intrauterine and perinatal forces with fluid-tissue responses. We are trying to catch a glimpse of a dynamic process, which, of course, is still going on as the self-correcting 'intelligence' of the newborn strives to normalize function after the rigors of the birth process.

In the newborn, the effect of holding the occiput with 'thinking, feeling, knowing fingers' is most appropriate, and often sufficient, to effect release of all body tissues almost precognitively. In the older infant, the strain pattern becomes more evident and it may need to be engaged-with more consciously.

Although one must always keep an open mind, it is helpful on beginning this work to consider some of the main scenarios that the birth process presents to the occiput (The birth process and its effect on the infant cranium, p.67).

Whether the force is applied centrally/posteriorly or more laterally, there will be compression of the condylosquamous and condylobasilar junctions on one or both sides. In bilateral compression with the force acting centrally from behind, the condylosquamous junction may overlap or the angle become more acute. Alternatively, the condylosquamous may be gapped with injury to the cartilaginous matrix. Both condylar parts will be driven forward into the basilar part. When the basilar part has absorbed as much compression as its fluid-osseous structure permits, it may tip upward anteriorly, or downward, or rotate on an anteroposterior (a/p) axis. Magoun (1976) describes this compression as a 'pincer' effect, because the two condylar parts may be driven medially into the basilar part as well as anteriorly. This creates a very compressed, dense feel to palpation. The basiocciput may also turn on an a/p axis, dropping one side and rising on the other. These effects have implications for the SBS patterns. In unilateral compression where the force is acting from a point lateral to the midpoint of the occiput, the lateral angle of the squama goes forward on the side of the compression, compressing the condylosquamous junction on that side and turning it anteriorly. The anterior aspect of the basilar part will turn away to the other side. To palpation, one condylar part feels more anterior than the other. The density of the 'pincer' effect is felt mainly on the side of anterior compression. On the anterior side the squama feels flatter. The opposite is true on the contralateral side, where the condylar part is posterior and palpable, and the squama more prominent. The child will prefer to lie with the head to the side of compression, and the head will side-bend to the opposite side.

Wales (1998) described the birth process in relation to the squama. For me this point of view provides a logical means of working out what has happened to the various parts. Under pressure from the forces acting on any portion of the vault, the squama will rotate in relation to those forces – clinically, we find the opisthion (the posterior midpoint of the foramen magnum) slightly off-midline. By visualizing the squama as turning on an axis passing forwards through the inion, it can be seen that the turning squama will push the posterior aspect of the condylar part laterally (and relatively posteriorly) on the side to which the opisthion has turned. The other parts 'knock-on' from there, within the restraints imposed by their cartilaginous junctions. On the side opposite, the condylar part is compressed into the basilar part, and also into the pit of the atlas (Fig. 8.12).

In sum, the following series of events occur:

- pressure on the infant's vault is dispersed and transmitted through the cranium towards the condyles, articulating with the pits of the atlas
- these forces are, in turn, dispersed or absorbed by the accommodative movements of the four parts of the occiput and the parts of the atlas, and also by the resilience and distortability of the cartilaginous matrices of both the occiput and atlas
- this accommodation produces shape change while minimizing compressive forces which would impinge on the cerebral contents

However, during and after this process, the distorting foramen magnum may impinge on vascular and neurological structures. This potentially serious danger for the child is normally averted by the flexible resilience of the cartilaginous cranial base to birth forces within normal limits. If the newborn arrives with its vitality intact, and if the stress has not been too great, the events of the neonatal period – a successful first breath, forceful crying and sucking – will 'blow out' the cranial bowl and normalize the occiput. But distortion often remains, to a greater or lesser degree, and skilled treatment by a pediatric osteopath is vital.

Effects of distortion of the foramen magnum

The reciprocal tension membrane (RTM)

Both the falx cerebri and the tentorium cerebelli attach to the occipital squama, meeting at the straight sinus in the center of the 'wheel' formed by the RTM. The venous sinuses lie

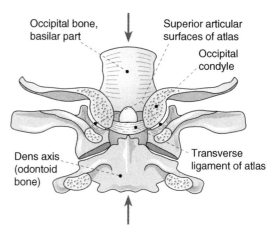

Figure 8.12 Compression of the condyles of the occipital bone. With permission, Henriette Rintelen, Velbert

in the dural 'sickles', meeting at the confluence of sinuses, which is located at the internal occipital protuberance. The dural 'tadpole' surrounding the brain and spinal cord is firmly fixed all around the foramen magnum. Disturbance of the parts of the occiput, with asymmetry and compression around the foramen magnum will cause strain in the other parts of the 'tripod' structure. Magoun (1976) described a tripod structure here with the falx cerebri and the two parts of the tentorium cerebelli as legs which meet at the straight sinus (Fig. 8.13). Altered tension in the tentorium and falx will literally reshape the cranial base. The 'reins' of the tentorium's anterior attachments will pull on the clinoid processes of the sphenoid and alter the sphenobasilar relationship at the SBS. The child's head may feel tense, unresilient, 'bony' and the child will be unable to be still.

Wales (1998) put stress on the fact that the tentorium cerebelli may lock the cerebellum down onto the brainstem in the posterior cranial fossa. The pyramidal (motor) tracts from the cortex sit directly on the basiocciput. If the tentorium has become locked down in this way, the medulla will sit low on the foramen magnum and pressure is put upon its ventral aspect, which adversely affects the circulation to the pyramidal tracts. As the child grows this pressure may increase. Potentially, the modulating influence of the cortex on the spinal motor centers may be lost, resulting in spastic cerebral palsy.

The dural 'tadpole' is firmly attached to the sacral canal at the level of S2 and below. Any alteration in the tensions or fulcrum of the cranial RTM will directly influence the sacral end of the 'core link'. Sutherland used this term to describe the relationship between the cranium and sacrum, reciprocally influenced by the dural connection. Early occipital compression is a frequent finding in patients with chronic low back strain. I have had several cases of older patients

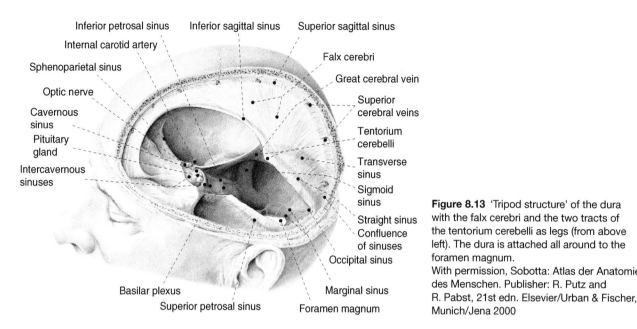

Inferior petrosal sinus   Inferior sagittal sinus   Superior sagittal sinus
Internal carotid artery
Sphenoparietal sinus
Optic nerve
Cavernous
sinus
Pituitary
gland
Intercavernous
sinuses

Falx cerebri
Great cerebral vein
Superior
cerebral veins
Tentorium
cerebelli
Transverse
sinus
Sigmoid
sinus
Straight sinus
Confluence
of sinuses
Occipital sinus

Basilar plexus
Superior petrosal sinus

Marginal sinus
Foramen magnum

Figure 8.13 'Tripod structure' of the dura with the falx cerebri and the two tracts of the tentorium cerebelli as legs (from above left). The dura is attached all around to the foramen magnum.
With permission, Sobotta: Atlas der Anatomie des Menschen. Publisher: R. Putz and R. Pabst, 21st edn. Elsevier/Urban & Fischer, Munich/Jena 2000

presenting with neck problems, which when successfully treated resulted in low back pain. Without an understanding of this connection, the back pain can be much more difficult to resolve. The occipitoatlantal compression clearly arose from the early pre-osseous stage, and the patient's compensatory pattern had to be re-built.

The relationships between the condylar parts, basilar parts and the atlas are so complex that we may be tempted to forget the importance of the squama. It cannot be overemphasized that the squama must be normalized so that the RTM can do its job of reorganizing all the bones of the neurocranium.

The vault

Since compression affecting the condylar parts is partly delivered via the vault, it is not surprising that freeing the vault bones, which are crowded down upon the cranial base, is essential to resolving occipital strains.

An important consideration is how the vault has adapted to strain affecting the cranial base. The RTM 'tripod' will draw the bones together into a 'best-possible' alignment, a little like the way a string-bag will arrange itself around different masses of shopping. The membranes will remain under tension, equalizing as much as possible.

This means that anything can happen. As Magoun (1976) said, 'the one factor which can be depended upon is the membranous'. Inconsistency between the vault and the base is common. Features of both flexion and extension patterns will be present in the face, the position of the mastoid processes, the squamal parts of the base bones, and the overall vault shape. Of course other patterns may be mixed in with

the main tendency. Vault/base inconsistency is an indicator of intraosseous strain in the base.

The condyles, the hypoglossal nerve and the jugular foramina

The basiocciput abuts the petrous temporal at the petrobasilar suture. If the basiocciput turns on its a/p axis, the petrous portion of the temporal will normally be carried with the basiocciput. It will therefore go either upwards or downwards; that is, into apparent internal or external rotation. The supraocciput, turning into the condylar part on one side, compresses the temporal parts in the region of the jugular foramen (Fig. 8.14). 'The condylar parts lesions of today are the occipitomastoid lesions of tomorrow'.

The jugular foramina, which are formed between the occiput and temporal bones on each side, transmit the 9th, 10th and 11th cranial nerves to the outside of the cranium. We should consider the 10th nerve (vagus) in cases of infants who vomit and cry after meals. The various forms of infantile colic are often associated with compression at the cranial base because of these relationships. The 12th (hypoglossal) nerve passes under the condyles in a canal formed in the cartilage joining the condylar and basilar parts. It is the motor to the tongue, and if tractioned or compressed, the child may be unable to latch on and suck properly. The 9th (glossopharyngeal) nerve's motor component contributes to swallowing by elevating the pharynx. Perhaps more importantly, its sensory fibres from the carotid body assist the hypothalamus in controlling respiration, blood pressure and cardiac output.

Torticollis (Ch.15) is a common condition which may be the result of muscular injury during birth, or of unilateral compression of one of the 11th (accessory) nerves. Its

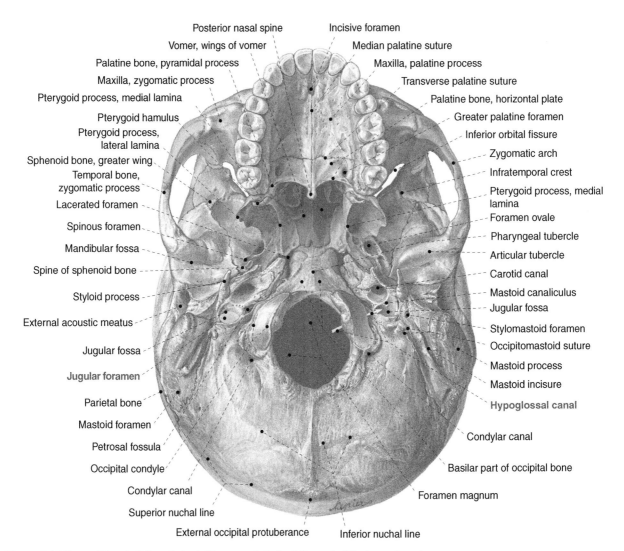

Figure 8.14 Base of the skull (from below). The *arrow* is in the left canal of the hypoglossal nerve.
With permission, Sobotta: Atlas der Anatomie des Menschen. Publisher: R. Putz and R. Pabst, 21st edn. Elsevier/Urban & Fischer, Munich/Jena 2000

nucleus arises in the first five or six segments of the spinal cord and its rootlets pass upwards through the foramen magnum to qualify as a 'cranial nerve'. It then joins the vagus nerve to exit from the cranium at the jugular foramen, where it can be compressed as described above.

The sigmoid sinuses issue into the internal jugular veins at the foramina, and these receive 95% of the venous blood from the interior of the cranium. Compression of these structures and their soft tissues will adversely affect every cerebral function. Distortion of the foramen magnum affects directly the medulla, cerebellar tripod and descending/ascending tracts carrying motor and sensory information to and from the rest of the body. The fourth ventricle and cerebellum may be affected.

Vascular injury and neurological damage are inevitable if distortion of the cranial bones and the membranes is severe and sudden. Fortunately, catastrophic injury is relatively rare. Usually, a slow adjustment takes place, and the consequences may be minimal, mild, or delayed until much later in life.

Sphenoid bone

The sphenoid (Fig. 8.15) is in three parts at birth: the body with the lesser wings on the midline, and the two greater wing–pterygoid units laterally. These three parts will unite during the 1st year. The two parts of the body, the pre- and post-sphenoid, unite shortly before birth. Prematurity brings with it many risks, but intraosseous compression of the sphenoid body – containing the pituitary gland, with its connections to the hypothalamus, the third ventricle and the midbrain – is one to remember in practice.

The 3rd, 4th and 6th nerves controlling the extraocular muscles pass through the superior orbital fissure which

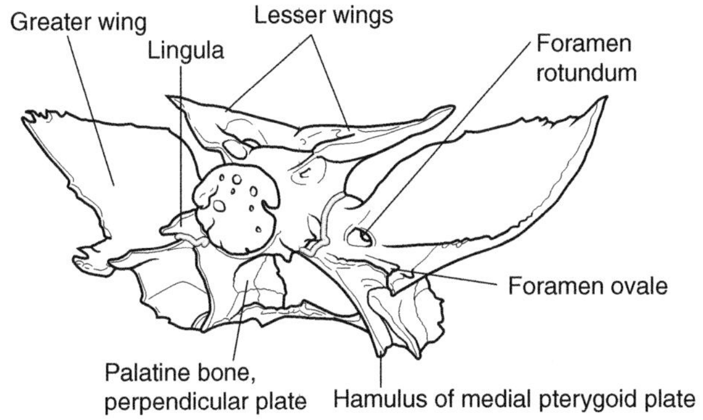

Figure 8.15 Os sphenoidale. **a:** from front. **b:** from back.

is formed around them and between the lesser and greater wings. Strain between the parts can cause congestion and trouble to these nerves, resulting in strabismus.

Case history

Barbara came to see me at only 11 days old. Her parents had noticed that her right eye failed to move laterally. She had been a face presentation with a long and difficult labor and was delivered after being 'half-turned'. She was 'floppy' for the first 1½ hours and did not cry for 15 hours. However, her only symptoms at presentation were the strabismus, restlessness and clinginess with inability to sleep.

In a face presentation the baby's face may be caught on the pubic brim, causing bruising and an inferior vertical strain. Such a strain brings the anterior of the tentorium down on the cranial nerves passing under it to the orbits; the 6th nerve, controlling lateral rectus, is particularly vulnerable. In Barbara this phenomenon was more pronounced on the right side, and the anterior dural girdle – continuous with the lesser wings – felt less mobile on the right and compressed at the anterolateral fontanelle. Rebalancing the vault, and the pelvis, immediately freed the right eye to move laterally, although weakly, in the first few weeks.

Normally the lesser wings develop in continuity with the pre-sphenoid. In Down syndrome the characteristic ocular shape is associated with non-union of the lesser wings with the sphenoid body. Committed treatment has been shown to bring a spectrum of functional improvements in these children. Colleagues tell me that in some Down children the eye shape itself has tended to normalize.

Intraosseous strain, distortion and compression between the main three parts of the sphenoid are of course possible in any young infant. Asymmetry between the two sides, palpable via the mouth and the area of the greater wing, will be associated with strains of the occiput and temporals, and will in turn determine the growth and development of the viscerocranium. Compression and/or asymmetry

of the pterygoid processes affects physiological motion of the sphenoid and impacts on the ability of the maxillae to expand and develop. In my experience the narrow palate and crowded mouth is as often associated with this type of intraosseous strain as with the classic extension pattern. The resulting effects on occlusion of the growing teeth will be compounded by strains of the temporal bone, affecting the mandible.

SBS patterns

The position and mobility of the sphenoid bone is largely determined by the combined influences of the occipital and temporal parts. As previously mentioned, the occipital basilar part may tilt forwards or backwards, rotate on an a/p axis or a vertical axis. These forces are communicated directly to the sphenoid body, which may rotate and/or tilt in turn, depending on its freedom in the field of motion. Next in line, the ethmoid, the greater wing-pterygoid units, the frontals (all to some extent preossified at birth) make their own compensations. In the posterior sphere, the petrous parts of the temporals follow the basocciput, while the squamous parts will be influenced by the rotation of the occipital squama. The familiar 'patterns' of function – both physiological and unphysiological – are initiated.

If the basisphenoid lags behind, or turns on the same vertical or transverse axis as the basiocciput, an unphysiological strain will result. This type of strain, in which there is a 'break' in the line of the longitudinal axis of the cranial base (and therefore in the shallow groove on which the brainstem sits) puts stress on the mechanism of primary respiration. If the basisphenoid turns on the same vertical axis as the basiocciput, a lateral strain results. If the basisphenoid turns on the same transverse axis as the basiocciput, a vertical strain is the result.

Torsion and side-bending rotation strains, which are more physiological, do not interrupt the central axis and seem easier for the organism to accommodate. One can easily visualize the effects on the brainstem lying upon the clivus.

When the 'patterns' involve intraosseous strain, the attachments of the reciprocal tension membrane to the rim of the foramen magnum will be affected. If the basisphenoid rotates in the same direction as the occiput on its vertical axis, into a side-bending rotation pattern, the effect would be a lateral strain. This would involve an unphysiological stress on the dural membranes.

The etiology of scoliosis

'As the twig is bent, so is the tree inclined', Sutherland (1990) wrote, expressing perfectly the idea that strains and distortion within the cranial base – and in its relationship with the atlas and axis – set the pattern, not only for the head shape but for compensations through the spine which ensure an erect posture. These compensations may lead to the characteristic 'S' or 'C'-shaped lateral curvature seen in the spine when viewed from behind.

A number of osteopathic writers have written in detail about scoliosis (Ch.15). Each gives slightly different emphasis. The important, and still radical, feature of all these analyses is that they differ from the classic orthopedic view that scoliosis develops from the ground up (short leg, pelvic torsion), often resulting from genetically or developmentally maintained structural factors such as wedged vertebrae. Instead, the spine and all the axial soft tissues are seen as being 'suspended' from a warped atlanto-occipital articulation. Certainly, this influence comes in far earlier than that of weight bearing. It should be remembered though, that SBS lesions may result in pelvic accommodation and that following a breech presentation, for example, primary lesions of the pelvis which lead to scoliosis may exist.

Scoliosis does, in my experience, cluster in families, but this persistence might be explained by the influence of the maternal occiput and temporals on the maternal sacrum and pelvis. The distortion of the maternal pelvis, in turn, shapes the baby's head, through the prenatal period and birth. This mirroring, in the female line, can continue for generations.

In the classic presentation of scolisis, there will be sidebending at the SBS, and rotation inferiorly on the side of the SBS 'bulge'. The atlas, articulating with the tilted occiput, must tilt the same way. The cervical spine and upper thoracic vertebrae follow, with compensation resulting throughout the spine in a scoliotic pattern.

Scoliosis affects every part of the body structure and function. On the membranous level, the Sutherland fulcrum shifts with the tentorium, which is altered by the position of the petrous temporals. The other two of the 'three diaphragms' – the respiratory diaphragm and the pelvic floor – as well as the thoracic inlet, accompany the scoliotic pattern; and they must be addressed along with other structural factors in any treatment of the infant. The whole fascial system and the system of muscular tensions throughout the body reflect the pattern expressed at the cranial base.

Osteopaths who work with adults know that scoliosis is common and usually well compensated. Carreiro (2003) makes the point that young children show asymmetries that do not develop into permanent scoliosis. This could be because asymmetrical or unilateral compression in the craniocervical junction has resolved spontaneously, or under treatment. Early intervention is of certain value in avoiding or minimizing the development of scoliosis.

Effects of strains within the sphenoid may be more subtle. In practice one sees the very compressed sphenoid associated with many problems on all levels. I have found endocrine problems (obesity, problems with the menses and ovaries) to be common later in life. These are often associated with strains within the sphenoid body. Although relatively undocumented, the nature of the 'knock-on effect' on adjacent bones of compression arising from the occiput can be imagined. The neurological and vascular connections of the anterior and posterior pituitary are affected by any turning of the sphenoid on an a/p, vertical, or transverse axis. The tentorium, attaching to the clinoid processes and continuing as the diaphragma sellae, can impose on the organ below or disturb the tracts communicating with the hypothalamus above. The petrous portions of the temporal can crowd into the tongue-and-groove articulation with the occiput and lock up the bony mechanism at the SBS.

Temporal bone

Relative to that of the occiput, the osteopathic literature on intraosseous strains of the temporal bones is sparse. The temporal bone (Figs 8.16, 8.17) arises from the otic capsule, the primitive organ of hearing, and until shortly before birth is in three distinct parts. At term the temporal is composed of two parts, the squama having united with the horseshoe-shaped tympanic 'ring' during the last few weeks of intrauterine life. The styloid process develops from two centers appearing just before and just after birth, the more proximal uniting during the first year, the distal not until puberty (if then).

The otic capsule, forerunner of the petromastoid part, develops early in intrauterine life. Its ossification centers (as many as 14) appear and ossify between the 5th and 6th month in utero, and the inner and middle ears are nearly adult size at birth. This puts a lot of emphasis on hearing as a

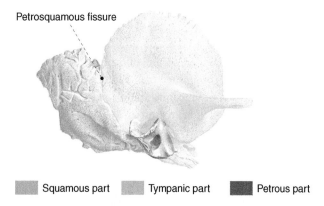

Petrosquamous fissure

Squamous part   Tympanic part   Petrous part

Figure 8.16 Os temporale in a newborn (from lateral). With permission, Sobotta: Atlas der Anatomie des Menschen. Publisher: R. Putz and R. Pabst, 21st edn. Elsevier/Urban & Fischer, Munich/Jena 2000

condition necessary to survival (or comfort?) of the fetus. We can only speculate about this.

The petromastoid part provides a roof, floor and medial wall for the ossicles and other sensory apparatus. The squama provides the lateral wall. Strain between these two parts before union at 1 year creates anomalies to palpation; for instance, a prominent, low ear with an anterior mastoid process and other signs of internal rotation. Some cases of hearing loss, although the loss is hard to recognize early, can be avoided by prompt treatment to an intraosseous strain involving the petrous contents.

The external auditory meatus, reaching into the petrous portion, will be warped, disturbing the relationships of the tympanic membrane, ossicles and eustachian tube. The condylosquamous junction of the occiput must accommodate. An apparently anomalous head shape bears all the signs, to palpation, of membranous strain (Fig. 8.18).

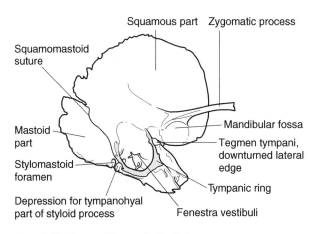

Figure 8.17 Temporal bone of lateral view.

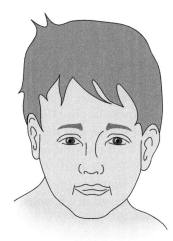

Figure 8.18 Anterior view of a child with an intraosseous strain of the left temporal bone: the squama is rotated externally and the petrous part internally. The left ear is lower and protudes.

Case history
A 6-year-old complained of headaches –which is not normal in young children. The birth history was unrevealing but his head had been severely molded. He had taken 2 days to latch on, and suffered from colic. He had had a history of sleep problems and night terrors, and now worried his mother because he seemed sad, withdrawn, and unsocial – in contrast to the rest of the family. He was having problems socially at school; an ENT hospital appointment was pending. To observation, there was marked ear asymmetry, with the left very prominent and the squama externally rotated; the rest of the cranium being consistently in an extension pattern. The foramen magnum was very narrow, the condylar parts sensitive to touch, and the SBS was compressed in a right lateral strain. The mandible was narrow and relatively forward as would be found in internal rotation of the temporals, slightly more on the left than the right. Intraosseous strain was also present between the greater wing/pterygoid units and body of the sphenoid, giving a narrow palate (as in an internal rotation pattern) and widely spaced eyes low at the corners (as in external rotation).

In fact, every aspect of primary respiration in this child was in a state of suspension. The entire CNS felt as if compressed into the posterior cranial fossa, the ventricles felt narrow and taut. Neither the diaphragm nor the sacrum was functioning properly. He responded very well to treatment, and by the third session had made breakthroughs in his schoolwork and interpersonally. Subsequently his adenoids were removed, but the headaches had already all but disappeared. Grommets were put in both ears, but his mother reported that the surgeon had reported 'not much fluid there'!

Ethmoid

At birth, the labyrinths of the ethmoid bone are already ossified. The perpendicular plate follows during the 12 months, the laminae of the cribriform plate during the 2nd year, and the crista galli between the 2nd and 4th year. They fuse as they ossify, completing the process by joining the lateral masses by year 6.

Consider the position of the ethmoid (Fig. 8.19) as the cockpit of the respiratory system, which underlies so many problems for children; for example catarrh, congestive conditions involving the eustachian tube (e.g. otitis media), asthma. These are often associated with either an overall extension pattern at the SBS, or an inferior vertical strain (sphenoid and ethmoid in relative extension, basiocciput in relative flexion). Compression of the SBS, and intraosseous

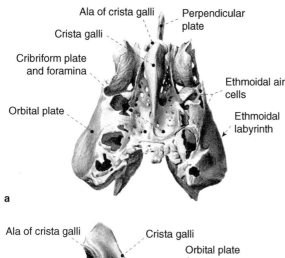

Ala of crista galli · Perpendicular plate
Crista galli ·
Cribriform plate and foramina ·
Ethmoidal air cells
Orbital plate ·
Ethmoidal labyrinth

a

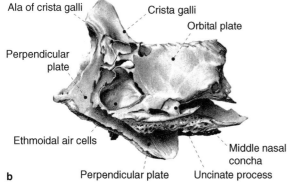

Ala of crista galli · Crista galli
Orbital plate
Perpendicular plate
Ethmoidal air cells
Middle nasal concha
b   Perpendicular plate   Uncinate process

Figure 8.19 Ethmoid. **a:** from above. **b:** from lateral.
With permission, Sobotta: Atlas der Anatomie des Menschen. Publisher: R. Putz and R. Pabst, 21st edn. Elsevier/Urban & Fischer, Munich/Jena 2000

compression in the cranial base, are virtually always present, along with inertia in the RTM. In the older child the external features of the nose may suggest underlying compression, 'scoliosis capitis' (deviated septum), or paradoxical ethmoid motion. This means motion out of phase with the spheno-basilar motion – palpation is the best guide. The infant may have difficulty feeding, owing to an inability to breathe at the same time.

Sacrum and coccyx

The sacrum ossifies from five segments, each containing five centers (Fig. 8.20a), which appear before birth in the manner of a typical vertebra. The paired 'costal' centers unite with each half-vertebral arch between the 2nd and 5th year (Fig. 8.20b). These join up anteriorly to the body of each segment, and posteriorly to each other, by 8 years of age. These completed segments are separated from each other by cartilage, both laterally and between the vertebral bodies. At puberty they begin to fuse, from below upwards, completing ossification between S1 and S2 by the 25th year

(Fig. 8.20c). Cartilage remains in the upper segments of some individuals.

Although we tend to speak only of 'the sacrum', let us look briefly at the coccyx, which is so functionally integrated with it.

The coccyx ossifies from three to five rudimentary vertebrae, each with one center. The process continues at a leisurely pace throughout childhood, in women completing by the age of 30. In later life it may fuse with the sacrum, especially in women.

This brief history of the sacrum and coccyx has considerable importance for osteopaths.

• It is vulnerable to compression perinatally, particularly in a breech presentation.

• It remains in a relatively flexible state throughout childhood and young adulthood.

• In young mothers under 25 years old, the sacrum is flexible. Under 30 years, the coccygeal segments may not be fully ossified. This flexibility seems designed to assist childbirth, but leaves the sacrococcygeal unit vulnerable to compression and molding.

The child who has been born bottom first, or feet first, will often have a very dense feel to the sacrum, and indeed inertia throughout the membranes. The baby will cry and squirm when the sacrum and pelvis are palpated. Sacral compression is much less visible than molding of the cranium, and is easily missed. Failure to recognize and treat it will hinder the reorganization of all the infant's tissues and its mechanisms for health and progress. Cranial strains will stubbornly persist. Function of the diaphragm will be restricted. Strain of the cranial base includes the ethmoid, and both primary and secondary respiration will suffer. The three parts of the innominate bone will be strained and hip dysfunction may result.

Persisting intraosseous compression of the sacrum, with a molded, unforgiving, inflexible feel on palpation, unquestionably underlies many of the problems we see as osteopaths. Fascial drag and inertia of the RTM are often very well compensated – until, much later, a further stress occurs and disturbs these compensations. The 'three diaphragms' (the pelvic floor, respiratory diaphragm and tentorium cerebelli) work together to ensure that circulation and drainage as far away as the cranium is affected. Chronic catarrhal states, endocrine problems, depression, glaucoma and other eye problems are just a few examples. Postnatal 'sacral sag' may be the result of the body's failure to make further compensations. In respiratory problems, we often see sacral extension, and a diaphragm held in exhalation, associated with a cranial base that is locked in extension or an inferior vertical pattern.

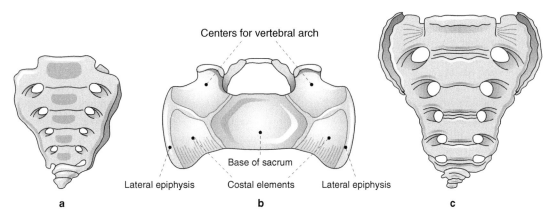

Figure 8.20 Os sacrum. **a:** sacrum at birth. **b:** sacrum seen from above. **c:** sacrum at the age of 25 years.

Treatment approach

Intraosseous strains and compression, as a result of traumatic forces or slow molding, are possible in any bone in the body, particularly in the years of childhood before ossification is complete. Their influence can be felt throughout the body structure and function, and it is therefore of paramount importance that they are recognized and addressed as early as possible. Encourage pregnant patients to bring their babies for checking as soon as possible!

Unification of the enlarging areas of ossified bone occurs in an orderly sequence. Ossification times are a partial guide to the plasticity of a bone receiving treatment; but Dr Wales reminds us that other factors play a part: the dates when the baby starts to raise her head, and to develop the postural muscles necessary for sitting up, arrive much earlier. After this time the myofascial system will start to express the intraosseous and interosseous pattern of the cranial base, from which it is suspended. At any age, much strain and tension can be released from the child's system by attentive treatment. But it becomes increasingly difficult to change the structure after the first few months.

Treatment approaches are best learned from a tutor, hand to hand. In general, W. G. Sutherland's rule applies: 'Know your anatomy, know your mechanism, the rest is easy.' A thorough knowledge and understanding of the principles of 'balanced membranous tension' and the 'fluid drive' are prerequisites.

With these principles in mind, here are a few thoughts:

- Remember the fluidity of bone; this is what molds and unmolds.
- Never exaggerate, or compress; remember what passes through the foramen magnum.
- A compressed occiput is sensitive. Approach slowly, unimaginably gently, and after making a leisurely

acquaintance with the mechanism through contacts elsewhere.

- Keep the mind on the whole, the fingers specific.
- Remember that all the parts of the occiput, and of the other cranial base bones, are adapting to the pattern.
- Remember the role of the RTM, the CNS, the fascia and the three diaphragms, and the pelvis in maintaining the pattern.
- The growth process is our friend. Encourage the parent to watch their babies for periods of increased appetite – you may 'catch the wave' of a growth spurt.

I like to treat infants under 3 months often, if needed perhaps weekly or fortnightly, but being careful not to over-treat in one session as their mechanisms are quick to tire. In children, the importance of the vitality of the individual in producing changes is particularly noticeable. Change can happen quickly in a fundamentally healthy child; but a child who has been seriously compromised by intrauterine stresses or a difficult birth may need fundamental treatment to support the fluid drive that empowers change. Such children need a particularly fluid, patient approach to osseous lesions. Above all, listen to the body – however hard it may be to 'hear' it – and trust the drive for health in the living child.

References

Allen R: Lecture on the condylar parts. Sutherland Cranial College 2001

Arbuckle B E: Scoliosis capitis. JAOA 70, 1988: 131–137, collected in Clinical Cranial Osteopathy, published by Feely R A, Cranial Academy (USA)

Carreiro J: An osteopathic approach to children. Churchill Livingstone, Edinburgh 2003

Frymann V: The collected papers of Viola M. Frymann, D.O. American Academy of Osteopathy, 1998

Handoll N: The osteopathic management of children with Down's syndrome. British Osteopathic Journal 21, 1998: 11–20 (posted on the web at www.cranial.org.uk)

Lay E M: Cranial field. In: Ward R C (ed.) Foundations for osteopathic medicine. Williams and Wilkins, London 1997

Magoun H G: Osteopathy in the cranial field. 3rd edn. Sutherland Cranial Teaching Foundation, Kirksville, Mo. 1976

Standring S: Gray's anatomy. Churchill Livingstone/Elsevier, London 2005

Sutherland W G: Teachings in the science of osteopathy Anne Wales (ed.). Sutherland Cranial Teaching Foundation 1990

Sutherland W G: Contributions of thought. 2nd edn. Ada Strand Sutherland and Anne Wales (eds). Sutherland Cranial Teaching Foundation 1998

Wales A L: in notes of personal tutorial taken by Susan Turner, 1998

AN OSTEOPATHIC APPROACH TO THE NEWBORN AND INFANT

(with adaptation for older children)

Susan Turner

'The inherent forces within the patient's body are more potent and accurate than anything you can safely bring to bear from outside. Let them go to work!' (Sutherland 1990).

This chapter discusses treatment of the neonate and infant, exploring the interrelationship of living anatomy and physiology. The word 'neonate' describes the infant from birth to 30 days, and in this chapter I will refer mainly to the infant at term. Some reference to premature babies will be found on p.208. Where appropriate, adaptations of this osteopathic approach to older children will be described at the end of this section (see p.209).

This section is designed neither to be prescriptive nor to presuppose what the osteopath might find in any individual. It is intended to foster an open listening that awakens the operator to the conditions present in the patient, from the point of view of the expression of the innate wholeness in living beings that is constantly at work to transform all that stands in its way.

Birth and molding

When we approach a newborn infant, she is in the process of recovery from intrauterine molding and labor with its compressive, rotational and perhaps tractional forces. The occipital condyles will often have been compressed into the anterior convergence of the atlas facets. The four parts of the occiput will have shifted position slightly to absorb these forces from above (via the cranial vault) and from below (via the spine and pelvis), and also perhaps from the medial squeezing of the birth canal.

The bones will have folded down, the brain with it, to permit an easier passage in birth. Sutherland (1990) described how the infant's first cry, which also necessitates the first breath, requires vigorous expansion of the thorax as the lungs inflate (see p.52). This fluctuates the cerebrospinal fluid (CSF) in the posterior cranial fossa, as the fluid that was squeezed into the birth canal in labor re-enters the head.

The first breath begins to unlock the atlanto-occipital and cranial compression from the inside. This also lifts the tentorium and with it the cerebellum, thus giving space to the brainstem and fourth ventricle, in whose floor are many physiological centers, including those that govern breathing and heart rate. Then the membranes including the falx cerebri and the tentorium and the CSF together reorganize and reposition the cranial bones. This is made possible since the dural membrane is developmentally continuous with the cranial periosteum. The fluids act on the unfolding process not only of the membranous bones of the vault but also of the four parts of the occiput that form the shape of the foramen magnum. They also act on the three parts of the sphenoid and the two parts of the temporal bones. The actions of suckling, crying and kicking also assist this process by producing a pumping action on the cranial and spinal dural membranes and sacrum via the CSF.

When the falx cerebri and tentorium begin to re-establish involuntary rhythmic motion, the venous sinuses in their folds and borders begin to express rhythmic three-dimensional shape change, providing a pump that allows venous drainage to clear the cerebral edema that often exists for the first 36 hours after birth. This drainage of the venous sinus system allows accessibility of oxygenated blood to the brain, to keep apace with the vastly increased levels of cerebral activity that follow birth. The fluids, membranes and bones can then re-expand and the brain and its ventricles take up their natural space, re-establishing the inherent motility that is an expression of health. Likening the brain to a motor Sutherland (1990, 1998) referred to a process analogous to 'ignition' within the ventricular system, as a key place for the re-initiation of inhalation of the primary respiratory mechanism and the postnatal expansion of the brain.

However, when it comes to osteopathic treatment, though the unfolding of the infant cranium and brain, together with the unlocking of the atlanto-occipital joint, are vital keys to neonatal recovery, it is not necessarily the head that is the first point of therapeutic contact. The head of the newborn is often sensitive and possibly traumatized, so there is good sense in starting by supporting that unfolding from the trunk and periphery. This way, we are setting up a similar cascade of events as happens in nature, where the natural expansion of the thorax and pelvis initiate cranial unfolding from within. This has the advantage that by the time we address the cranium itself, the inherent fluid forces are already at work and come to meet us to support our efforts. In a literal way we are using 'the powers within the patient's body' (Sutherland 1990).

This part of the chapter will describe how we may begin by making contact at the feet, palpating and where appropriate treating, from below upwards, to support the physiological shifts that are in process in the postnatal state. This is not a 'recipe', however, as the conditions that we find in the infant body on palpation will reveal what is required in terms of treatment and its sequence. The sequence described here may take two or perhaps three treatment sessions to complete, as we set the stage for nature to do the real work between sessions. Though each of the areas mentioned here needs to be checked for integrated function, it may be sometimes appropriate to treat only the areas that are the essential key to the unfolding of the body as a whole.

What is described here is applicable, with adaptation, throughout childhood.

When making contact with a newborn infant we have to take into account that we are meeting a being with an eventful history, whose frame of reference, neural wiring and anatomy is in many ways very different from our own. So we need to be careful not to make assumptions based on our adult experience of the world.

The infant is like a traveller who has arrived from another shore and needs to take time to adapt and settle to this new land. In addition she is probably in a process of recovery from that rite of passage that we call birth. The newborn is in a process of integrating dramatic physiological shifts from intrauterine to postnatal life, involving the heart, lungs, digestive, immune and musculoskeletal systems as well as the brain, sensorimotor pathways, cognitive, social and feeling functions. By understanding the particular anatomy and physiology of the infant, an osteopath is in a position to help ease the transition into postnatal life so that this newborn human may fulfil her potential for life present and future. The anatomy of the newborn needs to be seen not so much as a structure but as a process in continuity with the prenatal life as well as with the postnatal potential for what the child is yet to become.

The neonate neuromuscular skeletal system

At term, the infant only has 20% of her mature quota of muscle fibres. These are attached only to the periosteum; it is not until 2 to 3 months of age that tendinous attachments form through the periosteum to the bone itself (Carreiro 2003). On palpation the bones of the neonate more resemble periosteal sacs in which the cortex 'floats' than at any

other time in life. This particular quality has relevance for the way we approach osteopathic treatment. Sutherland's reference (1990) to bone as a 'fluid' is at its most literal at the neonatal stage. In health the bones of a neonate are vibrant with metabolic activity, breathing within themselves with a quality of resiliency.

For the last 3 months before birth and in the 1st year of the neonatal period, almost all red blood cell formation is by hemopoiesis in the bone marrow, which has been active since the 4th month of gestation. The bones have gradually taken over from the liver and spleen, which began hemopoiesis in the fifth gestational week. At birth, every bone is hemopoietic and it is only at the end of the 1st year that the fingers and toes cease to be so. The bone marrow is also active forming lymphoid cells at birth which will evolve into T and B lymphocytes, essential to the infant's immunity throughout life (Netter 1987).

The skeleton (Fig. 8.21) of the newborn has a much higher proportion of cartilage to bone than the older child. The bony components have not yet developed the tuberosities and moldings that they will have later in childhood through the stimulation of gravity and muscle activity. The most visible examples of these are the ischial tuberosities, greater trochanters and mastoid processes.

The development of the joints in utero and in childhood depends on movement, involving the stimulatory forces of both intermittent compression and tension. Continuous compression however produces bone atrophy. This is one reason why, osteopathically, we need to be sure that all parts of the body are free to shift and move in relation to one another. In order to grow, the bone forms at the periosteal surface and reabsorbs at the endosteal surface. This function of continuous remodelling of bone activates in the first year. The annual rate of bone renewal in the first 2 years is 50% as compared with only 5% in the adult. The postnatal stimulus of intermittent tension and gravitational compression, together with new movements, promotes especially active musculoskeletal growth in the first 2 years of life. This illustrates what a potent period these first 2 years are for osteopathic treatment. In periods of rapid bone growth the system is primed for change so that it is also receptive to making dramatic corrective changes. Rapid growth periods tend to make the joints vulnerable because of the high level of vascularity in the growth plates. We see this again in the growth spurt of teenage years. But it is also true that it is in periods of rapid growth that osteopathic treatment can be at its most effective for positive therapeutic change. For this and other reasons, potential problems can be averted by appropriate osteopathic care at this early stage of life. Sutherland often quoted Walt Whitman's words 'As the twig is bent so doth

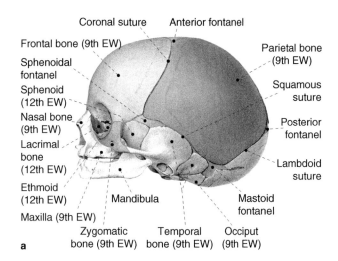

Coronal suture
Anterior fontanel
Frontal bone (9th EW)
Parietal bone (9th EW)
Sphenoidal fontanel
Sphenoid (12th EW)
Squamous suture
Nasal bone (9th EW)
Lacrimal bone (12th EW)
Posterior fontanel
Lambdoid suture
Ethmoid (12th EW)
Mandibula
Mastoid fontanel
Maxilla (9th EW)
Zygomatic bone (9th EW)
Temporal bone (9th EW)
Occiput (9th EW)

a

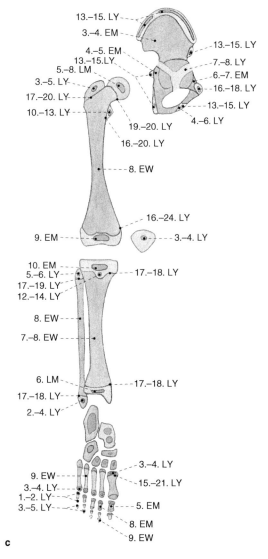

13.–15. LY
3.–4. EM
4.–5. EM
13.–15.LY
5.–8. LM
13.–15. LY
7.–8. LY
6.–7. EM
3.–5. LY
17.–20. LY
10.–13. LY
16.–18. LY
13.–15. LY
4.–6. LY
19.–20. LY
16.–20. LY
8. EW
16.–24. LY
9. EM
3.–4. LY
10. EM
5.–6. LY
17.–18. LY
17.–19. LY
12.–14. LY
8. EW
7.–8. EW
6. LM
17.–18. LY
17.–18. LY
2.–4. LY
3.–4. LY
9. EW
15.–21. LY
3.–4. LY
1.–2. LY
3.–5. LY
5. EM
8. EM
9. EW

c

Talus 7. month of embryonic life
Calcaneus 5.–6. month of embryonic life
Navicular 4. year of life
Cuboid 10. month of embryonic life
Middle cuneiform bone 2.–3. year of life
Intermediate cuneiform bone 3.–4. year of life
Lateral cuneiform bone 12. year of life

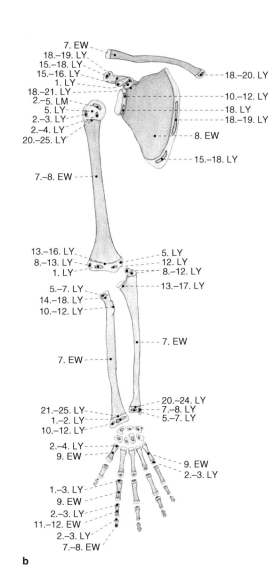

7. EW
18.–19. LY
15.–18. LY
15.–16. LY
1. LY
18.–21. LY
2.–5. LM
5. LY
2.–3. LY
2.–4. LY
20.–25. LY
18.–20. LY
10.–12. LY
18. LY
18.–19. LY
8. EW
15.–18. LY
7.–8. EW
13.–16. LY
8.–13. LY
1. LY
5. LY
12. LY
8.–12. LY
13.–17. LY
5.–7. LY
14.–18. LY
10.–12. LY
7. EW
7. EW
7. EW
7. EW
20.–24. LY
7.–8. LY
5.–7. LY
21.–25. LY
1.–2. LY
10.–12. LY
2.–4. LY
9. EW
9. EW
2.–3. LY
1.–3. LY
9. EW
2.–3. LY
11.–12. EW
2.–3. LY
7.–8. EW

b

Scaphoid 3.–6. month of life
Lunate 3.–6. year of life
Trapezium 3.–8. year of life
Trapezoid 3.–7. year of life

Pisiform 8.–12. year of life
Triquetrum 1.–4. year of life
Hamate 2.–5. month of life
Capitate 2.–4. month of life

Figure 8.21 Cartilaginous and bony components of the infant skeleton. Appearance of growth centers, closing of epiphyses: **a**: cranium; **b**: upper extremity; **c**: lower extremity. *EW*, week of embryonic life, *EM*, month of embryonic life; *LM*, month of life, *LY*, year of life. With permission, Sobotta: Atlas der Anatomie des Menschen. Publisher: R. Putz and R. Pabst, 21st edn. Elsevier/Urban & Fischer, Munich/Jena 2000

the tree incline'. By attending to the young sapling we support the potential for the mature tree to grow strong and straight.

Though the premature infant is hypermobile, the joints of the term infant have a relatively limited range of movement compared with a 3-year-old, since in a relaxed position the term neonate tends towards the flexed fetal position, slowly balancing extensor tone over the first year of life (Carreiro 2003). As mentioned above, only 20% of the adult muscle fibres are present at birth and no muscle tension should be evident, whether on palpation or on pulling the infant from supine to sitting. Areas of segmental paraspinal muscle tension may, among other reasons, indicate viscerosomatic irritation; for example from the heart (T2–T5 on the left), stomach (T5–T9 on the left) or lung (T2–T5), because the infant neuromuscular system is much more sensitive to afferent visceral influences than the adult. This very sensitivity necessitates care not to overtreat osteopathically as a little input goes a long way.

In the newborn infant limb movements are mainly reflex, as they are not yet under cortical control. The upper limb is more advanced than the lower limb. The development of volitional motor patterns is dependent on the development of motor pathways and myelination of the corticobulbar and corticospinal tracts. The development of the synapses of the brain in utero and the myelination of the long tracts begin just before birth and will continue throughout the growing years. The brain synapses continue to develop every time new learning takes place all through life.

The neuromuscular junctions are immature at birth so neuromuscular transmission is often unpredictable. At this stage the motor units overlap so that a muscle fibre or group may be innervated by more than one axon, which can make coordination between muscle groups chaotic. These two factors can particularly cause problems with the respiratory muscles in the first year. With maturation, the neuromuscular system is progressively remodelled until each muscle or muscle group will receive input from one axon only. Correspondingly on the sensory side, in infancy and early childhood pain is poorly localized and experienced as diffuse irritation or ache over a wide area, and will only become more specific as the nervous system prunes and matures.

The principle of balanced tension

The balance point

In *Contributions of thought* Sutherland (1998) writes how he learnt from Dr. Still, the founder of osteopathy, to engage the balance point from which the innate potency and intelligence of the body's self-corrective mechanism would bring about correction of a strain pattern from within. This approach has come to be called balanced ligamentous tension (BLT) when applied to the ligamentous-articular joints of the body and balanced membranous tension (BMT) when applied to the membranous-articular mechanism of the cranium, sacrum and interosseous membranes of the upper and lower limbs. Balanced fascial tension (BFT) uses the same principle when treating fascial planes and envelopes (e.g. of organs). Sutherland (1998) wrote: 'The ligaments, not the muscles are the natural agencies for this purpose of correcting the relations and positions of joints. Dr. Still's application of the technique is the gentle exaggeration of the lesion that allows the natural agencies to draw the bones into place. Dr. Still has taken my hand into his and allowed me to feel the lesion as it was being exaggerated and then as the natural agencies pulled the bones back into place.' He then went on to say that there is reason for applying this same principle within the cranium on the finer sutural mechanism, the main difference being a matter of scale. When working with the ligamentous articular mechanisms of the body we apply ourselves more like a mechanic; in the finer sphere of the cranium we apply ourselves more like a watchmaker where the reciprocal tension membrane, the CSF and the brain (the motor of respiration) are the agents of correction. We can see here how the 'gentle exaggeration of the lesion', which was Dr. Still's indirect approach, led to the development of the osteopathic inherent force techniques, such as fascial unwinding, functional technique and in Dr. Sutherland's case, balanced ligamentous/membranous tension. It is important to understand here that the term exaggeration means allowing the expression of the strained tissues only up to the point where all the connective tissue forces of compression, torsion, shear, and so on, balance each other out to a neutral point. It does not mean exaggerating the lesion strain beyond the balance point up to an indirect motion barrier; that is a principle that applies to fascial unwinding but not to balanced ligamentous, membranous or fascial tension. To work with a newborn infant safely it is necessary to have a clear palpatory sense of the balance point.

Balanced ligamentous tension (BLT)

The sequence of this corrective approach entails the following phases:

- Engaging the ligaments, membranes or fascia by placing that part in a position of ease, or simply matching the tone in the tissues.
- Supporting the inherent search of the joint ligaments for the balance point. This is the point at which the lesion

strain fully expresses itself and finds a harmonious balance within it.

- The tissues pause at a point of balanced tension. Here all connective tissue tensions are equally balanced in all directions so that there is a sense of poise and balance in a neutral field. The osteopath now simply supports the tissues and waits. This is the state in which there is minimum resistance to the self-correcting intelligence, to which the fulcrum within the state of balanced tension has aligned itself.

- Very often **a spontaneous** action such as a deep breath, an involuntary muscular movement or a strong inherent fluid drive in the tissues will come in to shift the balance fulcrum into a resolution phase. This involves a sense of the ligaments realigning the joint from within, concurrent with a sense of fluid reorganization of the tissues.

- A sense of health and integration returns to the tissues palpable as warmth, expansion, tissue breathing and rhythmicity, midline organization (whether on a limb or on the craniospinal axis). In the case of infants and children the bones are so fluid that a sense of remolding within the bones themselves often accompanies this resolution: in other words, engaging with the ligaments often addresses their continuity with the periosteum, which also facilitates intraosseous remolding.

The term 'engaging the tissues' means supporting the intelligent process that is always potentially at work. When an articulation is in a position of strain, the ligaments search for the balanced state from which the self-corrective process is able to realign the joint. In many cases, when our hands can match the tone quality of those tissues, this will be enough to activate them towards this healing cycle. To initiate this process, if we are receptive to the tissues in question they will normally guide our hands towards their position of ease. Sometimes, however, we need to help create the conditions for them to make the correction. This may require either giving more space by holding the joint components apart by just a hair's breadth, or by approximating (i.e. compressing a little), so as to paradoxically give the ligaments more slack, and therefore room to maneuver. Sometimes, also, we need to actively support the components of the joint in the direction towards which the ligaments are naturally moving it. The aim of 'engagement' is to enliven the natural tendency for the ligaments, membranes or fascia to explore for the balanced state; that is, that point from which there is minimum resistance to the inherent self-corrective impulse that is always at work within the body. It is also the state that expresses all components of the lesion but in which all connective tissue tensions balance each other equally in all directions. In

essence, having engaged the tissues, we support them in the direction they are seeking to move until they become poised in a state of balance and also ease. Then we wait and support this point of BLT until the tissue fulcrum shifts and the ligaments and fluids realign the joint. This is accompanied by a feeling of health and organization returning to the tissues. One caution that is often cited about using the indirect (exaggeration) approach on an infant applies to the occipital condyles, where insensitive exaggeration of the lesion that goes beyond the balance point can damage delicate neural structures that may already be compromised. This is why we need to have a precise appreciation of the balance point. This is also why, when assisting the decompression of the occipital condyles of the infant cranium, that direct disengagement is generally advised.

Wherever we are working in the body, it is important that we don't think of ourselves as actually 'doing a technique', but rather entering into a conversation with the tissues so that we are receptive to what the innate self-corrective mechanism of the body intelligence is seeking to do to resolve any strained situation. It is also worth remembering that the term 'exaggeration' is a misnomer since it means supporting the expression of the strain pattern to the balance point only, not exaggerating the strain beyond the balance point (Wales 1986–2004).

Balanced membranous tension (BMT)

In the membranous-articular sphere of the cranium, it is the dural 'sickles' that guide and limit the involuntary motion of the cranial bones, just as the ligaments do in the joints of the trunk and periphery.

The falx cerebri and tentorium cerebelli, which are continuous with the internal periosteum of all the bones of the neurocranium, function like an interosseous membrane for the modified sphere of the cranium.

In a well-balanced state, the involuntary motion of the whole cranium, the craniosacral axis, and by extension, the fascial system of the whole body, are organized around an 'automatic shifting suspension fulcrum', also called the Sutherland fulcrum. This functions towards the anterior end of the straight sinus, where the falces and tentorium meet. It minutely shifts position along the straight sinus, in synchrony with the shape change of the whole dural continuum, with each phase of cranial primary respiratory flexion and extension.

The intracranial and intraspinal dura function like a 'reciprocal tension membrane' (RTM) (Sutherland 1990), integrating the involuntary motion of all the bones of the cranium and also the sacrum as its lower pole of attachment. Because of the RTM all osseous components within the system move interdependently. All components need to be free to shift in relation to the Sutherland fulcrum. If even one bone is not free to shift it will act as a fixed fulcrum. When this happens, all other components of this mobile reciprocal tension system adapt their motion pattern around the fixed fulcrum, and the Sutherland fulcrum loses its free automatic shifting modality and also becomes functionally displaced.

Strain patterns that occur anywhere in the craniosacral axis will be palpable by their alteration of three dimensional shape, loss of tissue resiliency, and by their distortion of normal, biphasic symmetrical motion and midline organization. This is so whether the problem is in the sphenobasilar junction, within the sutures or is intraosseous; for example, in the condylar parts of the occiput.

The RTM, together with the CSF and the brain, 'the motor of primary respiration' are the 'natural agencies' of correction of the cranial bones (Sutherland 1998). The corrective principle of balanced membranous tension is essentially the same as balanced ligamentous tension, although on a much finer scale. We see a parallel situation in the osteopathic lesion of the cranium to that which we see in the ligamentous articular (joint) mechanism of the body as a whole. Within any distortion of shape or motion pattern, the membranes carry this pattern of strain, shifting the 'normal' fulcrum towards the area of the strain.

'Within the strain there is a point of balanced membranous tension. This is a fulcrum point, a relative point of stillness around which all the forces are gathered. When we bring all these forces into focus it goes through a stillpoint, a fulcrum point, a moment of stillness and then the fulcrum shifts back towards the so-called 'normal' pattern for that individual – towards the Sutherland Fulcrum. You have a correction for that particular day. Through this process, we are shifting the fulcrums within the cerebrospinal fluid and in the RTM' (Becker 1976).

To engage the principle of balanced membranous tension, the osteopath supports the motion pattern and three dimensional shape that the cranium most easily takes up. Torsion, side-bending, and so on, each have their characteristic shape. This is the external expression of the action and shape of the brain and the RTM within. Include the CSF in the picture. In the words of Magoun (1951): 'Allow the fluctuation of the fluid to guide the membrane to the point of balance.' This engages a refinement of the balance point, which is as far as possible from any motion barrier in any direction. At this point of balanced stillness within the membrane and the fluid, the system is at its most aligned to the innate therapeutic potency that is always present.

A whisper in the fluid subtly shifts the balance fulcrum, and then the membrane begins to reorganize, taking the bones with it. Freer biphasic motion is palpable through all tissue layers, bone, membrane, CNS, CSF, with less distinction between the layers than before. This effect is palpable throughout the body. Because the inherent therapeutic potency has been retuned by going through a BMT cycle, if any true sutural restrictions are still present, they will emerge more clearly than before and be receptive to resolution through fluid drive; that is, direction of the potency of the CSF or 'V' spread.

Just as the point of BMT is refined by acknowledging the potency of the CSF, so also is the therapeutic fluid drive maneuver enhanced by acknowledging the search of the sutural membranes for their balance point.

To release a suture or intraosseous strain through a fluid drive, the fingers are placed aside the suture, gently spreading it. The other hand directs a fluid impulse from the longest opposite diagonal position available. If a restriction is present there will be a sense of turbulence as the fluid drive meets the barrier. As this happens the palpating fingers may be aware of the sutural membrane squirming in the search for a balance point, as the suture expresses any shear, or any other pattern that is present. The potency of the CSF works most effectively when the strained suture is at its point of BMT. To quote Harold Magoun 'the cerebrospinal fluid is attracted to the field of the lesion' (Magoun 1951).

With regard to infants and children up to the age of 7 years, it is especially important to work within the balance point and never to exaggerate the pattern beyond it.

Position of the child

We need to be flexible when working with newborns, infants and children. Often we treat the child in a supine position on the treatment table, but other positions may be useful as well. It may be appropriate to have a parent close by. For example, mother and osteopath may sit opposite each other with the baby lying on a cushion between the two (Fig. 8.22a). The child can see her mother well, which will give her a good sense of security. This position makes it easy for the osteopath to treat the pelvis, thorax and cranium. It may also be useful to treat the baby in the arms of the mother; for example when being breastfed (Fig. 8.22b). It is also possible to treat the infant sitting on the practitioner's lap (Fig.8.22c; the photograph shows treatment of the diaphragm and sternum. This handhold can also be adapted for treatment of the umbilicus and abdomen).

Centering

Before you initiate a palpatory dialogue with your patient, it is important to just take a few moments of preparation. This

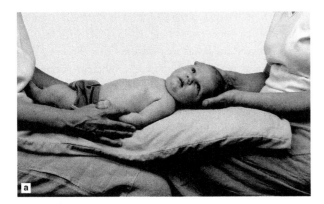

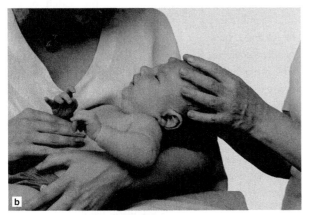

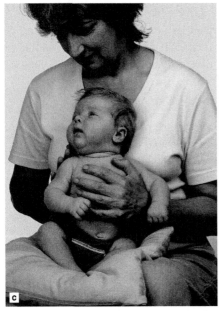

Figure 8.22 Different positions of the child in treatment. **a:** on a cushion between mother and osteopath; **b:** on the arm of the mother; **c:** treatment on the lap of the osteopath.
With permission, Karsten Franke, Hamburg

centering or grounding, will help to place you in the best possible state to expand the potential for sharpened perception.

The success of treatment is dependent on taking a little time to center and attune to the patient before engaging in palpation. Becker (1997) offers us steps to take to help find the mental attitude that will open our palpatory awareness, attuning us to the patient. His words, 'Accept the living mechanism in yourself and the patient. Life is always trying to express health', refer to the same living mechanism that breathes both patient and practitioner. This thought brings to me a sense of reposing within the breath of life and being supported by it.

To quote Becker (1997) again: 'the body is wiser than you are'. He sees the practitioner as assistant to the patient's 'inner physician'. This is practical advice, because placing oneself in this way allows for receptivity to the 'innate intelligence' within the patient's physiology. An approach that is too intent on 'doing' can inhibit the expression of self-healing in the patient's tissues. This may bring us to enquire, not only on what level the child's anatomy and physiology needs to be addressed, but also how her being seeks to be met. We need to find the interface where the patient's system is comfortable to be in communication with us. We could begin by sensing from our peripheral awareness what physical and environmental space the child naturally occupies. For example, does it feel as if the infant is comfortable to be mentally embraced at her skin, or about a meter around it? Often the newborn will not yet be fully identified with her physical body, so it is as if the metaphorical space in which the child needs to be held is as wide as the horizon, or even as vast as the starry universe. Finding the patient's natural symbolic dimension can make all the difference to the way the physical tissues receive our hands, and how the hands tune to more subtle factors (Jealous 1986–2005). By aligning our approach to the innate physiological intent towards health that is within the child we will be more effective than if we stay inflexibly with a plan or routine. It is helpful, however, to have an adaptable routine within which we remain constantly open to the needs of the patient's system.

A possible treatment sequence for the whole body

Having completed a full examination we are ready to approach treatment, but the process of gaining understanding continues as we treat because it is as the body both reveals and lets go of its strain patterns that it tells its full story. In treatment, although we may be addressing specific areas, it is important that the whole patient is encompassed in our awareness at all times.

The feet

Many infants are receptive to being greeted through contact with the feet so that they can initially register our presence and our touch without intrusion, taking time to get to know us. Starting our treatment at the feet we can gain much information here about the system as a whole, by taking time to sense how this infant would like to be met by us and by offering support in a safe space.

Positional talipes, bowed tibia or varus knees are often telltale signs of the way the infant lay in utero, and because of the pliability of the tissues at this stage, they often respond well to the appropriate osteopathic treatment. A certain number of cases will resolve spontaneously before the age of 3 years, but others will need osteopathic treatment.

Treatment of the feet

The child lies supine; you stand by the treatment table. The child may also lie on her mother's lap. Gently playing with the feet (Fig. 8.23), and moving the ankles into dorsiflexion, plantarflexion and circumduction, may reveal any anomalies or unequal fascial tensions that may have resulted from the way that the legs and feet were folded in utero.

In addition, the degree to which the legs and feet express primary respiratory motion (PRM) is revealing. Where there is poor expression of PRM in the feet we need to determine whether this is a situation affecting the body as a whole or just the lower half, in which case there may be tensions in the diaphragm and pelvis.

Please refer to p.209 for the adaptation of an osteopathic approach to the feet for older children.

The fibula

Fulford (1982) observed that when the first breath had not fully expanded the thorax and re-awakened the PRM after birth, the fibulae may express a 'wooden' quality. This may indicate that the infant may not have made the energetic shifts appropriate to postnatal life. Fulford described an energetic lemniscus (figure of eight) passing round the upper body, crossing over at the xyphoid and descending down the left fibula to return up through the right one. The left fibula is commonly strained at birth as it is dragged over the anterior angle of the maternal lumbosacral junction in descent.

When the fibula is in a position of strain at its articular ends and on the interosseous membrane, the lower limb exerts fascial drag on the hip, pelvis and diaphragm. This can indirectly influence the activity of the autonomic nervous system via the sympathetic chain ganglia that lie adjacent to the costovertebral junctions. The fibula like all infant bones should feel alive, resilient and 'breathing'. It should also feel aligned with the tibia. If on palpation the fibula expresses a hard quality, it may be in a position of strain in relation to the tibia and the connecting interosseous membrane. Either

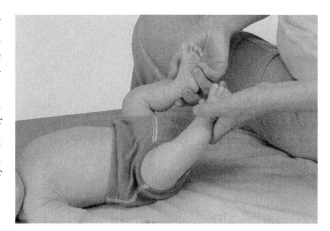

Figure 8.23 Testing foot mobility.
With permission, Karsten Franke, Hamburg

its proximal or distal end may be in an anterior position. The interosseous membrane between the tibia and fibula is part of the core fascia of the budding embryonic limb; close to it run the main arteries, veins and lymph vessels. When this membrane is sheared or in strain, it also interferes with venous and lymphatic return from the foot.

The tibia and fibula together form the ankle 'mortise and tenon' joint with the talus. The ankle mortise holds the talus so that it can function as a hinge joint. This enables the talus to support the developing arches of the foot. When, through tibiofibular strain, the ankle mortise is widened, the talus is unsupported and the tibiotalar joint functions then as a universal joint, so that there is insufficient tone in the ankle for the tarsal arches to develop (Wales 1986–2004). This is one of the factors in the development of flat feet if the situation is not resolved early in life. The tarsal arches do not develop until 3 years old, but in treating neonates we are thinking preventively so that the infants can fulfil their potential and lay the foundations for integrated future growth.

So for the functional integrity of the foot, knee, hip and trunk, the fibula needs to be aligned in its appropriate relationship to the interosseous membrane and tibia.

Treatment of the fibula

The child lies supine; you stand or sit to the side. Take each end of the fibula between the thumb and index finger and support the two ends towards the direction that the interosseous membrane guides the fibula (Fig. 8.24). Bear in mind the totality of the infant at the same time, thereby meeting the infant as she needs to be met within the treatment.

In approaching the fibula, it helps to hold the mental image of the bone as a periosteal sac in which its cortex floats. The periosteum of the fibula is continuous with the interosseous membrane, which in turn is continuous with

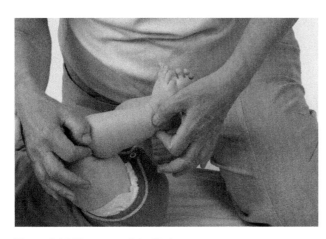

Figure 8.24 Treatment of the fibula.
With permission, Karsten Franke, Hamburg

the tibial periosteum. Another helpful image is to acknowledge the hydrophilic collagenous quality of the bone. This mental shift makes us more aware of the connective tissues (i.e. ligaments, membranes, periostium, etc.) as the guides of the osseous structure. It allows the fluid dynamic within the living bone to become more foreground in our awareness. We could ask the question: does it breathe? Is there a feeling of fluidity equally distributed throughout the whole bone? Or do we get an impression of unequal motion? Maybe one end feels dry, maybe the whole bone feels dry; or is it twisted forward or back at one end or the other? So whatever condition is found, support that fibula, matching the tone in the tissues with both your awareness and your hands.

The words, 'take it where it wants to go' may be a useful self-instruction here. In this way, you are supporting the search of the interosseous membrane to find the position of BMT. This is the state and position where all the conflicting pulls, compressions and shears are neutralized and equally balanced in all directions at a point of stillness. This is what is referred to as the 'balance point' or the point of balanced membranous tension. When the osseous elements are supported by their connective tissues in a 'neutral field' there is minimum resistance to the inherent self-corrective impulse that arises from within the living body. Often at this neutral point, a spontaneous deep breath will shift the fulcrum that suspends the joint or bone, and allow it to reseat in a more functional relationship within the body continuum. In the case of an infant, a sudden kick, wriggle, or cry will often be the agent of the shift. Support the fibula at the balance point for the interosseous membrane until a sense of fluid drive comes into the membrane and fills the fibula so that it starts to feel like a bag of fluid as it shifts its position into one of equal suspension at both ends. This will also have the positive effect of rebalancing the ankle mortise and be of

benefit to the developing foot and also the knee. When the fibula has balanced, changes may be observed in the fascia lata of the thigh and up into the pelvis, hip and even the diaphragm. By addressing the fibula, the positive shifts that have been made in the ankle and the knee will also have prepared the hip for our attention. For an osteopathic approach to the knee in an older child, please refer to p.210.

The hip

In the initial examination we may perhaps have already noted some functional asymmetries of hip movement. The infant acetabulum is formed by the cartilaginous meeting of the ilium, ischium and pubis. These fuse normally at the age of 13 to 18, but may not fuse completely until 25 years of age (Fig. 8.25). When addressing the hip of a newborn we need to keep in mind the fibrocartilagenous ring that deepens the socket and the capsular, ischiofemoral and iliofemoral Y ligaments, as well as the balance between the 'rotator cuff' and muscles of the leg.

The innominate is vulnerable to intraosseous strain from chronic intrauterine compression, difficult labor (particularly breech deliveries) or later traumatic events. Intraosseous strains can alter the shape of the acetabulum. This will determine the angle of orientation of the femur and the tensions in the origin and insertion of the 'rotator cuff' muscles of the hip and hip capsule. Still (1986) wrote about the effect a twist in the hip could have on the blood and nerve supply to the femur. If we look at the ligaments of the hip we see that a nutrient artery to the femur travels in the teres ligament between the center of the acetabulum and the fovea capitis of the femur. Other important arteries are the median femoral circumflex artery and the obturator artery, which can also be compromised by positional strains in the hip and give rise to ischemic changes in the femoral head and epiphyseal plate. Congenital hip dysplasia is the most obvious problem related to intraosseous strains of the hip joint in the neonate, but in the absence of an overt problem we need to be alert to intraosseous strains as a preventive measure. In my experience later development of Legg-Calve-Perthes hip (see Ch.15, Perthes disease), irritable hip or slipped capital epiphysis (see Ch.15) very often appear to show a pre-existing intraosseous strain both within the innominate and in the femoral neck. The teres ligament is the functional fulcrum of the hip and it is helpful to keep this in mind when supporting the realignment of the hip joint.

Strains in the hip and pelvis can also give rise to compensatory changes in the developing spine and thorax where they may interfere with thoracic respiration and venous and lymphatic return through the posterior part of the diaphragm.

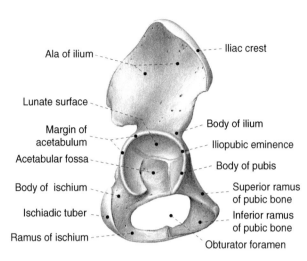

Figure 8.25 The innominate bone of a 6-year-old child. The three parts, ilium, ischium and pubis meet in a Y-shaped cartilaginous union at the acetabulum and fuse at the age of 13–25. With permission, Sobotta: Atlas der Anatomie des Menschen. Publisher: R. Putz and R. Pabst, 21st edn. Elsevier/Urban & Fischer, Munich/Jena 2000

The function of the hip influences the mechanical balance of the whole leg, and therefore the development of gait. Carreiro (2003) observed also that the myofascial continuity between the hip and abdominal pelvic cavity can associate hip strains with reflex visceral dysfunction and vice versa.

It is worth noting that placing babies in a prone position when awake enables the development of the hip extensors and external rotators, thereby preparing them to crawl. This also stimulates the suboccipital muscles to normalize occipital squama asymmetries, so countering plagiocephalic tendencies. The current thinking on sudden infants death syndrome (SIDS) encourages mothers to place babies on their backs to sleep, but it is not stated clearly enough that, when they are awake, they should frequently be placed on their front to assist symmetrical development of the cranium and spine.

Treatment of the hip joint

We can address the hip of the newborn in any position: supine, supported sitting or side-lying. It is helpful to be adaptable about the position in which we treat.

Taking the supine position as an example, with you sitting to the side of the treatment table. Place the middle finger of one hand under the sacrum to gently stabilize it while the other hand surrounds the upper femur (Fig. 8.26).

Feel the relationship of the femoral neck and head to the acetabulum and sense through the piriformis muscle and related tissues to the sacrum. Gently explore for the position of ease by subtly changing the position of the femur until

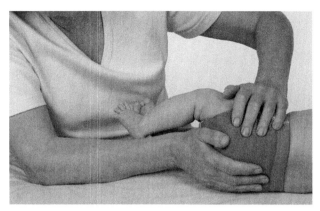

Figure 8.26 Treating the hipjoint.
With permission, Karsten Franke, Hamburg

there is a feeling of balanced tension within the hip capsule. Keep in mind the image of the tripartite acetabulum, the joint capsule and the femur as three fluid sacs organized around the teres ligament as the functional fulcrum of the hip. Wait for fluid activity to take the ligaments to the balance point followed by spontaneous reorganization of the joint. Throughout this process your hands and consciousness support and match the tone and tempo of the tissues. If tissues do not engage in this search, then this is a good indication that either this part of the body is not ready for change, that the primary problem is elsewhere or that there is an intraosseous strain between the three components of the acetabulum. If tissues do not respond, be also alert to the possibility of hip pathology.

For an adaptation of an approach to the hip for older children, please refer to p.211.

Treatment of intraosseous innominate strains

With the child supine or side-lying, stand or sit to the side of the treatment table, contacting the upper femur, ilium, ischium and pubis together, with both hands, with your thumbs crossed over the region of the greater trochanter for orientation to the acetabulum (Fig. 8.27).

To support the resolution and remolding of intraosseous innominate strains that have distorted the Y-shaped cartilaginous union in the acetabulum, it helps once again to acknowledge them as three periosteal sacs filled with fluid in relation to the periosteal sac of the femur and the articular capsule of the hip.

Observe any fluctuant movement within the tripartite innominate until the fluid fluctuation within the osseous elements organizes itself around a fulcrum, concurrent with a sense of stillness. When a more organized pattern of inherent motion returns and unifies the expression of involuntary motion within the three parts of the innominate, the stage is

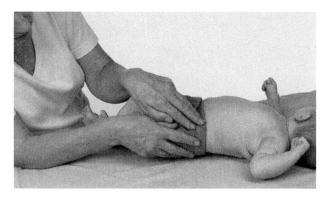

Figure 8.27 Treating an intraosseous strain of the innominate bone.
With permission, Karsten Franke, Hamburg

set for the body to continue the corrective process (modified from the approach of Jealous 1986–2005). It is always useful to address both innominates. Even if only one side had been strained, when the strained side is realigned, the opposite side will have to readapt to this change also.

The pelvis and sacrum

Wales, who was a student of Sutherland, would advise that before approaching the head directly, it is often helpful to prepare the resolution of cranial membranous-articular strains in the newborn by releasing bilateral structures from the midline; that is, from the spine and the sacrum. The release of the sacrum from the pinching of the ilia frees it to respond to the movement of thoracic breathing. It also allows the sacrum to respond to primary respiratory motion so that it is better able to function as the mobile lower pole of attachment of the reciprocal tension membrane. It now has the freedom to shift on the continuum of the spinal and cranial dura.

The neonate's sacrum is largely cartilaginous, and its five segments are separated by inter-vertebral discs. It is therefore common for intraosseous strains to occur between the segments from intrauterine molding or from traumatic forces during labor and in early life (see Ch.8, Intraosseous strains). Embryologically, the S1 and S2 segments are derived from the induction of the notochord. The S3 segment and below, including the coccyx, are derived from the primitive streak. S2 articulates with the ilium and so allies itself to the gravitational support function of the spine. Below S2, the segments are suspended and are more associated with the coccygeal tail, which is completely cartilaginous at birth. It is interesting to note on palpation a difference of quality between the articular area of S2 and the suspended quality of the lower segments S3–S5. Although the S1 and S2 segments ossify by the age of 6 to 8 years, the lower segments do not complete their ossification until the age of 25 (see p.178). If

we perceive the sacrum, holding this mental image of a segmented cartilaginous structure within its periosteal sac, our palpatory awareness will be open to the possible intraosseous activity patterns within and between the individual sacral segments.

The neonatal sacroiliac joints are C-shaped with the apex facing anteriorly. The sacral surface is concave and formed of hyaline cartilage, the iliac surface is convex and formed of fibrocartilage. In the neonate the surfaces are smooth but they gradually roughen with weight bearing and markedly so at puberty (Carreiro 2003). All the adult sacroiliac ligaments are present at term, although they will remodel with the eventual stimulus of weight bearing from sitting and then standing. The neonatal pelvis is more vertical than the adult and shows no gender difference. The sacrum sits higher in the ilia until the child walks, when it descends between them.

The forces of intrauterine molding and labor can exert compressive strains upon the sacrum and coccyx, wedging the sacrum tightly between the ilia and limiting its nutation and counternutation with involuntary flexion and extension. The involuntary motion of the sacrum has a reciprocal relationship with that of the cranium through the intraspinal dura. Also the anterior and posterior longitudinal spinal ligaments link it to the periosteum of the basiocciput, and the ligamentous chain of the supraspinous and interspinous ligaments with the occipital squama. Because of this connection, fixation and side bending or rotational strains of the sacrum may restrain the natural postnatal unfolding of the cranium. Wales (1986–2004) related an observation of Sutherland that upward tractional forces such as exerted during forceps may draw the sacrum superiorly within the pelvis so that the child delays sitting because of discomfort. Nowadays we could say the same about ventouse delivery. Pelvic strains may also cause local visceral problems like constipation because of disturbance to the neural, vascular and lymphatic relationship to the involved tissues. Still (1986) observed that delayed bladder control could be associated with strains in the pubic symphysis. Particular attention should be paid to the examination of all the components of the pelvis, hips, lower spine and pelvic floor following breech delivery.

Freeing the sacrum from restriction by the ilia

To release the motion of the sacrum so that it can move freely between the ilia, we have a very simple maneuver that is useful beyond expectations. That is to hold the two ilia of the supine infant with the fingers wrapped around the medial border of the ilium, and extremely gently hold the ilia laterally, just to the degree where the sacroiliac ligaments give their first hint of resistance (Fig. 8.28).

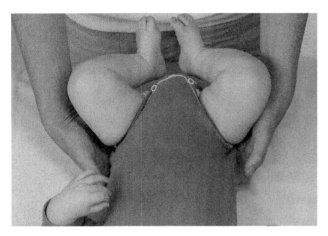

Figure 8.28 Freeing the sacrum from restriction by the ilia. With permission, Karsten Franke, Hamburg

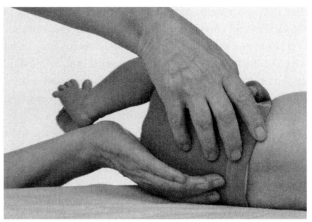

Figure 8.29 Unilateral treatment of the iliosacral joint. The infant usually lies fully supine. Here he is positioned on his side to show the practioner's hand position. With permission, Karsten Franke, Hamburg

The difference between too much and too little lateral distraction might be that of a hair's breadth. The image of 'giving space' is a helpful one here. In doing this, we are waking up the ligamentous sheets of the sacroiliac area, by alerting them and also providing a little extra room to maneuver. The ligaments will begin to explore for the balance point, the neutral field. Initially this feels as if the ligaments are beginning to exaggerate any pattern of strain that may be present. The paradox here is that in fully expressing the distortion pattern the tissues are seeking the point where all the stresses and pulls, compressions and shears balance themselves out in a neutral field within the composite pattern of the pelvis. In expressing the strain pattern they find a balance within it. Having found the point of balance, gently hold the balance, supporting the innominates until the fulcrum shifts within the pelvis. As the tissues release there may be an impression under the hands of more space, so the ilia move more freely and symmetrically on the sacrum. The sacrum also responds by taking on a softer and more motile quality with more ample expression of primary respiratory flexion and extension.

If this resolves on one side only, then we may work unilaterally holding the sacrum with the middle finger of one hand, holding the innominate on the side of the restriction with the other hand (Fig. 8.29). Sense what support these tissues need in their effort to free themselves, with the attention more on the ligaments than on the bones. If lateral distraction does not work, perhaps very gentle approximation will be what is required for that restricted relationship to unhitch itself. If this is still resistant, this pattern may require resolution in another area of the body, or may be due to an intraosseous strain in the three parts of the innominate or between the five parts of the sacrum. At the balance point the underlying strain pattern of the structures under our

hands reveals itself more clearly and in a more precise detail than could be discerned by motion testing. Because of this, this process is diagnostic as well as therapeutic. This maneuver will help the sacrum to integrate with both primary and thoracic respiratory motion. Because of this, the reciprocal tension membrane (i.e. the dural continuum) will be more available to assist the resolution of any strains within the sacrum itself.

Treatment of the sacrum and coccyx

The child lies supine, while you sit at the side. If we now support the supine sacrum and coccyx with the middle finger we can observe by the way it moves under our palpating hand whether there is a quality of hardness or fluidity. Does it move around its physiological primary respiratory transverse axis running horizontally through the lamina of S2, or around other axes (e.g. anteroposterior or vertical), taking it into side bending or rotation? Having ascertained this, we may look a little deeper. A useful image in approaching the infant sacrum is to acknowledge it as a five segment structure, mainly cartilaginous, and therefore hydrophilic and pliable, floating in a layer of subperiosteal metabolic water within its periosteal sac. The cartilaginous coccygeal segments are suspended within their ligaments. We may also acknowledge the presence of the filum terminale, corda equina and sacral autonomics, including the ganglion impar at the coccyx. The palpating hand experiments with the quality of contact that the tissues require, so as to match their tone quality. When matched, the sacrum begins to be guided by its dural attachment (as part of the reciprocal tension membrane at its second segment), and move towards its natural position of balanced membranous tension. As it does this, other strain components between the segments of the sacrum and coccyx may reveal themselves. The conversation between the supporting hand and the tissues may reveal what quality of support or space is needed. This helps fluid resolution to take place both within the sacrum and coccyx, and positionally for the sacrum as a whole, in relation to the dural membrane and the pelvic floor.

An alternative hold that is useful for addressing the individual sacral segments and coccyx is to approach the supine patient from the side with your fingers as near as possible to each segment (Fig. 8.30).

The sacrum carries the parasympathetic supply to the pelvic floor and the restoration of normal sacral motion may have a beneficial effect on sphincter activity of the bladder and bowel. As mentioned above, it is also important to check the pubic symphysis, if there are problems with the bladder in children. To engage the pubic symphysis in a corrective process towards balanced tension, make contact with finger and thumb on each pubic ramus, sensing the corrective principle that is sought by the tissues.

The diaphragm, 12th ribs and posterior abdominal wall

Dr Sutherland said: 'The Crura of the diaphragm have more influence on physiology than almost any other structure' (Wales 1986–2004). The previously mentioned principle of freeing midline from bilateral structures has an important application in our approach to the 12th ribs. Through their relationship with the arcuate ligaments, which are continuous with the crura, the 12th ribs hold a key position in the interface between the diaphragm and the posterior abdominal wall. Strains in the 12th ribs can distort the arcuate ligaments and vice versa. For full thoracic respiration it is

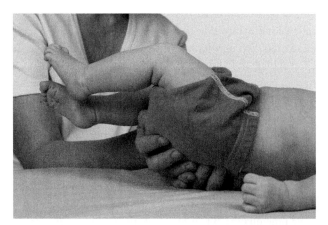

Figure 8.30 Treating the sacrum. The infant usually lies fully supine. Here he is positioned on his side to show the practitioner's hand position.
With permission, Karsten Franke, Hamburg

important that the 12th ribs are free to be moved with the rest of the thorax. During treatment, it must be remembered that the newborn infant's ribcage is much more horizontal that that of the adult. In the newborn infant the relationship of the lower ribs to the quadratus lumborum muscles is particularly important in breathing, as infant breathing is almost entirely diaphragmatic.

The respiratory movement of the 12th ribs is also essential for the rhythmic flow of lymph in the thoracic duct where it enters the thorax under the right median arcuate ligament. Thoracic respiration is responsible for 50% of the lymph movement in the thorax, and diaphragmatic movements especially are essential for enabling the lacunae on the undersurface of the diaphragm to absorb abdominal fluid, the gut being the largest lymphoid organ in the body. The efficiency of the terminal lymphatics, whose role is to maintain extracellular–intracellular fluid balance throughout the body, depends on lymphatic return through the thorax. This has great relevance to the vulnerable infant immune system.

Diaphragmatic motion is often compromised in the new born, whether it be from the stress of labor and delivery, or from poor thoracic expansion in the establishment of the first breaths.

In the view of Still, as quoted by Sutherland (1990), restriction of motion at the diaphragmatic crura could impede the descent of aortic blood through the diaphragm, causing back pressure that could damage the valves of the heart. This has relevance for the infant, since the newborn is still in the process of reorganization of the circulatory pathways within the heart and their stabilization. It is the change in relative circulatory pressures between the right and left heart that closes the atrial septum, as a result of the full expansion of the lungs with the first breaths. This process takes days and sometimes longer to become stable, so the postnatal reorganization of the heart compartments is extremely sensitive to alterations in the balance of circulatory pressures. In addition to this, congenital cardiac anomalies are more common than is generally known, being 13 in every 1000 infants (Lissauer and Clayden 1977). Because of this, the release of residual diaphragmatic and thoracic tensions will contribute greatly to the creation of optimum conditions for neonatal physiology.

Also the physiological motion of the organs of elimination (i.e. lungs, liver, kidneys and colon), is enhanced by the rhythmic motion of the posterior abdominal wall through thoracic respiration and suffers when this is inhibited. Radiographic studies have shown that where the crura are hypertonic this may, in some cases, restrict the passage of blood through the renal artery and occasionally alter the blood pressure regulation in the kidneys (Panicek et al 1988).

In infants and young children, the fascia from the inferior surface of the diaphragm contribute to the phreno-esophageal ligament of the esophagus as it lies between the thorax and abdomen. This, together with the diaphragmatic crura plays the role of a functional sphincter at the lower esophagus, which means that the tone of the diaphragm has a significant part to play in gastro-esophageal reflux (Carreiro 2003; see Ch.12).

It is also interesting to note that in infants and young children, freeing the lower ribs and crura can help to normalize an autonomic nervous system that may have retained the stress of birth or other traumata.

The rhythmic respiratory pulling and releasing of the crura on the anterior longitudinal ligament also aids fluid perfusion to the vertebral bodies and discs and also moves the blood in Batsen's venous plexus that drains the spinal cord. Because it is valveless, this plexus is dependent on diaphragmatic motion for movement of the blood within it, especially in the infant.

The motion of the crura is also important for trophic function of other paraspinal structures. It follows that it is important to recognize and treat hypertonicity of the crura and arcuate ligaments. One indication of diaphragmatic hypertonicity acting on the crura and arcuate ligaments is a short flexion curve between the level of T12 and L2. The infant spine should not have any marked curve so this is a useful indicator. Freeing the 12th ribs will begin to allow the crura to move appropriately with thoracic respiration to re-establish the pumping function that is essential to the health of all the tissues of the body.

On the upper surface of the diaphragm the middle clover leaf of the central tendon is continuous with the pericardium, which also has ligamentous connections with the pleura of the lung (Panicek et al 1988). The pericardium is continuous above with the aortic arch and with the pretracheal fascia, which are suspended from the basiocciput and sphenoidal pterygoid plates by the pharyngobasilar fascia. There is therefore a fascial tube continuous from the cranial base to the diaphragm, blending with the superior, middle and inferior constrictor muscles. The freedom of motion of this 'tube' will influence the health of the organs within and around it, especially the thyroid and thymus glands, the vocal chords and eustachian tubes. Because of this fascial connection, emotional and physical shocks that register in the diaphragm, pericardium or in protective postures of the thorax will also be seen in the cranial pattern and the pelvis. It was not for nothing that Still (1992) spoke of the diaphragm as the 'great piston shaft in the engine of life' attributing to it the words, 'by me you live and by me you die'.

Treatment of the 12th ribs

To release the 12th ribs we can simply work as we did with the pelvis. The child lies supine and you sit to the side, cupping the area of the floating ribs bilaterally with each hand. It should be remembered that the rib cage is more horizontal in an infant than in an adult. Synchronizing with each breath we can gently encourage the 12th ribs laterally, only as much as the tissues will naturally yield on each outbreath, without creating any resistance or recoil in the tissues (Fig. 8.31). The secret of 'less is more' is that if we exert such minimal lateral movement that the tissues do not resist or recoil against us, we will be at our most effective. In an older child the 12th ribs may be addressed one side at a time. One hand lies under the 12th rib, with the middle finger parallel to it, and is sensory in function. The other hand lies under the first hand and is active in function.

Another secret here is to think of the structures on the outside (i.e. the ribs) as handles to access the internal body, so that in a real sense we are 'finger surgeons'. If our focus is on the arcuate ligaments anterior to the 12th ribs, our hands will engage the whole posterior abdominal wall in the release, and with it the organs in the area. A tissue conversation is required, as always, in which we are receptive to whatever quality of contact or interaction the tissues need, rather

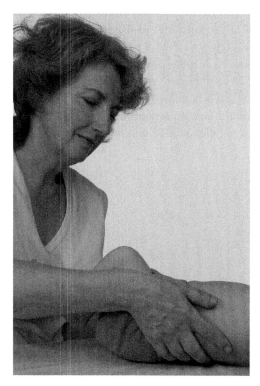

Figure 8.31 Treating the 12th rib.
With permission, Karsten Franke, Hamburg

than doing a technical procedure. When the 12th ribs have released, they should feel as if they respond to the motion of breathing rather than tethering the whole thorax. Because of the relationship of the medial arcuate ligaments to the psoas muscles and the lateral arcuate ligaments to the quadratus lumborum, there may also be beneficial effects to the legs, hips, pelvis and respiratory system.

Any individual rib strain that may be found in the thorax will be easier to release if the 12th ribs and the first ribs are free to shift. These are potent places physiologically, but they are also potent structurally.

Treatment of the diaphragm

There are many ways to release the diaphragm. In practice, a strain in the umbilicus and in the diaphragm are often mutually interdependent.

Face the supine patient with the radial border of your hands gently resting around the costal rim, which is more horizontal in a baby than in an older child or adult (Fig. 8.32). Visualize the hands directing a fluid drive up under the inferior surface of the diaphragm.

This may focus your awareness, guiding your hands to mirror and support any strain patterns that may have arisen from weakness of the first inhalations when breathing was becoming established, or from shock or anxiety during delivery. The contact is gentle as it is easy to bruise the internal organs through inappropriate pressure. The fluid drive may focus at a particular area of the diaphragm, forming a fulcrum or a neutral field around which it can release and reorganize. Sometimes the response is such a big thoracic inhalation that it is as if the first breath is being taken again in a way that was perhaps not possible the first time around. It is always interesting after this maneuver to check the body as a whole to realize how much more spaciousness and

freedom of motion is present throughout – in the pelvis, the respiratory excursion of the thorax, and in the primary respiratory expression of the cranium and in all tissues. For more detail on fluid drive techniques, refer to Magoun: *Osteopathy in the cranial field*, 1951.

An alternative hold is to hold one hand at the back of the diaphragm along the lower ribs while the other hand senses along the linea alba between the xiphoid and the umbilicus. Find the point of most significant relationship to the diaphragm and do a fluid drive from that point. You will know when that point is found because the diaphragm is most responsive to treatment from that point.

Another comfortable hold for both the osteopath and infant is with one hand enveloping the diaphragm anteriorly and the other posteriorly (Fig. 8.33). This often gives a good three dimensional picture of the diaphragmatic dome and of its quality of function. Also, because it is so comfortable, it encourages the tissues to relax and release.

A further method of treating the diaphragm which is comfortable for both infant and older child, is for the child to sit on your knees, facing away. The child could also be standing whilst you kneel behind. In this way the child may like to be looking at a toy or book on the treatment table. Fold the ulnar border of the hands bilaterally around the costal anterior border, gently adapting to the position of ease of the diaphragm and supporting the softening of the tissues on each outbreath, acknowledging the connections both above and below. As the diaphragm eases it may express torsional or other patterns, which you match, as the tissues seek a point of balanced fascial tension followed by release and relaxation. In addition, the solar plexus has the opportunity to normalize its activity. This position can also be adapted for engaging the umbilicus, linea alba and abdominal contents, by supporting

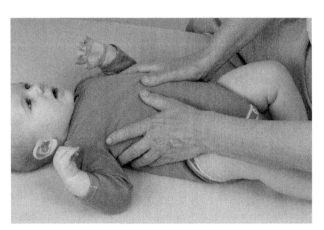

Figure 8.32 Treating the diaphragm with fluid drive.
With permission, Karsten Franke, Hamburg

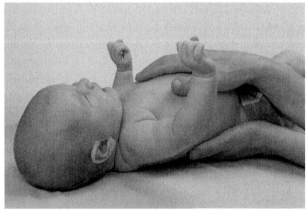

Figure 8.33 Treating the diaphragm with anterior-posterior contact.
With permission, Karsten Franke, Hamburg

the whole peritoneal sac with one or both hands. It is also a good position for engaging the sternum and abdomen.

The umbilicus and liver

Both the umbilicus and the liver are important structures to check, and treat if appropriate, in the neonate. For a more detailed description and method of treatment please refer to pp.219 and 220.

Thorax and ribcage

One of the pieces of advice that Sutherland gave was that if we free the spine from the bilateral impingement of the ribs before addressing the spine itself, we will have an easier job to do (Wales 1986–2004). We have already seen the effect of releasing the 12th ribs, but we can apply this same principle to all the ribs. With the exception of ribs 1,11 and 12, the ribs articulate with the sides of the vertebral bodies, each one with a hemifacet on the vertebral bodies above and below. On account of this dual attachment between vertebral segments, when the ribs become strained on their articular facets they can act as wedges, limiting segmental intervertebral movement.

The costovertebral junctions can significantly influence the function of the autonomic nervous system. The sympathetic chain ganglia float on the rib heads anteriorly. To function appropriately they need freedom of motion on thoracic respiration, so that they are rocked with each inbreath and outbreath. If a rib or group of ribs are strained on their vertebral attachments, this contributes to segmental facilitation which feeds into the autonomic nervous system systemically. Segmental strain that facilitates local neural activity and organ function also registers somatic stress to the brain. Raised autonomic stress, of which somatic stress is one possible component, has been shown to reduce the efficiency of the immune system (Cotman et al 1978).

The infant respiratory system is vulnerable in various ways:

• In the neonate, thoracic movement is somewhat disorganized because the ribcage is so pliable that it provides very little mechanical resistance. The respiratory accessory muscles, for example the quadratus lumborum, are especially important in stabilizing the ribcage on inhalation. It is, however, this very pliability of the ribcage that allows for dramatic growth in the lungs in the first 2 years of life (Carreiro 2003). Any factor that limits the pliability of the thorax may also limit the dramatic alveolar growth spurt during those first 2 years.

• Another reason for the disorganized movement is that the neonate has not yet developed neural organization to the level of specific segmental control, since single neurones govern a relatively large area, with overlap.

• The balance between abdominal and thoracic pressures is not used as much in neonate breathing as it is later on in childhood. Overall, because of poor mechanical effectiveness, the neonate requires more effort to breathe than slightly older children.

• Another factor that makes the respiratory system of the neonate vulnerable is that there is no cough reflex. Also, neonates are obligate nasal breathers, so that if the infant has a chest infection or a cold, there is a further complication. This is that hypoxia, or raised levels of carbon dioxide, do not raise respiratory activity as they will later in life, but rather they depress it.

This respiratory vulnerability may be problematic since throughout the first year of life the lungs, like the gut, are being exposed to substances from the external environment. The immune system is educating itself, testing out whether each new substance is 'friend' or 'foe', mounting frequent immune responses that manifest as snuffles, which cause congestion in the bronchial and nasal passages. This is exacerbated by the shape of the infant's nasopharynx (Fig. 8.34), which is narrowed by flexing the head on the chest or by sleeping prone, partly because there is no supralaryngeal space as yet.

The arrangement of the neonate nasopharynx is useful in breast feeding as it allows suckling and breathing simultaneously, but it may also make the infant vulnerable to compromised breathing in certain circumstances. Propping the

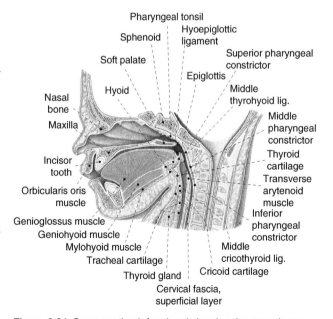

Figure 8.34 Cross section infant head showing the nasopharynx. With permission, Sobotta: Atlas der Anatomie des Menschen. Publisher: R. Putz and R. Pabst, 21st edn. Elsevier/Urban & Fischer, Munich/Jena 2000

supine infant's head on a pillow, for example, is contraindicated because it narrows the dimensions of the nasopharynx. Cranial base strains can also exacerbate the narrowing of the nasopharynx, as can asymmetrical fascial pulls into the thorax, diaphragm and abdomen (Carreiro 2003).

The neonate sternum is cartilaginous and segmented like an anterior midline reflection of the vertebral column (Fig. 8.35). These segments can express individual motion and sometimes we find shears or rotation patterns between the sternal components, just as we do in those of the sacrum. This can interfere with the integrity of the anterior midline of the body. Where there has been difficulty or stress in the expansion of the thorax when the first breaths were taken, we may find the anterior ribcage tight, as if anchored to the diaphragm interiorly by the fan shaped transversus thoracis muscle and by the pericardial attachments to the sternum. The transversus thoracis is active in the expulsive action of coughing to draw the sternum down towards the diaphragm. In older children and adults, following bronchial infections, retained tension in this muscle may persist, altering the posture of the thorax; but this pattern is responsive to osteopathic treatment. The thymus gland is almost the same size as the heart in infancy. Its size is seen as a testament to its importance in developing an adequate population of T-lymphocytes for lifelong immune efficiency. If the manubrium and sternal body are tethered from fascial drag from within the thorax or below, this will restrict blood flow within the thymus gland and reduce its functional effectiveness. Restricted sternal movement also drags the anterior attachments of the upper ribs and clavicles inferiorly, retarding the flow of lymph through the thoracic duct into the left subclavian vein. This will not only retard fluid interchange at an interstitial level throughout the body, but, within the thorax

itself, it will slow down lymph drainage from the lungs. This is especially relevant at the neonate stage where the lymphatics play a vital role in the absorption of excess lung fluid following birth. Stresses in the diaphragm and tension in the transversus thoracis muscle may contribute to this problem.

Pulmonary diseases like pneumonia, or scar tissue associated with heart surgery early in life, commonly exert fascial drag extensively through the body. The effect may be seen in the asymmetry of the pelvis and legs, sometimes extending into the neck and cranium. For this reason, torticollis has been shown in some cases to follow heart surgery, and locking of the involuntary motion cycle of the temporal bone into internal rotation may follow pneumonia on the side affected.

So restraint upon motion of the infant thorax may arise not only from external compressive causes but from the internal organs; for example the pericardium, pleura, lungs and heart. Loss of free motion of the anterior thoracic fascia will tend to pull the upper thoracic vertebral group into kyphosis. The integrity of the thoracic inlet is physiologically important from various points of view. The upper two thoracic segments and their attendant ribs and costovertebral junctions exert vasomotor influence upon the head via the ascending sympathetic nerves and cervical ganglia. The brain dramatically raises its demand for oxygen at birth and therefore for arterial blood; but any restriction upon the mobility of the upper ribs, clavicles and upper thoracic spine may inhibit both arterial flow to the head and also its venous drainage. Recovery of the brain from the cerebral edema that accompanies 65% of births in the first 36 hours (Amiel-Tison and Stewart 1994) depends on the mobility of the venous sinuses within the reciprocal tension membrane. The secretion and renewal of CSF is itself dependent on cranial venous drainage. So the vascular influence of the upper thoracic segments is of note. During birth the upper ribs, clavicle or shoulder may be injured, especially if there is any problem with the restitution phase of labor.

Treatment of the middle ribs

If we wish to release the middle ribs, probably the easiest position is to sit behind the head of the supine infant. Our hands cradle the ribcage bilaterally and gently suggest spaciousness to the costovertebral articulations by drawing the hands very slightly laterally (see Fig. 8.36). This will allow the costovertebral and costotransverse ligaments to go through their own process of reseating the costovertebral relationship. Freeing the costovertebral articulations will have a beneficial effect on the sympathetic chain ganglia, enabling them to be rocked by the motion of thoracic respiration.

In cases where the first breath was taken before the delivery of the thorax, costovertebral compression may persist unless

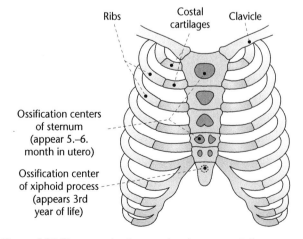

Figure 8.35 The neonate sternum showing segmentation. With permission, Henriette Rintelen, Velbert

this pattern is addressed. Likewise, after ventouse or caesarean delivery strains may persist in the diaphragm, which acted as a stabilizer to counterbalance traction through the neck.

Treatment of the thorax

It is also helpful to keep in mind the whole three-dimensional shape of the ribcage as if viewing it from the inside. We may then find that the ribcage as a whole begins to explore for a three-dimensional balance point. When the containing structure reaches a point of balance, the contents of that container also have an opportunity to experience balance. So, in doing this we are setting the stage for the thoracic organs (i.e. the heart and lungs) to make their own appropriate accommodative changes too.

Integration of thorax and thoracic organs

Holding the chest of the supine child in its three dimensional expression as described above may lead us to sense the relationship between the heart and the lungs. We may silently ask the question whether the lungs feel 'flat-packed' or whether they have expanded as fully as they needed to on their first inhalation when they originally established thoracic breathing. We may also ask the question whether the heart and lungs have completed their interaction in a way that is appropriate to postnatal life. It is the rush of blood into the neonatal heart from the newly expanded lungs that closes the atrial septum, and it is the raised oxygen saturation that maintains the closure of the ductus arteriosus. The stabilizing of the neonate heart in its new postnatal design is in a process of completion over the first hours and days, running parallel with the stabilizing of pulmonary breathing. The two organs are interdependent. This silent recognition, acknowledgement and support of the state of the tissues and organs by the osteopath enables the physiology to perceive how it

may have deviated from its matrix and allows it to realign with its blueprint for health.

Treatment of the sternum

To engage in the resolution of any mismatch between the two sides of the sternum, or between the segments, particularly at the manubriosternal joint, a comfortable position is with the child either supine (Fig. 8.37a) or supported on your knees, facing away (Fig. 8.37b). If an older child wishes to stand, you can kneel behind her with your hands wrapped around the front of her chest.

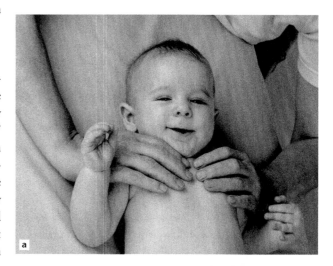

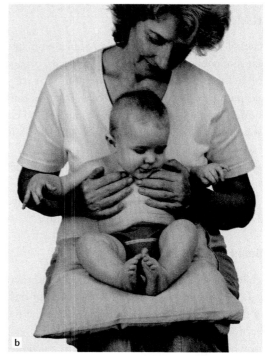

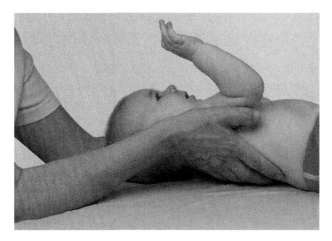

Figure 8.36 Treating the middle ribs.
With permission, Karsten Franke, Hamburg

Figure 8.37 Treating the sternum: **a**: supine; **b**: sitting up.
With permission, Karsten Franke, Hamburg

As the osteopath matches the natural motion tendency of the sternum, the influence of the pericardium may reveal itself as part of the sternal pattern. Likewise if the child has a history of coughing or respiratory distress, a sternal pattern of axial compression and inferior tethering may be evident due to retained tension in the transversus thoracis. Matching the tone (i.e. 'gathering together') of this axial compression will approximate the origin and insertions of the muscle, thus enabling relaxation to occur, followed by the natural expansion of the anterior thorax.

Once these fixating influences are freed from the sternum, the manubrium may then be receptive to a gentle lift in a cephalad direction. This is a very gentle variation of the lift of the manubrium described in Ch.3, p.25. It restores fascial glide to the anterior throat tissues. This is particularly relevant if the umbilical cord was wound tightly around the neck in delivery. This is beneficial to thyroid circulation since the thyroid arteries and veins enter and leave the gland from above, because of the embryological descent of the thyroid from the back of the tongue (Moore 1988). Because of this historical circulatory U-turn, the thyroid is intolerant of any fascial drag from the thorax. The tissues of the throat, larynx and eustachian tubes all function better when their natural fascial glide is restored, and this may be relevant in cases of recurrent infections in this area. These anterior fascias can also exert drag on the cranial base and face, predisposing to problems of sinuses, ears and dental occlusion as the child grows.

The clavicle and shoulder joint

The clinical significance of clavicular dysfunction is apparent in such commonly seen conditions as torticollis, plagiocephaly, ear and upper respiratory tract infection, Erb's palsy and thyroid problems. In addition, clavicular fractures can happen during delivery, and in less severe injuries the clavicle will absorb intraosseous strain. The full range of motion of the shoulder joint is partially dependent on sternoclavicular joint movement so the clavicle needs to be checked carefully.

Sometimes babies are born with one arm up, so the hand and head have to be delivered together. This can engender strains in the shoulder joint and in the upper ribs.

Treatment of the clavicle

The child lies supine; you sit at the head of the treatment table. To address the clavicle, we can take hold of each end with a finger and thumb, and gently move each end towards its direction of articular ease (Fig. 8.38).

It may be helpful to visualize the clavicle as a periosteal sac of hydrophylic collagen, and therefore fluid, and to see the bone with its ligaments (sternoclavicular, coracoclavicular,

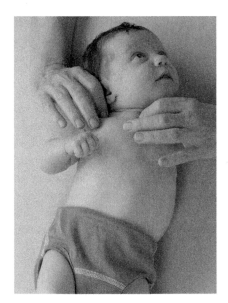

Figure 8.38 Treating the clavicle.
With permission, Karsten Franke, Hamburg

acromioclavicular and costoclavicular) as a continuum of that periosteal sac. Finding the position of ligamentous ease will free its articular ends enough to allow intraosseous reorganization within the bone. At this point there is often a sense of fluctuant activity within the bone, followed by homogeneity as if the bone 'breathes' rhythmically and evenly throughout its length. For adapting an approach to the clavicle for older children, please refer to p.211.

Treatment of the shoulder joint

For treatment of the shoulder joint the infant lies supine, but an older child may sit, with you at the side. Place your middle finger on the coracoid process of the scapula, with the index finger on the humeral head and thumb in the axilla. Place the middle finger of your posterior hand on the scapular spine, with the index and thumb also on the humeral head and axilla, respectively. The glenoid fossa is then between your two middle fingers (Fig. 8.39).

My preference for dealing with shoulder strains is to once again relate to each bone as a periosteal sac of fluid, since collagen is hydrophilic. If we visualize the scapula as a periosteal sac of hydrophilic substance continuous with the articular capsule of the shoulder joint, which is in turn continuous with the periosteal sac of the humerus, we then have three connected fluid sacs. It may also be helpful to acknowledge the embryological tissue memory of the shoulder joint as the limb bud whose impulse arose from the C7 notochordal level. By doing this we are supporting the reconnection of the area in strain with its embryological blueprint for health

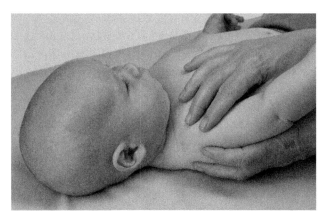

Figure 8.39 Treating the shoulder joint.
With permission, Karsten Franke, Hamburg

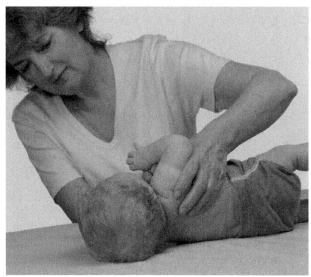

Figure 8.40 Treating the scapula.
With permission, Karsten Franke, Hamburg

and perfect organization. This is reminding the body that its memory of health is a stronger imprint than that of the strain pattern. We give support and observe the inherent motion within the tissues until a sense of balanced stillness is followed by reorganization within the joint and within the bones themselves. This way of working was shown to me by J. Jealous, adapted from an approach he received from his teacher Ruby Day, who was a pupil of Dr. Sutherland.

The scapula

Spinal and upper rib problems may be maintained by their interrelationship with the scapula. The scapula has a myofascial relationship with the shoulder, upper ribs, occiput and each vertebra to the sacrum. The upper thorax, shoulder girdle, upper ribs and spine down to T4 are best considered as one unit of function. A scapula that is poorly seated on the body wall alters the angle of the glenoid fossa and may contribute to an upper limb or shoulder problem.

Treatment of the scapula

The easiest way to myofascially release the scapula is to have the child side-lying and take the scapula in one or both hands, depending on the size of the child (Fig. 8.40).

Allow the myofascial field of the scapula to move it through a series of ease points until it finds a poised neutral position. Following the point of balance there is an unravelling and then resettling of the scapula with a softening of the whole shoulder girdle, especially the trapezius and supraspinatus. This also has a beneficial effect on the neck, upper ribs and whole spine.

Elbow, radius and ulna

Treatment of the interosseous membrane

If there are any strains in the forearm or elbow itself we can address the forearm similarly to the way we addressed the lower

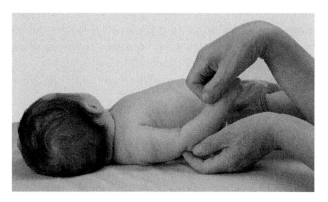

Figure 8.41 Treating the interosseous membrane of the forearm.
With permission, Karsten Franke, Hamburg

leg; that is by balancing the interosseous membrane between the ulna and the radius. The infant is supine, or sitting if older; you sit next to the treatment table. Take hold of the proximal ulna with one hand, and the distal radius with the other (Fig. 8.41) and gently feel which way they tend to move as they guide your hands towards the position of balance for the interosseous membrane. It is, as always, from this point of balance that the shift will take place and resuspend the two forearm bones in relation to each other. Arm strains are less common in newborns than strains of the leg, but we need to be open to their possibility, particularly if the delivery of the arm or shoulder was complicated in the delivery process. Ligamentous continuity between the humerus, ulna and radius, forming the composite elbow joint, means that addressing the forearm bones will begin the resolution of elbow strains.

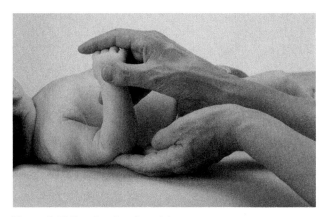

Figure 8.42 Treating the elbow joint.
With permission, Karsten Franke, Hamburg

Treatment of the elbow

Where the elbow needs more attention, the operator may address it by holding the distal humerus with one hand whilst with the other engaging the 90° flexed elbow joint, with fingers around the olecranon process. The elbow ligaments may be engaged either by gentle distraction or approximation until they guide the joint to the balance point from which release and resolution unfolds.

Another possibility is to hold the wrist with one hand instead of the humerus (Fig. 8.42).

The newborn spine

Having introduced ourselves to the child from the periphery and having freed any restrictions in the process, the spine or the core becomes more naturally amenable for both diagnosis and treatment. The newborn infant spine should not have any evident spinal curve, only a very mild continuous C-shape that is barely discernable, with no vertebral groups having prominence. If a short flexion curve is observed at the thoracolumbar junction, this indicates that the diaphragm is hypertonic, with its posterior attachments at the crura pulling upwards on the upper lumbar vertebral segments via the anterior longitudinal ligament (Wales 1986–2004). The work already described releasing the diaphragm and 12th ribs should have accessed the crura and begun to give more length and freedom of motion to this area.

Sutherland (1998) advised regarding the treatment of the spine that it is helpful to attend first to the structures anterior to the spine itself. The anterior longitudinal ligament runs down the anterior aspect of the vertebral bodies. The radiate rib ligaments, the pleura, mesenteries, crura, prevertebral fascia and longus colli muscle all attach to it. Remembering Sutherland's words that it is the ligaments rather than the muscles that are the agents of articular correction, we should

consider the anterior longitudinal ligament which, with the posterior longitudinal ligament, forms a stocking or tube surrounding the vertebral bodies from the sacrum to the basi-occiput. In addressing vertebral strains the engagement of this ligamentous stocking is useful. So when attending to the infant spine it is helpful to allow the anterior longitudinal ligamentous stocking to become foreground in one's awareness, the bones taking second place. In this way we can engage with the spinal ligaments so that they can more easily guide the vertebral segments to the position of composite balanced tension, from which they can realign and reintegrate.

Another consideration with respect to the infant spine is to acknowledge how it formed embryologically. The center of each embryological segment was originally where the nucleus pulposus develops. So, from an embryological point of view, one segment encompasses the lower half of the vertebra above, the top half of the vertebra below, and centers around the disc. This means that in resolving a vertebral strain, it is more accurate to think of harmonizing an embryological segment within itself than breaking a restriction between two vertebrae.

Yet another aspect to keep in mind is that the neurospinal axis has developed in alignment to the notochord. This embryological organizational axis has relevance throughout life as a reference for the self-correcting mechanism within the spine and its sphere of segmental influence.

The newborn spine has in general undergone a degree of axial compression either from delivery or from intrauterine molding. Because this quite often remains unresolved, it is important to be aware of potential osteopathic dysfunction. The infant spine is highly responsive to afferent influences from the visceral organs (Carreiro 2003), which may be palpable in the spinal segments, paraspinal muscles and overlying skin.

Treatment of the spine

To address the thoracic spine, you may sit to the side of the supine patient, supporting each spinous process with the fingertips (Fig. 8.43) or, as is my preference, sit behind the supine infant's head and bring your hands under the body so that the child's spinous processes rest along the third ray of your hand; that is along the third finger, the palm, and between thenar and hypothenar eminences. Your other hand supports the occiput, including C1 and C2 (Fig. 8.44).

Gently support the spine as if slightly lifting it towards the ceiling until there is a sense of engaging with the anterior longitudinal ligament, which is of course the most anterior part of the ligamentous stocking of the whole spine. If the tone of the spinal tissues, and particularly their stocking, is supported and matched precisely by your hands, then that ligamentous stocking starts to guide the spinal segments, exploring

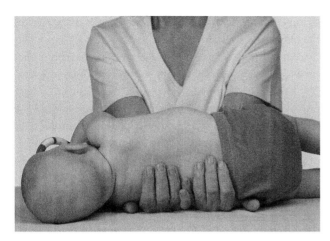

Figure 8.43 Treating individual spinal segments or groups contacting the spinous processes. For treatment the baby lies supine, in this photo he is side-lying for demonstration purpose only.
With permission, Karsten Franke, Hamburg

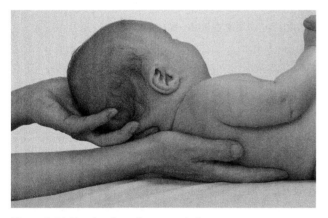

Figure 8.44 Treating the spine as a whole.
With permission, Karsten Franke, Hamburg

the hidden pattern within it. For instance, if in birth there was much axial compression, the spine may begin to express a sense of axial bunching under the supporting hands. Then each segment begins to arrange itself within the stocking in a way that is revealing of the subtler components of the hidden pattern programmed in the tissues. This may be side bending, rotation, side shift, flexion, extension, and so on.

The spinal stocking arranges the whole vertebral group at a composite neutral. If we wait with this neutral at the moment of stillness, what will follow will be an unravelling and reorganizing, lengthening and warming of that whole vertebral group.

If the strain patterns, registered in the longitudinal spinal ligaments, do not have an opportunity to release at this stage, then this may well be one of the factors that programmes the spine to grow into kyphosis or scoliosis later on in childhood, particularly in adolescence. This simple maneuver enables

the child's spine to release the axial compression forces of birth and intrauterine molding and reveals the hidden story of the force factors that are held in the tissues. In the composite neutral or balance point for the spinal group, it is as if we are offering a mirror to the body of the pattern that it is holding. The body's intelligence can then perceive how far it has deviated from its embryonic blueprint for health and perfect organization so that its response is to realign its structure to its original blueprint, first expressed physically in the embryonic notochord, rather than continuing to align itself to the pattern of distortion. This is relevant following intrauterine molding and birth. It is also relevant throughout the growing years of childhood.

When we are working with the transitional areas (i.e. the cervicothoracic junction and the thoracolumbar junction), we need to include the prevertebral fascia and the crura in our ligamentous reference so that, as we engage with the anterior longitudinal ligament, we also take these into the picture.

The same principle of engaging the anterior longitudinal ligament may be applied to individual segments. Contact is best made on the laminae for the cervical and thoracic area and on the spinous processes for the lumbar segments. Contact should be made with both the vertebra above and below the strained intervertebral relationship. The principle of exaggeration to the point of balance as guided by the inherent exploration of the anterior longitudinal ligament is effective.

Occasionally, the segments respond better to direct action: Sit by the supine patient, on the side to which the vertebral body has rotated. Hook your fingers around the spinous process and draw it gently towards you, just up to the point of ligamentous resistance, and hold until the vertebra naturally derotates. This approach is as relevant to the older child, especially after a trauma such as a fall.

Special considerations for the neck

The neck of the newborn may have been subjected to many traumatic forces: it may have suffered the effects of a tight cord around it, or perhaps axial compression, rotational or tractional forces from a complicated delivery. One of the aims of treating the spine is to normalize neural activity both somatically and viscerally. In treating the infant neck we need to consider, therefore, the somatic and visceral relationships, with the aim of normalizing the sympathetic and parasympathetic nervous system activity, as well as lymphatic and circulatory function throughout the cranial and cervical region. The superior cervical ganglia lie anterior to the transverse processes of C2 and C3 and send branches to C1–C4. They are closely interrelated with the joints and fascial planes of the neck, so dysfunction in the cervical joints and fascial planes can disturb the activity of these ganglia. The heart, eyes, ears, throat and sinuses can be made more vulnerable to infection or other types of dysfunction by raised sympathetic activity in the cervical ganglia. This may be a contributory factor in irritable and unsettled babies. The superior, middle and inferior (stellate) ganglia all arise from the cell bodies of T1 to T4. Therefore the upper thoracic segments exert strong neural and vasomotor influence on the head as well as on to the brachial plexus, heart and lungs.

Just as the crura exert significant influence on the thoracolumbar junction mechanically and physiologically, so too do the prevertebral fascia similarly affect the neck, cervicothoracic junction and cranium. The prevertebral fascia originate on the anterior aspects of the bodies of T2 and T3 to attach to the inferior surface of the basiocciput just anterior to the anterior longitudinal ligament. Sutherland (1990, 1998) saw the prevertebral fascia as a 'check ligament' limiting head/neck hyperextension and exerting mechanical influence on the basiocciput. The longus colli muscle spans the same area, and when it retains hypertonicity it may prevent the development of normal cervical lordosis. Somatic dysfunction in the neck can maintain cranial base strains and vice-versa.

The axis has many muscular and ligamentous connections with the skull, including a direct dural one which bypasses the atlas, giving a strong reciprocal influence between C2 and the tentorium and falx cerebelli. Rotation and sidebending at C2 may be compensatory to the lower neck, thorax or pelvis. The atlas is also of interest because of the tendency of the occipital condyles to become wedged bilaterally or unilaterally in its articular facets through the axial, rotational and medial forces exerted on this joint in labor (see p.69). The convex occipital condyles tend to slide into the anterior convergence of the concave atlas facets. If they remain wedged there, this may exert a medially compressive influence on the four parts of the occiput that form the borders and therefore the shape of the foramen magnum. This may strain the transverse ligament of the atlas, and in extreme cases lead to anteroposterior narrowing of the spinal canal with adverse effects on the circulation of the spinal cord and medulla (Sutherland 1990). Medial compression of the condylar portion by the atlas facets limits lateral intraosseous expansion of the squamous occiput and tentorium, and with it the temporal bones. This tends to impede venous drainage from the jugular foramen in the occipitomastoid suture. Venous drainage is essential to dispersing potential edema in the neonate cranium, so this has great clinical relevance. Koslov (2005), who practices osteopathy in Siberia where it is routine to scan the spine of every newborn infant using ultrasound, observes a strong correspondence between colicky, crying babies (see Ch.11) and somatic

dysfunction of the upper cervical spine that is detectable on the ultrasound scan.

Lasarowa (2005), a doctor and DO in St. Petersburg, has shown in recent studies that in cases of adenoid hypertrophy (see Ch.13, Adenoids) osteopathic treatment had a high rate of success so that surgery could often be avoided. She found that an unresolved atlanto-occipital joint compression was commonly associated with compensatory hypermobility of C2, resulting in tension of the falx cerebri, which in turn tended to pull back on the ethmoid and restrain the natural growth and expansion of the face. Such a restriction of the face appeared to contribute to stasis and tissue change within the adenoids and facial sinuses. This was reversible in many cases, once the tissues were free to express motion.

Sutherland (1990) viewed the occiput, C1 and 2 as the craniocervical junction and a composite universal joint. The neck proper begins from C3 downwards and maybe treated as described above. (see Treatment of the spine).

Treatment of the atlanto-occipital joint

Sit behind the supine child and place a fingertip on the posterior tubercle of the atlas. With the other hand very gently draw the occipital squama back minutely without flexing the cervical spine (Fig. 8.45). This rolls the occipital condyles posteriorly from the anterior convergence of the atlas facets into their posterior divergence. Holding the posterior atlas tubercle steady prevents the atlas moving posteriorly with the occiput and has the effect of freeing the joint. It may sometimes take about 30 seconds before the ligaments activate and the occiput floats free. When this is completed there is a palpable sense of intraosseous expansion of the occipital squama, as the cerebrospinal fluid finds space to fluctuate in its cysternae and float the brain, lifting the dural sickles (i.e. the tentorium and falx cerebri). As this happens the cerebellum is able to lift

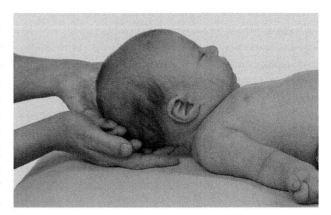

Figure 8.45 Treating the atlanto-occipital joint.
With permission, Karsten Franke, Hamburg

free from any crowding of the brainstem, allowing normalization of function within the physiological centers in the fourth ventricle (Sutherland 1990).

Treatment of the axis

It is often at this point that the axis will be amenable to release its pattern also. When supporting the axis towards its position of balanced ligamentous tension, it is also useful to hold the occiput, acknowledging the relationship between the tentorium and dural attachments at C2. This engages the ligaments externally as well as the dural membranes internally. Because of the continuity of the dura, a therapeutic change may follow throughout the cranium, spine and sacrum.

Specific anatomy of the newborn cranium

As discussed in the chapter on intraosseous strains, the neonate cranium has no formed articulations except for the temporomandibular and the atlanto-occipital joints. The sutures are just thickened membranes at the periosteal borders of the cranial bones. As Carreiro (2003) observed from her dissections, the external and internal dural layers are easy to see in the infant as a bag anchored to bony plates that have grown within it during embryological development. The internal dural layer has been folded by the growing brain to form the falces and tentorium.

Specific features of the dural arrangement

The neonate dural arrangement differs in emphasis from that of the adult. The most noticeable feature is the anterior transverse septum, which is a thick bilateral dural fold running coronally towards the vault from the lesser wings of the sphenoid (see p.49). This functional dural 'hoop' plays a part in the delicate balance of mechanical forces that organizes the embryological development of the vault bones within the dural envelope. It represents a dural fold between the frontal and temporal lobes; that is, between the anterior and middle cranial fossa. As the brain grows postnatally the anterior transverse septum will recede in relative size and importance as the lesser wings of the sphenoid grow and ossify within it. In delivery, the anterior transverse septum may have an important function in restraining the molding of the cranium so that the more delicate falx cerebri and tentorium do not tear.

The relatively tough and small 'sickle' of the falx cerebelli may serve a similar function for stabilizing the four parts of the occiput by restraining it from too much adaptive distortion. A study of the interior surface of the occipital squama shows how the falx cerebelli molds the bone into a 'v'-shaped ridge that spreads laterally around the posterior border of the foramen magnum as it blends with the periosteum. The neonate dissections of Hagopian (2004) revealed that the dural membrane of the cranium attaches firmly to the periosteum at the foramen magnum and at C2 and C3, with looser attachments to the vertebral bodies until sacral segment 2, where the periosteal attachment is once again firm. This supports the observation of Sutherland (1990) regarding the attachments of the 'reciprocal tension membrane'.

Histological studies show that no subdural space exists except where it has been forcibly separated; for example by a bleed (Haines et al 1993). There is tissue continuity between the scalp, the bones in the periosteal envelopes, the internal dura, arachnoid membrane, subarachnoid space, pia mater and the brain with its ventricles. This implies that the rhythmic shape change and tone quality that we palpate on the outside of the head reflects the motility of the brain and its meninges and fluids on the inside. It also means that any release of compression or distorsion of the container can positively affect the spatial environment of its contents and their physiology.

Another feature of the neonate meningeal system is that the venous sinuses are relatively large, being formed in the folds and borders of the dural-periosteal continuum. This allows for venous drainage to be possible even during the folding down of the cranium during labor. Effective venous drainage is also essential for recovery postnatally, because of the need to disperse cerebral edema. The newborn's upper and lower tentorial layers, which originate from the cerebral and cerebellar mesenchymal spheres respectively, are less firmly adhered to one another. Therefore, with the torsional forces of labor a functional 'shear' between them can result and this can maintain intraosseous strains of the occiput. This is not a shear in a gross sense but, on palpation, may sometimes be perceived as a minute loss of true apposition between the two surfaces. Because of their reciprocal influence, any intraosseus strains of the four parts of the occiput may need to be addressed as a functional unit together with this tentorial pattern within one treatment session. As the brain grows in the 1st year of life, the two layers of the tentorium will become more firmly adherent.

Specific features of the cranium

There are six fontanelles at bregma, lambda, pterion, and asterion which allow for overlap and folding during birth (see Fig. 8.7, p.167). The fact that the skull is in parts may make for vulnerability but it also makes huge brain growth possible in the first 6 years.

The occipital squama and partes laterales (condylar parts) do not fuse fully until 3 years of age; the condylobasilar junction does not fuse fully until the 8th year, after which time brain growth proceeds more slowly (see Fig. 8.9). The three parts of the atlas and the upper two sacral segments also complete their fusion in the 8th year.

The temporal bone at birth is in two parts – the squama and the petrous (see Fig. 8.16). The tympanic ring fuses with the other two parts at 7 months in utero, though it is still possible for it to express intraosseous distortion at birth. Any intraosseous strain between the three parts may be a factor to consider in recurrent ear infections (see Ch.13, Otitis media). In the neonate the temporal bone has no mastoid process at birth to protect the seventh cranial nerve as it exits from the stylomastoid foramen. The external auditory meatus, ossicles and tympanic membrane reach adult size before term. The external auditory meatus faces inferiorly and at birth the eustachian tubes are horizontal. The carotid artery enters the temporal bone vertically; at birth it is not yet enclosed in the bony carotid canal with 90° turn from a vertical to a horizontal and anterior direction (Carreiro 2003). The petrous portion of the temporal bone has the same relationship to the occiput and sphenoid as a rib does to its thoracic vertebral segments (Wales 1986–2004). Distortion of the occipital condyles from birth can also distort the position of the temporals, and the shape of the occipitomastoid suture with its jugular foramen. This may adversely affect the function of the glossopharyngeal, vagus and accessory nerves, and also the venous drainage from the cranium. The temporal bones directly and indirectly may mechanically affect all the cranial nerves apart from the olfactory, optic and hypoglossal nerves, partly because of their influence from the tentorium. The vasa nervorum that surround the cranial nerves are sensitive to compression or traction, so impingement either in their foramina or by soft tissues such as the meninges can alter their function. It is worth noting that the foramen magnum, the superior orbital fissure, the hypoglossal canal and the jugular foramen all form around blood vessels and nerves that lie either between bones or between parts of bones that had not yet fused at birth. For this reason distortions that are not resolved postnatally may begin to create physiological disturbance as the child grows.

The sphenoid is in three parts at birth. The greater wing–pterygoid plate units are joined only by cartilage to the lesser wing–sphenoid body unit (see Fig. 8.15). The superior orbital fissure forms between the two parts so the nerves and blood vessels passing through it are vulnerable to distortion. The pre- and post-sphenoid body, that together form the sella turcica, normally fuse by 7 months in utero, though radiographic studies of even full-term infants sometimes show them to be unfused at birth. The sphenoid bone has a strong relationship with function of the eyes. The optic foramen is in the base of the lesser wing. When subjected to compression from the two hemifrontal bones, the plasticity of the lesser wing can cause the optic nerve and ophthalmic artery to become functionally disturbed. This is seen especially when the frontal area has undergone particular compressive force in delivery. Alteration of the sphenoid position makes cranial nerves II–VI vulnerable as they pass though its fissures and foramina. This also changes the position of origin of the extraocular muscles on the common tendinous ring and alters the tension balance between them, with implications for strabismus. The greater wings exert strong influence on the shape of the orbit. The cavernous sinus sits on the 'fault line' between the greater wings and the sphenoid body, and distortion may alter venous drainage from the eye.

At birth the ethmoid (see Fig. 8.19) sits between the lesser wings, giving the impression that the falx cerebri blends with the periosteum of the sphenoid as well as the crista galli of the ethmoid. As the brain grows in the 1st year of life the ethmoid and anterior falx will be drawn anteriorly, and a 'bony bridge' will form between the lesser wings (Carreiro 2003).

The viscerocranium

The pterygoid plates of the neonate sphenoid are short and face laterally, indicative of the vertically short dimension of the middle face. The maxillary sinuses are only perceivable as slits, and the frontal and sphenoid sinuses are not present at all. Only the ethmoid sinuses are functional at term having developed with the relatively large size of the orbits and eyes. The maxillae carry unerupted teeth and their horizontal portion is close to the orbital floor. The movements of the mandible and tongue are mainly forwards and back, to allow for suckling. Vertical movement will only develop with more complex vocalization and the development of the teeth and chewing action. The temporomandibular joint of the term infant is angled anteriorly because there is at birth no vertical mandibular body.

The very short vertical dimension of the infant face is consistent with the flatter dimension of the cranial base. The angle of the clivus is 30° in the infant as compared with 50° in the adult. Consistent with this are the horizontal nature of the eustachian tubes and the absence of the supralaryngeal space. The development of the supralaryngeal space will later be necessary for the faculty of speech, but during the 1st year the particular shape of the nasopharynx (see Fig. 8.34) makes it possible for the infant to suckle and breathe at the same time.

The brain and ventricles

When considering the cranium and its contents, Sutherland (1990) drew attention to what he called the 'ventricular bird'. The body of the bird is represented by the third cerebral ventricle, the wings by the lateral ventricles and the tail by the

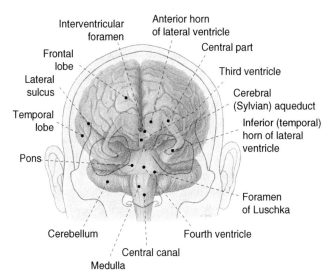

Interventricular foramen

Anterior horn of lateral ventricle

Central part

Frontal lobe

Third ventricle

Lateral sulcus

Cerebral (Sylvian) aqueduct

Temporal lobe

Inferior (temporal) horn of lateral ventricle

Pons

Foramen of Luschka

Cerebellum

Fourth ventricle

Central canal

Medulla

Figure 8.46 The 'ventricular bird' (frontal view). With permission, Sobotta: Atlas der Anatomie des Menschen. Publisher: R. Putz and R. Pabst, 21st edn. Elsevier/Urban & Fischer, Munich/Jena 2000

fourth ventricle and central canal (Fig. 8.46). He likened the inherent motion of the ventricles to that of a bird in flight. The spreading of the 'wings' and the lifting and widening of the third ventricle 'body' on primary respiratory inhalation correspond to the flexion phase of the sphenobasilar junction. The folding of the 'wings,' narrowing and dropping of the 'body' correspond to primary respiratory exhalation and extension of the sphenobasilar junction. He also likened the 'breath of life' within the brain to the ignition spark of a motor car engine, literally 'the spark of life'. Although primary respiratory motion has been present since the first cell, the 'reignition' of the brain's 'spark' and its ventricles should express itself in inherent motion after birth, with the first breath. Often the babies that are brought to osteopaths are those in whom the motion of the 'ventricular bird' may be less evident, where perhaps the brain has not found the way to completely unfold postnatally and reset itself appropriately to the demands of postnatal life (see p.52).

An osteopathic approach to the infant cranium

When we place our hands on the infant cranium, and indeed on the body as a whole, we may feel that three-dimensional shape change that we call flexion/extension or primary inhalation/primary exhalation; its living motion transmitted through all tissue layers – membranous, fluid, neural and osseous. We need to ask whether all tissues seamlessly express this rhythmic motion of life, breathing in every cell and between every cell, or whether any tissue layer puts a

brake on this expression of life through the body. The question then becomes not how do we correct these strains and lesions, but how do we support this body so that these tissues can fully express life? This seeking of health, as opposed to looking for lesion strains, is important throughout the whole body, but particularly in the sensitive area of the cranium. Seeking the quality of dynamic health sets the lesion strain in a contextual relationship with the Life impulse that is infinitely greater than anything that resists it. To quote Sutherland (1990): 'Dr. Still taught the principle of letting the hands light gently on the vault, wrist, foot or any region, and settle into the contacts, so as to be aware of the action within so as to feel what is going on. The living action is perceptible if your hands are quiet and your attention is on what is there to be felt. Grasping vigorously stops the motion of what you want to feel because you have interfered with it. If you do not interfere the motion within carries your hands enough to register in your proprioceptive pathway.' When palpating the infant cranium Sutherland's words (1990) pertain: 'Carry this always in your mind. How do these membranous tissues resist the fluctuation of the Tide?' It may be that the membranes and the bones within them resist the inherent motion of Life expressed through the brain and its fluids. This may be due to traumatic inertia (see p.68) or compressive forces being retained in these connective tissues. Related to this, a hard quality of the cranium upon palpation may be associated with fluid engorgement through poor venous drainage, since restricted involuntary motion of the RTM limits the flow of venous blood through its folds and borders. Postnatal cranial unfolding involves both a physiological and bioelectrical awakening, and with it a dissolving of the restraining influences imposed on the brain by its container. The work already described on the body and atlantooccipital joint will often have initiated reorganization of intraosseus strains in the four parts of the occiput, allowing the fluctuation of the cerebrospinal fluid to engage corrective unfolding from within.

The occiput

To support a process of intraosseous release of the condylar parts there are various approaches. The simplest is to 'carry the parts away from the area of trouble' (Sutherland 1990). The area of trouble in this case is either the medial compression of the condylar parts onto the posterior basiocciput at the condylobasilar junction, or the squama onto the condylar parts at the condylosquamal junction. This is an extremely potent area physiologically if one considers the neural and vascular structures contained by the foramen magnum and posterior cranial fossa. The urgency and ability to suckle immediately after birth is one of the prime indicators that the central and peripheral nervous systems have adjusted appropriately to life outside the womb. Where this is not so, it may also suggest crowding of the hypoglossal nerves as they pass laterally through either of the occipital condyles. The condyle is formed by two-thirds condylar part and one-third basiocciput, so the inability of the tongue to engage a strong suck may indicate generalized crowding or distortion of the occipital components. This is often associated with loss of occipital-temporal motion at the jugular foramen, with limited cranial venous drainage and possible irritation of the vagus and glossopharyngeal nerves. The occiput and temporal bone control the shape of the posterior cranial fossa with their cargo of pons, medulla, cerebellum and upper spinal cord, and give passage to the main arterial and venous pathways of the brain. They also exert strong influence on the tentorium and the cranial nerves.

As mentioned before, it is very important to have a precise appreciation of the balance point in this area as insensitive exaggeration of the lesion in this area that goes beyond the balance point can damage delicate neural structures that may already be compromised. Therefore, when assisting the decompression of the occipital condyles of the infant cranium, direct disengagement is generally advised.

Release of intraosseous strains of the occiput

The infant is preferably supine, the osteopath sits behind the head and places an index and third finger as close as possible to each pars lateralis or condylar part, close to the opisthion (Fig. 8.47).

With the aim of giving a sense of spaciousness to both the anterior and posterior borders of the condylar parts, very gently draw the tissues posteriorly up to the first hint of resistance and hold them at this point. The force required is merely a suggestion, since it is most effective to stay below the level that would evoke tissue recoil. With the other hand place a finger very lightly on the hairline area of the metopic suture, and with it direct an impulse through the CSF towards the foramen magnum.

A sense of a fluid axis may naturally emerge between the directing hand and the occiput. Observe any chaotic fluid activity around the foramen magnum as this is diagnostic of the precise area of greatest compression. Observe whether the center of the turbulence is more towards the right or left, and more anteriorly at the condylobasilar junction or more posteriorly at the condylosquamal junction. Wait for this fluid activity to become still, followed by a sense of opening, softening and reorganization of the occiput, palpable as an intraosseus breathing and resiliancy.

As the four parts reorganize around the foramen magnum, observe the response of the occipital squama. Any compressive rotation of the condylar and basilar portions will be reflected in the squama; and so it will also respond as they release. Because the occipital squama holds a key position in the role played by the reciprocal tension membrane in guiding the motion of the cranial base and vault, this will have a global effect. When the occipital condyles and squama begin to unfold, this allows the natural CSF fluctuation to flood the cysterna magna, expanding the internal space. As the parts decompress, the fluid lifts the cerebellum and tentorium so that the 'membranes go to work to release the bones' (Sutherland 1990) from within. When this inherent action is at work, recovery is already under way. Even if sutural overlaps are present, it is astonishing to see how many steps nature will take between treatment sessions, following one tiny change. Once this process is at work the course of treatment becomes clearer, since the fluid action itself becomes the guide, highlighting areas that resist inherent physiological motion and indicating the part the osteopath needs to play. The activation of the CSF fluctuation in the posterior cranial fossa, which allows the tentorium to lift and enables the cerebellum to lift

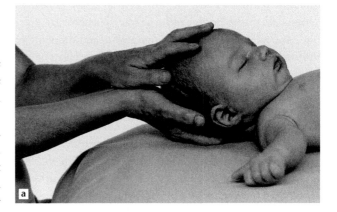

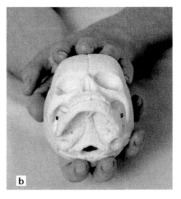

Figure 8.47 a: Treating the occiput; **b**: demonstration of finger position on plastic skull.
With permission, Karsten Franke, Hamburg

free of the brainstem, also permits the expansion of the fourth ventricle. Since the 'ventricular bird' is one unit of function, the third ventricle may also respond by lifting and widening. With it, the pituitary at its base rises and the sphenoid turns towards flexion. As the fluid fluctuation and reciprocal tension membrane begin to move together, any areas that are not free to shift may become evident, particularly where spontaneous fluid turbulence is observed.

If sutural overlaps or ridging do persist after one or two treatment sessions, they will often respond well to direction of the potency of the CSF, as described for the occipital condyles above. The index and third fingers of the receiving hand gently spread the suture, whilst the fingers of the other hand direct the fluid impulse from the longest opposite diagonal position on the cranial sphere.

Fronto-ethmoid junction

A common site of anchoring of the reciprocal tension membrane after birth is at the frontoethmoid junction, particularly if the frontal area has undergone compressive force, either in intrauterine molding or during labor. The nasal and lacrimal bones are suspended from the frontals, and limitation of an inherent motion in this area may predispose the infant to blocked tear ducts or sticky eyes. If this situation makes its presence felt, it may be helpful to manually acknowledge any fluid axis between inion and ethmoid and augment the fluid drive towards this complex and delicate area.

The approach is similar to that described for the fluid drive to the condylar parts. Again, the infant lies supine, with you sitting behind her head. One hand is at the occiput and two fingers of the other hand lightly contact both sides of the glabella (Fig. 8.48). The difference is that the fingers contacting the frontoethmoid area are listening rather than active,

simply observing the way that the tissues move towards a balance point. As Magoun (1951) wrote: 'the potency of the cerebro-spinal fluid is attracted towards the field of the lesion'. This is especially so when the tissues are at the point of balance and in their neutral field. The falx cerebri is an infolding of the dural layer lining the internal periostium of the two hemifrontals and parietals, so that when the 'ethmoid bell' (Sutherland 1990) is free to move with the falx cerebri, the frontal bones, frontal lobes and facial mechanism may all be better able to express primary respiratory motion.

Reorganization of the relationship between cranial vault and base

Quiet listening hands contacting the 'fluid bones' of the vault may then sense the relationship between the cranial vault and base, through the dural hoops; that is, the anterior transverse septum, tentorium and falx cerebri. The infant lies supine; you sit behind her head. Hold the vault gently, with your thumbs crossed above the vault, to act as an external fulcrum (Fig. 8.49). It is then possible to induce the merest suggestion of a lift of the membraneous vault away from the cranial base to give space to its delicate contents, but without any hint of medial compression when working with an infant or young child under 4 years of age.

The fluctuant action of the CSF guides the whole modified sphere to its neutral – balanced – state, followed by

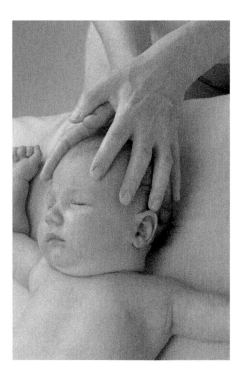

Figure 8.49 Contact on the vault for reorganization between the cranial vault and base.
With permission, Karsten Franke, Hamburg

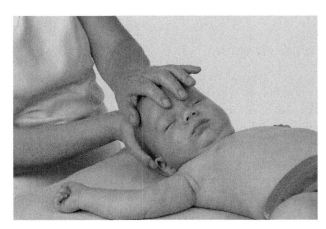

Figure 8.48 Fluid drive of fronto-ethmoidal area.
With permission, Karsten Franke, Hamburg

reorganization of the vault and base together in alignment with its embryonic matrix. In the words of Sutherland (1998): 'When the Breath of Life enters the fluid at a moment of Stillness, see a transmutation occur.'

The perfect end point for the treatment is when all tissue layers, bone, membrane, fluid and neuronal, lose their sense of distinction, as if they express the primary breath as one continuum through every cell.

Conclusion

By restoring freedom of motion to the body as a whole before approaching the treatment of the cranium, we have initiated the process that happens in nature where the expansion of the thorax at the first breath stimulates the unfolding of the postnatal cranium and the sacrum. The freeing of primary respiratory motion in the sacrum stimulates the dural pump within the cranium; the restoration of pulmonary respiratory movement at the diaphragm, thorax and anterior neck releases fascial drag from the cranium and supports its PRM. The cascade of events involving the fluid unfolding of the cranium and brain are already in process, supporting the accessibility of the cranium to osteopathic treatment. In this way we will have reduced the time that we need to spend on the cranium directly, respecting the sensitivity of the child in this sphere.

Sutherland (1990, 1998) said, 'the purpose of an osteopathic treatment is to effect a more efficient fluid interchange across all tissue interfaces'. For the living body to fully express health there must be freedom of neurotrophic, vascular and lymphatic flow. It necessitates a freedom to shift in all parts of the body, macroscopic and microscopic, with reciprocal balance between all the fascial compartments, with freedom to express innate rhythmicity. In engaging in an osteopathic treatment, we are seeking to set the stage for health to take over and re-establish innate balance with the hope that that individual may express his or her true potential for present and future life.

Specific aspects in the treatment of the premature newborn

This section of the chapter has in the main been addressed to the term infant. With premature infants, either at the incubator state or later, there are special considerations.

The child has left her natural container, the uterus, earlier than she was ready to, so first of all we need to take special care to sense how the infant seeks to be held, both metaphorically and in terms of physical contact. Having lost the normal containing boundary ahead of time, we need to sense how we can offer the sense of boundary that the baby needs in order to feel safe enough to let go and heal.

When called to treat a premature baby in a hospital incubator, the osteopath often has to operate in a position of discomfort, negotiating the edge of the cot, and having limited contact with the child's body. Particular care must be taken to remain non-invasive, spacious, receptive, still and not to overtreat, as infants at this early stage are easily overstimulated. In the early stages of prematurity the tissues will feel more like the undifferentiated mesenchyme than in a full term baby.

Shock

Shock is almost always present in the premature and may be the first thing that needs to be addressed. Often this seems to be received through the umbilicus, affecting it and the surrounding tissues, especially the peritoneum. Shock may also complicate the mother–child bond (see Ch.4, pp.38–39, Ch.5, p.73).

Treatment of shock

There are many approaches to shock. My preferred approach is to place an open receptive hand over the area where the shock is focused, such as the umbilicus, pelvis, diaphragm or sternum, while the other hand cradles the back, and to feel the relationship between the two hands; that is, to appreciate the tissue quality and activity between my two hands.

Shocked tissues often express a vibratory quality like a tremble, too fine to be seen from the outside. With one's presence and also hands, the osteopath supports the infant in a sense of being enfolded in an aura of safety and warmth, once again respecting the metaphorical containing boundary in which the baby seeks to be held. Sense the greater rhythm of the tide as expressed in the natural world, and hold the awareness of both frequencies at the same time, until the fast vibration of shock in the tissues is absorbed into the ample life-supporting rhythm of the tide.

Respiratory system

After the hospital stage one of the areas in need of attention will be the respiratory system. Appreciation of the lungs as a pair of structures which float in order to perform their function, tethered at their hilus, can be a palpatory revelation for those who only think of respiration in terms of the diaphragm and ribcage. In health, the functional fulcrum for lung movement appears to be situated at the bifurcation of the trachea to the main bronchi, and this should be free to automatically shift. It often feels fixed and rigid when the infant has been ventilated. Where there has been a pneumothorax or chest drains there will be marked asymmetry.

Treatment of the respiratory system

To address these strains the osteopath may simply support the two sides of the thorax of the supine infant, sitting behind the baby's head, thinking of support to the lung field, as well as its 'container'. Sense the space or containing boundary that the lung field needs and simply be present to the way the life spark within is seeking to express itself and unfold these lungs. An anterior-posterior contact may also be useful.

In this situation it is important to engage with the potency for life and health in the tissues. Is it possible to sense the time in intrauterine life when the fetus expressed that health? If the quality of that expression before the subsequent trauma can be accessed and met, the shock pattern can transform within the context of the fundamental pattern of health.

Strains resulting from intubation

The strains or deformations of the facial structures resulting from intubation or even nasogastric tubes present their own complications. Paying attention to the integrity of the midline structures of the face in relation to the lung fields will often arouse the potency to reveal problems. It may be helpful to view the whole airway from nasopharynx to bronchi and beyond from the inside (i.e. the shape of the space). This can be illuminating and give rise to spontaneous therapeutic changes (Armitage 2004).

Adaptation of BLT approaches to older children

The foot

When the ankle mortise is widened by misalignment of the fibula in relation to the interosseous membrane that binds it to the tibia, the talus can slip anteriorly. This will weaken the ligamentous support of the foot. The talus also tends to slip forward when the ligaments and ankle bones remain in a position of strain; for example inversion following a sprain. This pattern may remain for years, even decades. Because of the importance of the tibiofibular relationship in maintaining the integrity of the ankle mortise, it is important to address this relationship (see p.187) before attending to the talus.

Treatment of the talus

For the treatment of the talus the child sits with legs hanging over the edge of the treatment table; you sit in front. To aid realignment of the talus, clasp the calcaneus with the palmar surface of one hand and, with the wrist on the sole of the foot, ease it towards dorsiflexion. The palmar surface of your other hand covers the dorsum of the foot, contacting the

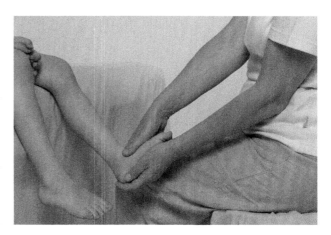

Figure 8.50 Treating the talus.
With permission, Karsten Franke, Hamburg

anterior surface of the talus between the base of the thumb and index finger (Fig. 8.50).

In this position the talus can be gently eased into the space that is opened up by the dorsiflexion of the foot via the calcaneus. As the talus is being eased posteriorly, be alert to the way the ankle ligaments respond (because they often retrace the pattern of old or new injury) before the talus comfortably reseats in the ankle midline. Old injuries such as inversion or eversion sprains may reveal themselves before releasing. This will allow the ankle to strengthen, changing the pattern of recurrent ankle injury and articular instability that frequently follows a sprain.

Treatment of Chopart's joint

The interface between the hind foot and forefoot is referred to as Chopart's joint. It is one curved joint plane between the talus and the calaneus proximally, and the navicular and cuboid distally. In flat feet the navicular and cuboid may have descended at their medial side so that the tarsal arch loses its integrity (see Ch.15, Flat foot).

For the treatment the child sits on the treatment table, with legs hanging; you sit in front. To address this joint surface, approach the foot from the lateral side so that one hand holds the talocalcaneal surface and the other the navicular-cuboid surface (Fig. 8.51). The two surfaces are approximated with sensitivity until the ligaments begin to exaggerate positional dysfunction, up to the point of BLT. Following the point of stillness the ligaments begin to reverse the pattern by lifting the medial aspect of the tarsal arch. In this case you may see fit at this point to actively further encourage the lifting of the arch.

Treatment of the cuboid

The cuboid contributes to the lateral support of the tarsal arch. You may actively lift the medial aspect of the cuboid as

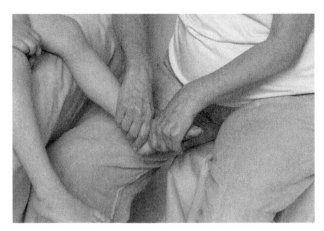

Figure 8.51 Treating Chopart's joint.
With permission, Karsten Franke, Hamburg

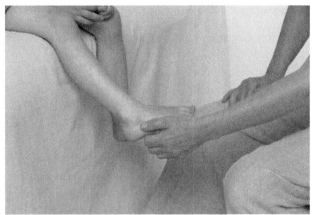

Figure 8.52 Treating the cuboid.
With permission, Karsten Franke, Hamburg

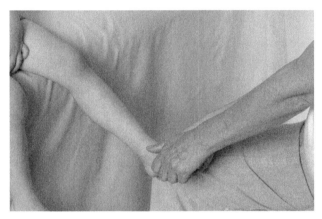

Figure 8.53 Tarsal arch lift.
With permission, Karsten Franke, Hamburg

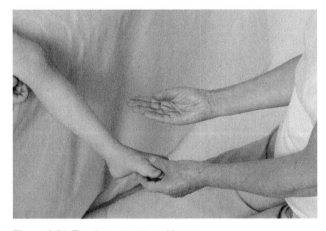

Figure 8.54 Treating a metatarsal bone.
With permission, Karsten Franke, Hamburg

follows: with the patient sitting, and leg hanging, hold the cuboid between the thumb on the dorsal surface of the cuboid and the side of your index finger on the plantar surface, turning it so as to lift the medial aspect (Fig. 8.52). The weight of the foot and leg will provide the precise amount of traction necessary for the size of the patient, providing the space for the cuboid to lift and reseat through ligamentous action.

Tarsal arch lift

Sit facing the seated patient, and hold the upper and lower surfaces of the tarsal arch with both hands (Fig. 8.53). The weight of the leg and the ankle provide traction from beneath, while the fingers lift the arch so that the second cuneiform may rise. The thenar surfaces of your hand assist by rolling the sides inferiorly.

Treatment of the metatarsals and the toes

The child sits with legs hanging over the treatment table; you sit in front. With the weight of the ankle once again providing traction from behind, the metatarsal heads can be lifted by the palmar surfaces of your hands, whilst the distal ends of the metatarsals are counterbalanced by the your thumb on the dorsum; in other words, from above (Fig. 8.54). The ligaments are engaged here by a combination of leverage and suspension.

Stubbed toes and compressed metatarsals can be addressed by simply suspending the foot from the toe to allow the tendons, plantar fascia and joints to release.

The knee

It is not common for infants to need osteopathic attention to the knee at the newborn stage. As the child gets a little older the BLT principle may be applied with contact on both tibial and femoral components of the joint, followed by finding the balance point of the patella and on its ligaments and bursae.

When a child is old enough to sit, the knee can be most effectively treated flexed at right angles. The child sits on the treatment table with legs hanging down. Sit facing the patient and gently approximate the ligaments and articular capsule of her knee by lifting the tibial plateau towards the femoral surface (Fig. 8.55). This approximation slackens the ligaments just enough to allow them to express their natural tendency to guide the joint towards the position of balanced tension. As this happens the pattern of strain; for example twist, shear or compression, may reveal itself. Support the tissues at the point of BLT, remaining alert to the moment when the ligaments 'pull the bones' into realignment (Sutherland 1990).

To integrate the patella let the child deposit her extended leg on your knee. Gently lift the patella at right angles to the extended leg, being receptive to the direction in which the ligaments, including the sub-patella bursa, are guiding it towards a balance point (Fig. 8.56). Support it at this point of stillness until it realigns. Improved tissue motion quality, warmth and a sense of midline realignment of the limb indicate that resolution is in process and that the stage is set for the healing process to continue.

The hip

Once the child begins to walk, mechanical forces begin to form the greater trochanter, which provides a good handle for engaging the hip joint.

With the patient supine, stabilize the sacrum with one hand. The fingers of your other hand need to roll behind the greater trochanter and gently draw the femoral head and neck away from the acetabulum, but only to the minute degree that enlivens the exploratory action of the ligaments and capsule of the hip. Support the tissues as the joint finds its point of balance within the expression of its strained position; this is followed by spontaneous realignment.

As an alternative to using the principle of disengagement, the principle of approximation may be useful according to the conditions present in the tissues. The child may sit up or lie on the side with her hips flexed. This unwraps the spiral arrangement of the ligaments (as does the sitting position), which can be helpful when addressing the hip. Contacting the lateral aspect of the greater trochanter, gently approximate the hip within the capsule with sensitivity to the point where the ligaments begin to respond and enliven their exploration for the position of BLT (Fig. 8.57). From this point a spontaneous reorganization of the joint is made possible. Beware of compressing painful and inflamed tissues.

The clavicle

The child sits on the table. Sit down facing her and, taking a thumb contact under each end of the clavicle, ask her to lean towards you with her back straight, just to the point where

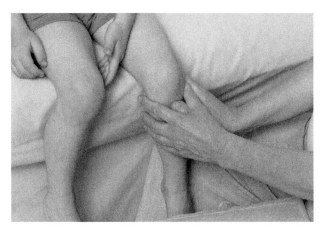
Figure 8.55 Treating the knee.
With permission, Karsten Franke, Hamburg

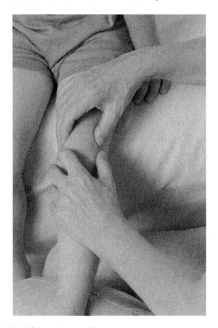
Figure 8.56 Lifting the patella.
With permission, Karsten Franke, Hamburg

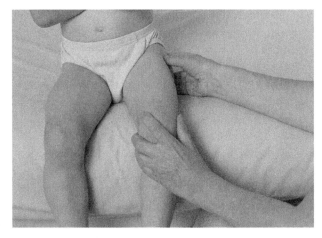
Figure 8.57 Treating the hip joint with the child seated.
With permission, Karsten Franke, Hamburg

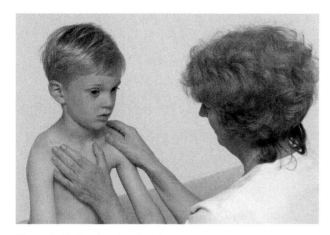

Figure 8.58 Treating the clavicle.
With permission, Karsten Franke, Hamburg

your two weights balance each other like a card house, so that you each feel supported and with no sense of muscular strain or instability (Fig. 8.58).

This engages the clavicular ligaments at either end. Then ask the child to turn her opposite shoulder posteriorly just a few degrees while you hold the clavicle stable. This slightly stretches the sternomanubrial ligaments and has the effect of lifting the clavicle superolaterally relative to the patient's trunk. This activates the ligaments and allows them the space to reorganize their articular relationship at either end. Often, the coracoclavicular ligament emerges as a fulcrum around which the clavicle see-saws before it resettles. Maintain support while asking the child to sit up and take back postural control. Then repeat on the other side. Balancing of the clavicle is especially beneficial for the fascias of the neck and for venous drainage of the thyroid.

The neck

Usually the child lies supine, with you sitting behind the head. To address the neck of a child who is old enough to enjoy carrying out instructions, the point of balance can be augmented by postural cooperation. For instance, to address a sidebending-rotation strain to the left of C3–C4, contact the laminae of both vertebrae concerned with your fingertips and move them towards the position of ease, which will be towards left sidebending. Acknowledging the anterior and posterior ligamentous stocking will allow the ligaments to 'take over' and refine the balance point in its various components. Once the balance point is found the patient can bring the trunk into relationship to this balanced state by raising the left shoulder, but only as far as the balance point is augmented, and no further. This adds power to the fulcrum, the balance point, from which segmental reorganization happens spontaneously. Once relaxation and release have taken place,

postural cooperation is then relaxed and the neck naturally straightens. According to Hildreth (1942) Dr. Still would take the joint through its full range of motion once release was achieved.

Other ways of supporting the balance point with postural cooperation are to raise the shoulders to augment an extension dysfunction of the neck and lower them for a flexion dysfunction. Active respiratory cooperation can also help. For example, holding inhalation augments a flexion strain of the neck, and holding exhalation augments an extension strain. The correction happens as the breath is finally let go. These efforts may be made in reverse for the thoracic region.

The atlanto-occipital joint

As in the treatment of the atlanto-occipital joint of the infant, the older child lies supine on the table; you position yourself behind her head. With one hand you stabilize the occiput and you place the middle finger of the other hand on the tubercle of the atlas. Again, in a child who is old enough to enjoy carrying out instructions, the point of balance can be augmented by postural cooperation. You may wish to ask your patient to tuck in her chin without flexing her neck. This draws the occiput posteriorly as your middle finger, which is situated on the tubercle of the atlas, prevents the atlas from moving with it, so the occiput can float freely into the posterior divergence of the atlas facets.

Bibliography

Amiel-Tison C, Stewart A: The newborn infant – one brain for life. Les Editions Inserm, Paris 1994

Armitage P: Personal Communication 2004

Becker R: Life in Motion. Stillness Press. Portland, Oregon 1997

Becker R: SCTF lecture (transcript). USA 1976

Blechschmidt E: Ontogenetic basis of human anatomy. North Atlantic Books, California 2004

Carreiro J: An osteopathic approach to children. 1st edn. Elsevier, Edinburgh 2003

Clemente C: Anatomy CD. 3rd edn. Urban & Schwarzenberg, Munich/Baltimore 1987

Crelin E S: Functional anatomy of the newborn. Yale University Press, Newhaven 1973

Dove C: Occipito-atlanto-axial-complex. In: Manuelle Medizin. Springer, Berlin 1982

England M: A colour atlas of life before birth. Wolfe Medical Publications, Weert, Netherlands 1983

Fryman V: Relation of disturbances of craniosacral mechanisms to symptomatology of the newborn, study of 1250 infants. In: Feely R (ed.): Clinical cranial osteopathy, selected readings. The Cranial Academy, Meridian, Idaho 1988

Fryman V, Carney R, Springsall P: Effects of osteopathic medical management in neurologic development in children. Journal of the American Osteopathic Association 92 (6), 1992

Fulford B: British School of Osteopathy, SCTF course lecture, London 1982

Goldbloom R: Pediatric clinical skills. Churchill Livingstone, New York 1992

Grant J C B: Method of anatomy. 7th edn. Williams and Wilkins, Baltimore 1965

Hagiopian S: Personal communication 2004

Haines D E, Harkey H L, al-Mefty O: The 'subdural' space: a new look at an outdated concept. Neurosurgery 32, 1993:111–120

Hildreth A G: The lengthening shadow of Andrew Taylor Still. Osteopathic Enterprises, Kirksville, Mo. 1942

Holle B: Motor development in children, normal & retarded. Blackwell Scientific, Copenhagen 1976

Jealous J: Personal communications 1986–2005

Koslov V: Personal communication 2005

Kuchera M, Kuchera W: Osteopathic considerations in somatic dysfunction. 2nd edn. Greyden Press, Colombia, Ohio 1994

Lagecrantz H, Slotkin T: The stress of being born. In: Larsen W (ed.): Human embryology. 2nd edn. Churchill Livingstone, New York 1998

Lasarowa L: Personal communication. St. Petersburg 2005

Lee P: The primary respiratory mechanism beyond the cranio-sacral-axis. Journal of the American Osteopathic Association 2001

Levene M: Jolly's Diseases of children. Blackwell Scientific, Oxford 1991

Lissauer T, Clayden G: Illustrated textbook of pediatrics. Mosby, Spain 1997

Magoun H: Osteopathy in the cranial field. The Journal Printing Co., Kirksville, Mo. 1951; reprinted 1997 by SCTF USA

Magoun H: Entrapment neuropathy of the CNS. Academy of Applied Osteopathy Yearbook 1967

Miller A: Lymphatics of the heart. Raven, New York 1982

Moore K: Essentials of human embryology. Blackwell Scientific, Toronto 1988

Netter F: The CIBA collection of medical illustrations. Vol 8: The muskuloskeletal system. Woodburne R, Crelin E, Kaplan F (eds) CIBA-Geigy, New York 1987

Nilsson L: A child is born. Delacorte, New York 1990

Panicek, Benson, Gottlieb, Heitzmann: The diaphragm – anatomic, pathologic and radiographic considerations. Radiographics 8(3), 1988

Pottinger F: Symptoms of visceral disease. 6th edn. Mosby, 1944; reprinted by Parker Chiropractic Research Foundation, Fort Worth, Texas 1984

Still A: Philosophy of osteopathy. American Academy of Osteopathy, Indianapolis 1995

Still A: Osteopathy – research and practice. Eastland Press, Seattle 1992

Sutherland W: Condylar parts of the occiput – the hole in the tree. Free, Mankato, Minn. 1945

Sutherland W: Teachings in the science of osteopathy. SCTF, Fort Worth, Texas 1990

Sutherland W: Contributions of thought. 2nd edn. SCTF, Fort Worth, Texas 1998

Wales A: Personal communications, 1986–2004

Wilson P, Millar E: Internal Medicine: An Osteopathic Approach. Osteopathic Annals Insight, 1979

Zitelli B J, Davis H W: Atlas of pediatric physical diagnosis. Mosby Gower, New York 1987

TREATING THE VISCERA WITH THE PRIMARY RESPIRATORY MECHANISM

Noori Mitha

Although many children with abdominal complaints are seen in our practices, little has so far been written concerning osteopathic treatment of the abdominal organs in children. However, some useful remarks on this subject are to be found in the writings of Sutherland (1990, 1998) and Barral (1989). This section will discuss the special features of pediatric anatomy and physiology that are of relevance for diagnosis and treatment.

In the osteopathic treatment of children, especially as it relates to the viscera, our approach must always be particularly careful and considerate. The child's health can be favourably influenced by appropriate treatment; in contrast, a heavy-handed approach may exacerbate existing lesions or possibly trigger them in the first place. It is therefore advisable to work with the primary respiratory mechanism (PRM) because this method gently and respectfully addresses the pediatric patient and is tailored entirely to the child's needs and her potential for change at a particular moment in time. Various ways of working with the PRM were described at the beginning of this chapter.

Two additional treatment approaches that can be used with good success will be described here: working with motion present and balanced tension – in both cases as these relate to the viscera. The practical use of these treatment principles will then be illustrated with four examples. The description of the treatment principles and techniques is based on the published work of Sutherland (1990) and Becker (1997).

Special characteristics of organ topography in the newborn

At birth the entrance to the esophagus is located at the level of C3/C4. It does not attain its final position at the level of C6/C7 until about the age of 12 years. At birth the gastric cardia is already situated at the level of T11. In newborns the stomach is initially round and positioned transversally and only has a capacity of 30–35 ml. It is not until the child grows older and taller that the stomach assumes its subsequent elongated shape, attaining a capacity of 1.5–2 L in adulthood.

The liver in the newborn occupies two-thirds of the abdominal space. It thus protrudes by as much as 3 cm below the right costal margin. In the neonatal period, in relation to height, the liver is also considerably larger than in adults and may protrude by up to 2 cm below the left costal margin (Fig. 8.59). In contrast to the situation in adults, it should therefore still be palpable in the newborn.

The position of the small intestine at birth is already the same as that in the adult. The adult small intestine differs merely in terms of length. The initial length in the newborn is about 3 m and this increases to as much as 7.5 m by adulthood. In the course of this growth the number of villi shows an approximately threefold increase.

The large intestine in the infant has already gained its ultimate position. However, the taeniae and haustra designed to optimize peristalsis do not become fully developed until the 4th year of life. The caecum is fully mobile by the 2nd year of life and may therefore be a source of palpatory confusion because its position may be variable. In many cases it can be palpated in the upper right quadrant of the abdomen or in a central position instead of in the lower right quadrant.

Relative to height, the sigmoid colon is considerably longer than in adults; its loops may extend up to the transverse colon and liver. In the newborn it merges with the rectum initially at the level of L3, and later in adulthood at the level of L4/L5.

The urinary bladder lies completely within the abdomen, and the uterus also largely occupies an intra-abdominal position, in contrast to the situation in adults.

Instructions on palpating and treating organs

Immediately after birth the abdominal muscles of the newborn are still poorly developed. They offer virtually no resistance to finger palpation. Consequently, examination and treatment should be performed with the utmost delicacy so as to avoid excessive compression of the organs, which may result in injuries such as bruising or perforation. Barral (1989) recommends deferring examination and treatment based on the mobility of the child's organs until the patient is at least 7 months old, and even then only with extreme caution. Up to that time he considers treatment using the motility model to be more advisable and safe.

Immune system of the gut

Whilst in the womb the fetus receives immunoglobulin G (IgG) from the mother by transplacental transfer. These immunoglobulins are important in conferring immunity to microbial infections and protecting the child for the first 3 months of life. The child receives IgA with the breast milk, something that is particularly necessary for immunity to viral diseases.

The child's immune system matures during the first year of life. A significant proportion (approx. 80%) of adaptive immunity stems from contact between antigens and immune structures in the gut. The gut mucosa, together with that of the respiratory tract, forms by far the largest surface area through which the child is directly in contact with the outside world.

The immune system of the gut is divided into different areas:

- Bacterial colonization with symbiotic organisms: these suppress pathological organisms and thus fend off the

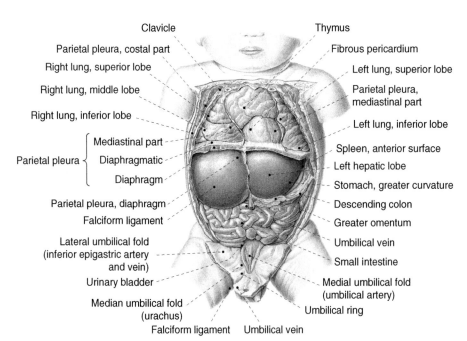

Clavicle
Parietal pleura, costal part
Right lung, superior lobe
Right lung, middle lobe
Right lung, inferior lobe
Parietal pleura { Mediastinal part
Diaphragmatic
Diaphragm
Parietal pleura, diaphragm
Falciform ligament
Lateral umbilical fold (inferior epigastric artery and vein)
Urinary bladder
Median umbilical fold (urachus)
Falciform ligament   Umbilical vein

Thymus
Fibrous pericardium
Left lung, superior lobe
Parietal pleura, mediastinal part
Left lung, inferior lobe
Spleen, anterior surface
Left hepatic lobe
Stomach, greater curvature
Descending colon
Greater omentum
Umbilical vein
Small intestine
Medial umbilical fold (umbilical artery)
Umbilical ring

Figure 8.59 Position of the liver and spleen in a newborn.
With permission, Sobotta: Atlas der Anatomie des Menschen. Publisher: R. Putz and R. Pabst, 21st edn. Elsevier/Urban & Fischer, Munich/Jena 2000

toxic substances produced by them. Colonization builds up slowly during the early years of life and it is not until the age of 3 to 5 years that adult levels of microbial metabolic activity are achieved.

- The mucosal immune system (GALT=gut-associated lymphoid tissue) consisting of Peyer's patches, mesenteric lymph nodes, lymphocytes and solitary follicles located on the mucosal surface. The mucosal immune system becomes active shortly after birth.

- The intestinal epithelial cells which, with their tight junctions, grant passage only to molecules of a certain size. As a result they are specifically able to accommodate antibodies via specific transport cells, known as M-cells. These are then confronted with the GALT and an immune response ensues.

The gut of the unborn child is sterile. The immune structures located in the fetal gut do not come into contact with antigens until the time of birth. The child's first exposure to bacteria – from the mother's vaginal flora – occurs on her journey through the birth canal. The newborn is colonized by other bacteria, such as streptococci and lactobacilli, as a result of skin-to-skin contact with the mother.

Particular importance attaches to the physiological *E. coli* which colonize the child's colon and constitute an important barrier against invading pathogens. In addition, a normal microflora helps to supply the child with the necessary folic acid, biotin, vitamins K, B1, B2 and B6 by a process of biosynthesis (Fig. 8.60).

Yeast-like fungi, such as *Candida albicans*, also take up residence in the child's gut soon after birth. In small numbers (up to a total bacterial count of 10^2) these are harmless, but because of the high sugar content prevalent in today's diet they proliferate excessively in many children. Sugar provides a good nutritional basis for yeast-like fungi. Furthermore, without subsequent treatment to restore the physiological flora of the gut, administration of antibiotics may lead to fungal overgrowth because many antibiotics also kill off the symbiotic organisms in the gut, with the result that they can no longer suppress fungal organisms.

Prior to osteopathic treatment of the viscera it is therefore important to elicit information about previous infections and their treatment and about dietary habits. To facilitate a complete recovery, advice on diet (see Ch.10) and on the restoration of healthy gut flora is often indispensable.

Maturation of the autonomic nervous system

To be able to assess visceral complaints in children it is important to be familiar with the various developmental phases of the autonomic nervous system.

Organized motor activity along the entire digestive tract is required to move food from the mouth to the anus. This depends on the proper functioning of the enteric nervous system. By the end of the first trimester of pregnancy the fetus has already started to swallow amniotic fluid. After birth, in order for food to be ingested, the actions of sucking, breathing and swallowing have to be finely tuned. Usually, even a term newborn requires several days before this process unfolds in a coordinated manner (Carreiro 2003).

Peristaltic motions of the gut can be identified by ultrasound from week 26 of pregnancy; however, these movements are still weak and lack organization. Organized peristaltic waves, similar to the pattern seen in adults, are not identifiable until several months after birth.

Research has demonstrated that the length of the peristaltic cycle increases simultaneously with the length of the child's sleep cycle. This in turn permits more thorough digestion and absorption of nutrients from the diet. This prolonged peristaltic cycle also correlates with changes in the electroencephalogram (EEG). It is therefore suspected that the maturation of the digestive tract plays a major role in the development of the central and enteric nervous systems (Carreiro 2003).

Sphincter function develops only gradually. Neuromuscular coordination for bladder control should be fully developed between the 2nd and 3rd year of life. Anal sphincter control has usually fully matured by the 4th year of life at the latest.

Visceral pain sensation may be diffuse in preschool children. Because their somatic sensory system is still immature,

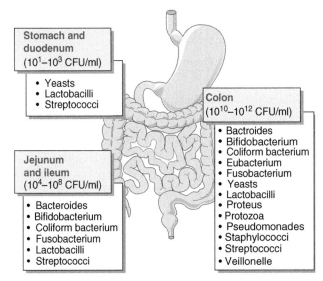

Figure 8.60 Microbial colonization of the gastrointestinal tract. CFU, colony forming units.
With permission, Henriette Rintelen, Velbert

Stomach and duodenum
(10^1–10^3 CFU/ml)
- Yeasts
- Lactobacilli
- Streptococci

Jejunum and ileum
(10^4–10^8 CFU/ml)
- Bacteroides
- Bifidobacterium
- Coliform bacterium
- Fusobacterium
- Lactobacilli
- Streptococci

Colon
(10^{10}–10^{12} CFU/ml)
- Bactroides
- Bifidobacterium
- Coliform bacterium
- Eubacterium
- Fusobacterium
- Yeasts
- Lactobacilli
- Proteus
- Protozoa
- Pseudomonades
- Staphylococci
- Streptococci
- Veillonelle

younger children are usually unable to state precisely where their pain is located. Extra-abdominal pain is often projected into the abdominal cavity; pneumonia or tonsillitis, for example, may be perceived as stomach pain. From the age of about 3 years upwards children's pain reporting is often overlaid by a psychological component. Concerns, apathy and anxieties may then trigger abdominal discomfort of uncertain etiology and children report them as such. We should therefore never rely solely on information volunteered by the child; instead we should always conduct a comprehensive examination of the viscera and body as a whole in order to discover the root cause of the pain.

The body's internal environment is determined by the autonomic nervous system (ANS), which consists of the sympathetic and parasympathetic divisions and the enteric nervous system. The ANS has a decisive influence in maintaining the body's homeostasis (Wilson-Pauwels et al 1997).

At least 10% of school-age children suffer from recurrent abdominal pain. In turn, an underlying cause can be identified in only about 10% of these cases (Hull and Johnston 1996). In my experience many of these children are suffering from autonomic dysregulation caused by a variety of stress factors of a psychological and physical nature. School-age children in particular are often exposed to a heavy burden of pressure in terms of their schoolwork. When factors such as excess noise in the classroom, stress at home, and an absence of peace and quiet for study and relaxation are added into the equation, then somatic reactions may result from psychological stress. Physical stress factors also include poor diet such as caffeine-based drinks, fast-food products containing colouring agents and flavour enhancers and, in allergic patients, contact with allergens. The reminder from Jealous (2004) that we need to 'recognize the role of the autonomic nervous system in health and disease' becomes increasingly important in this context. Osteopathy can be employed to influence functional abdominal pain and to prevent the development of disease. This can be achieved, for example, with the aid of techniques to regulate the ANS, as described below (and also in Ch.12, Nervous (functional) stomach ache).

Osteopathic diagnosis of the abdominal cavity

Osteopathic diagnosis involves meticulous history-taking and inspection as well as auscultation, percussion and careful palpation of the abdominal cavity. The next step is to monitor the expression of involuntary motion in the area to be examined. A gentle and non-invasive way of sensing, which usually leads to a therapeutic process, is to monitor organ movement or lesion patterns in the inhalation phase

of involuntary motion. This is called monitoring motion present. In this type of diagnosis care must be taken that we do not induce any movement at all.

Perceiving with the aid of motion present is different from diagnosis using motion permitted. When testing using motion permitted, the movement potential and restrictions of structures are tested to their limit of movement. This can also be unpleasant because painful movements may possibly be provoked or induced.

To palpate the motion present of the involuntary motion, place your hands as close as possible over the organ in question with a light, soft contact. Here you should simply be aware of the expression of involuntary motion of this tissue in the inhalation phase under your hands but do not follow the motion. Following the motion may already induce an additional movement and thus possibly produce a change in the free expression of the organ.

Although it may be reduced, the involuntary motion of the organ is also always present even where a lesion exists. This motion can be used as a reference system for our treatment. Information concerning the nature of the lesion can be obtained from the amplitude strength and the expression of the involuntary motion.

Practical hints

During osteopathic diagnosis of the viscera using involuntary motion, attention should be paid to the following characteristics since they provide clues to the type of lesion, its possible cause and how it may be treated:

- How does the organ move, what are the preferred directions of movement?
- What is the quality of this movement? Is it vital, hesitant, exaggeratedly strong, fast or slow?
- Is there a fulcrum around which the organ moves and where is it?
- What is the condition of the organ? Do its tissues have a good or poor blood supply? Does it feel dry or congested?
- What is its elasticity and tissue tone?

Osteopathic diagnosis using involuntary motion requires a particular method of 'observing' that is very similar to the way we might look at a painting. We can take most of it in if we choose to stand at the correct distance. If we move too close to the painting and concentrate on details, we will lose the overall impression. Only if we maintain sufficient distance can we recognize the overall relationship of the individual parts of the painting. In the same way, looking too closely at a lesion so that we focus too much on the details has a disruptive effect on the involuntary mechanism, and the involuntary motion eludes our attempts to sense it. Sometimes we then have the feeling of sensing nothing at all.

Furthermore, it is helpful to view the involuntary motion not too intensively but rather to allow part of our awareness to wander a little and also to note other things around us. The involuntary motion then generally expresses itself more clearly. This method of observing and monitoring is also known as 'palpating with divided awareness' (see p.160).

Our ability to sense during palpation improves the more we achieve an inner stillness. Involuntary motion is sensed most clearly if observed from a sufficient distance and received without evaluation. The information received can and should be evaluated afterwards and not during palpation.

> ### Case history
> Two-year-old Tim was brought to my practice because of frequent diarrhea without an infectious etiology.
> His condition had been investigated by a pediatrician using allopathic medical methods, but the findings were inconclusive. Tim was conspicuous for his restless behavior. He was also often aggressive towards others. His own pain threshold was higher than normal.
>
> There had been birth-related complications; because delivery was arrested Tim had to be delivered by vacuum extraction. As an infant he was very restless and cried a lot. His fidgety behavior meant that his mother had problems breastfeeding him and she gave up after a few weeks. Tim was fed with hypoallergenic milk formula.
>
> Cranial examination revealed the following findings: SBS torsion left, SBS compression, and anterior position of the left occipital condyle with possible irritation of the left vagus nerve. Examination of the abdominal cavity showed a general increase in abdominal tension, restlessness in the region of the coeliac plexus, and a tensed diaphragm. The small intestine showed preferred movement into the exhalation phase of involuntary motion. The tissues of the small intestine felt irritated, slightly swollen and restless. In general, the involuntary motion lacked force and had a fairly rapid rhythm. This was evidence that the body was heavily occupied with compensating for the previously detected lesions.
>
> The aim of osteopathic treatment was to regulate the autonomic nervous system by releasing the cranial lesion patterns and normalizing the mobility of the small intestine.
>
> After a few treatments Tim became calmer and generally more sociable. However, his diarrhea showed little improvement although the restrictions detected initially were released and the involuntary motion increased in vitality. Irritation of the tissues of the small intestine was

still detectable. They still felt slightly edematous and poorly perfused. Irritation of this type is commonly encountered in cases of food intolerance. Therefore targeted naturopathic therapy was recommended to support the symbiotic organisms in the gut, and advice was given to avoid cow's milk. The tissue quality of the small intestine then improved noticeably and Tim's diarrhea ceased.

Principles of osteopathic treatment of the viscera

Treatment using motion present

For treatment using motion present, direct your awareness to the organ to be treated and sense the pattern of lesion. After you have identified how the body has organized itself in order to compensate for a lesion, direct your awareness to the expression of health. The body has an inherent power and tendency to heal itself. More than a century ago Dr. A.T. Still (1902) stated that our object should be to find and support health, not to fight disease. Monitoring along these lines seems to provide the body with the necessary framework to implement change.

As you observe and monitor the involuntary motion of the area to be treated while maintaining an appropriate inner distance, the involuntary motion will usually calm down after a period. The body enters a therapeutic process – often also referred to as the still point – during which the tissues undergo reorganization. After some time you will sense the resumption of involuntary motion. It is often then found that both local tissue quality and the overall expression of the PRM have improved.

Treatment using balanced tension

The body often only needs awareness in order to treat itself, as described above for treatment using motion present. The body's innate intelligence knows best what change or what correction is most useful for it, and you should allow it the freedom to implement the treatment. Sometimes, however, this process does not begin spontaneously of its own accord. In these circumstances treatment can be induced and supported using the principle of a balanced tension technique.

Principle of balanced tension

By definition, a tissue lesion involves a change in mobility and/or function. The tissue is no longer able to move freely in all directions. In this altered state the body no longer functions in an unstressed manner as before. Because of the unbalanced tissue tensions and tractions both the blood supply and venolymphatic drainage are impaired. Often the body lacks the strength to free itself unaided from this situation.

Within this state there is a position in which all the tensions and tractions acting on the tissue layer to be treated are in balance; the forces cancel each other out. This state is termed the point of balanced tension (PBT). This PBT can be identified for specific tissues; for example as balanced ligamentous tension (BLT) for the ligaments, balanced membranous tension (BMT) for the membranes, and balanced fluid tension (BFT) for the fluid tissue components. This PBT can usually be found by going into ease with the tissue – as far as the point where the different tissue forces and tractions are in balance. Once the body, with our assistance, has found a PBT, the inherent self-correction tendency within the body is activated. In this position of balanced tension the neurological proprioceptive feedback from the tissue is kept at a comparatively low level and the body has the opportunity to reorganize itself. The involuntary motion quietens and generally passes through a still point. The treated tissue or organ finds its way back to a more favorable position from which it can function in greater harmony with the rest of the body. The body is now less stressed and the involuntary motion expresses itself more freely and clearly than before. Blood flow in the tissue is improved and the entire treated region has a more vital feel to it.

Treatment with balanced tension is very well suited for infants and children. It can be used to treat any body structure, with both a global a local approach. It is respectful and gentle in application because the osteopath follows the PRM entirely, does not overstep the limits of movement, and works with very minimal finger pressure so as to receive as much palpatory information as possible (see previous section, An osteopathic approach to the newborn and infant).

Techniques for treating the viscera

Treating the peritoneum

Mothers often come to the osteopath bringing infants suffering from colic. In these cases it is very helpful first to treat the peritoneum as a whole. Many aspects should be considered as possible triggers for complaints of this kind. Particularly prominent in this context are autonomic overstimulation, psychological stress and food intolerances.

The treatment of the peritoneum described below acts to relax and regulate the autonomic nervous system and makes subsequent local examination and treatment of the abdomen easier. This technique is also very effective in older children suffering from functional abdominal pain. The treatment is a variant of the technique that Anne Wales called the 'turkey bag'.

Method

Perform treatment with the child in the prone position; gravity then acts as a cooperating supportive force and the visceral organs with their peritoneal lining are freely accessible in your hands. Infants may also be carried in a reversed cradling position if they are too restless when placed prone on the treatment table (Fig. 8.61).

Place the palms of your hands next to each other under the child's stomach, with your little fingers touching. As far as possible, your hands should have no contact with the bony structures of the pelvis or thorax so that you can devote yourself entirely to information from the peritoneum and not from the bones. In infants the treatment may also be performed using one hand.

With your hands relaxed, use your fingers to palpate the area of the peritoneum and sense the expression of involuntary motion in the inhalation phase.

While doing this, direct your awareness to the two layers of the peritoneum – the parietal and visceral peritoneum – and their points of attachment to the diaphragm and pelvic floor. You may sense how the visceral peritoneum lines the organs and how the two peritoneal layers move in relation to each other (Fig. 8.62).

After a time the peritoneal motion will calm down and usually go through a still point. The tissue reorganizes itself and the organs are able to reorient themselves in their peritoneal lining. A little while later you will again sense the involuntary motion. Generally, the expression of the involuntary motion will now be more vital and have better symmetry. The autonomic nervous system regulates itself, causing abdominal wall tone to become normalized and to feel uniformly yielding. The movement of the two peritoneal layers in relation to each other will generally have improved.

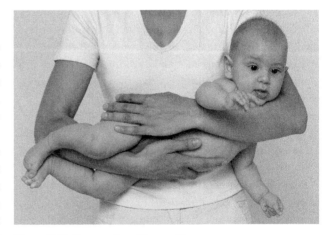

Figure 8.61 Reversed cradling position.
With permission, Karsten Franke, Hamburg

Treating the umbilicus

During history-taking it is of interest to establish whether any umbilical cord complications occurred before or during labor. The umbilical cord is a robust, tensile structure. A variety of situations may produce fascial lesion patterns involving the umbilicus: in utero, for example, traction on an excessively short umbilical cord may result in premature detachment of the placenta, thus impairing the supply of oxygen to the baby and constituting a medical emergency. Later on, in the infant, this lesion can still be palpated in the umbilical region. During labor the umbilical cord may also have been coiled around the child's neck or body or have been too short.

The umbilicus has connections to the urinary bladder and liver via the urachus and the teres hepatis ligament. Its attachment to the liver creates a fascial connection with the diaphragm. A direct connection to the peritoneum is also formed by the medial, median and lateral umbilical folds (Fig. 8.63). Consequently, traction on the umbilical cord can be transmitted as far as these structures and cause pain and sensations of tautness in the entire abdomen and, via the attachment to the diaphragm, also impair breathing.

Barral (1989) observed that there is often a restriction at T4 if the umbilical cord was cut before it had stopped pulsing. As a result a recoil pattern may also be triggered in many cases. The area surrounding the umbilicus then feels tense and as if it has recoiled after a shock.

Method

Perform treatment of the umbilicus with the child supine.

Palpate around the margin of the umbilicus to locate the softest and most yielding point. Place one middle finger over this point, with the palm of your hand resting lightly on the abdomen. Place your other middle finger over the first and induce a slight movement in the direction of ease.

Your awareness should be both on the umbilicus and on the fasciae and ligaments connected to it. Seek and hold a PBT until the involuntary motion comes to rest. Tissue reorganization takes place during the still point. You will sense the involuntary motion again after a time. Then slowly release hand contact (Fig. 8.64).

Treating the neck and umbilicus

If the umbilical cord was positioned around the baby's neck during delivery, it may easily have compressed the neck, and especially the larynx, if traction was exerted. As well as having adverse physical sequelae such as disorders of swallowing

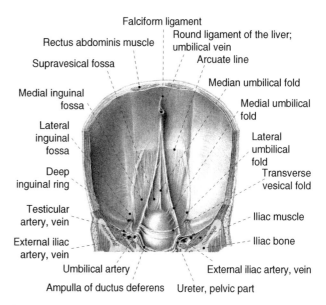

Figure 8.63 Fascial continuity from navel to liver or diaphragm and bladder (front abdominal wall in a newborn, from back). With permission, Sobotta: Atlas der Anatomie des Menschen. Publisher: R. Putz and R. Pabst, 21st edn. Elsevier/Urban & Fischer, Munich/Jena 2000

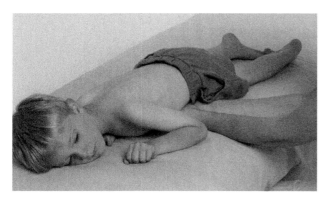

Figure 8.62 Treating the peritoneum.
With permission, Karsten Franke, Hamburg

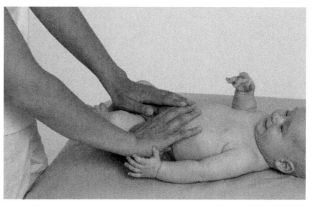

Figure 8.64 Treating the umbilicus.
With permission, Karsten Franke, Hamburg

and later of speech, this may also result in long-term impairment on a psychological level. One expression of this, for example, may be an anxious frame of mind in which affected individuals often put their hands to their neck as a reflex action and dislike wearing tight scarves or collars. In such cases it is advisable also to treat the neck and larynx in addition to the umbilicus.

Method

Lightly from behind, place the fingers of one hand round the side of the child's neck and place the fingers of your other hand in soft and open contact over the umbilicus and monitor the expression of involuntary motion, paying particular attention to the inhalation phase. Because memories are sometimes stored in the tissues, this technique may make the child agitated if the treatment perhaps acts as a reminder of the difficult circumstances around her birth. I recommend that you warn the mother in advance and ask her to maintain body contact with her child during treatment to give the infant a sense of security (Fig. 8.65).

If necessary, the larynx can also be treated afterwards using a BLT technique.

Treating the liver

Following immunizations, drug administration and infections it is generally advisable to examine the liver and to treat it, where necessary; in such situations special demands are placed on the liver's detoxifying function and osteopathy can support this activity. If drugs capable of crossing the placenta were administered during pregnancy and/or labor, treating the liver of the newborn may stimulate the excretion of these substances. In neonatal jaundice osteopathic treatment can support hepatocyte maturation and erythrocyte breakdown.

In my own practice I sometimes see foster children whose natural mothers were alcohol- or drug-dependent during pregnancy, causing the children to be exposed to these substances in utero. Immediately after birth many of these children need to undergo withdrawal. In this context, osteopathic treatment encourages toxin excretion by the liver, supports the hepatocyte regeneration and improves general tissue quality.

Barral (1989) emphasized the importance of treating the liver in chronic infections, chronic fever, digestive disorders, low muscle tone and dehydration. Treatment of the liver is most effective if the diaphragm, hepatic portal vein and proper hepatic artery are first released from any restrictions. This guarantees optimal venous drainage via the inferior vena cava and a good blood supply to the liver via the vessels supplying it.

Method

Perform treatment of the liver with the child in the supine position. Sit at the child's right side and span the liver using both hands. Place one open hand under the right costal arch and the other hand gently over the ventral costal arch. The fingers of both hands point in direction of the spinal column.

Monitor the involuntary motion of the liver, paying particular attention to the fibrous capsule of the liver, its ligamentous attachments, the arterial supply to and venous drainage of the organ, and the hepatocytes (Fig. 8.66).

Wait until the involuntary motion of the liver has come to rest. This is followed by a still point and tissue reorganization. Once the involuntary motion has clearly resumed, it is generally more powerful and symmetrical, and the drainage and perfusion of the liver are improved.

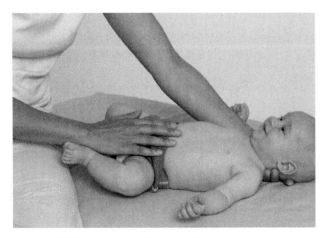

Figure 8.65 Treating the neck and umbilicus.
With permission, Karsten Franke, Hamburg

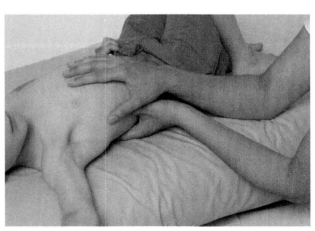

Figure 8.66 Treating the liver.
With permission, Karsten Franke, Hamburg

Bibliography

Barral J-P: Visceral manipulation. Eastland Press, Seattle 1989

Becker R: Life in motion. Rudra Press, Portland, Ore. 1997

Carreiro J: An osteopathic approach to children. Churchill Livingstone, Edinburgh 2003

Hull D, Johnston D I: Essential pediatrics. 3rd edn. Churchill Livingstone, Singapore 1996

Jealous J S: Emergence of originality. Course transcript 2004

Moll R, Schain-Emmerich U: Allergiekost für Mutter und Kind. Econ & List, Munich 1998

Netter F: Netters Pädiatrie. Thieme, Stuttgart 2001

Rapp D: Ist das Ihr Kind? 4th edn. Hamburg, Promedico 2000

Schöllmann C, Zimmermann K: Interstitielle Mikroflora und Immunsystem. Materia Medica, Forum Medizin, Stockdorf 1997

Stadelmann I: Die Hebammensprechstunde. Eigenverlag, Kempten 1994

Still A T: Philosophy and mechanical principles of osteopathy. Hudson Kimberly, Kansas 1902. Reprinted by Osteopathic Enterprise, Kirksville, Mo. 1986

Sutherland W G: Teachings in the science of osteopathy Anne Wales (ed.) Sutherland Cranial Teaching Foundation 1990

Sutherland W G: Contributions of thought. 2nd edn. Ada Strand Sutherland and Anne Wales (eds) Sutherland Cranial Teaching Foundation 1998

Wilson-Pauwels L, Stewart P, Akesson E: Autonomic nerves. B C Decker, London 1997

9

Psychological aspects

Christine Conroy, Susannah Booth, Renate Sander-Schmidt

DIAGNOSING AND TREATING EMOTIONAL FACTORS

Christine Conroy

Osteopaths working with involuntary motion are fairly adept at 'reading' the body. We know that it is not only the amplitude of motion, whether there is normal or excessive motion or no motion at all, but also the quality of that motion which brings diagnostic information through our palpating hands to our awareness. When treating infants and children, that diagnostic palpatory skill is extremely important, since these patients do not usually explain their symptoms in detail.

The more we palpate involuntary motion, correlating that palpatory experience with known clinical, environmental, traumatic and emotional history, the more understanding we acquire. We become connoisseurs and even surprise ourselves at the precision of our discernment of what happens in the patient at that point in time when we engage our attention with the tissues. We become aware of areas of health and discomfort, the probable cause and when this is likely to have occurred. Endless nuances of the expression of involuntary motion reveal the natural history of the individual.

When all is well, we perceive peaceful, rhythmic fluid motion evenly throughout the tissues and in the space around the patient. This, however, is rare. There is almost always some remaining asymmetry or oddity of motion, so we continue to 'feel around' for information. When we feel we have treated all of the tissue or fluid based lesions that we have found; when we feel we have reached the limit of our clinical competence and have even referred to colleagues for a second opinion, we may still have a crying baby. We can give up or we can look further into the living physiology for other clues to the cause of the infant's distress.

What makes each of us unique as human beings? It is the combined effect of everything we have encountered since our arrival on earth and how we have each adapted or compensated for it until this point in time. This includes the effect of our culture, social status and education, our acquired or rejected values from parents, teachers, peers, idols, our traumatic history (both physical and emotional), and our soul's longing.

How do we know we are having an emotion? It is also a physical experience. Our feelings are expressed as internal disturbance; for example, as butterflies in the stomach with anxiety, a 'lead weight' in the abdomen with disappointment, neck/shoulder tension when overwhelmed by life's demands, or we are trembling with anxiety. Those things we can feel in ourselves can be perceived in others as subtle variations in the expression of 'primary respiratory motion'.

A baby is just the same as an adult, but his life story is short and the environmental imprint upon it is thereby limited. It is worth a gentle enquiry of the infant's carers about circumstances which may be disturbing the baby emotionally. When no information is forthcoming, it is useful to have a palpatory skill that can reveal the information to you from the anatomy and physiology of the patient.

Emotional patterns of disturbance

Some variations in the expression of involuntary motion appear as 'patterns' of disturbance in babies. These patterns do not necessarily respect anatomical boundaries or embryological fluid fields. They are a particular combination of quality and amplitude of involuntary motion. These patterns occur also in adults and have qualitative consistency. They may be called emotional patterns.

Emotional patterns of involuntary motion may accompany voluntary motion; for example the unilateral raising of a shoulder while inclining the head to the same side in anguish, holding the breath, bilateral internal rotation of the lower limbs with shyness. Such distortions of physique and involuntary motion patterns are often the only clue to unexpressed emotion. When the connection between the patterns of involuntary motion expression and the emotions that patients feel is made, it begins to make sense.

Recognizing and acknowledging an emotional 'lesion' while engaged with primary respiratory motion brings about an immediate change in the quality of motion in exactly the same way as all therapeutic transmutations. Diagnosis becomes treatment the moment that the problem is seen. When we sit in stillness and observe, the 'lesion' starts to unwind, though it may take some time or repeated treatment for full resolution to occur.

Our acknowledgement of patients' feelings, with a few kind words, and a compassionate disposition are of value in a clinical situation. Indeed, this is often sufficient to allay minor anxieties and many symptoms. Unacknowledged emotion often results in treatment reactions.

Emotions as etiological factors in osteopathic lesions

Emotions are part of our everyday life experience. They motivate or stultify our behavior. There are almost always emotions present in ourselves as well as in our patients, whether we pay attention to them or not. We may not notice some feelings because we are directing our attentions at our thoughts and plans. We may notice but not express our emotions for reasons of social impropriety or deny their existence for fear of disapproval.

In clinical practice, we become increasingly aware that our patients' emotions can be both etiological and maintaining factors in presenting conditions. There seems to be enormous variability in the degree to which osteopaths acknowledge emotion in our evaluation of cases, our approach to treatment, our prognoses and in the advice given to patients.

Unless we are educated in psychotherapeutic skills, it is not within our remit as osteopaths to engage in the processing work necessary to help our patients to resolve their emotional problems. Where there are frank clinical psycho-emotional conditions we refer patients for appropriate help. But emotion is a significant variable in clinical presentations and can account for inconsistencies in our clinical findings and therapeutic effectiveness. They are often covert etiological and maintaining factors in presenting cases.

As infants and young children are not necessarily able to communicate their feelings, it can be useful to be able to detect emotional factors in symptomatology with one's own palpatory skill. To read these emotional patterns it is important that we center ourselves and are still enough to perceive primary respiration. We are then no longer in an intellectual state, but in a 'feeling state', where the world of subtler phenomena becomes revealed to us. As Dr. Sutherland said in a phrase borrowed from the bible: 'Be still and know'.

Examples of covert emotional etiology

• Patients with musculoskeletal pain which began 'for no apparent reason', whose symptoms we cannot satisfactorily account for within established osteopathic or pathological paradigms.

• A baby who constantly cries and whose mother is distressed.

• Patients who take a very long time to get better, if they get better at all.

• Patients who always get symptoms in particular life situations; for example:
  – a baby who always wheezes when visiting a tense household.
  – a man who has a fall or strains himself or has an accident whenever he is decorating the house. His wife loves decorating. He hates it.
  – a child who always gets a headache on Wednesdays, the day a disliked teacher is in charge.

• Children with 'bad posture': the strict mother of a child with 'bad posture' was observed raising her hand as if to strike her son's head in reprimand for a perceived misdemeanour. He cowered deeper into his kypholordotic posture, which was presumably how his posture had developed.

• Patients presenting in clusters, for example:
  – more children develop aches and pains around the time of examinations or when performance results are awaited.
  – teachers from the same school appear in increased numbers when a school inspection is due.

• Acute onset conditions following a life trauma, for example:
  – the death of a loved one.
  – the feeling of abandonment when a family member leaves home permanently.
  – moving house, moving school, etc.

Examples of covert emotional maintaining factors

• Patients with vague musculoskeletal pains, which 'move around'. Once a symptomatic area is treated, the patient tells you that the pain has moved to another area and then another place altogether.

• Patients who leave your practice relieved of pain and full of gratitude, only to return over and over again with that pain re-created for no apparent reason.

• 'Gifted' children, like musicians or dancers with recurrent pains unrelated to strain or injury may not share their parents' ambitions for their lives.

• Children with very strict or exacting parents present with myriad symptoms.

• A child with a recurrent pain in the neck who reveals that his teacher is always breathing down his neck.

• Patients with apparently similar conditions who report enormously variable levels of pain. The ones who have more pain are often the ones carrying more emotional weight.

When we recognize and acknowledge the emotional component of structural dysfunction in our patients, it may solve a lot of mysteries.

Babies' feelings

A baby lives primarily in the feeling state; at an instinctive level. A baby's world is small. To a breastfeeding infant the world is no bigger than the arms, breast, lap and face of his mother. The atmosphere of that world is determined by his mother's feelings.

A loving attentive mother imbues the baby's world with peace. An anxious mother imbues that world with anxiety. Similarly the baby perceives the emotions or mood of other people who hold him. As a mother's mood changes, so does her facial expression, the tone of her voice, the way she handles the baby and, some say, even the sweetness of her milk. The baby feels and reacts as we all once did.

As the baby grows, so too does his world and therefore the range of his 'antenna'. The baby feels his environment; the room he is in, the 'vibe' of a throng, the atmosphere of changing surroundings during a journey and so on.

Any threat to the mother's well-being is a threat to the baby's survival. If entering a certain environment is associated with the mother's distress or anxiety, this feeling is transmitted to the child, who will react in a particular way. Mostly infants will cry. Older children may panic, have a tantrum or go missing. The child will react in the same way whenever his mother feels the same emotions or enters a similar environment. That environment may, for example, be your osteopathic practice.

Identifying emotional patterns in involuntary motion

In adulthood instinctive awareness is preserved. That awareness, however, may be eclipsed by emotions developed from past experiences or our thoughts and plans. When there is fear in the air, everyone feels fear. Do you ever wonder whether the feelings you have arose from within yourself or from without? Most often we assume that if we feel something, then the feeling arizes from within ourselves.

In a clinical situation working with the involuntary mechanism, we are in the 'feeling state'. When we feel an emotion do we assume we have strayed from our neutral observation position? Do we disregard them because they fail to fit in with our clinical diagnosis, treatment plan or prognosis? What if those feelings are part of the information we are seeking?

Feelings in a treatment room pose a dilemma. How can we distinguish whether the feelings present are our own, the patient's or those of other persons in the room; the parents, for example? It is always helpful to be aware of our own emotions at the start of a working day and to be vigilant about projecting the nature, scale and weight of our emotions onto our patients. It is important to find a neutral emotional state from which to work, to check out our emotions throughout the day and to keep bringing ourselves back to neutral. This increases our objectivity of perception. From a neutral position we can better observe subtle changes in the expression of involuntary motion in all or part of a patient's anatomico-physiological body, particularly when they spontaneously remember something or express emotion during treatment.

When physical trauma is releasing, there is almost invariably an emotional component. The patient may re-experience shock or terror or the stress they were feeling at the time the trauma took place. They may weep. The pattern of their breathing may change. They may curl up a limb or other body part in the pattern of the trauma. Their involuntary motion will certainly change.

Notice how the patterns of those emotions are part of, or coexist with inter- or intraosseous strains, fascial drag, membranous inertia or the turbulence of fluid motion. In this way you will build up your palpatory and perceptual library. As with all perceptual skills, they take time to develop. We observe and observe for as long as it takes. Slowly understanding comes.

Emotional awareness exercises

Exercise 1

Sit quietly for a while and bring yourself to peace. Center yourself in the way you would before starting a treatment. Become aware of primary respiratory motion within yourself. Notice its rate, amplitude and quality.

Now recall a situation when you felt excited. Remember as much as you can about yourself and the circumstances at that time to help you to feel that excitement again. When you really feel excited redirect your attention to primary respiratory motion within yourself. How is it now? Notice whether the rate, amplitude and quality has changed in both the inhalation and exhalation phases. Did the space around you feel different? If so, in what way? Which part of your body or the space around you was most affected by this feeling? Make a note of the particular quality of excitement.

Allow the memory to fade and wait until a neutral is reached and then wait again for biphasic involuntary motion re-establish itself.

Perform the same exercise again and recall a situation in which you were terrified. Make a note of the changes in the expression of primary respiratory motion within and around yourself. Compare this with the quality of excitement.

You can repeat this exercise with delight, anger, disappointment, apathy, jealousy, sadness, rejection, feeling forlorn, bewilderment and so on. You will recognize that these feeling states have a characteristic feel to them. I call it a hallmark.

Exercise 2

Take a partner who is willing to be your model.

Sit quietly for a while to bring yourself to peace. Be aware of any emotions within yourself. Wait until you have come to a true neutral. Prepare yourself in the usual way before placing your hands upon the model. Anywhere will do. An anteroposterior hold at the diaphragm is a good place. Become aware of primary respiratory motion within your model.

Ask the model to recall a time when they were excited and direct them through the exercise points as described in Exercise 1.

Notice how the expression of primary respiratory motion has altered in rate, amplitude and quality. Notice changes in the space around them. Make a note of your observations. Then wait for a normal rate and rhythm to be re-established.

Repeat the exercise with other emotions. Two or three emotions are plenty for one practical session. You can try more on other occasions.

Compare your objective findings with your previously noted subjective observations. Are there similarities? What are they? What is the hallmark of each emotion?

Case histories

Case history: Wyn

Wyn, a healthy, fresh-faced local horsewoman, called for a treatment during the early stages of labor for her first baby. She was on her way to the hospital with her friend Val, a mother of two and the appointed 'wise-woman' of the situation.

I had treated Wyn once during her pregnancy and she was in good shape. During this treatment I was balancing fluid. I focused my attention on optimal function within her pelvis; sacroiliac, sacrococcygeal and lumbosacral articulations, the pelvic floor, diaphragm and psoas muscles. I was also looking at the midline of the mother, the womb and the baby; a useful prenatal treatment.

All was balancing well. Wyn had settled into a deep neutral and I was waiting for all of the automatic shifting motion to settle down. Val was sitting in on the treatment. She had been mostly silent then suddenly said out loud, 'It doesn't matter what you do, Wyn. It's going to hurt like hell. You just have to get through it.'

Under my palpating hands there was an abrupt change in the quality and pattern of the motion present. There seemed to be a sudden absence of motion around her midline, a column of hardness around the midline and a spiky quality in the space around her. She felt like a thorn apple without a core, save for the fluid turbulence around her solar plexus. Shock, fear and foreboding. I was shocked, too. The treatment seemed to have been arrested. After a little time I retrieved a personal state of stillness and focused on that part of her that was healthy. I maintained my hand contact while telling a few stories of ladies who had quite a different experience; particularly of one lady I once knew who had described her birthing experience as 'like a jolly good defecation'.

Wyn laughed uncertainly. Miraculously, I did not have to start the treatment again. She soon re-entered a deep neutral before the gentle inhalation-exhalation rhythm re-established itself and the treatment was finished.

Case history: Haf

Haf was 3 months old when I met her and her mother Lowri. She had been born by caesarean section after a long hard labor, with her mother's cervix only dilating 6 cm. Haf was reported to have been irritable for a couple of days after birth and 'hyper alert' since then. She resisted sleep and woke several times a night when she was breast fed. Breastfeeding was always a very long, slow process.

The baby's tissues had a wide-awake, 'alert' feel to them. I recognized this feeling as like being on the 'lookout' in a threatening situation.

At the first treatment Haf responded well to balanced fluid tension techniques. She came to neutral. Not for long, apparently. At the next meeting Lowri reported that Haf's hyper-alertness remained.

Lowri had a high-pitched voice and always spoke in a hurried, breathless way. She hardly ever stopped talking when I was treating Haf, except when I asked her to. She was constantly explaining to me that she does everything to ensure the baby's peace and comfort. In her efforts to get the baby to sleep, she creeps around the room, refuses to play the radio or television and forbids any noise in the house. Haf, she said, was always awake, alert, and watching her. Sometimes she also cried.

Recognizing that it was difficult for me to breathe when Lowri was talking, I also noticed that it took some time to center myself in this force field before I could treat the baby. What effect was Lowri's disposition having on Haf? Haf always dozed off during treatment and Lowri said how wonderful it would be if I could come to their house every evening and do the same thing.

While maintaining my hand contact on Half's head, I explained to Lowri that it was not so much the outer silence in a room that assisted a baby to rest, but the inner silence in those close by. In order to treat Haf, I had to first ground, center and silence myself and that the peace within me was bringing the baby to peace.

Lowri was doubtful and apparently unaware of the disturbance that her own anxiety might create. As if by divine providence, a medical textbook fell from the top of my wall-mounted bookshelf, dislodged a picture hanging nearby and both came crashing to the floor.

Haf did not stir or make a sound. I did not budge, and Lowri was sitting in silence.

Case history: Joanne

Joanne was 16 years old. She complained of pain around the left patella and behind the left knee. The pain was reported to have begun about 18 months earlier but for no apparent reason. There had never been any swelling or redness, nor any loss of movement. Also there had never been any trauma to the lower extremity.

She had visited her GP, who offered no diagnosis, but did offer anti-inflammatories, which were ineffective. A referral was made to an orthopedic surgeon, who X-rayed and MRI scanned the knee and found nothing abnormal. She reported that nothing in particular aggravated the pain but she noticed it more when her knee was straight and sometimes when 'running about'. Walking and swimming did not affect the pain.

When I examined her, there was a vaguely positive compression test of the left lateral meniscus area. The lower extremity was held in hyperextension. The popliteus muscle was hypertonic and the lateral thigh muscles were very slightly hypertonic. The patellofemoral joint was normal. While palpating involuntary motion, I got no further diagnostic clues.

Lacking etiological information, I made a tentative diagnosis of a possible meniscal problem and set to work in addressing the symptomatic tissues with a functional/BLT/BFT approach to treatment. When I had finished, I shared my observations with her father, who had accompanied her to the practice, and suggested that an arthroscopic investigation might reveal something.

Her father replied with anger and impatience that he had no time for the orthopedic doctor, he was useless. As his neck and shoulders tightened, his face reddened. He raised his hand and pointed his index finger at me as he spoke. He complained that the stupid man had even offered to operate on the knee with no diagnosis. Joanne's father had apparently left the surgeon's office in disgust.

I felt a little scared of his ferocity and was privately trembling. My discomfort had begun during his intense scrutiny of my working on his daughter. Joanne's father calmed down a bit as I explained that arthroscopy is both an investigative and therapeutic procedure. 'Well, why didn't he explain that?' he asked me. I shrugged my shoulders non-commitally. As they left my office, I breathed out.

The following week, Joanne and her father returned. Her knee had been symptom-free for 4 days. A couple of days earlier she had had a severe left low back pain, which had come on acutely while in bed. She reported that she 'couldn't move' and had called her sister for help. It was still there now, 'a bit'.

On examination, there was nothing remarkable about the knee. No positive meniscal test. There was a fascial drag from her left innominate superiorly, fading around her left lower ribs, which created a mild left sacroiliac misalignment. Bewildered about the etiology, I set to work. The sacroiliac was brought to balance very quickly leaving nothing obvious left to do, so I 'looked around'.

Joanne's father was scrutinizing. I was trying to stay in neutral and to resist the tension emitting from him, while explaining to Joanne that we sometimes fear that we cannot move but usually we can. We get locked in fright. Joanne was beginning to relax.

Her father suddenly offered information that he kept a good household. He had standards, he did not permit his children to run around, not even in the street. His children must sit at the table at mealtimes and must say their prayers before they eat.

Joanne's mechanism changed under my palpating hands. The involuntary motion stopped abruptly in the whole left lower quadrant of her body. She retracted her hyperextended left leg superiorly, as if she were wincing. The space around her had developed a 'buzz'.

And there it was, the etiology. Joanne told me her knee was hurting. I remembered that she noticed the pain most when she was running around or keeping her leg straight; that is when she incurs the wrath of her father.

It is difficult to suggest to someone like her father that the cause of Joanne's problem might be her reaction to him. I feared that she would be reprimanded or subjected to the further tyranny of a shouting father telling her to 'relax'.

The next time her father brought Joanne for treatment, he waited in the waiting room. His confidence in me had apparently grown since Joanne was complaining less. There had been only one occasion of knee pain since we last met and that was while Joanne was standing near to her father while being reprimanded by him. I asked her: 'How were you feeling then? ' 'I just wanted to run away', she answered. I helped her realize that she was tensing her leg in these situations and that she could choose not to. That she would soon be an adult and everything would change. She smiled and then rushed into the waiting room shouting to her father, 'I am cured!' I hear she has had no further knee pain since then.

> ### Case history: Sally
>
> I first met Sally when she was 3 months old. She was brought by both of her parents, an apparently contented, easy going couple. Being near them was comfortable and warm. She was their fourth child. They had heard about cranial osteopathy being useful sometimes for crying babies.
>
> The labor had been induced on the calculated due date, since the ultrasound scan had revealed that the baby was large and the mother had a history of hemorrhaging badly.
>
> The first stage of labor was described as 'slow' and the second stage had taken 7 minutes exactly. Sally was born with a narrow head in the lateral dimension. There had been a good primal scream and Sally had never stopped screaming since that moment, except when she was asleep, which was not often enough. This was the sole symptom.
>
> Sally's head was now very wide across the lateral dimension of the vault and very narrow around the cranial base. After engaging with the involuntary mechanism, the head felt immensely compressed throughout, most especially at the cranial base and the atlanto-occipital joint. It reminded me of a balloon with its base squeezed into a tight ring. After releasing the occipital condyles from the atlantal facets, I allowed the fluid within the cranium to come to balanced tension. Sally screamed for about 5 minutes and then abruptly stopped.
>
> When I saw Sally again 10 days later her parents reported her to be a different baby. She had not screamed at all, but she had cried when hungry only. Her mother felt she was 'quite normal'. It seemed too good to be true, so I checked the involuntary mechanism. The compression I had previously noticed did not seem to be there, save for some restriction of motion in the diaphragm, the tent and other transverse membranes, which I attended to. Just to be sure that was true, I decided to check the baby again in 3 weeks time.
>
> On the third visit her parents reported again that Sally had not screamed at all. Her head had assumed a more normal shape. Full of pride and enthusiasm, I took hold of the baby in order to check the involuntary motion. Sally screamed at once.
>
> I was startled, confused and a little irritated. Thankfully I realized very quickly that what was disturbing Sally was me! I had not centered myself and invaded her. I backed off and talked to the baby directly: 'I'm sorry, did I startle you? Now let's start again. May I have another look?' Sally stopped screaming. After centering myself, I gently reapplied my hands. Sally remained peaceful as I directed my attention here and there within the involuntary mechanism. I could find little to treat, save a little tension around her left diaphragm.

At 4 months old, Sally was happy and well.

A CHILD'S WORLD

Susannah Booth

For the osteopath assessing a young patient, acknowledgement of the child's world may provide an insight that changes both the diagnosis and approach in treatment. For example, the inability for a 2-year-old to cope with any change to routine or environment may not be autistic in nature. Rather, this may relate to the difficulties the child has in adjusting to having an increased awareness of the outside world.

Furthermore, the phenomenon of quantum mechanics suggests that it is possible for there to be an effect on an object merely by observation. If this holds true for osteopathic treatment, then it would seem important when working with the immaturity and constant growth associated with childhood to make the child's consciousness central to this process.

How then is it possible to understand a child's world? Firstly by observation; by watching how the child seems to interact and experience the world and gaining an idea of what he is trying to achieve.

Obviously, some clues may come from noting the outward behavior, which in itself is a complex interaction of a child's increasing abilities, awareness, experience and character. Further clues may manifest themselves through a child's creative activities such as in drawings, as these often symbolize the child's inner experience and feelings.

By looking at the various stages in a young child's development, his world is seen to evolve in many different ways.

Sensation before and after birth

During pregnancy, the child's world is at one with his mother. Erich Blechschmidt (1978) described the flowing fluid-like formative movements of embryogenesis. It is within this process that, with growth, the child's character appears to gain expression, becoming more distinct from the mother's.

At birth, the bonded mother and child begin a process of separation from the moment of the first breath. This awakening triggers the need to fully unfold and expand into a physical helplessness created by gravity.

Steiner (1923) suggested a newborn's world as being one where children are 'sleeping' in their consciousness, 'dreaming' in their emotions and are most 'awake' in their willing. This is sufficiently powerful to provide the means for survival and even the ability for preterm infants to will physiological function out of immature structures.

Jaffke (1996) described small children as being like eyes, which allow impressions to enter and pass through, liken-ing will to being something that is used 'to take hold of and assimilate the world through the senses'. From this, it becomes understandable why some infant's distress with colic pain can be so severe. Sleep allows respite from a world of constant sensation.

Each day the process of unfolding, initiated at birth, continues as the child grows.

The child starts to lift himself up

The child's visual axis provides the fulcrum for orientation within the world, allowing him to strengthen flexor tone and gain control of his head. Later, using the axes of his limbs and spine enables the dexterity and strength to grasp and move against gravity. After a year of continuous practice begins the ability to lift the body upright. From this position there is a developmental surge of proprioceptive activity in the feet and the start of a journey to map the details required for spatial awareness.

The osteopathic concepts of midline, center of gravity and suspended automatic shifting fulcrum are all interwoven in the child's task of lifting himself upright. Without a midline, there is no orientation for movement to progress from; there is no acquisition of a sense of gravity and no ability to correctly adjust the suspension of the body's fulcrum and maintain balance.

Looking at early children's drawings: so often large circular movements are made which are hardly contained by the paper itself (Fig. 9.1). Strauss (1988) suggested that these relate to the life processes and formative processes within the young child's own body. She also suggested that the vertical lines drawn 'reflect the child's experience of standing upright' and that the symbol of a cross 'documents standing in space' (Fig. 9.2).

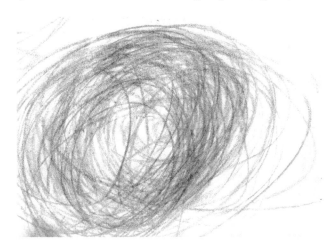

Figure 9.1 Large circular movements reflecting the formative and life processes within a young child's body.
With permission, Rosie Runciman, London

The child starts to speak

The milestone of speech comes only after walking has been accomplished. Steiner (1923) suggested that the equilibrium between the movements of the legs and the movements of the hands and arms creates the physical and psychical balance for the child 'to stand within the universe' and speak. Whilst this may hold for the normally developing child, for an autistic child the experience of being centered and being in contact with the outside world can create considerable distress.

Developing a sense of self

Following the explosion of vocabulary at around 18 months, the 2-year-old child starts to become aware of his sense of self. The change in consciousness of the outside world that this brings frequently creates the sudden need to be controlling and resistant to change.

Strauss (1988) linked the drawing of the circle with the experience of the ego and, later, in the 3rd year, the drawing of 'I-forms' (the point or cross within a circle) with the child's sense of ego and of the world about him (Fig. 9.3).

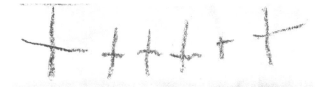

Figure 9.2 The symbol of the cross documenting the experience of standing in space.
With permission, Rosie Runciman, London

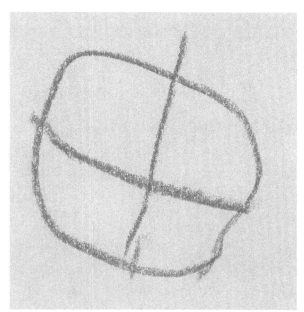

Figure 9.3 A cross within a circle representing the child's sense of ego and the world about him.
With permission, Rosie Runciman, London

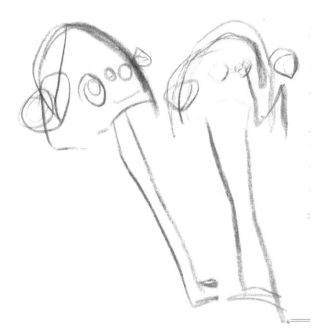

Figure 9.4 'Pillar' people drawn at the age of 2–3years showing a developing sense of gravity.
With permission, Rosie Runciman, London

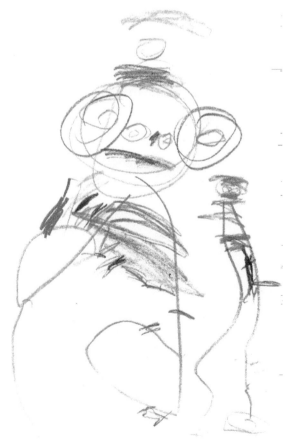

Figure 9.5 'Ladder motif' suggestive of a changing awareness of segmental growth and motion.
With permission, Rosie Runciman, London

Drawings of people or trees, Strauss (1988) believes, illustrates the child's awareness of the forces working within his own organization. The 'pillar' people (Fig. 9.4) drawn at the age of 2 to 3 years seem like static pedestals as the child is developing his own sense of gravity. Later drawings of people evolve this process by becoming grounded and symmetrical, growing a 'ladder motif' through the torso (Fig. 9.5), with limbs and large fingers being added like 'organs of perception' (Fig. 9.6).

The picture of the house which appears in the drawings of slightly older children represents the relationship of the child to the world about them, evolving from 'head' people within circles (Fig. 9.7), perhaps an unconscious memory of the

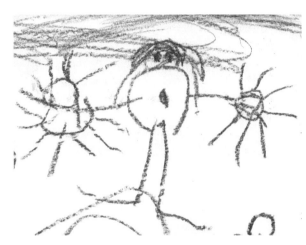

Figure 9.6 Open hands with large fingers representative of a child's constant exploration and appreciation of the world.
With permission, Rosie Runciman, London

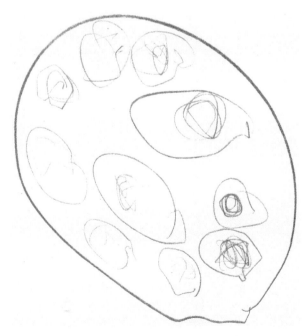

Figure 9.7 'Head' people in circles as precursor of a house.
With permission, Rosie Runciman, London

Of course whilst children's drawings are helpful to deepen ones understanding of their view and hence our own ability to observe this more carefully, it is not a necessary requirement of an examination to have a collection of our small patient's drawings. More, it is the development of an appreciation of the child's awareness, response and interaction with their world as they take on the challenge of growing up which should be central to the work of a pediatric osteopath.

Bibliography

Blechschmidt E, Gasser R: Biokinetics and biodynamics of human differentiation. Thomas Books, Springfield, Ill. 1978

Jaffke F: Work and play in early childhood. Floris Books, Edinburgh 1996

König, K: The first three years of the child: walking, speaking, thinking. Floris Books, Edinburgh 2004

Steiner R: Lectures given in Dornach, Switzerland, April 15–22, 1923, reported by Steffen A, The Library of the Anthroposophical Society in Great Britain, London

Steiner R: The child's changing consciousness and Waldorf education, Lecture II, Dornach, April 16, 1923. Rudolf Steiner Press, London 1988

Strauss M: Understanding children's drawings, Rudolf Steiner Press, London 1988

UNEXPECTED INTERACTIONS

Renate Sander-Schmidt

'... what is essential takes place neither in the one participant or the other, nor in a universe that includes them both as well as everything else; instead, in the most precize sense, it takes place between the two of them, in a dimension that is accessible only to them' (Buber 2000).

This chapter is intended to shed yet more light on both internal as well as external factors to which the osteopath is exposed in the course of therapeutic activity – especially as it relates to children and infants. Although this outline cannot lay claim to completeness or systematic coverage, a number of factors that are influential in this context will be described as illustrative examples. The idea of writing on this topic arose from the body psychotherapy experience of an osteopathic practitioner who felt inexplicable fatigue as a result of her work, even though she found this to be helpful and rewarding.

The ability to help others and to support them in their healing often has the implicit corollary that the individuals delivering this help lose sight of themselves. They are 'touched' by what happens in the treatment, and yet they fail to recognize that their reactions to being touched are also rooted in their personal experience of life. In this setting it is inevitable that 'blind spots' will also be addressed. The term 'blind spots' covers all those things that have shaped and determined us,

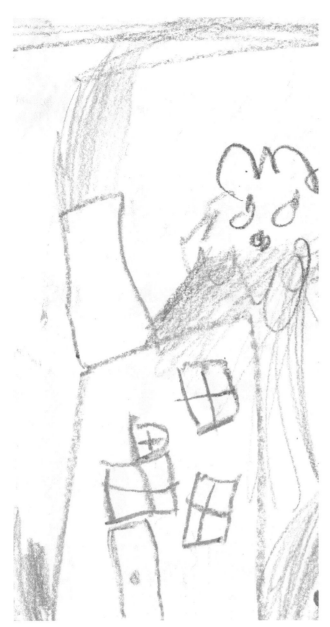

Figure 9.8 A completed house suggestive of the 4-year-olds' maturing sense of themselves within the world, the world about them and their connections.
With permission, Rosie Runciman, London

embryonic state, to houses with doors, windows and chimneys which connect the child to the world (Fig. 9.8).

It is important to remember that a child's outlook and requirements in relation to the physical world differ to that of the adult. From infancy to adolescence, each stage of childhood development has its own characteristics, which are shaped by the formative and life forces within. The three major achievements of the first three years – learning to walk, to speak and to think – were described by König (2004) as 'an act of grace in every child'.

even if we are unable or unwilling to recall them. And yet all this is stored in our bodies and it is only with difficulty or in part that it has access to our conscious mind.

Our body memory reaches back to our time in the womb. 'The primary senses – and hence the first psychological representations in terms of body memory – are already formed in the first 4 weeks' (Reiter 1999). 'They are the aspects that are often problematic for us' (Janus 1997). If these are touched by the treatment, we deny them at the expense of strength and energy, which are then no longer available to the therapist and hence to the treatment.

The osteopath as part of the treatment process

During and after the treatment, you should definitely take space and time to heed your own emotions and feelings and to respect them. This includes physical reactions, such as sudden tiredness or pins and needles in your neck, and consciously perceived feelings such as annoyance or pleasure. Depending on what governs your approach, there may also be a noticeable change in tension; for example, in that your touch becomes firmer without any identifiable reason, or there may be a shift in the quality of intuition, possibly recognizable in that there is a sudden change in inner closeness to or distance from the patient. These signals indicate that you are part of the treatment process. They also make it plain that during the treatment process we therapists are exposed to external as well as internal influences.

External influences

Apart from the information communicated by the patient, external influences include the setting, and this refers in particular to the working atmosphere. Thus, for example, the presence of accompanying adults or siblings may be helpful or disruptive for the osteopath. In the latter case it is entirely possible that the osteopath may become caught up in the complex web of a family conflict, or may sense transferred reactions to a family conflict on the part of the child who is to be treated. In such cases, attempts should be made to reach a solution with the adults to ensure that next time the child is treated alone or that the sibling is looked after elsewhere during the treatment session. Once an appropriate solution has been found, the osteopath can then give undivided concentration to the treatment.

It is important to ensure a setting in which it is possible to remain concentrated on and devoted to the patient. Sometimes a period of experimentation is required to discover the external setting that works best.

Internal influences

Internal influences refer to those reactions that reflect our personal life experience and its conscious and unconscious processing; in other words the patterns and life attitudes that we, as therapists, have developed against the background of our own personal life history. Because as therapists we always react against the backdrop of our personal life experience, this means that there is also always an appeal to our own history. It is not possible to exist without a history, without being shaped by experiences and intentionality. We are bound by this, at every moment. There is a constant appeal to our own history, even if we are not aware of this and actually do not want this to happen.

If the start of the child's course of osteopathic treatment is viewed from this premize of different influences, we can see that some complications are possible.

The treatment situation
Start of treatment

What happens at the start of treatment? The child is brought to the appointment by the parents or a carer. The adults accompanying the child will arrive with desires, fears and expectations that are communicated both verbally and non-verbally. These signals are always picked up by the osteopath, and the unspoken messages will usually be just as perceptible as those that are put into words. The parents will describe what is wrong and hope to receive help for themselves and the child.

It can be extremely helpful to notice how you yourself feel at this point in time. You may become restless or tired or feel extremely well. It is important to sense how you respond emotionally to the situation by listening to what your own body is saying. The body responds involuntarily to the signals communicated before these are consciously picked up.

An example will illustrate this: while the parents are outlining their reasons for coming to you, your own back starts to ache. The possible causes of this may be as follows: you sense that the parents' expectations of you as the osteopath are unreasonably high. Or the relationship between parents and child is charged with tension. Perhaps the child is also under excessive strain. At this moment, however, it is clear that your own body is reacting to something that is not accessible to your conscious mind at that point in time. It is not at all a question of changing something here or of looking for a solution to this perhaps tension-charged situation. The first and most important step is to sense how your body is reacting to the situation, and to heed the expression of the emotional reaction and to take this seriously as information.

This information is additional to your specialist skill, and such knowledge is incorporated into the treatment without you consciously being aware of it.

Your own body wants to help you to assess the atmosphere in which the treatment is performed so that you can adapt to it. For example, in an atmosphere that is very much shaped by agitation and tension, it may be advisable to proceed more slowly, and to introduce breaks so as not to have to keep on working against the agitation. Possibly, however, you may be accustomed to working more quickly in the presence of agitation and to making much more effort than necessary because this is the pattern that has developed on the basis of your own life history experience. This helps to explain why it can be difficult to sense and accept the cooperation of the body because it is simultaneously a question of personal patterns and the often painful history of their development.

Examination

Let us consider further what happens before a treatment starts. History-taking is followed by the physical examination. The picture is now considerably expanded through the medium of touch. At the moment when you touch someone, that is, when your hands become an additional source of information, it is not uncommon for something else to become perceptible apart from what can be picked up through talking and observing. The picture of the patient's energy status may change. Your hands comprehend something that was previously inaccessible. Communication between patient and osteopath is widened out. During history-taking, for example, an infant may appear to be quite calm when viewed from the outside. However, when you touch the child, you may perhaps sense great agitation and simultaneous rigidity. The message the infant is communicating is: 'I am really agitated but I can't move.' Through touch the osteopath is able to comprehend what is happening with the child.

And you are influenced and possibly irritated by this 'comprehension'. Once again this is an interaction which cannot be planned, which is born of the moment.

A vivid experience recounted by an osteopath may serve as an example of such involvement. She reports: 'It happened as we were saying goodbye at the end of an infant's treatment. It had been a good session. I was moved by my contact with the young child. Its father lovingly took the child in his arms, the child snuggled into him and the father held the child close. It looked good. Suddenly I was overcome with feelings of jealousy. It was as if I had been struck rigid, and I was hardly able to say goodbye. It was exceedingly unpleasant for me and it has been very much on my mind.' As she reviewed the

account, it turned out that the intimate contact between father and child had reminded the osteopath of her longing for closeness that was not reciprocated by her own father – something that she had buried deep within herself. Therefore images and emotions surfaced so suddenly at this moment when she had been 'softened' by the treatment and was open. This example clearly shows what often happens unseen without our being aware of it. Beneath the protective armor of professionalism, which in this case was probably pierced by the particular situation of saying goodbye, such moments of contact often lead to restrictions in the osteopath's system that are so difficult to understand if we assume that only the patient – but not the osteopath – is touched by the treatment process.

And this example is informative for another reason. It indicates that painful and sad experiences of your own can be awakened, especially in good moments. The capacity to empathize and to 'resonate' opens the door for your own inner, wounded and neglected 'child'. It is good to recognize and understand this if you work with children and infants. If we do not remember how we felt and reacted in early childhood, then our image of the child is shaped by notions that we want to have. Surprising conclusions that surface in memory work, such as 'And to think that was so important!' or 'Just imagine that children can experience such a wealth of emotions!' open up a different avenue to the real child who is being treated. Often it is a small movement, a small change in breathing, a small contact from inside or outside that opens up the way to such resources, but also the way to remembering past experiences.

Relevant results from the fields of infancy research and prenatal research

At this point we will refer to the fields of infancy research and prenatal research, where results from the past two decades in particular have considerably broadened our understanding of physical data transmission, developmental and relational needs, the experiential world and the child's capabilities during this early period, and have thus fundamentally altered our thinking. As a result, entirely new possibilities have emerged for perceiving and understanding non-verbal messages and contact.

Already before birth the child has experiences and sensations (Janus 1997). He reacts and makes contact (Dornes 2001). The fetus is active, discriminating, and able and wanting to relate. 'Today through the medium of film we are able to observe how during diagnostic amniocentesis the unborn child recoils alarmed and intimidated from the needle or moves inquisitively towards it. As we watch we can experience how, when the mother is frightened, the child also becomes motionless or, when the mother is worried, the child also withdraws into a corner of its uterine home' (Häsing 1994, Janus 1997). From as early as week 6 onwards pain reactions have been demonstrated in unborn children (see p.30).

The body language of the recoiling child can be interpreted roughly as follows: 'I feel threatened and I need a safe place. I'm searching for this by drawing back.' The body language of the inquisitive child can be understood to mean: 'Oh, so what's this then?'

To conclude this section, I have selected another example from an extraordinary childbirth situation that very clearly depicts the active, discriminatingly sensing and reacting child. 'On one occasion the gynecologist told a pregnant woman that he would give her one hour so that she could discuss with her baby how it should engage its head, and he showed her with his clenched fist what he meant. ... The head of the baby about to be born engaged in the birth canal within the stipulated time period. ... If in the interim the mother's thoughts wandered off somewhere else, the baby would move and virtually call her back' (Hidas 2001). The unborn child obviously needed the full and devoted attention of the mother in order to do what had to be done. Without her total child-centered attentiveness, and hence support, it was not possible for the child. The thoughts that distracted the mother prevented the child from continuing his activity.

The child's cooperation in treatment

Two important thoughts to emerge from the aforementioned examples will now be taken up: first, a newborn child – even an unborn child – 'knows' a very great deal and provides a wealth of information, if we are prepared to heed it. Second, the child relies on the fact that due note should be taken of this information and his knowledge about what he needs and his body wants to do.

A child is able and willing to cooperate in treatment, providing information about what he wants to do, what he lacks and what he needs. For example, in the treatment situation you might pick up the following messages: 'You have touched me in a way that makes me anxious.' Or: 'Your attempts to touch me are too fast or too slow for me.' Perhaps also: 'You won't find me, touching me that way.' The child communicates these things. Even though he is so tiny that he cannot express these messages in words, the child lets the osteopath feel how he perceives her touch. It may easily happen that this information is overlooked if special attention is not paid to it.

It may also happen that you subconsciously disregard it because you might interpret the messages as rejection or as criticism of your own efforts. And yet in reality it is an invitation to make further tactile proposals and to pay heed to the child's reaction. The child relies on the fact that proper note be taken of what he communicates. He requires time and space to be able to continue with what the treatment has stimulated, escorted in an attentive and careful manner.

In the childbirth example quoted by Hidas (2001) the unborn child – through his movements – is saying to the mother: 'Your attention is elsewhere and not with me; you have gone away. This makes me restless and I can't concentrate on engaging if you're not there. Then I become anxious. I need you to be with me, otherwise I won't manage to engage my head.' The child is also saying: 'It's not a bad thing that you were distracted for a moment, but you must respond when I ask you to come back, I need your full attention.' After the interruption the child continues with his engagement activity as soon as the mother notices the increased movement and focuses her attention back on the child.

Although the mother-child and therapist-child relationships are entirely different, what has been said above can be transposed to the osteopathic treatment situation: the child is able and willing to influence the treatment, and often to a greater extent than we may think. The child will let us know if something is not right. The osteopath's desire to understand the child can then perhaps be imagined as follows: 'I will now start to treat you. I know that I cannot do everything correctly and that I will perhaps sometimes misunderstand you, or be inattentive or move too quickly. But I presume that you will then let me know. Although we are different, we will set out together on this search. I will take care to ensure that I repeatedly allow you time and space for your signals and for what your body wishes to do. Sometimes I will do this by looking at you, and sometimes I will listen to my own inner voice to hear what my body has understood from your signals. We will then see whether perhaps you need a rest, whether perhaps I am doing too much and you are not getting a chance to do enough. It may also be that you need something entirely different, or I need to find out whether we are already in contact at all.'

It is this process of searching together that engenders in the patient a feeling of being supported and valued. This feeling creates the space that the organism needs in order to be able to unfold its wisdom with the help of the treatment. This is also the space where both parties can develop confidence in their own searching movements.

For the osteopathic practitioner delivering the treatment this state of searching together is healing too, in the sense of lightening the load because the concept of treating and helping is also often associated with a tendency to assume too much responsibility. In the supervision of a treatment, for example, an osteopath discovered that her left hand felt devoid of energy and strength. Aside from the memories that were awakened by this discovery, questions also arose that were linked directly with the treatment: has this hand perhaps been over-exerted because it assumed too much responsibility for the treatment process? Did it perhaps try to 'put something right' without recognizing and accepting the cooperation of the patient? Or did it not want to notice that the patient had ceased cooperating, for whatever reason? At what point had the osteopath lost contact without consciously realizing it? It was a surprise for her to discover that her hand had lost its strength and energy. Initially it was almost embarrassing for her to detect a restriction in her own system and also to have overlooked it. However, it is illusory to believe that we can sense everything because we are always trapped in our own system. If we are accustomed to assuming more responsibility than necessary, we tend to miss signals through which our body might make us aware of things that are not quite right in our contact with the patient or ourselves. We do not then wish to see our own limitations and the limitations of the other person that are present in that moment. It is as if we are blind and we need someone from outside who will try to understand our body language.

Returning to the treatment situation, the following questions might arize, for example: did I continue treating when you already couldn't go on or you needed time? Did I want to mobilize more or faster than your body could cope with? Because even a small touch can have a major effect, especially if it is a good touch. Integration requires time and space. 'If I perform a minor change, the change – when viewed from the outside – is hardly visible. I only noticed the difference when I had the same procedure performed on me. I felt how a tiny change has repercussions on the whole body' (Herz 2003).

From the perspective of searching together, messages concerning inability and unwillingness, fending off or even rejection become valuable information that a treatment process needs in order to be shaped. This approach may perhaps require rather more time but it is more likely to lead to the hoped-for outcome. The child is involved as a whole person and is supported in his appropriate development.

Self-reflection

In psychotherapy it is self-evident that concern for our own history, lessons learned from our own experience, and self-reflection are helpful and necessary sources of professionalism and self-regulation. However, it has not always been remembered – and this is still the case – that osteopathy also always treats the whole person and therefore engages and places demands on the osteopath as a whole person.

And yet, once effort, stress, difficulties and exhaustion in the treatment setting are considered from this perspective, much that is experienced may perhaps become more understandable. It can be classified and thus acquires meaning, and this in turn benefits the work. To promote self-care and the work, it is helpful when thinking about the treatment also to think about yourself as therapist.

Bibliography

Buber M: Das Problem des Menschen. 11th edn. Gütersloher, Gütersloh 2000

Dornes M: Der kompetente Säugling – Die präverbale Entwicklung des Menschen. 10th edn. Fischer, Frankfurt 2001

Häsing H, Janus L (ed.): Ungewollte Kinder – Annäherungen, Beispiele und Hilfen. 1st edn. Rowohlt, Hamburg 1994

Herz, A von: Vom Lastenschleppen zur Körperkommunikation. In: Dr. med. Mabuse, no. 142, March/April 2003

Hidas G: Mutter-Fötus-Bindungsanalyse. In: Fedor–Freyberg P (ed.): Internationale Zeitschrift für pränatale und perinatale Medizin, Vol. 13, no. 1, 2, Mattes, Heidelberg 2001

Hoffmann-Axthelm D. (ed.): Schock und Berührung. 1st edn. Transform, Oldenburg 1994

Hüther G: Biologie der Angst – Wie aus Streβ Gefühle werden. 3rd edn. Vandenhoeck & Ruprecht, Göttingen 1999

Janus L: Wie die Seele entsteht – Unser psychisches Leben vor und nach der Geburt. 1st edn. Mattes, Heidelberg 1997

Montagu A: Körperkontakt – Die Bedeutung der Haut für die Entwicklung des Menschen. 7th edn. Klett-Cotta, Stuttgart 1992

Reiter A: Pränatale Inhalte im bildnerischen Ausdruck. Internationale Zeitschrift für pränatale und perinatale Medizin, Vol. 11, no. 4, Mattes, Heidelberg 1999

Stern D: Tagebuch eines Babys - Wie ein Kind sieht, spürt, fühlt und denkt. 1st edn. Piper, Munich 1993

Questions about nutrition often crop up tangentially during osteopathic treatment of children and counseling of young parents. The nutritional building blocks that children receive in their diet help to determine the success of osteopathic treatment. Only children eating a healthy diet will be able to develop a healthy musculoskeletal system and healthy organs and remain unscathed in the face of infections and the demands imposed by the outside world. The following chapter provides practical tips on infant and child nutrition.

PHYSIOLOGICAL ASPECTS

Astrid Fischer

Human beings have two 'shells' that serve to protect us from the environment: the first is our outer covering of skin, and the second is the mucosa of the gastrointestinal (GI) tract, the surface area of which is much larger than that of our skin. In nutritional terms, the GI mucosa also acts as a barrier to everything that we consume in our diet, and it decides what should enter our bloodstream and what should not. Under normal circumstances the GI mucosa is colonized with symbionts – bacteria of many different types that live with us in a symbiotic relationship. If our diet is balanced we provide these symbiotic bacteria with a good milieu for growth. In return they produce vitamins for us, protect our sensitive mucosa from pathogenic organisms and break nutrients down into even smaller constituent parts. As a result we are enabled to absorb nutrients more efficiently because excessively large molecules might possibly provoke an allergic reaction. In addition, these symbionts provide our immune system in the intestinal mucosa with a 'training partner'. Through its contact with these physiological bacteria there, our immune system is able to practise in preparation for a real emergency. This would happen, for example, if these bacteria were to penetrate to another undesirable location, an eventuality that would lead to illness.

In a vaginal delivery, during her passage through the birth canal, the baby first comes into contact with these symbionts, which then colonize the intestine of the neonate. If the mother's vaginal flora is intact, the baby's gut will be exposed to lactobacilli and bifidobacteria during the birth phase. The second group of bacteria with which the baby comes into contact during the birth process originates in the mother's anal region. As well as further bifidobacteria, these chiefly comprise enterobacteria and enterococci. Children born by caesarean section often experience greater difficulty in building up a healthy balance of intestinal symbionts. If the neonate is ultimately breastfed by the mother, she comes into contact with the protective bacteria of the skin – lactobacilli and streptococci.

EFFECT OF NUTRITION ON THE IMMUNE SYSTEM

Astrid Fischer

The development of a well-functioning immune system can be decisively encouraged or discouraged by the nutrition that is chosen for the child at a given age. The immunoglobulins present in breast milk constitute an important source of protection for the child against infections. In the older child a diet that is too rich in protein promotes a putrefying or alkaline milieu in the gut and causes a shift in intestinal symbionts, a condition known as dysbiosis, which leads in turn to a weakening of the immune system. Children are then particularly prone to infections, especially tonsillitis, otitis, bronchitis and diarrhea. Dysbiosis also encourages the development of allergies that are often already present in the parents. This allergic disposition is usually passed on genetically to the child.

In the event of recurrent infections prescription of antibiotics is not uncommon, and these medicines may further compromise the already unstable symbiosis in the intestine. Antibiotics kill not only the pathogenic bacteria but also those that are necessary for intestinal symbiosis. This signals the start of a vicious circle of further infections and allergies unless the symbiotic bacteria in the gut are restored again by dietary means and, where necessary, with pharmacological support, a process known as symbiosis regulation.

A compromised intestinal milieu also encourages the growth of fungi, such as *Candida albicans* and molds, which can only be tolerated to a minimal extent by our intestinal flora. Fungal overgrowth ushers in increasing problems: thrush and genital fungal infections, flatulence and stool irregularities, a tendency to headaches through to migraine, concentration disorders, and again a greater propensity to allergy to other foods and different kinds of trigger (pollen, house dust, etc.). Some of these conditions may not be observed immediately during infancy but we prepare the ground for them by possibly making unwise decisions in the choice of early nutrition.

NUTRITION FOR BABIES

Astrid Fischer

Breast milk

Even before her baby is born, the mother-to-be will already be asking herself the first questions about nutrition: these will revolve around the issue of whether or not to breastfeed. Basically, with a little relaxation and practice, almost every mother will be able to breastfeed and so nourish her baby in the best possible way. Sometimes, in addition to practical tips from the midwife or an experienced mother, the new mother will also need a great deal of encouragement and support from other therapists (see Ch.3, Osteopathic support when breastfeeding).

Breast milk is the optimal food during the baby's initial months of life. During every developmental phase in this initial period the mother's breast milk is perfectly adapted to the changing needs of her baby. As a personalized 'natural cocktail', breast milk supplies optimal nutrients in balanced proportions that are ideally suited to the baby's growth requirements and metabolic capabilities. Maternal immunoglobulins are passed to the baby in the breast milk, and during the initial months of life these immunoglobulins confer protection against infectious diseases and allergies. In addition, human breast milk has a lower protein content than any other mammalian milk.

Colostrum is yellow and sticky and contains plenty of protein and abundant minerals and is particularly rich in immunoglobulin A (IgA), which is especially important for protecting the intestinal mucosa. Colostrum is produced during the first 3 to 5 days after birth. Transitional breast milk is more watery and already resembles mature breast milk. It is adapted to meet the baby's growing energy requirements. Mature breast milk develops from day 14 after delivery onwards. Compared with colostrum, it has a higher fat and carbohydrate concentration but contains relatively little protein. Overall, the volume of mature breast milk production is greater than that in the previous stages.

A frequently cited argument against breastfeeding is based on the possible contamination of breast milk with toxins. Every day we consume toxins with our food and these are stored in fatty tissue. These may be passed on to the baby via the breast milk, especially in cases where the mother loses a great deal of weight after childbirth. Nevertheless the benefits of breastfeeding clearly outweigh any possible exposure to toxins. A mother who eats healthily before and during pregnancy and who recognizes the importance of organically produced fruit and vegetables will be laying down a good foundation that will do much to ensure her breast milk is largely free from any contaminating substances.

Cow's milk

Aside from not knowing which food or additives have been fed to the cows that are the source of the milk, feeding a baby with cow's milk has a number of decisive disadvantages: doing so may lead to accelerated weight gain and ultimately to obesity. Its excessively high protein content encourages the development of putrefying processes in the gut and hence of dysbiosis. Excessive contact with foreign proteins may also result in the development of allergy to these proteins. Cow's milk allergy is the commonest form of allergy today. Among other things, it triggers reactions such as cradle cap, atopic eczema (neurodermatitis) and allergic bronchial asthma.

Some babies are fed from birth with bottle formula made from dried powder. It should be kept in mind here that this is also manufactured on a cow's milk basis and may also lead to cow's milk allergy. In the immature or allergic child, animal or plant protein constituents are insufficiently digested, causing large protein particles to enter the bloodstream. The immune system identifies these as non-self and develops specific antibodies to them. In some infants this exaggerated immune response may result in an allergy to all foods that contain the protein in question.

In all such cases it is therefore advisable to switch to hypoallergenic milk (HA formula) because this has been specially processed. As a result of hydrolysis the foreign protein from various sources (whey, casein, soya protein, bovine collagen) has been moderately or extensively broken down so that the body can tolerate it better. The higher the degree of hydrolysis of an HA formula, the smaller the probability that allergy will ensue in the at-risk baby because the process of hydrolysis renders the protein 'unrecognizable' by the body's immune system. Despite scientific research, however, it is still disputed whether cow's milk products treated in this way can in fact prevent, delay or attenuate an outbreak of allergic illness. HA formula should not be used in cases where milk allergy is present.

In cases of genuine milk allergy an extensively hydrolyzed special formula (semi-elemental formula) should be given in which the protein constituents have been even more extensively broken down. This product is very expensive, has a bitter taste and is used exclusively to treat severe gastrointestinal disorders, as well as severe allergies. It is prescribed by a physician in the context of treatment and is available from pharmacies only.

Alternatives to breast milk and cow's milk

As alternatives to breast milk or cow's milk during the first 5 months of life the following other types of milk may be used:

- **Mare's milk** is very similar in composition to breast milk. It is low in fat, rich in vitamins, rich in unsaturated fatty acids and contains bifidobacteria and lactic acid bacteria that make it particularly well tolerated by the gut. Unfortunately, mare's milk can usually only be obtained deep-frozen and it is very expensive.
- **Sheep's milk** also offers a good alternative for families living in the countryside where it can generally be obtained fresh.
- **Goat's milk** is available in powdered and fresh form in health food shops as well as supermarkets. Special milk powder for babies is also commercially available.
- **Soy milk** is also available in formula form for infants. If the parents have any soya allergy this milk should not be used.

For babies who are intolerant to animal protein there is a product based on carob seed flour that can be given from the age of 4 months onwards. This is free of soya and milk protein.

After the age of 5 months consideration may be given to feeding with plant-based milk:

- **Rice milk** is very well tolerated by people with allergies, is rich in minerals, but contains little fat and protein. These can be added in the form of almond puree, for example.
- **Oat milk** is also very rich in minerals and can be used like rice milk.
- Nowadays there is a large range of **soya milk products**. However, in many people they can cause an allergic reaction (according to the German Allergy and Asthma Association, in about 30% of cases). Therefore, they should only be used if the parents have no soya allergy, and even then only with caution.

Adding other foods from the age of 5 months

From the age of 5 months onwards babies may also be given additional solids. In this area too we repeatedly encounter questions and uncertainties. There follows some concrete advice on choosing the right foods.

Solids

- Ideally, food should be farmed organically so as to have as few toxins as possible and high vitamin content.

- Puréed food should always be freshly prepared and finely blended.
- A new food can be added each week. However, variety is not essential during the first year of life.
- Suitable vegetable types include carrots, fennel, potatoes and sweet potatoes, as well as cauliflower and kohlrabi.
- To the baby's diet add rice and other gluten-free cereals such as millet and maize in the form of flakes. From the age of 7 months oats, barley, quinoa and buckwheat can also be added.
- Suitable fruit varieties include apples, bananas and pears.
- Almond and sesame purée can be used as a source of fat and protein.
- Meat – ideally from organic farms – may be added from the age of 9 months, but then only once or twice weekly. Wherever possible, sausage products should be avoided because the quality of the meat used is an unknown factor.
- Fish may also be given once or twice a week, but as an alternative to meat.
- Sugar, salt and spices should always be avoided.
- Heating in the microwave oven destroys important ingredients. In particular, avoid heating milk and drinks in plastic bottles because constituents from the plastic may leach into the drinks.

Drinks

The following are suitable:

- Water – non-carbonated with a low nitrate and sodium content
- Fennel or rose-hip tea
- Highly diluted fruit or vegetable juices (e.g. carrot juice); however, sensitive skin reacts to fruit acid, which also encourages dental caries.

Suggested schedule for adding solids

From the age of 5 months onwards slowly start to replace the milk feeds in sequence; the ideal pattern is to replace one milk feed about every 4 weeks.

It is best if vegetable and fruit meals are freshly prepared at home. In this way the ingredients are known and the vitamin content is best preserved. However, ready-prepared jars containing organic ingredients are also available that can be fed to babies.

Vegetable-potato purée

From the age of 5 months a vegetable-potato purée can be introduced for lunch. Start with spoonfuls of one vegetable, such as carrot or pumpkin, so that the baby can get used to eating from a spoon, and increase the amount each day. When the baby eats the whole portion, switch to vegetable with potato. Introduce just one new food into the dietary schedule each week. As a maximum, no more than two types of vegetables plus potatoes should be given at each meal. Salt and spices are not needed.

The best vegetables to use are those varieties that are rich in nutrients and well tolerated, e.g. carrots, pumpkin, fennel, courgettes, cauliflower, spinach, broccoli or kohlrabi. Suitable oils include those made from rapeseed, soya, sunflower or maize germ.

Recipe

Cook 1000 g vegetables and 500 g potatoes in 400 ml water, and purée with a stick blender, add 16 teaspoonfuls of oil and mix thoroughly. For babies up to the age of 8 months, make up finely puréed portions of about 190 g per meal; for babies aged 8 months or older the portions should be about 220 g and puréed slightly less smoothly. Portions may be frozen and can be used for up to 2 months if stored at −18ºC.

Milk-cereal mix

From the age of 6 months replace the evening feed with a mix of milk and cereal. To prepare, use either powdered milk (as for bottle formula), full milk containing 3.5% fat or preferably the alternatives to cow's milk listed earlier. The recommended cereals include pure flakes, ideally whole grain products such as oat flakes.

Fruit-cereal purée

From the age of 7 months that baby may be given a milk-free fruit and cereal purée in the afternoon. Locally grown fruit varieties such as apples, pears and peaches (depending on the season) are suitable. Give bananas in moderation only and avoid feeding them to children with a tendency to colds and bronchitis because they encourage mucus formation. As the cereal component give preference to pure flakes (e.g. spelt flakes). Take grated apples or pears or bananas mashed with a fork and mix with spelt flakes and water.

Eating the same food as the rest of the family

From the age of 12 months children can eat the same food as the rest of the family. To begin with, if necessary, the meals can still be puréed or mashed. However, meals should not be heavily spiced.

NUTRITION FOR TODDLERS AND SCHOOLCHILDREN

Astrid Fischer

Even after they are no longer babies, children should still have a diet that is as natural and as unprocessed as possible. However, the ideal of a sugar-free, wholefood diet should not be taken too dogmatically. If children are given sweets as an occasional treat they will naturally take them in their stride. On the other hand, to label sweets as 'totally off-limits' may fuel an exaggerated desire for them, because anything that is forbidden tends to have particular appeal for most children.

For the parents of school-age children the whole subject of diet can develop into a real challenge in terms of sugar, fast food and soft drinks. Here we should remind parents of the saying 'You are what you eat' and constantly encourage them to give their children food that is as wholesome and as natural as possible. What is true for infants and preschool children also applies for older children: as well as causing obesity, white flour and sugar also lead to problems with concentration and to overgrowth of intestinal mucosa with intestinal fungi, and this sets in motion a spiral of infection and allergy and thus disturbs the child's natural balance. In Germany, one child in every five is currently overweight and diabetes mellitus among children is on the increase.

As a thirst-quencher, water should be the first choice for younger and older children, supplemented by unsweetened herbal or fruit teas or diluted fruit juice. Something a little different is acceptable for special occasions, if requested. If the variety and quality of the daily diet provides a balanced, healthy foundation, the body is well able to cope with little 'extras'.

A healthy foundation is created, for example, by:

- Vegetables – either raw or freshly prepared.
- Fruit – a varied selection according to the season.
- All sorts of cereals as whole grains that can also be coarsely ground or milled.
- Meat and fish, but not more than two or three times a week; fish should be preferred to meat because it contains omega-3 fatty acids and the protein is more easily digestible.
- As beverages – water, unsweetened herbal or fruit teas, diluted fruit juices, e.g. apple juice mixed with water, and these can also be consumed at mealtimes.
- Dairy products such as cheese, quark (curd cheese) and yoghurt; however, these should be considered as side dishes and not as basic foods because calcium requirements are not covered by dairy products alone, but also by fruit, cereals, fish and meat.

The following are best avoided:

- Refined white flour and white flour products.
- Any products containing refined sugar, e.g. sweets, biscuits, jams and marmalades, soft drinks.

Nutrition and concentration disorders

A deficiency of various substances such as vitamin C, magnesium and calcium can lead to restlessness and inattention. An imbalanced diet that contains too much sugar, refined white flour and hydrogenated (hardened) fats may produce a deficiency in essential fatty acids and in vitamins and minerals. Studies conducted by Schoenthaler (1982) showed that the intellectual performance of poor students was markedly improved by reducing their dietary content of food colorings, artificial flavourings, food additives and sugars.

Sugars and refined flour also increase the requirement for essential fatty acids, which are important for the ability to concentrate. The key essential fatty acids are omega-6 and omega-3 fatty acids. They:

- increase the postsynaptic potential of the nerve cells, causing a clear improvement in learning and concentration abilities. Therefore they are helpful in the area of ADHD therapy.
- lower triglycerides and are therefore effective in the prevention of arteriosclerosis and coronary heart disease.
- have an anti-inflammatory effect that is important in the treatment of rheumatism and, for example, in the treatment of psoriasis.

Omega-6 fatty acids are particularly abundant in seeds, and in oils from sunflowers, maize germ, evening primrose and sesame; omega-3 fatty acids are plentiful in fish varieties such as salmon, tuna, mackerel, herrings and sardines. Linseed oil and walnut oil are also good sources.

TESTING FOR FOOD INTOLERANCE

Teresa Kelly

Depending on the age and level of cooperation of the child, there are two methods that are particularly suitable when testing for food intolerance.

Muscle test (kinesiology)

In the older child a simple muscle test (kinesiology) using pressure on the outstretched arm has proved useful. The child stands and holds one arm in 90 degree abduction. The therapist exerts caudal pressure on the child's forearm, initially without testing a food in the process. Then the foods in question are placed in the hand of the child's non-abducted arm, and muscle strength is again tested in the abducted arm. If the strength is equal to the original test, the food is not a problem. If however the muscle strength is weaker, the food being tested is 'weakening' the child's system.

Involuntary motion

In the younger child monitoring of the involuntary motion (IVM) is a suitable method of testing for food intolerance. To begin with, monitor the quality of expression of the IVM either from the cranium or from the central thorax. I personally gain a better impression via contact at the thorax. Then place the food in question either in the child's hand or on the child's abdomen and monitor the change in the quality of expression of the PRM. Its amplitude and quality may remain unchanged or a negative response may perhaps be obtained, such as the mechanism becoming heavier or shutting down. The PRM may also become weaker, with a resultant decreased, weaker amplitude of the IVM.

This method can also be used to test the correctness or appropriateness of a homeopathic remedy. If a specific strain pattern is palpated through the body prior to the test, this pattern may 'be lifted' or 'become lighter' if the remedy is correct. The strain pattern may be accentuated if the remedy is not appropriate.

This method of testing is quite subjective and although osteopathic practitioners may differ in their use of language to describe the effects of the food/remedy, the outcome invariably is the same. With practice, it becomes a very effective tool in the testing of intolerances of many food groups.

Bibliography

Brehmer G: Aus der Praxis einer Kinderärztin. Rowohlt, Hamburg 1988

Elmadfa I, Leitzmann C: Ernährung des Menschen. 3rd edn. Ulmer-UTB, Stuttgart 1998

Friedrichsen K, Meyer K: 1 x 1 der Babyernährung. Haug, Stuttgart 1998

Graf FP: Homöopathie und die Gesunderhaltung von Kindern und Jugendlichen. Spangsrade, Spangsrade 2003

Moll R, Schain-Emmerich U: Allergiekost für Mutter und Kind. Econ & List, Munich, 1998

Rapp D: Ist das Ihr Kind? 4th edition, Promedico, Hamburg 2000

Stadelmann I: Die Hebammensprechstunde. Published privately, Kempten 1994

Schoenthaler S J: The effect of sugar on the treatment and control of antisocial behavior: a double blind study of an incarcerated juvenile population. International Journal of Biosocial Research 3, 1982: 1–19

Waskow F, Mühlenz I: Kinderernährung. BeltzKiwi, Munich 2002

Section **2**

11

Accommodation difficulties of the newborn

Clive Hayden

THE BIRTH PROCESS

The newborn infant faces many challenges on his entrance into the world, and his ability to cope successfully with the transition from the more muted sensations of the amniotic world into the sharper, sensory-rich atmosphere of his new life depends a lot on how well he copes with the ordeal of labor and delivery. Prior to the birth, events in the pregnancy are also very relevant to the health of the fetus, and his strength and fortitude in coping with the forces and stresses of birth (see Ch.4, Behavior and living space of the unborn child). There are many conditions that may present in early infant life that are directly attributable to trauma experienced by the infant during the birth process, but there are also conditions such as infantile colic, some types of cerebral palsy and developmental difficulties that may have their causative roots in conditions experienced by the fetus in utero. For example, one of the proven causative factors in infants suffering from infantile colic is stress during pregnancy, labor or postnatally (Hogdall et al 1991). During labor the fetus relies on anaerobic respiration, in which glycogen is metabolized to provide vital oxygenation to delicate neuronal tissues during times of hypoxia (Carreiro 2003). Apparently a 'diving-seal reflex' exists in which the circulation to the vital centers of the nervous system and central organs is maintained, whilst being reduced to peripheral limbs and structures. The metabolism and heart rate also slow down. Stress may interfere with this process, causing essential energy reserves to be used rapidly. This reduces the capacity of the fetal adrenal glands to respond to extra demands by producing norepinephrine (noradrenaline), which is part of the metabolism of glycogen production. The end result is that the fetus has a reduced physiological reserve and is less able to cope with the physiological demands of the labor.

At the moment of birth or soon after, the infant takes his first breath and initiates a whole sequence of extensive physiological changes (see Ch.5, p.52; Ch.14, p.297). These changes enable the lungs to expand and the infant pulmonary circulation to become established, so changing the circulatory routes within the heart. Exhaustion of the adrenal response by prenatal stress sustained by mother or fetus during difficult deliveries appears to have implications in reducing the success of the first breath/physiological changeover at birth.

Another factor that also directly affects the state of the infant during birth is the effect of analgesic medication given to the mother during the labor (see p.57). Sedation of the infant and mother appears to have many implications in infant care and recovery (Odent 2001). The unresponsive, sedated newborn infant appears less likely to experience the critical windows of development in the first 24 hours because his recovery from the birth process has been retarded. This may impair the start of a healthy relationship developing between mother and the infant, and subsequently between that developing child and society in general. The negative effect of hospital care routines on the relationship between mother and infant has been well documented (Klaus and Kennell 1982). It appears that interruption of the normal contact time between mother and infant in the first 24 hours after birth may result in detectable differences in the development and behavior of 2-year-old infants and even later. Differences in the speech of 5-year-old children who missed the vital window of bonding contact with the mother in the first 24 hours have also been found.

Part of the immediate accommodation of the infant at birth is the development of the special senses: sight, sound, smell, taste and touch. These enable the infant to communicate, recognize the mother and father and commence the process of gaining knowledge about his new environment. An exhausted, depleted or traumatized perinatal infant appears to be less able to take these first important sensory steps.

THE UNSETTLED NEWBORN
Definition

The unsettled infant is attempting to convey a need, but instead of talking uses behavior to draw the attention of the parents. Thus the unsettled newborn may experience trouble settling down in a variety of different ways: sleeping, feeding or disruption of his digestive functions. He may be generally irritable, tend to cry a lot and be very hard to pacify.

Etiology and pathophysiology

In the immediate postnatal period, especially the first 48 hours, the infant is effectively in a 'postoperative' recovery state (Odent 2001). He has just undergone a major physical experience, and been exposed to high levels of opiates, either as naturally produced endorphins or analgesics administered to the mother during the labor. In addition, in most labors, extremely high levels of epinephrine (adrenalin) will have been experienced that have created huge 'highs' for the infant and mother. The exception perhaps being the elective caesarean, in which the normal triggers and hormonal inducements for the onset of labor have not occurred.

Even with a normal vaginal presentation, the pressures on the baby's head, spine and body are huge (Amiel-Tison et al 1988). A study of 40 cases on the pressures on the human fetus during labor have shown that the fetal head is subjected to 2.2 to 3.5 times more pressure than the intrauterine part of the body (Furaya 1981). This pressure doubles in the second stage of labor, and procedures such as vacuum extraction increase the pressures on the fetus in the birth canal markedly. Also the manual extraction in a caesarean birth leads to increased and uneven pressure on the head (see p.65).

The after-effect of enduring the pressures of the uterine contractions may result in physical pain and discomfort felt by the infant after the birth.

Once the first 2 to 3 days have passed, the swelling, bruising and molding should reduce. It should now be possible to gain an indication of how the infant has been generally affected by the experiences of labor. Sometimes it may take up to 2 weeks for the infant to recover. It may well take the parents, particularly first-time parents, all that time to realize that their newborn infant does seem to be crying excessively, is feeding poorly, is excessively flatulent and does not sleep well compared with other infants of a similar age.

We must always consider the possibility that irritability could have other medical causes, for example an acute infection, and refer to the family's doctor if appropriate.

Clinical signs and symptoms

If we think of the general pressure sustained during birth combined with the focal pressures on the infant head in the maternal pelvic birth canal, it is not surprising that the infant often appears very swollen, bruised and misshapen. This is a normal edematous reaction to trauma, but perhaps is also a good indication of the severity of the pressures that have been experienced during the labor. The most visibly affected areas are the face and cranium, which may appear puffy and swollen; the eyes being reduced to mere slits. However excessive pressures causing reactive edema may have been experienced on any part of the infant's body or limbs.

What must be considered is that the visible effect of edema on the face or cranium will also have occurred within the cranium, and the delicate meninges and central nervous system may also be undergoing a period of cerebral edema, with all the consequences of raised intracranial pressure. The normal venous drainage routes through the veins and sinuses of the cranium and neck will struggle to clear the backlog of accumulated fluid and congestion, taking time to reduce the edematous load from all the tissues of the head and face.

Often the infants who have shown signs of edema will also undergo a period of sensitivity to excessive stimuli. Bright lights, loud noises, sudden touch (especially to the head), will cause the infant to easily startle and cry. If the experience and pressure of the labor have resulted in a legacy of pain and discomfort for the infant, then he will readily cry, often for long periods at a time. These delicate and irritable infants must be handled with care, but this reactive time will normally ease within the first few days.

Diagnosis

In the early days of the newborn, apart from the ability to demonstrate gross movements of body, spine and limbs indicating an intact motor control, and the ability to respond to the presence of the parent, there are some common indicators of the physical comfort, well-being and health of the baby.

Mostly the processes of sleeping, crying, feeding and digestion will be the functions that can be readily monitored. The unsettled infant may present signs in any or all of the categories.

Medical diagnosis

Medical examination will generally have screened for major pathologies.

Osteopathic examination

Commonly, the osteopathic examination of the newborn is reduced to the most important aspects, or distributed over several visits, to avoid stressing the child further. Careful palpation of the tissues with the help of the involuntary mechanism usually turns into treatment. It takes time for the molding pressures and physical strains experienced by the infant to become clearly palpable to the trained hand. On quiet passive palpation, the initial tactile impression is usually one of a static, inert quality to all tissues, whether in the infant cranium or through the body and limbs. The tissues may have a puffy edematous quality, or may be static because of a sense of shock due to intense physical compression.

Treatment

The infant's central nervous system is immature at birth and has a limited capacity to respond to excessive levels of stimulation without rapidly fatiguing. Too much stimulation to any infant, such as caused by too many visitors, too much noise, too many journeys and being picked up and put down too often, will cause the infant to rapidly tire. As a personal opinion, this is often the reason why there is an unsettled evening period when the infant is irritable and tired, and is more likely to cry and 'be difficult'. Unfortunately for the father this is often the time when he comes home from work, full of expectation of seeing his baby again, only to find relative chaos and tension in the house as the mother tries to cope with the needs of all family members, including an irritable baby. With irritable infants a time of relative quiet, minimal amounts of general handling and intervention, especially by visitors, will help them to recover from birth.

For the infant who is already unsettled and difficult to console, the reaction to fatigue can be that much greater, with increasingly high levels of distress and discomfort being demonstrated. Appropriate advice to new parents of an unsettled infant is to limit or control if possible the general level of 'noise' and business in the household through the day – and also then to notice how busy days affect the temperament and behavior of their baby afterwards.

Allopathic medical treatment

By and large the medical care of the infant will revert to a 'watch and wait to see how the infant settles' type of approach, with the emphasis on parental management, and advice on feeding and routines, and so on.

Occasionally these infants may require sedation, especially if there is any indication or aberrant cortical activity, such as fits or seizures.

Osteopathic treatment

Osteopathic palpation and observation of the effects of primary respiration in the tissues usually turns into treatment. My own preference is to play a very calm 'waiting game'. At some point the soft fluid-filled tissues of the newborn will start to show an organized pattern of motion. Where this manifests is impossible to guess because the tissue changes are very subtle. We must be alert but passive and watch as the expression of life motion shows itself in the tissues. It is generally not appropriate to be working on specific physical strains and compressions sustained by the infant, but every infant will differ in his state and vitality, and it is important to be very alert to every need of the child.

At this time, treating an infant who cries frequently will help to settle him, and assist in his general recovery. Care must be taken not to initiate compressive approaches, as the risk of hematoma to these delicate newborns is still high.

Prognosis

The mild and moderately irritable child will usually respond positively to osteopathic treatment within 48 hours. However, predicting how the infant will behave after treatment is difficult, and advice is usually given to parents to prepare them for different reactions.

The baby may relax so well after the treatment that he literally falls into a deep sleep for most of the next 24 hours. The infant is usually catching up with much needed rest and just needs to be raised to be fed and changed. Alternatively, and in particular if the bony/membranous parts of the infant cranium are irritable, even the most delicate and fluid techniques will induce an exacerbation of the irritable behavior of the infant for 2 to 3 days after treatment. Parents are encouraged to phone for advice if they are uncertain. But unless the infant is unduly distressed, allowing a few days to pass in this case will almost always be enough time to let the infant settle. There are exceptions, and it is always advisable to check the baby again if uncertain.

SLEEPING DIFFICULTIES
Definition

When trying to assess sleeping difficulties we must first consider what are normal sleep requirements. It is quite difficult to determine what the normal sleep requirements are for a newborn. It appears from available textbooks that probably 16–18 hours would be the normal for this age, but suggestions have been made that colicky infants sleep less and are subject to more frequent wakening at night. Although the difference was found to be not significant between colicky infants and normal controls (Lehtonen et al 1994), parents of colicky babies will commonly report that their child appears to be restless whilst sleeping and appears to wake readily and frequently.

Delayed sleep refers to difficulties in getting the infant to relax and settle down to sleep. Other children may present in practice waking up a lot at night.

Etiology and pathophysiology

From experience and observation in practice it seems that these infants are still in a state of physical and neurological excitability, a legacy of the difficulties they may have experienced during the labor and/or prenatally.

The problem of waking up a lot at night may be exacerbated or perpetuated by the inexpedient behavior of the parents; for example picking the child up and carrying him around until he has fallen asleep again, or playing with him at night. Also changing nappies after feeding at night may keep the child from falling asleep again quickly.

Clinical signs and symptoms

Infants who suffer from delayed sleep and children who wake up a lot possibly do not get enough sleep at night.

An infant who has problems settling down to sleep tends to 'nap' or have shorter spells of sleep during the day. He is usually also more easily disturbed by noises, even trivial ones. The infant takes a long time to settle in the evening and because he is over-tired becomes more fractious. The infant may appear to be generally very alert, and capable of maintaining himself in a permanent state of arousal. It seems that the infant is always aware of what is going on around. Parents do tend to think at first that this is an indicator that this child is bright, alert and intelligent, which may be initially gratifying for them. However the difficulties of getting their baby to settle to sleep without having constantly to wait by the cot, or to continually breastfeed to comfort, reassure and settle means that the parents soon become aware of the reality of the demands and difficulties of the bedtime battle.

Sometimes the infant appears to be fighting or resisting sleep. He may be just drifting off to sleep when he will startle, waking suddenly and often crying again as well. This is the time when the patience of the parents may be sorely tested, as they have to start the process of soothing the infant once more. It is no wonder that thoughts that the infant is attention-seeking often intrude into the parents' minds.

It appears from personal observation that the infant who suddenly awakes with a start is hyper-alert, and the one who frequently wakes up crying is also showing signs of fear. This almost always relates to a time of fetal distress or extreme difficulty experienced by that baby during labor. These signs of fear may be manifested as crying, fists being bunched and tense, the infant looking wide-eyed and looking all around. He may appear fearful and show general signs of sympathetic arousal. The infant is literally still reliving the distress and trauma experienced during the birth, and may take some time to get over it. Settled sleep patterns are the inevitable and understandable casualty of such a difficult start to life outside the womb. When the infant does sleep, the sleep will be restless and more likely to be in the REM sleep level. It is normal that a breastfed baby will wake every 4 hours or so to be fed. Often irritable children will, however, not settle into a deep sleep but wake every 1 or 2 hours, taking their time to get back to sleep again. They may need to be comfort-fed to enable them to sleep again. Such behavior in my view is understandable and appropriate; the infant has undergone a stressful and difficult time and needs continual reassurance for some time afterwards.

Diagnosis

Diagnosis of sleeping difficulties may be made through the case history or by your own observations. It is important to ask when and how long the infant sleeps, and how often he wakes, both at night and in the day.

Osteopathic examination

Once the initial 2 to 3 days have passed the approach to the treatment of the infant will differ. All normal cautions about pathologies and risks of intracranial hemorrhage are still appropriate, but it becomes possible for a more objective assessment of the types of strains and pressures endured by the infant to be made.

It is still imperative that this evaluation is not rushed. The infant already has a story to tell your enquiring hands which will gently unfold. My own approach is to cradle the infant's head very gently whilst he is lying on a pillow on my lap facing me. Using a very gentle, guiding contact pressure, the infant will slowly and gradually assume and move towards the position he held during the first stage of labor. Slowly the twists and turns that he experienced will unfold, showing the osteopath and parents precisely the maneuvers that he had to perform to make his way through the birth canal. This is a means of starting to release the physical strains associated with the compression experienced during the birth process.

After this, attention to some of the more specifically compressed parts of the body and cranium may be needed; especially the occipital condyles, frontals, shoulders, cervical spine, diaphragm and pelvis. These can be examined in a systematic way (see Ch.7, Examination of the infant and toddler; Ch.8, An osteopathic approach to the newborn and infant, p.180).

Treatment

Advice may include a discussion of sleeping arrangements (dark, quiet, appropriate room temperature). After the 6th month, feeding at night is not strictly necessary if the infant is healthy and developing well. Behavioral therapy recommends a gradual solution: when the child cries commonly at night, the parent gives his or her attention after waiting a minute, then waiting a bit longer each night; and also staying a shorter time successively.

Sleeping position

The current medical advice to parents is for babies to be put in a supine position when preparing them for their sleep. The reasons for this are the reported increased risks to infants of Sudden Infant Death Syndrome when lying prone or face down.

However for some infants it appears that this may not be the most comfortable or natural position for them to go to sleep in. The supine position puts pressure on the occipital bone, which is often very sensitive as it is the focal point for much of the molding pressure of the birth process. Some of this pressure seems to be directed onto the tentorium cerebellum through the inion process of the occiput, with possible associated pressure on the venous sinuses draining the skull via the transverse and sigmoid sinuses.

The baby may be restless and slow to settle, with the parents often finding that their baby has managed to wriggle and turn onto a favourite side by the morning. Parents may find that when putting the infant to bed, sleep will come easier if the infant is placed in their most comfortable position to start with.

Most adults will relate to the fact that they have a preferred position to lie and sleep in. This may be on one side, with one leg flexed or drawn up at the hip; or they might prefer to lie on their front or curled up in a very fetal flexed position. Our chosen position accommodates the strains and distortions in our own bodies. Our bodies are rarely symmetrical, and to the trained observer postural twists, strains and positional anomalies of the limbs are readily observable. When we find our most comfortable position, our musculoskeletal tissues can relax, so reducing the afferent somatic neurological input into the central nervous system.

It appears that when the brain activity is allowed to diminish, sleep becomes possible, or certainly a deeper restful sleep occurs when 'the body is quiet'. When uncomfortable it seems much more likely that we remain in the REM (rapid eye movement) level of light sleep, which does not appear to be so restful.

The central nervous system is considered to be extremely sensitive to physical pressure. The neurological responses to raised intracranial pressure are well documented. In my opinion, sleep patterns may be disturbed by undue pressure on the cranium when we sleep in an uncomfortable position, so diminishing the depth and quality of sleep. In a similar manner, the compressive effects of the molding patterns on the infant cranium and body during labor appear to lead to a level of irritability of the meninges, with consequent afferent excitation of the central nervous system.

Allopathic medical treatment

Sometimes sedatives may be given to the child.

Osteopathic treatment

Osteopathic treatment arises from the osteopathic examination and palpation of the effects of primary respiration in the tissues. As mentioned above, mostly the very compressed parts of the body and cranium may be in need of treatment; especially the occipital condyles, frontals, shoulders, cervical spine, diaphragm and pelvis.

Case history

Thomas, an extremely active 3-year-old, had always slept poorly since birth, needing constant reassurance. The birth had been difficult, as he had presented in the birth canal as an occipito-posterior (OP) presentation (see Ch.5, Difficult delivery, The birth process and its effect on the infant cranium). There had also been signs of fetal distress. In my opinion this is often associated with fearful behavior and unsettled sleeping patterns.

His head appeared to be very wide in the coronal plane, and there were also indications of a plagiocephalic parallelogram pattern of head distortion. Observation of these distortions of the cranium often reveals either the right or left side of the occipital squama to appear flattened and pushed anteriorly, whilst one of the frontal bones also appears to be flattened or pushed posteriorly.

Treatment of this lively child was difficult, as the degree of molding compression apparently sustained during the birth proved to be extremely resistant to cranial techniques. He had to be treated initially in a less-than-ideal sitting position because he would not lie down. Eventually he was persuaded to lie down on the treatment table, with his mother lying alongside him. Now a more direct palpatory contact could be made with his cranium. His cranial base displayed no movement pattern at all, as the right occipital condyle appeared to have been compressed anteriorly, locking the right occipitomastoid suture. The left frontal was also compressed medially and posteriorly, so creating a 'right lateral-shear' strain pattern through the cranial base.

An appropriate condylar release technique was employed, described by Lippincott as the 'Basion Technique'. That night Thomas slept soundly for the very first time, and although apparently still a very active boy, has not required any further treatment since. In my experience, this case is not unusual.

Prognosis

My experience in practice is that sleeping difficulties in infants and children reliably respond to osteopathic treatment. This is also true for all ages! I feel that the treatment works by primarily releasing and relaxing the somatic musculoskeletal tissues of the body, which in turn diminishes the afferent neurological input into the central nervous system. This helps the infant to settle and improves the sleep pattern.

IRRITABLE INFANTS AND COLIC

Definition

Infantile colic is a common cause of paroxysmal abdominal pains with resultant distress and excessive crying in a large number of infants. It is a widely reported multifactorial condition thought to affect infants up to the age of 3 to 4 months. To date, the causes and current treatment strategies for the control of this multifactorial condition remain largely unresolved and to some extent controversial. Infantile colic may be considered to be a behavioral condition, with no apparent associated pathology. It was originally thought to only affect infants under the age of 3 months (Illingworth 1954). Infantile colic has been found to affect 15–40% of all infants. These figures seem confusing as the range is so wide, but the variation in the figures may indicate the severity of the condition. Thus the 40% may indicate mild colic and 15% indicates a more severe colic condition.

Etiology and pathophysiology

Current medical physiology suggests that undigested lactose enters the lower intestine where it ferments, causing gas (Marieb 1998). In the gut, a negative osmotic gradient is established that pulls water into the gut lumen from the surrounding tissues. This results in an expansion of the intestinal wall, which when allied to the gas fermentation creates considerable pressure and pain. The expansion of the gut lumen stimulates rapid peristalsis, giving loud stomach sounds (borborygmi) and eventually explosive flatulence.

Undigested lactose being propelled into the lower intestines before properly being broken down by lactase dehydrogenase enzyme may be due to an irritable nervous system overstimulating the peristaltic action of the intestines, thus causing rapid peristaltic contractions.

Another cause may be an inability to secrete lactase dehydrogenase enzyme, causing lactose intolerance. Studies have shown that up to 24% of older children are apparently unable to digest lactose, suggesting perhaps a similar percentage of infants (Webster 1995).

By using breath hydrogen testing Miller (1989) found that 62% of all colicky infants suffered from incomplete lactose digestion. This perhaps indicates that all types of animal lactose, including human breast-milk, may be indigestible to some children. It appears that the rate of gut motility is normal and unaffected in lactose intolerant infants, meaning that undigested lactose takes a more normal time to reach the lower intestine where it then ferments.

Liebman (1981) conducted a study on the relationship between allergic response and infantile colic. Exhaustive blood tests including immunoglobulin E (IgE) tests were conducted and the rates of atopy in the general population were compared, but were not found to be any greater than normal. So it was concluded that infantile colic was not an allergic manifestation and the fermentation of lactose in the lower gut was not considered a sign of the allergic response. More recent testing of IgAs indicate that allergens may indeed be part of the etiology of infantile colic.

There is no clear consensus of agreement in the debate of the cause of infantile colic as to whether cow's milk or human milk are likely causes of colic – literally, this is an area in which no researchers can agree. Evans et al (1981), Hyde et al (1983), Carey (1984), Thomas et al (1987), Miller et al (1991), Rautava et al (1993) and Gurry (1994) have all produced important definitive studies but it has been difficult to replicate the results of the various studies, and replication of results has to remain a reliable authentication of any study.

Infantile colic has been found to have a higher incidence in infants of Afro-Caribbean origin (Liebman 1981). This could be an indication that genetic predisposition may play a role.

Another indication of genetic involvement is that it has also been shown that if you have had one colicky child, you are more likely to have other colicky children (Wessel 1954, Hogdall et al 1991). This is not a categoric statement as it has been stated that stress within the family is a factor; the problem is that stress is often very hidden, on the surface everything seems perfect (Relier 1996).

Interestingly, the pattern of symptoms of infantile colic has similarities with the diurnal, circadian rhythms of production of the gut activator and inhibiting hormones, melatonin and serotonin. The peaks and troughs of production of these hormones coincide with the times of increased symptoms of infantile colic (Weissbluth et al 1992). The rationale for not accepting this as a cause of infantile colic is that if these hormones were responsible for the symptoms of infantile colic, then all infants should be equally affected, not just the reported 15–40%.

Stress in the individual is recognized as accelerating the rate of gut peristalsis (Rautava 1993). These rapid peristaltic contractions due to stress may have many origins, as stress from many causes in pregnancy, labor and postpartum can have an effect on the incidence of infantile colic (Hogdall et al 1991).

- **Antenatal stress:** stress in pregnancy that affects the fetus may be a result of hypoxic events suffered by the mother, such as asthma. Fevers and undue pressures in normal life may also serve to lower the oxygen available to the fetus because the mother requires more oxygen to meet her metabolic needs. Long-term prenatal stress of the mother is not buffered by the placenta after a while and may make the infant more prone to colic because it will set the level of excitability of the autonomic nervous system in the child at a higher level (Nathanielz 1999, Relier 1996; see p.34).

- **Labor stress:** osteopathic theory contends that probable molding compression of the hypoglossal canal and jugular foraminae in the base of the skull from the forces of birth are a possible cause of infantile colic (Magoun 1976). However it appears that the delivery type does not affect the incidence of infantile colic (Stahlberg 1984). But the central nervous system (CNS) and its meningeal coverings appear to be extremely sensitive to mechanical pressure, so that a possible hypothesis is that the molding effects of the birth on the cranial casing may cause the CNS to react in a stressed way and thus cause the speeding up of gut motility.

- **Post-partum stress:** the first-born is more likely to suffer from colic. The reason for this may be because the first labor is usually longer, more stressful and difficult (Stahlberg 1984). Also, first time parents tend to be a lot more nervous than the second or third time around, plus the change in life circumstances is greater, which may also be stressful for the whole family.

Research shows that stressed parents may be responsible for some aggravation of the symptoms of colic, but it seems quite natural that they will be upset and bothered if their child is crying so dramatically. Family size tends to be small where there has been a very colicky child, and who can wonder! The colicky infant tends to be more temperamental than normal (Wessel 1954, Hogdall et al 1991, Forbes 1994, Gurry 1994, Rautava et al 1993, 1995).

Clinical signs and symptoms, differential diagnosis

Excessive colicky crying is defined as crying frequently and for an extremely long duration, without identifiable cause, during which an otherwise healthy infant of between 2 weeks and 3 months of age is difficult to console. Peak incidence is at 6 to 8 weeks. It is paroxysmal in nature and thought to occur more likely in the evenings. 'Stiffening, drawing up of the legs over the abdomen, and the passage of flatus are common although not invariable accompaniments' (Miller and Barr 1991). The abdomen appears extended in many babies and the child seems to be in pain or discomfort. These symptoms are usually seen as tummy ache, but usually there are no objective signs linking the symptoms to the intestinal tract. However, parents often say that defecation and passing wind seem to relieve

symptoms; also symptoms seem often to improve with being carried around, being cradled and given attention.

Crying is the most commonly used criterion of measurement, but infantile colic behavior is not characterized solely by crying. In my study it was found that some infants were clearly uncomfortable, were writhing, restless and flatulent when asleep or awake but not crying.

A stressed irritable CNS may be one of the main etiologies of infantile colic, causing as a secondary effect rapid peristaltic contractions of the intestines. Observations suggest that these infants produce symptoms of colic from 30–75 minutes after a feed. Loud stomach sounds (borborygmi) will be audible and palpable as soon as the milk enters the digestive tract. The infant will also start to show increasing signs of discomfort, commencing the behavioral activities of writhing and squirming, and starting to draw his knees up to the stomach and perhaps stiffening and arching his back.

Differential Diagnosis

In differential diagnosis you need to consider

- **'Normal crying':** Infantile colic shares some similarities with normal crying, peaking in the evening, but the **amount of crying** is so much greater than normal crying (300–600%), that the two states should not be confused. (Hill et al 1995, Lehtonen et al 1995).

- **Painful pathologies:** Infections like, e.g., otitis media or pyelonephritis, or invagination.

- **Cerebral damage:** Children show a true opisthotonus posture which will be maintained a longer time.

- **Lactose intolerance:** A personal observation suggests that infants who are lactose intolerant but have a normal rate of gut motility are at first relatively quiet after a feed. They tend to produce signs of discomfort after approximately 90–120 minutes when the undigested lactose starts to ferment in the large intestine. Signs and symptoms are the same as in colic due to rapid peristaltic contractions; i.e. they start drawing their knees up, etc., and you can hear and palpate borborygmi.

- **Gastro-esophageal reflux (GER)** (see Ch.12): This is a condition in which pain and discomfort and a burning irritation in the distal end of the esophagus is caused by ineffective closure of the cardiac sphincter of the stomach. This sphincter acts in conjunction with the left crus of the diaphragm to close the entrance to the stomach and prevent the painful regurgitation of the acidic gastric juices into the esophagus. Incompetence of the cardiac sphincter causes the gastric acids to leak upwards, irritating and burning the esophageal membrane. Infants affected by

GER tend to experience pain and discomfort on feeding or soon after. The pain may be eased by a change in feeding position; for example the child may experience more discomfort feeding on one breast than the other, or when held along the mother's left arm rather than the right. The infant's symptoms may well be relieved by propping him upright. Reflux is often accompanied by positing, in which small amounts of milk are continually vomited. This suggests an incompetence of the cardiac sphincter of the stomach, but may simply be the result of over-feeding. However, just before the baby posits he may grimace in discomfort and cry, because of the pain and burning irritation in the lower esophagus. There may be an associated cough in which a simultaneous bronchospasm is triggered through the MALT (mucosal associated lymphoid tissue) network of embryologically associated tissues.

Diagnosis

'Colic' is diagnosed if the excessive crying happens at least on 3 days a week, lasts longer than 3 hours/day and lasts at least 3 weeks. To exclude organic causes a medical and neurological examination is necessary. Beware: psychologically unstable parents may be pushed towards abuse by an excessively or permanently crying child. Be on the lookout for signs.

The time of onset of symptoms is one of the main criteria of differential diagnosis: borborygmi occurring immediately on ingestion of food indicate that the gut is over-alert and primed and ready to overreact. Lactose intolerance will present approximately 90 minutes after a feed. However, other facts and signs must also be considered, such as family history of proven lactose intolerance, or reports that certain family members will not eat or drink fresh milk such as on breakfast cereals, but may eat yoghurts and cheese. The latter two foodstuffs may be digestible for a lactose intolerant person because the bacterial action in their manufacture has already commenced the breakdown of the milk itself.

Allergies will be indicated frequently by associated changes in the skin of affected infants. The facial skin and scalp is a very good indicator of allergic manifestation, being part of the mucosal associated lymphoid tissues (MALT) which also make up the mucous membranes of the gut and lung systems. Rashes may be seen on the face, which will rapidly appear on feeding; the skin may become dry and scaly in various parts of the body; cradle cap may also be an indicator of an allergic response and there may be outright signs of atopy or eczema.

Medical diagnosis

Laboratory testing of fecal matter is perhaps one of the most reliable indicators of true lactose intolerance. Examination of the stools may show small white 'grains-of-rice' indicating undigested milk. Normal allergic screening is not always successful as the infant is not reacting to the lactose in an allergic manner, but he simply does not have the enzyme capability to break lactose down.

There are laboratories in the UK who will perform a pin-prick blood test, screening for allergies. Other laboratories can conduct an analysis of the hair, and kinesiologists will also generally be able to help to identify the causative reagents.

Osteopathic examination

In my experience there are often palpable changes in the tissue quality of affected infants. The fascias feel more tense and have a spiky, irritable unfluid quality. This latter quality may interfere with the response of the infant to osteopathic treatment, and in particular delay the release and resolution of birth trauma and strain patterns that are also affecting the health and disposition of the infant.

Reflux irritability of the esophagus may result in a tension of the esophagus that is palpable from the pharynx. In particular it will pull the occiput into a cranial base extension pattern, owing to the attachments of the pharynx onto the pharyngeal tubercle of the inferior surface of the basiocciput.

Treatment

Most important is putting the parents at ease and advising them that very often the child will settle down in a few weeks time, as there is a natural tendency for infantile colic to improve with time. If the parents are put at ease and can keep in control of the situation then the infant will also benefit from a calmer atmosphere. Often the situation also improves if parents do not let the child cry a long time, but carry and cradle him, play or give him a pacifier.

A low allergen diet in the mother has been shown to alleviate the symptoms of colic in the breastfed infant (Hill et al 1995). It is useful to advise mothers to avoid brassicas (cabbage, broccoli, cauliflower, lettuce, etc.) and bananas, and to reduce the amount of coffee consumed. The brassicas contain natural alkaloids that all infants find difficult to digest, and bananas are a very complex food that infants also find difficult to digest, being high in potassium and containing epinephrine (adrenalin), dopamines and many complex carbohydrates.

Some children seem to be allergic to cow's milk. If they are bottle-fed, using lactose-free formula or one where the casein has been hydrolyzed appears to help these infants.

For other alternatives see Ch.10, Nutrition.

Allopathic medical treatment

Many questions have been raised over the years about the medications available.

Anti-spasmodic medications may be effective in pacifying this sort of irritable gut (with rapid peristaltic contractions), although their effectiveness overall has generally been shown to be variable. Response to this medication may possibly be considered a retrospective differential diagnostic tool. Back in the 1950s and 60s it seemed that antispasmodic medication was the effective treatment of choice, but there were some unwelcome side effects reported, and so some of the available prescriptions were withdrawn (Illingworth 1985).

Regarding the treatment of gastro-esophageal reflux see p.273.

Osteopathic treatment

It seems that cranial osteopathic treatment may be an important non-drug approach to alleviating or controlling the symptoms of infantile colic (Hayden and Mullinger 2006). However, infantile colic is a multifactorial condition, which means that the condition will generally respond to our treatment approach but that we should be aware that the underlying cause, such as lactose intolerance, might still persist at a lesser subclinical level.

Osteopathic treatment has the potential to release many of the focal strains acquired from birth that may create a hypersensitive, irritable system. This includes molding pressure on the fetal head during the birth process. It appears that osteopathic treatment relaxes the infant by releasing many of the musculoskeletal and physical strains acquired during the birth process, so helping to reset the resting tone of the body. In the majority of infants this appears to be effective in settling down the colic.

In my experience, osteopathy also seems to help those children who have a more excitable autonomic system (perhaps due to prenatal stresses).

A long-held and generally popular view held by osteopaths is that a specific manipulation to a single structure, such as easing the pressure on the vagus (cranial nerve X) in the jugular foramen of the occiput, is responsible for the improvement gained by osteopathic treatment of a colicky child. In a retrospective analysis of the anatomical cranial base patterns of the treated group of children in a study by Hayden et al (2002), no single pattern (i.e. left condylar part compression or right lateral shear pattern) seemed to predominate. What was indicated in the greater percentage was that the births had been difficult, and the trauma levels and strains experienced by the infants had been correspondingly greater too.

The emphasis in osteopathic training is that we should use diagnostic palpation to differentiate between various strains and restrictions in the body. In some infants it may be appropriate to release compressive patterns that have caused restrictions in the sensitive meninges and layers of the scalp; but in others the strains may primarily influence and distort the thoracic tissues and diaphragm, perhaps resulting in reflux symptoms. In others infants, however, compression and restriction of the ligamentous and muscular balance of the segments in the cervical spine may be implicated. These are just some of the physical aspects that may be encountered, which makes it difficult to be prescriptive in our treatment approach.

Gastro-esophageal reflux

Personal palpatory observations are that the dysfunction of the cardiac sphincter of the stomach may be associated with the twists, strains and compressions of the thorax and shoulders acquired during the birth process. This can affect the integrity and function of the diaphragm in general, and the crura of the diaphragm more specifically. Releasing the strain patterns in the thorax is a primary consideration in restoring the integrity and function of the diaphragm. But equally lower extremity, pelvic or sacral strain patterns may act through the quadratus lumborum and psoas muscles, the iliac fascia and the spinal structures to upset the balance of the integral components of the diaphragm.

Also apparently implicated are the tensions generated through abdomen and umbilicus via the ligamentum teres onto the diaphragm, especially if the umbilical cord had been wrapped round the infant's neck. Liver enlargement, congestion and turgor will also affect the balance and function of the diaphragm. Spinal lesions, especially in the lower thoracic spinal segments, will also affect diaphragm function, either directly by interfering in a biomechanical way or by interference with the autonomic supply from the sympathetic and parasympathetic spinal ganglia.

Prognosis

Mostly the excessive crying peaks at the 3rd month and then gradually gets less; rarely it lasts up until the end of the 1st year.

A randomized prospective controlled preliminary study of infantile colic in 28 infants that was performed as part of an MSc research project in 2001 showed a highly significant 11% ($p < 0.002$) improvement in the sleep patterns of the babies in the test group, who were treated osteopathically, compared with a non-significant <2% ($p > 0.05$) improvement in the control group. Moreover, parents reported that the treated infants also enjoyed a better quality of restful sleep (Hayden 2006). A surprising fact borne out by the study undertaken in 2002 is that some of the infants who were clearly lactose intolerant (family history, etc.) also seemed to benefit from osteopathic treatment.

I am not sure of the overall success rate that can be claimed for osteopathic treatment. Many babies are better for treatment, but some still show some signs of discomfort or excessive wind. This may be due to the various levels of severity of infantile colic.

In treating young infants we are aiming to release the physical tensions created by the discomfort and distress experienced to date, and in doing so we also help the carers – the immediate family. By easing the discomfort in a young infant we are also helping them to develop a more positive attitude to life, not soured by intense abdominal pains associated with feeding. Further research has shown that children who suffer from colic early on are more likely to have behavioral and social problems 3 years on. They are more emotionally reactive and have more tantrums; do not sleep as well and are more often fussy eaters. In addition they do not concentrate so well at school because they sleep less. It is important, however, to consider the whole psychosocial picture, and in doing so perhaps we can see better the importance of appropriate osteopathic treatment.

Treatment of the twists and strains of the thorax and shoulders, and from abdominal strains and pressures is effective in treating reflux. However, where there has been prolonged esophageal irritation and burning, it may take 1 to 2 weeks for the signs of the reflux to subside. Rarely do the signs disappear immediately. Infant Gaviscon medication will help to give more immediate relief but will not solve the real cause of the problem.

VOMITING AND REGURGITATION

Definition

Occasional vomiting is not rare in the newborn. First you need to check whether the baby is really vomiting, or whether it is just a little bit of milk coming back out of the mouth. We differentiate between:

- **regurgitation** of small amounts of feed
- **real vomiting** of larger amounts with signs of vegetative disturbance like feelings of nausea, increased salivation, pallor, sweat and tachycardia.

Serious signs are persistent vomiting, loss of weight and failure to gain weight.

Etiology and pathophysiology

A common cause for regurgitation is overfeeding, especially if when bottle-feeding the baby the hole in the teat of the bottle is too large, or the child swallows air and is not burping enough. The diaphragm in small babies is less able to compress the cardiac sphincter on inhalation and so reflux is more common, especially if the stomach is very full (Carreiro 2003).

Allergy can be another common cause of vomiting in the bottle- or breastfed baby.

A bottle-fed infant's allergic response to formula feeds is easier to quantify than the response to breast milk, in that the formula can be more readily changed away from a cow's milk formula to a goat or animal-free formula. The improvement is usually immediate (see Ch.10, Nutrition).

For the breastfed infant, close consideration of the family history of allergies will often yield important clues as to the causative reagent. There may be a variability to the vomiting of the feed in the breastfed infant. Some feed will be vomited but not others. This is due to the changes in the maternal diet, in which the reactive food may or may not be eaten by the mother.

Clinical signs and symptoms, differential diagnosis

The child vomits smaller (regurgitation) or larger amounts. With an allergic reaction to ingested food copious amounts of vomit are often produced. The vomit is profuse and gushes forth, but does not tend to be projectile, although parents will often report it as projectile. The reaction to the allergen may also be accompanied by other signs of allergy: rashes around the mouth; scaly cradle cap on the scalp; redness and swelling of the tongue; excessive oral and nasal mucous production which may result in phlegm draining down to the lungs and bronchi, giving a chesty rattling cough that is worse in the morning; areas of patchy dry skin on the face or body; or a family history of allergic sensitivity.

Differential diagnosis

In vomiting that is not acrid/bilious think of:

- gastro-esophageal reflux (GER) (see Ch.12)
- gastroenteritis: usually also presents with diarrhea and fever
- raised intracranial pressure: e.g. hydrocephalus
- severe systemic infections: like meningitis, sepsis, urinary tract infections, pneumonia
- pyloric stenosis: (see Ch.12, Pyloric hypertrophy)
- intolerance of food
- metabolic disease (in rare cases).

With acrid/ bilious vomiting think of:

- necrotizing enterocolitis
- intestinal obstruction.

Diagnosis and differential diagnosis

The following facts need to be determined by the case history and observation: when did the vomiting/regurgitation start? What kind of vomiting and how often? What does the substance look like? Does the child still gain weight? Observation may also point to major indicators of allergies, such as skin rashes and redness, or dry, flaky skin.

Medical diagnosis

Laboratory tests include blood count, cross-reacting protein (CRP), electrolytes, tests for metabolic acidosis or alkalosis. Generally there are raised IgA levels.

Skin tests may also provide positive reaction to the suspected allergens.

A sonogram of abdomen and CNS to exclude pathologies.

Osteopathic examination

As always, a complete osteopathic examination of the whole body and cranium is undertaken.

In my experience it is especially useful to note the tone and weight of the esophageal and gut tissues before feeding commences. This is achieved with quiet passive palpation. Personal observations are that if one continues palpating while the feeding starts, the central esophageal tube through the mediastinum becomes turgid and heavy with the stomach feeling tense, and there is a feeling of reactive edema in the peritoneal cavity.

Treatment

Important to note is the documentation of weight gain, to see if the curve is normal or below. If no pathology is found and children gain weight, parents need not worry overmuch. It may also be of help to lay children on their back with the thorax propped up a bit after feeding, not immediately on their stomach.

Appropriate advice on an exclusion diet should be given to the mother of the breastfed infant. For example the mother may be encouraged to eliminate a major food group from the diet for one week, for example cow's milk, and monitor the behavior of the baby. After a week a challenge can be made in which the mother reintroduces that foodstuff and the infant's behavior is monitored over the next couple of days. In this way a clear indication may be gained of the cause for the allergic response. This is not foolproof, but is a useful way of determining what the cause for the allergy may be.

Osteopathic treatment

Techniques that aid lymphatic drainage of the viscera will usually help to minimize the allergic edematous response. Fluid management techniques will help to promote tissue drainage. Also releasing musculoskeletal strain patterns will assist to decrease the general irritability of tissues, and help to calm the irritable child.

Prognosis

In case of allergy, the allergic response should diminish rapidly once the offending food (even second-hand through breast milk) has been eliminated from the infant diet. As a personal observation, the homeopathic therapeutic approach is also effective in dealing with the tendency for the infant or child to react in a particular way. This may improve the effective longer-term treatment to allergies.

Careful osteopathic treatment will also help to quieten and settle the infant or child, which in conjunction with dietary management may minimize the allergic response fairly quickly.

Bibliography

Amiel-Tison C, Sureau C, Shnider S: Cerebral handicap in full-term neonates related to the mechanical forces of labor. Baillières Clinical obstetrics and gynaecology 2(1) 1988

Apley J, Naish N: Recurrent abdominal pains, a field survey of 1000 school children. Archives of Disease in Childhood 33, 1958: 165–170

Carey W: Colic: primary excessive crying as an infant environment interaction. Pediatric Clinics of North America 31(5), 1984: 993–1005

Carreiro J: An osteopathic approach to children. 1st edn. Churchill Livingstone, London 2003

Evans R, Ferguson D, Allardyce R, et al: Maternal diet and infantile colic in breast-fed infants. Lancet 1, 1981: 1340–1342

Forbes D: Abdominal pain in childhood. Australian Family Physician 23(3), 1994: 347–357

Furaya H, Hashimoto T, Kokuho K, Kino H, Fukamauchi K: Pressures on the human fetus during labor, intrauterine and on the fetal head. Nippon Sanka Fujinka Gakkai Zasshi 12, 1981: 2173–2181

Gurry D: Infantile colic. Australian Family Physician 23,1994: 337–346

Hayden, C, Prashad D, Molinari C, Patel S: Towards an understanding of the role of osteopathy in the treatment of infantile colic. Abstract published in Journal of Manual and Manipulative Therapies, October 2002: 69

Hayden C, Mullinger B: A preliminary assessment of the impact of the cranial osteopathy for the relief of infantile colic. Complimentary Therapies in Clinical Practice 12, 2006: 83–90

Hill D, Menahem S, Hudson I, Sheffield L, Shelton M, Oberklaid F, Hosking C: Charting infant distress: an aid to defining colic. The Journal of Pediatrics 121(5) 1992: 755–758

Hill, D, Hudson I, Sheffield L, Shelton M, Menahem S, Hosking C: A low allergen diet is a significant intervention in infantile colic. results of a community based survey. Journal of Allergy and Clinical Immunology 56(6), 1995

Hogdall C, Vestermark V, Birch M, Plenov G, Toftager-Larsen K: The significance of pregnancy, delivery and post-partum factors for the development of infantile colic. Journal of Perinatal Medicine 19, 1991: 251–257

Hyde D, Guyer B: prevalence of infant colic. Archives of Disease in Childhood 560, 1983: 559–560

Ilingworth R: Three-Month Colic. Archives of Disease in Childhood, Jan 1954: 165–174

Illingworth R.S: Infantile Colic revisited. Archives of Disease in Childhood 60, 1985: 981–985

Klaus M, Kennell J: Parent-infant bonding. 2nd edn. Mosby, 1982

Klougart N, Nilsson D, Niels D, Jacobson J: Infantile colic treated by chiropractors, a prospective study of 316 cases. Journal of Manipulative and Physiological Therapeutics 12, 1989: 380–387

Lehtonen L, Korhonen T, Korvenranta H: Temperament and sleeping patterns in colicky infants during the first year of life. Developmental and Behavioral Pediatrics 15(6) 1994

Lehtonen L, Korvenranta H: Infantile colic–seasonal incidence and crying profiles. Archives of Pediatric Adolescent Medicine 149, 1995: 533–536

Liebman W: Infantile colic, association with lactose and milk intolerance. JAMA 245(7), 1981

Lothe L, Lindberg T, Jakobsson I: Cow's milk formula as a cause of infantile colic, a double-blind study. Pediatrics 70, 1982: 7–10

Marieb E: Human Anatomy and Physiology. 4th edn. Cummings, 1998

Magoun H: Osteopathy in the cranial field. 3rd edn. Journal printing Company, Kirksville, Mo. 1976, p.226

Miller J, McVeagh P, Meer G. et al: Breath hydrogen excretion in infants with colic. Archives of Disease in Childhood 64, 1989: 725–729

Miller A, Barr R: Infantile colic, Is it a gut issue? Pediatric Clinics of North America 38(6), 1991

Nathanielz P: Life in the womb- the origin of health and disease. Promethean Press, New York 1999

Odent, M: The scientification of love. Free Association Books, London 2001

O'Donovan J, Bradstock A: The failure of conventional drug therapy in the management of infantile colic. American Journal of Diseases of Children 133, 1979: 999–1001

Rautava P, Helenius H, Lehtonen L: Psychosocial predisposing factors for infantile colic. BMJ 307, 1993: 600–4

Rautava, P, Lehtonen L, Helenius H,. Sillanpaa, M: Infantile colic, child and family three years later. Pediatrics 96(1), 1995

Relier, J-P, Influence of maternal stress on fetal behavior and brain development; Biology of the Neonate 69, 1996: 165–212

Stahlberg M: Infantile colic, occurrence and risk factors. European Journal of Pediatrics 143, 1984: 108–111

Thomas, D, McGilligan, K, Eisenberg, L, Lieberman, H, Rissman, E: Infantile colic and type of milk feeding. American Journal of Diseases of Children 141, 1987

Webster R, DiPalma J, Gremse D: Lactose maldigestion and recurrent abdominal pain in children. Digestive Diseases and Science 40(7), 1995: 1506–1510

Weissbluth L, Weissbluth M: Infantile colic: the effect of serotonin and melatonin circadian rhythms on intestinal smooth muscle. Medical Hypotheses 39, 1992: 164–167

Wessel M, Cobb J, Jackson E, et al: Paroxysmal 'fussing' in infancy, sometimes called 'colic.' Pediatrics 14(5), 1954

12

Pathology and treatment of the gastrointestinal tract

Tajinder K Deoora, Clive Hayden

By far the commonest symptom picture presented in any pediatric clinic is that related to abdominal pain. When asked where the pain is, the young child will often point to the tummy, generally in the umbilical area. However, this pain may be of any origin, coming from the teeth, ears, respiratory tract, kidneys or elsewhere. Such diverse symptoms as a baby that is inconsolable, or one that has difficulty in sleeping or is vomiting, constipated, lacking in appetite, has a variable temperature, or bloating, or a child that is not thriving, may or may not be related to the contents of the abdomen. It is therefore vital to appreciate a wide differential diagnostic picture before concluding that the symptoms are purely related to the domain of the gastrointestinal area.

One of the tenets of osteopathy is that the body has a constant dynamic interaction with its environment. We utilize air, food and water from the external environment for our physiological processes, whilst our activities take place in response to social and gravitational factors. As far as the gastrointestinal system is concerned, it provides a very large surface area for the interface between the internal and external environments. It is exposed to the external environment in the fluids drunk and foods eaten. When these interactions are considered along with congenital and genetic influences, emotional and behavioral patterns, weaning, pollutants and vaccinations, it is not surprising that the variety and complexity of the presenting complaints is so great.

The digestive system in some respects may be thought of as the 'initial brain' in the sense that the stomach of the newborn baby is more developed and with greater obvious function than the brain. So, whilst the gut can already function to digest, the brain of an infant is only at the stage of responding by crying or gurgling. It takes the brain of a newborn baby 3 years to develop speech fully and yet the stomach is quite capable of assimilating complex foods. In addition, it has also learned to respond as part of the endocrine and immune systems of the body.

The gut can also be considered to be the 'emotional brain'. The child's response to any emotional upsets may be read as gastrointestinal (GI)-related symptoms. Factors such as anxiety, insecurity or even a focus for 'grounding' or 'centering' oneself are generally considered to be at the umbilical area, which is often seen in many cultures as the center for personal power. This is not surprising when we consider that, as a developing fetus, we gain nutrition and energy from the umbilical cord.

EMBRYOLOGICAL DEVELOPMENT OF THE GASTROINTESTINAL TRACT

Tajinder K. Deoora

The endodermal gut begins as a 4 mm tube during the 4th week when the embryo folds two ways – from top to bottom and laterally. This primitive gut forms as the blind-ended foregut and hindgut, and has a midgut that is open to the yolk sac via the vitelline duct. The proximal foregut will continue to form the tongue, pharynx, pharyngeal pouches, larynx and the respiratory tree. The caudal foregut in the meantime will go on to form the esophagus, stomach, duodenum, liver and biliary passages as well as the pancreas and the spleen. The midgut will form the small and large intestine and the hindgut will form the rectum.

Esophagus and stomach

To begin with, the primitive abdominal gut is a straight tube that hangs in the peritoneal cavity by a dorsal mesentery. The trachea and esophagus are separated from each other by the formation of the tracheoesophageal septum. The growth and downward migration of the heart and lungs enables the elongation of the esophagus and it reaches its final relative length by the 7th week. By the 70th day, it contains a ciliated epithelial lining, which in the 5th month gives way to stratified squamous lining. The external muscles of the super-ior third and the smooth muscles of the inferior one third of the esophagus are supplied via the vagus nerve (10th cranial nerve).

During the 5th week the stomach appears as a spindle-shaped swelling of the foregut that is anchored to the posterior abdominal wall by a dorsal mesentery. In the meantime, the duodenum gives off a bud that develops into the liver, thus creating a ventral mesentery. In this way, the posterior part of the ventral mesentery attaching the stomach to the

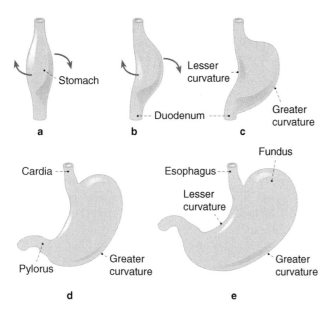

Figure 12.1 The development of the stomach and the changes in its position. **a:** Spindle-shaped expansion of the ventral intestine in the 5th week. **b, c:** Torsion of the stomach around its longitudinal axis as the result of uneven growth (development of anterior and posterior wall), 1. torsion of the stomach) and formation of the greater and lesser curvature. The arrows show the direction of torsion. **d, e:** During further growth 2. torsion of the stomach around the sagittal axis.
With permission, Henriette Rintelen, Velbert

liver becomes the lesser omentum, whilst the anterior part forms the falciform ligament.

The primitive alimentary tract is attached to the posterior abdominal wall by the dorsal mesentery. No ventral mesentery develops below the umbilicus – it is present only in the foregut region and attached to the anterior abdominal wall above the umbilicus.

At the 6th week of gestation the stomach and the gut begin a series of rotation and migration processes that eventually reach their final position at the 20th week. The stomach descends until the 51st day from C7/T4 to L2. This is the final position also seen in an adult.

Because of this descending of the stomach and the liver, and the body wall and other organs continuing to grow at different rates, the stomach and its dorsal mesentery undergo a 90° rotation (first stomach rotation) in a clockwise direction about its long axis during the 7th and 8th week. This brings the left side forward and the right side faces dorsally (Fig. 12.1a,b). In the adult you can see these changes in position in the autonomic innervation. The left vagus innervates the front wall and the right vagus the back wall.

In the meantime, the dorsal mesentery folds onto itself to the left to form the omental bursa. This expands sideways and upwards to lie between the stomach and the posterior

abdominal wall; thus facilitating the movement of the stomach. It is stopped from expanding cranially by the development of the diaphragm. The rotations of the stomach force the duodenum to bend into a 'C'-shape.

The dorsal part of the stomach grows faster so that the greater convex curvature (curvature major) facing downwards develops. The lesser, concave ventral curvature (curvature minor) which faces upward develops more slowly (Fig. 12.1c).

The second rotation of the stomach of 30° takes place around a sagittal axis. The cardia thereby sinks and moves to the left, the pylorus is lifted and is positioned on the right side. The whole stomach is shifted to the left (Fig. 12.1d,e). At birth the pylorus sphincter is weakly developed.

Caused by the change in position of the stomach, the liver is shifted into the right upper abdomen and the spleen to the left side.

Gastric pits appear in the mucosa of the 7-week-old embryonic stomach, and gastric glands bud off by the 14th week. By 5 months enzyme secretion is possible but the production of hydrochloric acid (HCl) occurs much later. Also by 5 months, peristaltic waves occur along the stomach.

Intestines

Duodenum

The duodenum is composed of the end of the foregut and the upper part of the midgut. The stomach grows so fast, bulging dorsally, that the duodenum has to move ventrally. It lengthens and forms a C-shaped loop ('duodenal C'). The stomach rotates around its longitudinal axis to the left, forcing the duodenum to rotate to the right and move to the dorsal abdominal wall. The meso of the duodenum and the parietal peritoneum then meld and the duodenum now lies in its secondary retroperitoneal position.

Jejunum, ileum

The jejunum and the ileum develop from the midgut. By the 5th week the growing ileum lengthens much quicker than the abdominal cavity itself and the umbilical loop is formed directly behind the duodenum (Fig. 12.2a). The superior mesenteric artery growing from dorsal to the gut is the axis of this loop. The cranial part of the umbilical loop forms the lower part of the duodenum, the jejunum and a part of the ileum. The caudad part forms the lower part of the ileum, the caecum with the appendix, the ascending colon and the right two thirds of the transverse colon.

The tip of the umbilical loop remains connected to the yolk sac via the ductus omphaloentericus. A remnant of the

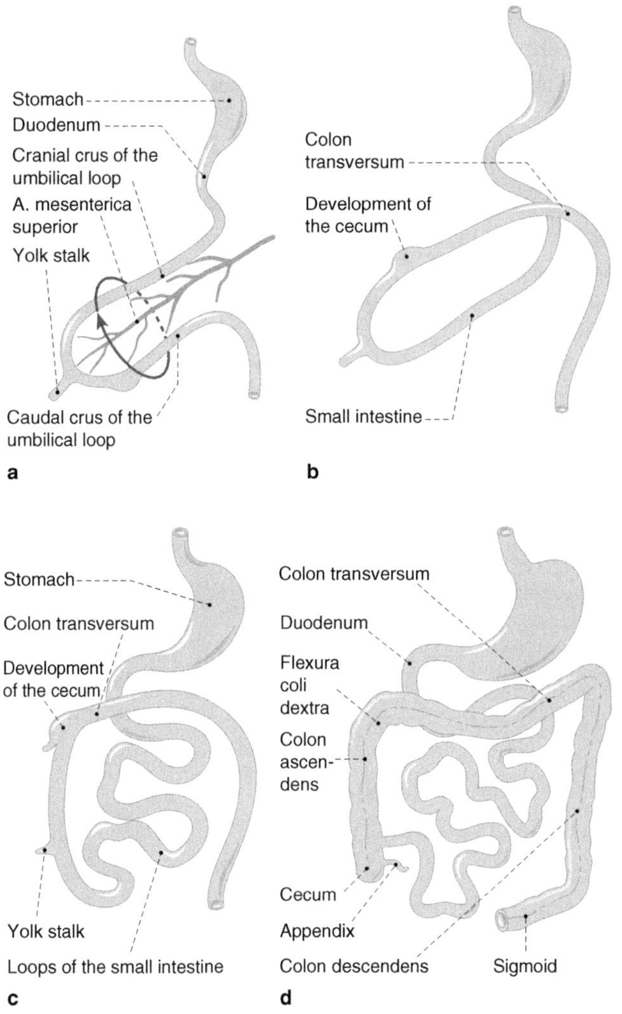

Figure 12.2 Development of jejunum and ileum. **a:** Umbilical loop before torsion with the A. mesenterica superior as the axis. The arrow shows the anti-clockwise rotation; **b:** The umbilical loop after anti-clockwise rotation by 180°; **c:** Position of the umbilical loop after rotation by 270°. The jejunum and ileum create a large number of loops. Although the large intestine increases in length, it does not participate in the formation of loops. **d:** The final position of the intestinal loops.
With permission, Henriette Rintelen, Velbert

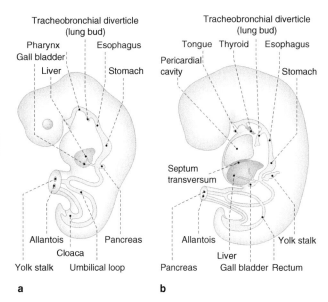

Figure 12.3 Development of the liver. **a:** In the 4th week the liver is sufficiently developed for the first liver cell trabeculae to form. The gall bladder is present as an appendage; **b:** in the 6th week the liver grows caudally to the abdominal cavity. The mesenchyme between the liver and pericardial cavity condenses (septum transversum) and commences the development of the diaphragm. The gallbladder develops.
With permission, Henriette Rintelen, Velbert

Here, in order to place the GI tract in the correct abdominal place with its associated mesentery, the midgut rotates an initial 180° counter-clockwise around the axis of the superior mesenteric artery (Fig. 12.2b). In the meantime, the GI tract in differentiating into its different structures elongates and forms loops so that the top of the loop comes to lie to the left and the bottom comes to lie to the right. The rotation is completed by the 8th week.

At the 10th week, the intestinal loop re-enters the abdomen and undergoes a further 90° counterclockwise rotation (Fig. 12.2c); the complete rotation of the intestine amounts to 270°. By the 11th week the intestines have completed the process of returning to the abdominal cavity and the caecum comes to rest against the dorsal abdominal wall in the final position (Fig. 12.2d).

Liver

During the 3rd week the liver makes its appearance as ventral bud from the area that goes on to form the duodenum. This sacculation is the hepatic diverticulum and it differentiates at the top end into glandular tissue and bile ducts (Fig. 12.3a).

The liver bud pushes its way into the mesoderm of the transverse septum, which is the site of the future diaphragm.

yolk sac can remain called Meckel diverticulum. It can be the site of mucosa inflammations or duodenal ulcers.

The umbilical loop, and particularly the cranial part, grows rapidly lengthwise and in circumference. The mucosa is formed leading to a fattening of the loop. The cranial part is folded into loops, owing to the developing intestine. This continued lengthening takes place along with the increasing pressure from the growth of the other abdominal organs, especially the liver. Consequently, through its development, much of the midgut is forced to herniate at the umbilicus and move external to the abdomen.

By 6 weeks the liver, gall bladder and the pancreas have been formed (see Fig. 12.3b). Over several weeks their position and morphology continues to change.

In the area between the ventral abdominal wall and the growing liver the transverse septum becomes drawn out to a thin membrane called the falciform ligament and between the liver and foregut (stomach and duodenum) it forms the lesser omentum. The umbilical vein is to be found in the free margin of the falciform ligament of the liver. It obliterates to become the teres hepatic ligament after birth. The bile duct, the hepatic portal vein and the hepatic artery run along the free margin of the lesser omentum. The ventral mesentery into which the liver bulges as it grows becomes the capsule of the diaphragm (of the visceral peritoneum) except cranially where the liver remains attached to the diaphragm (area nuda). The bottom end becomes the gall bladder and cystic duct.

The growth of the liver is so rapid that by the 10th week it contributes to 10% of the total fetal weight. From the 2nd to the 7th month, the liver is actively involved in blood cell differentiation. This activity ceases after birth, although this capacity can be reactivated later in life in dire emergencies.

By the 5th month, the meconium (cells forming the first feces) gains a greenish-yellow color due to bile secretion.

Neurological development

The gut is fairly immature at birth and remains so until about 2 years of age. This is in part due to the developing neurological influence. The neural components of the developing distal colon are the mesenteric and submucosal plexuses. During the 5th to 7th weeks of embryonic life the intramural nervous system develops as cells of the neural crest migrate into the walls of the colon. As a result the Auerbach and Meissner plexuses see the development of the parasympathetic ganglionic cells. At full term, they are immature and remain this way until about 2 years of age, and this means that the motility of the GI tract is not fully functional. As the plexuses mature by 5 years of age, so too does the function of motility. At full term, the gastrointestinal tract is 400 cm long, formed primarily of smooth muscle except at the proximal esophagus and the anus where voluntary control is through striated muscle.

Anomalies of the midgut

These are primarily related to a glitch in the rotation processes or in the fixation of the intestines to the abdominal wall.

Omphacoele

This congenital fault occurs at the 10th week when the intestines fail to migrate to the abdominal cavity. Since the umbilicus does not close completely this causes the abdominal contents to herniate out. Large defects may contain the liver and spleen as well as the abdominal contents.

Umbilical hernia

Here the intestines return to their abdominal cavity, but then herniate through an imperfectly closed umbilicus or through a defect in the linea alba. The hernia reaches its full size at the end of a month after birth and protrudes with increased abdominal pressure as in crying or coughing. It tends to reduce after 3 to 5 years.

POSTNATAL DEVELOPMENT OF THE GI TRACT
Tajinder K. Deoora

The GI tract of the premature infant and term infant are different and, in turn, there is also a difference in the toddler and adult. This is due to:

- activity and concentration of the transport systems
- activity and concentration of digestive enzymes from the GI tract
- permeability of the gut wall
- insufficient pancreatic enzymes
- autoregulatory mechanisms not yet being well established, or even being absent in the premature infant.

Whilst the wall of the GI tract in an older child and adult has mucosa that forms a protective barrier against the ingested external materials, term newborns and premature infants have a degree of permeability to macromolecules. In premature infants the levels of small protein, carbohydrate (eg, lactalbumin, lactulose and mannitol) present in the plasma are higher than those in the term baby and higher in term baby than in the adult.

Maturation of the baby's gut wall is stimulated by feeding, and breast milk has a greater influence on this than formula does. This is because colostrum and breast milk supply immunoglobulins (IgA) to protect against microbial infection. It also encourages mucus secretion by stem cells in the gut wall, which increases the impermeability of the gut wall.

Specialized cells, together with a portal venous system and lymphatics, are involved in the absorption of food. The small intestine has villi to increase the surface area for absorption as well as providing a multitude of enzyme systems. Where there is an absence in this development of villi, malabsorption occurs, resulting in coeliac disease, which may in turn be responsible for growth lag in a child.

Where there has been hypoxia of late pregnancy or during birth, or necrotizing enterocolitis, the microcirculation of the intestinal villi can also be affected. This can have consequences upon the absorptive function of the villi and therefore to the growth delay.

Defence mechanisms

To protect the mucosa from its own digestive enzymes and bacteria there is a rapid turnover of epithelial cells, production of mucous and a specialized immunological system.

The GI tract contains the largest lymphoid organ and microbial reservoir of the body and contains vast populations of myeloid and lymphoid cells. It has a microbial ecosystem (1–1.5 kg in the adult) and this has a major influence on the development and functioning of the intestinal immune system, and vice versa.

The mucosa of the GI tract is involved in both humoral and cellular immunity via the gut associated lymphoid tissue (GALT). These are localized collections of immune cells scattered throughout the mucosal layer of the GI tract. The GALT interacts with the lymphoid tissue in the lung, breast, skin and genitourinary tract as part of the mucosa associated lymphoid tissue (MALT) complex, thus allowing for rapid communication of immunity and antigenic information between these systems.

Medication such as phenylbutazone slows down the turnover of epithelial cells in the stomach whilst corticosteroids can alter the composition of the protective mucous covering; thereby predisposing it to peptic ulceration.

The coordinating mechanisms of digestion

The primary role of the gastrointestinal system is to digest, extract and absorb nutrients from the foods and liquids taken in. To achieve this there are different mechanisms involving secretory, motor, absorptive, endocrine and immune pathways. These are also age dependent and weaning is a part of this process of maturity of the gastrointestinal system.

The neurological control mechanisms for maintaining functions of abdominal contents are from vast bundles of nerve plexus within the walls of the gastrointestinal tract and from the autonomic nervous system (ANS) coming from the spinal column through plexuses situated in front of the lumbar spine at the level of the diaphragm. In addition, the 10th cranial nerve influences the intestines' function by relaxing the sphincters and thus increasing gut motility.

The control and coordination of motility and secretion is under the influence of the autonomic hormones gastrin, secretin and cholecystokinin-pancreozymin. In addition, the process of digestion and assimilation of food occurs via enzymes not only within the gastrointestinal tract, but also from the gall bladder, liver and pancreas.

The plexuses influencing the function of the GI tract are situated at different levels of the bowel wall – subserous, myenteric, submucosal and mucosal. Essentially, the parasympathetic plexuses of Auerbach and Meissner lie in the intestinal walls. The motor cells are connected with the central nervous system (CNS) through connector neurons from the vagus, which is excitatory and so increases peristalsis and secretion of gastrin from the stomach. This is in turn produces acid and pepsin to digest proteins. The sympathetic plexuses on the other hand are inhibitory and come from the motor cells in the superior mesenteric ganglion, receiving fibres from the greater splanchnic nerves in the T5–T9 thoracic segments. This same ganglion also supplies vasoconstrictor nerves to the vessels of the small intestine.

The autonomic trunks, through which visceromotor reflexes occur, lie on the anterior border of psoas major, vertebral bodies and intervertebral discs; each trunk has four ganglia. The prevertebral plexuses are the coeliac, intermesenteric, superior hypogastric of which the coeliac or solar is the biggest. It lies behind the stomach, at the junction between the T12 and L1. It encircles the coeliac trunk and is known as the solar plexus because its branches radiate like the sun to virtually all the surrounding organs and their coverings.

The intestinal tract from the stomach to the rectum receives sympathetic information from T5–L3. The stomach itself receives from T5–T9, mainly T5–T7, so a visceromotor reflex presents as spasm in upper portion of the left m. rectus abdominalis. The small intestine receives from T5–T9 mainly T8–T9, whilst the colon receives from T10–L3. Owing to these visceromotor reflexes, pain from the small intestine can manifest in the umbilicus, whilst reflex pain from the stomach can manifest in the epigastrium.

The colon receives supply from the both parasympathetic and sympathetic agents. The parasympathetics supply the ascending and descending colon from the vagal fibres from the solar plexus, whilst the sigmoid and rectum receive from the cord through the pelvic nerve and plexus hemorrhoidalis. The rectal reflexes occur through the sacral plexus.

ANATOMY OF THE INTESTINAL VISCERA AND ABDOMINAL CAVITY

Tajinder K. Deoora

Although the gastrointestinal tract (GI tract) begins at the mouth and ends at the anus, its organs are contained primarily within the abdominal cavity. The tonicity of the muscular abdominal wall serves to support and hold in place the movable abdominal viscera. In children up to 3 years of age this tone is generally lacking, giving the appearance of a protruding 'stomach' and this means that the contents easily fall forwards.

The abdominal cavity is bounded in front by the abdominal wall. This is enclosed above by the xyphoid process, 7–10 costal cartilages, and below on each side by the iliac crests, anterior superior spine, inguinal ligament, pubic tubercle, pubic crest and pubic symphysis. The abdomen is formed by the diaphragm above, the lower six ribs laterally, along with the iliac crests and abdominal muscles, whilst the lumbar vertebral bodies bound it posteriorly and inferiorly by the pelvis and pelvic floor.

The abdominal cavity contains the organs of the GI tract that are held within the peritoneal sac. The GI tract is mesothelial in origin and is formed of double layers separated by serous fluid. The thicker, outer parietal layer contains sensory innervation. It cannot be enlarged but is readily deformable and lines the abdominal wall. The thinner and elastic visceral layer seems to have no innervation and loosely covers the viscera and except for the liver and spleen; it is not attached to the organs.

The double layers of peritoneum enclose the organs, allowing them to interconnect with the body, or to just hang within the abdomen. Because of this enclosure, organs such as the stomach, liver, spleen, jejunum, ileum, transverse and sigmoid colons are referred to as being intraperitoneal. Since the esophagus remains in the mediastinum, it does not acquire a mesentery. Retroperitoneal organs such as the kidneys and pancreas lie against the posterior abdominal wall and are only covered by the peritoneum anteriorly. When they pass from one organ to another or to the body wall, they are referred to as the peritoneal ligaments, except for the suspension to the stomach, where they are known as the omentum. Apart from their supportive function, these ligaments are important in providing conduits for blood vessels, nerves and lymphatics to and from the abdominal viscera. Due to the flexibility, fluidity, strength and vast looping of the ligaments, the GI viscera can respond to the postural changes of the body. They can slip, slide, roll and flop in the upright or resting positions as well as during activity. So, if the child is on all fours, the viscera will shift relatively forward within the sliding surfaces of the peritoneum. For example, the liver will slide forwards over the colon whilst the tone of the abdominal wall and the pull of the enclosing peritoneum will limit this.

The GI viscera are separated from the thorax and bounded above by the diaphragm. This dome is attached bilaterally to the 6th to 12th ribs, and posteriorly its crura are attached to the 3rd and 4th lumbar vertebrae. Through the diaphragm pass the esophagus, aorta, vena cava and the thoracic duct,

as well as the motor and sensory nerves of the abdominal organs. Each dome of the diaphragm rises to the level of the 5th rib in the midclavicular line. This means that although the viscera are below the diaphragm, the upper viscera are also contained within the thoracic cavity. As a result, the abdominal contents are constantly under the mechanical influence of the respiratory movements of the diaphragm.

Organs of the GI system have a degree of pressure within them as well as between them and this helps to hold the organs in place next to each other. The combination of these pressures enables an equilibrium between the internal environment of the viscera and the external environment; that is, pressure from gravity, weight as well as tension from the abdominal wall and the descent of the diaphragm upon inhalation. So, not only does each organ have its own inherent rhythmic motions as well as peristaltic motility but it is also able to slide and glide relative to its neighbours and in response to the total bodily movements.

DIARRHEA

Tajinder K. Deoora

Definition

Diarrhea refers to an abnormal frequency and liquidity of the fecal matter, so that the stool is watery or semi-formed.

Etiology and pathology

Although diarrhea is a common symptom with several important causes of disease in infancy and early childhood, it is also a natural process of the maturing GI tract. As the baby grows, there is a strong tendency to learn about the environment by putting objects into the mouth. This resultant exposure to microbes enables the GI tract maturation of its wall and immune function, changing bowel habits and intestinal bacteria.

The age of the child who has diarrhea is an important factor when considering differential diagnosis. Neonates and infants and older children suffer less with diarrhea than do babies between the ages of 4 months and 3 years. This is because during these times, the baby is growing, gradually getting more independent in terms of weaning/food and movement. As the baby is discovering and investigating her environment, she is exposed to a great number of microbes for the first time. Since the GI tract has the greatest population of microbes and also the largest lymphatic function of the body, the GI tract often responds with diarrhea when it meets this external environment.

In babies that have suffered with perinatal hypoxia, there is a higher incidence of GI complications including malabsorption and diarrhea. Premature infants and newborns are particularly vulnerable to gut ischemia, owing to the structural nature of the microcirculation of the villi, and as a result the tissues lose their ability to absorption and perfusion.

The causes of acute diarrhea may include:

- infectious gastroenteritis: due to viruses (e.g. rotaviruses), enteropathogenic *Escherichia. coli (E. coli)*, *Salmonella* spp, *Campylobacter jejuni*, *Yersinia enterocolitica*, *Shigella* spp., *Giardia lamblia* or *Entamoeba histolytica*; usually associated with fever
- food poisoning: sometimes with copious vomiting
- food intolerance
- appendicitis
- extra-intestinal infections, e.g. otitis media, pyelonephritis
- hemolytic-uremic syndrome: with oliguria, bloody diarrhea
- pseudomembranous enterocolitis due to *Clostridium difficile* following antibiotic therapy, usually with fever.

Causes to be considered in chronic diarrhea include:

- post-infectious malabsorption
- cow's milk protein intolerance: with failure to thrive, vomiting
- food allergy
- lactose intolerance: with flatulence and abdominal pain, thrives normally
- fructose malabsorption: with flatulence, thrives normally
- cystic fibrosis
- coeliac disease: with failure to thrive, distended abdomen
- Crohn's disease, ulcerative colitis: blood and mucus in feces, with abdominal pain, extra-intestinal symptoms, failure to thrive
- irritable bowel in the preschool child
- overflow encopresis: history of constipation.

There are generally two types of mechanism involved in producing diarrhea:

- Where there is a failure to absorb water and fluids normally, thereby causing an osmotic imbalance (**osmotic diarrhea**).
- When there is an excessive secretion of fluids and electrolytes by the small or large intestine (**secretory diarrhea**).

These mechanisms are useful in differentiating the origin of diarrhea and hence its management. The two types can be assessed according to the amount of sodium and potassium present in the fecal matter. Reduced feeding or fasting reduces the volume in 'osmotic diarrhea', whereas it has no effect on the volume in 'secretory diarrhea'. More commonly, however, there is a defect with reduced absorption and increased secretion in the GI tract. Usually, infectious and inflammatory agents stimulate water and electrolyte secretion from the small intestine and colon. This results in the secretory type of diarrhea.

Infections

Many acute infectious diseases begin with GI tract symptoms, of which diarrhea is the most common. Making diagnosis is quite difficult in the early stages of the illness. Conditions such as pneumonia and meningitis will often present with vomiting and diarrhea prior to the onset of fever, rapid breathing and marked listlessness. Once the vomiting and the other symptoms cease, then the diarrhea may be attributed to GI causes.

Viruses or bacteria such as toxigenic *E.coli*, *Clostridium difficile* and cholera cause infections in the intestinal tract. The mucosa becomes very irritated so that its secretions and motility are increased manifold. This has the effect of moving the infectious agent towards the anus, whilst flushing it at the same time.

Diarrhea due to infectious agents is often preceded by high temperature. Blood and mucous are present in the stools with severe infections, owing to injury to the intestinal and mucous producing walls. Dehydration is a serious and common complication, and in a young baby this may also be complicated by convulsions. It should also be remembered that in a fever, the child will lose fluids through the skin and the lungs, thus adding to the dehydration.

Local infection of the GI tract resulting in gastroenteritis leads to diarrhea that is acute and lasts until the infection is arrested. Diarrhea may also be related to an infection elsewhere in the body, as in otitis media. This is accompanied with additional symptoms, such as pain in the ears or discharge from the ears. The young infant will often rub her ear as well. The mumps virus can also result in diarrhea, but this will be associated with enlarged parotid glands. Teething in babies is another cause of runny bowel motions. It is often accompanied with a runny nose and slight fever.

Maldigestion

Problems with maldigestion, such as infantile lactose intolerance or milk allergy, are leading causes of osmotic diarrhea. Ingestion of non-absorbable substances such as magnesium and sorbitol preparations in laxatives can also result in watery, acidic diarrhea.

Malabsorption syndromes

Malabsorption syndromes are related to some sort of physical dysfunction within the GI tract. When there is a disorder of intraluminal digestion, as in Crohn's disease, there is a resultant inflammation of the part of the bowel affected. If the terminal ileum is affected, the bile acids cannot be reabsorbed. Instead they pass into the colon and are lost as feces. In the colon they interfere with water and electrolyte absorption, resulting in diarrhea. This loss of bile cannot be compensated for by liver synthesis.

Chronic and intermittent diarrhea may be also related to ulcerative colitis, especially in the older child, and this may lead to malabsorption of nutrients and loss of protein, thus leading to weight loss and reduced stature.

When there is a disorder of transport in the mucosal cell, the mucosa becomes damaged. This can be affected in a generalized manner as in coeliac (allergy to gluten), tropical sprue, Crohn's or the mucosa can be affected in a specific manner. Therefore, the mucosa is normal but lacking a particular enzyme that aids the digestion of a certain nutrient; for example lactase for lactose or intrinsic factor for B12 absorption.

As a result there is a lack of adequate absorption of nutrients and proteins and so the child fails to grow and thrive. There is a loss of weight and energy. The abdomen may be distended and there is often steatorrhoea, diarrhea, anemia, and deficiency of vitamins, as can be seen by the sore tongue, angular stomatitis, and dry and atrophic skin.

Diet

In babies and young children, excessive sugar in the diet that is greater than the digestive capability can often result in diarrhea. The young pancreas is sometimes not mature enough to handle the excessive sugar, which begins to ferment in the stomach, especially when mixed with cow's milk. The diarrhea will take a few days to develop. Prior to that, the abdomen will bloat and the distension causes griping pains, the stools smell foul and may cause irritation of the anus.

Mechanical causes

Mechanical factors do not play a huge role in early infancy, but become more common after weaning. As the child is exposed to unsuitable food that the GI tract is not yet mature to handle, such as food with large and tough fibrous residues, or ones that produce excessive gas such as cabbage, corn, unripe fruit or rough breads, the intestinal lining may be irritated. Milk, that has large proteins, or soya, may be another cause for this irritation, as well as foods with preservative and coloring. Once the offending food has been eliminated from the system, the diarrhea subsides.

Reduced motility of the colon means there is less activity and so the fecal matter can run through quickly resulting in loose bowel motions. The cause may lie in the influence locally of the myenteric plexus and hormones and also the spinal somatovisceral reflexes as well as the influence from the autonomic nervous system (see p.261).

Psychogenic factors

Diarrhea can be a reaction to psychological pressure or stress that disturbs the balance of the autonomic nervous system. The loose bowel motions may be associated with a loss of appetite and the child appears nervous and often fidgets.

Signs and symptoms

Diarrhea is often the chief symptom of a disease and is the cause of severe ill health and sometimes failure to thrive in the child. It refers to the abnormal frequency and liquidity of the fecal matter in that the stool is watery or semi-formed. This is often associated with other symptoms, such as acute and griping abdominal pain, bloating, fever, nausea, feeling unwell, listlessness or fatigue. These symptoms may precede the diarrhea.

The stools are in general composed of fecal matter to begin with, but very quickly become watery and colored green or greenish yellow due to the fatty curds and bile acids. In mild cases blood and mucous are absent, but in severe cases, where there has been damage to the intestinal wall, there may be blood and or mucous within the watery stools.

The severity, duration, frequency, times of occurrence, associated phenomena and the behavior of the child often give clues as to the origins of the diarrhea. In severe cases, the baby is very restless and discomfort in the abdomen is manifested by drawing up of the legs and crying inconsolably. Although the baby might be thirsty, she may refuse to feed.

Diagnosis

The case history can be complemented by inspecting the stools. Intestinal gurgling may be heard in the case of gastroenteritis when the abdomen is auscultated.

Allopathic medical diagnosis

The stools are tested for pathogenic organisms, parasites, chymotrypsin and pancreatic elastase.

Clinical laboratory diagnosis consists of hematology, erythrocyte sedimentation rate (ESR), cross-reacting protein (CRP), creatinine, iron, transferrin, ferritin, calcium, phosphate, transaminases, cholestasis enzymes, electrophoresis, immunglobulins, total IgE, and gliadin and endomysium antibodies. A sweat test and H_2 testing with lactose and fructose may also be performed.

Further diagnostic measures include ultrasound investigations, fecal fat, determination of zinc, folic acid and vitamin B_{12} in the blood, allergy testing, small intestinal biopsy, colonoscopy with biopsy, plain abdominal X-ray, fractionated gastrointestinal passage, and colonic contrast enema.

Osteopathic examination

The osteopathic examination consists of percussion and palpation of the abdomen and evaluating the according nervous plexi. Then the involuntary motion of the organs is checked (see pp.216, 217). The associated structures, such as the lumbar spine segments, the thoracic segments, the diaphragm and the pelvic floor, are also examined and possible restrictions treated.

Therapy

Allopathic medical treatment

The treatment given will be determined by the underlying cause.

In acute infectious enteritis the crucial and most important intervention is the provision of adequate rehydration to compensate for fluid and electrolyte losses. An oral rehydration solution is administered in cases where there has been weight loss of 5–8%. Intravenous infusion of fluid and electrolytes should be implemented in patients simultaneously presenting with recurrent vomiting, weight loss $\geq$ 8% or pH $\leq$ 7.1.

Early realimentation should also be attempted in order to prevent mucosal atrophy and achieve rapid recovery. Breastfed infants should continue breastfeeding and also receive a rehydration solution. After 6-hour intensive rehydration, non-breastfed infants should receive their infant formula diluted (initially 1 part milk to 2 parts water, then 2 parts milk to 1 part water). In preschool and school-age children realimentation should be built up gradually, starting with foods rich in carbohydrates (e.g. sweetened rusks, apples). Carrots in any form are also suitable. Controlled studies have shown that probiotic lactobacilli reduce the duration and severity of acute diarrhea. Motility-inhibiting drugs are obsolete in a pediatric setting and 'special dietary products' have no proven benefit and are therefore not recommended.

Osteopathic treatment

The treatment depends on the individual situation and the symptoms the child presents. The following areas should be considered when treating diarrhea.

- function of the autonomic nervous system
- mobility of the lower thoracic spine
- muscle tone of the pelvic floor
- function of the small intestine and the large intestine.

Case history

Alice was a very inquisitive curious 1-year-old baby who had been suffering with diarrhea for about a day. Her mother mentioned that she had become listless and clingy prior to the diarrhea starting. She was now also mildly feverish, her watery stools were yellow and very smelly. She had learnt to crawl very early on and was into just about everything.

Observation

As Alice lay in her mother's arms, she was not interested in engaging with toys, conversation or anything else. She was tired, and for a normally active baby she just wanted to remain quiet. Her birth and previous medical history related nothing of consequence and she had no abnormal reactions to her inoculations.

Examination

Alice's hands and feet were cold, as was the skin over the back and shoulders. However, her abdomen felt hot, and there was an increased tone over the abdominal wall, especially in the area of the left side of the diaphragm and in the lower abdomen and the lower right quadrant. There was mild perspiration over Alice's forehead and the pulse was thready and marginally raised.

There was an increased tone of the muscles of the thoracic erector spinae muscles, especially between the T8–T12 vertebrae and also in the neck, especially over the C3, 4, and 5 regions. The membranes of the reciprocal tension system also felt hot and irritated, whilst the abdominal mesentery felt like a wet sponge that displayed very little in the way of the inherent rhythmic motions of primary respiration. However, there was excessive borborygmy and this was associated with the griping pains in the stomach. There was a degree of axial compression within the spine, and the sacrum was not moving freely within its innominate neighbourhood. This was reminiscent of a fall onto the sacrum with a force that had shot up the spine and into the cranial base. The frontals were being dragged anteriorly and downwards towards the abdominal fascias, and the lower ribs were not able to fully display their inspiration phase.

On further questioning, Alice's mother explained that about 3 weeks earlier Alice had got very adventurous, as she was now trying to walk around the furniture, and had landed heavily on her bottom. This explained the axial compression. In addition, Alice had been to a birthday party and had eaten foods that were new to her. This, added to the fact the she was also playing with her friend's toys, meant further exposure to bugs.

Diagnosis

The history and examination suggested an overload (through new foods) on her developing digestive system along with a mild infection of her GI tract.

Treatment protocol and aims

- To release spinal axial compression (from the effects of the fall).
- To release the rigidity of the lower thoracic and upper lumbar spinal column and the T8–T12 vertebrae.
- To calm down the abnormal rigidity of the abdominal walls.
- To reduce the tone in the cervical spine especial at the C3, 4, and 5 levels (corresponding to the nerve supply and hence the trophic function of the diaphragm).
- To release the lower ribs and thoracic diaphragm.
- To ensure synchronicity of all four diaphragms, that is, cranial, thoracic inlet, thoracic and pelvic floor.
- To rebalance the cranial and spinal reciprocal tension membrane, especially at the cranial base and frontals.
- To correct the anterior fascial drag and allow the sacrum to have free function between the innominates.

Having achieved the above, the circulation improved and the heat of the skin over the abdomen, thorax, hands and feet soon normalized. The respiration and pulse rates were also much calmer and Alice simply dropped off to sleep.

Parental input

The parents were advised to stop feeds until the diarrhea had stopped. They were to ensure adequate water and hydration salts were given and to sponge her with lukewarm water if Alice got too hot.

As bacteria were suspected, in spite of the symptoms subsiding, another osteopathic treatment was given the next day. This time the mother was instructed to very gently massage the middle back with baby oil mixed with a few drops of camomile.

Once Alice started to feel better and the diarrhea had stopped, Alice could go back to her previous diet, but to avoid cow's milk and sugar initially. She was back to her normal routine within a few days.

Prognosis

The prognosis depends on the cause of the diarrhea. Diarrhea responds well to osteopathic treatment, especially if nutritional aspects are considered and the diet changed as necessary.

CHRONIC CONSTIPATION

Tajinder K. Deoora

Definition

One of the most frequent and often distressing conditions to present in the pediatric osteopath's practice relates to emptying of the bowels. Normal bowel patterns are variable in all children, but the term 'constipation' refers to the hardness of stools as a result of a prolonged time between bowel motions and often an insufficient defecation.

There is a great variation in the number of times of regular bowel motions amongst normal populations and also in different age groups. Amongst all the different factors, diet appears to play a huge part in bowel patterns. Breastfed infants tend to have greater number of bowel movements, producing a stool with each feed and opening the bowels two to three times per day. Bottle fed infants on the other hand tend to produce fewer stools; a bowel motion every two to three days is not uncommon. In general, the range for a normal bowel pattern may vary from between five times per day to as few as once every third day. Whilst the odd digression is fine, a bowel motion beyond four days is considered as constipation.

Etiology and pathogenesis
Formation of feces

The formation occurs due to absorption of water and electrolytes from chyme in the large intestine. Three to four mass propulsive movements per day caused by the gastrocolic and duodenocolic reflexes move the chyme. Most of the absorption occurs in the proximal half of the colon and sigmoid. The remaining matter is about three-quarters water and one quarter solid, which is composed of dead bacteria, fat, inorganic matter, undigested roughage, tiny amounts of protein, and constituents of digestive juices, such as bile pigments. The derivatives of bilirubin give the fecal matter its brown color. The rectum is the storage area for the fecal matter, which is expelled as stool when sufficient distension leads to an urge to defecate, thereby causing relaxation of the internal anal sphincter. The external anal sphincter is made up of striated or voluntary muscle so that one can control opening of the bowels.

The defecation reflex

As the feces enter the rectum, its wall is distended, thus activating the myenteric plexus and the awareness of a need to defecate. This initiates peristaltic waves in the descending colon, sigmoid and rectum, thereby moving the feces towards the anus. Here the peristaltic wave causes the myenteric plexus to send inhibitory signals to the internal anal sphincter, which cause it to relax. Simultaneously the urge to defecate from the conscious cortex sends signals to the external sphincter, which voluntarily relaxes, enabling defecation.

The myenteric pathway by itself, however, is a fairly weak reflex. It is fortified by another type of reflex in order for effective defecation to occur. This is a parasympathetic reflex from the sacral segments of the spinal cord so that when the nerve endings in the rectum are stimulated, signals go first into the spinal cord and lower bowel and anus via the parasympathetic fibres (hypogastric plexus) in the pelvic nerves. This intensifies the motility and relaxes the internal sphincter, thereby re-enforcing the intrinsic myenteric reflex into such a powerful force of evacuation that it empties the bowel from the splenic flexure of the colon to the anus.

These parasympathetic signals from the pelvic nerves also initiate other factors that strengthen defecation. Upon entering the spinal cord, they bring about the closure of the glottis, deep inspiration and contraction of the abdominal wall so that there is an increased pressure within the abdominal cavity and the fecal contents can move downwards. Simultaneously, the pelvic floor relaxes downwards and outwards on the anal ring in order to evaginate the feces.

Motility

Digestion and absorption occurs through the process of motility of the GI tract under the influence of the myenteric plexus and hormones. Due to this process, about half of a semi-solid meal leaves the stomach within 30 minutes; as the alimentary absorption is completed and absorption begins.

In the small intestine the slow wave of the longitudinal muscle fibres in the duodenum is greater than that in the ileum. In the colon, motility occurs via segmentation, whereby contraction rings produce slow mixing of feces but no propulsion and therefore there is a maximum absorption of water and electrolytes. Propulsion produces mass movement and this causes elimination of feces. All activity of the colon is increased after eating – hence the need to defecate. In diarrhea the colon is quiet, whilst in constipation it is active by segmentation and hence providing active resistance to flow along lumen.

Etiology

Primary (idiopathic), chronic habitual constipation may be caused by:

- diet: along with other factors this appears to be a key element in digestion and bowel evacuation; low fluid intake and low-fibre diet lead to constipation

- insufficient exercise/physical activity

- incorrect toilet training leading to fecal retention (see below, Functional causes)

- adverse situational and psychological factors

- perianal lesions: anal fissure, perianal inflammation.

Secondary constipation due to organic causes is rare:

- **Hirschsprung's Disease (Megacolon congenitum):** This onset of constipation is from birth, with a lot of abdominal pain, and failure to thrive is common. The stools, when present, are small, ribbon-like and there is a tight anal tone. In very severe cases there may even be vomiting of the fecal matter. Congenital deficiency of ganglionic cells in the myenteric plexus in a segment of the sigmoid colon is usually the cause of constipation. The aganglionic portion of the colon results in a lack of the defecation reflexes as well as reduced or absent peristaltic motility. The affected colon becomes small and spastic due to the absent or reduced parasympathetic control from the enteric nervous system. In the meantime, the fecal matter accumulates in the area proximally causing it to distend, sometimes to a diameter of as much as 7–10 cm, causing a megacolon. On radiographic examination, the diseased portion of the colon appears normal, whilst the proximal or originally normal portion of the large intestine appears greatly enlarged.

- **Volvulus and Malrotation:** Obstruction to the passage of intestinal contents resulting in acute abdominal pain and constipation can stem from any number and combination of volvulus (twisting of the intestines), and malrotations may occur during the complex developmental phase of rotations, elongation and looping of the GI tract.

- Stenosis is a partial occlusion, whilst atresia is a complete occlusion, of the intestinal lumen, thereby causing obstruction. This seems to occur more commonly in the duodenum. Others may be a result of volvulus, malfixation or strangulation that results in impaired blood supply to the GI tract and hence absent bowel motions below the obstruction.

- Imperforate anus and anorectal anomalies. The passage of feces is physically blocked because the anus is improperly formed or absent. The abdomen of the neonate is greatly distended, the feeds are immediately vomited and the vomitus may even contain fecal matter. In the West the incidence is 1:5000 newborn infants (Moore and Persaud), but this may be higher in certain cultures. During a recent trip to Kanti Hospital in Kathmandu in 2004, we saw a high number of cases of this and Hirschsprung, where the osteopathic care was given postoperatively.

- Spinal cord lesions: chronic constipation can result from congenital, traumatic or infective spinal cord lesions
- Cow's milk intolerance
- Cystic fibrosis
- Hypothyreosis
- Dysregulation of the electrolytes
- Side effects of medication, e.g. opiates.

Functional causes of constipation

In functional constipation, the onset is generally after 2 years of age, encopresis is common but there is no failure to thrive. The stool size tends to be large and there is a history of issues around bowel training. Infants are rarely constipated and in fact part of the early process is controlling defecation, which means inhibiting the natural defecation reflexes. When the natural urge to defecate is habitually repressed, the defecation reflexes themselves become weaker and chronically retained fecal matter overstretches the colon, making it atonic.

On examination, the degree of abdominal distension is variable; there are large amounts of stools with no transition zone. The distension from the retained fecal matter causes a relaxation of the internal sphincter.

There is often an underlying emotional component, which must be considered. The parental anxiety adds to the tension within the constipated child, and straining in the older child may well be an attempt to retain the stool and hence regain empowerment.

Osteopathic considerations and treatment

Cases of chronic constipation seen in a pediatric osteopathic practice tend to be primarily functional in origin, although it often accompanies and may even aggravate any pre-existing systemic condition.

Any osteopathic treatment protocol for the child presenting with chronic constipation should include all aspects of the neuromusculoskeletal system related to proper bowel function. Factors that result in an improper flow of the nervous, venous, blood and lymphatic fluids, as well as the mucous fluid inside the bowels, must be considered. In addition, the mechanical 'comfort' of the bowels and their position

within the thorax, abdomen and pelvis needs to be carefully assessed. As a result, although the problem lies in the bowels, in effect we need to look beyond at the integration picture of the whole body. The long loops of bowels together with their eternal mesenteries have not yet established a harmonious synchronicity with their surroundings. There is often an axial compression throughout the spine and in the pelvis as a result of labor. I often find that in babies with a posterior presentation there is an area of flexion through the lower thoracic and upper lumbar spine. This not only affects the attachments of the diaphragm and its function but also the posterior attachments of the mesenteries. As a result of this axial compression, the length of the GI tract does not 'match up' with the body. This leads to slipping and sliding into uncomfortable positions, thus compromising the function especially of the large bowel. The treatment here is aimed at reducing the axial compression of the spine and allowing the bowels together with their mesenteries to find a position of alignment within the abdominal and pelvic cavities.

Of special note is the functional relationship of the bowel in the pelvic area. Just at the level of S3 the sigmoid colon becomes the rectum and runs in front of the sacrum and coccyx. As it passes through the pelvic floor, it narrows and turns on itself to become the anal canal. Here the pelvic floor muscles support the anus and contribute to the external anal sphincter so that one can consciously contract the pelvic floor muscles to lift and tighten the anus. In a child, the sacral and coccygeal segments are not yet united and so can be considered as separate 'vertebrae'. Any intraosseous strain within these segments as a result of birth will affect their relative positions and therefore result in a twofold effect:

- The position of the rectum and anal canal will be similarly affected so that, at the level of the pelvic floor, the altered angle of the anal canal compromises the fecal outflow. In addition to this, the muscles attached to the sacrum and coccyx forming the pelvic floor, which contributes to the support of the anus and its external sphincter, will be also be affected. They may become overstretched on the side that deviates away from the midline, thus affecting the position of the anal canal.

- The defecation reflexes are via the pelvic nerves from the lower sacral segments. Any intraosseous strain within the sacrum will not only affect the nerve supply but also the blood supply and venous and lymphatic drainage mechanisms to the bowels.

Continuing along the lines of a neurological point of view, the effects may originate from any bony and articular lesions that contribute to the nerve supply of the GI tract. The parasympathetic supply, for example, comes from the vagus. This may be affected at its exit at the jugular foramen between the occiput and petrous temporal bone, and therefore any cranial base compression needs to be checked. Equally, the areas affecting the sympathetic outflow from the spine, primarily from T4 to T8 need to be free. Additionally, since the hypothalamus region is the seat of metabolic activities, it should be ensured that the sphenoid is not restricted in its natural, rhythmic motions.

Since the movements of the diaphragm so intimately influence the motions and functions of the gastrointestinal viscera, this too needs specific attention in chronic constipation. A poorly functioning diaphragm has an indirectly predisposing and precipitating effect through:

- mechanical movements upon the GI network
- congestion within the lymphatic mechanisms via the cisterna chyli
- liver and gall bladder functions, which are necessary for digestion and resorption, especially of the fats of the diet. The imbalance of enzymes released by these organs maintains any existing constipation
- the hepatobiliary venous tree, when the blood is not flowing completely freely, adds to the general state of congestion of the bowels.

Therefore, all the bony areas of attachment, from the lower six ribs to the 3rd and 4th lumbar vertebra at the back, and the xyphoid and costal attachments at the front, must be kept fully functional. Additionally, since the nerve supply of the diaphragm comes from the 3rd, 4th and 5th cervical segments, these should be addressed. The diaphragm developed in the neck and began its descent with the advent of lungs, thereby pushing the stomach and coeliac trunk in front and dragging the phrenic nerves behind it.

Signs and symptoms

The abdominal discomfort that comes from constipation is usually associated with a whole host of other symptoms such as cramps, flatulence, bloated stomach, and poor appetite due to a feeling of fullness. With chronic constipation, impaction, hemorrhoids and anal fissures may develop and bowel motions may be accompanied with pain and bleeding upon straining. Other complications are an overflow of diarrhea resulting from leakage around the fecal mass, the soiling adding to the distress of the parents and the child. Another complication of constipation is encopresis, which is soiling by formed stools. This occurs in children beyond the normal age of expected toilet training, generally about 4 to 5 years of age. The retained fecal mass stretches the internal sphincter so much that the child does not feel the need to defecate. Where the child has developmental and or neurological delay, as in cerebral palsy or autism, bowel incontinence is common and toilet training is very difficult.

The child may also complain of other, seemingly non-related symptoms such as headaches, irritability, lethargy or sinusitis. Since the body is not eliminating waste products in the normal manner, the disturbed metabolism causes a build up of toxins and finds other ways of eliminating them from the body. Therefore, chronic constipation seems to bear a causal relationship with sinusitis, glue ear, eczema and other skin afflictions and it may exacerbate any existing chronic constitutional disease.

Intestinal blockage (ileus) produces acute constipation. The abdomen is hard, and tenderness and guarding can be elicited. Auscultation reveals an absence of bowel sounds. The child must be examined for the possible presence of an organic pathology and referred immediately for medical treatment.

Diagnosis

In order to differentiate between the organic and functional causes of constipation, a careful history must be taken. This must include the birth history as well as familial tendencies towards bowel habits, diet and emotional status. In an infant born at full term, meconium should be passed within the first 24 hours of life. Constipation in a neonate may be functional but obstipation is likely to be of organic origin.

Enquiries should also be made concerning enuresis and urinary tract infections because these are commonly associated with constipation. In a full-term newborn passage of the meconium should occur within 24 hours. Infrequent or suppressed defecation in newborns may be of functional origin but is usually due to organic factors.

Allopathic medical diagnosis

Investigations include abdominal palpation, which will disclose meteorism and palpable hard masses of fecal matter, inspection of the anus and a digital rectal examination to assess sphincter tone, rectal ampulla dilation, and presence of fecal matter. Ultrasonography will provide information concerning rectal dilation, any displacement of the urinary bladder, and urinary transport disorders. A plain abdominal X-ray will also reveal fecal masses and extensive enlargement of the colon.

To rule out an organic etiology, a rectal biopsy should be performed in patients with onset of constipation in early infancy, failure to thrive, vomiting, fever or lack of success with conservative therapy to exclude Hirschsprung's disease, or spinal MRI should be performed if an innervation defect (such as tethered cord) is suspected.

Osteopathic examination

On palpation of the abdomen, the tension of the abdominal wall itself is usually low. On slightly deeper palpation, there will be found to be areas of hypertonicity, usually at the left iliac fossa, and in older children who have been constipated for months or years, the lymph nodes tend to be large and swollen. The descending colon feels dilated, lacking in tone and sags within the pelvis. There is often a hypertonicity of the diaphragm, especially over the right upper epigastrium, usually over the gall bladder and sometimes the liver as well. Patches of cold areas over the abdomen indicate reduced blood flow to the area of the bowel and general stagnation. This is also indicative of the lack of vitality and potency through the GI organs.

From a mechanical comfort point of view, when neonates are presented with functional constipation, there are several aspects that contribute to the lack of comfort of the bowel sitting within its given places. The position of the organs within the thorax, abdomen and pelvis should be examined so that a holistic view of the body is possible.

Treatment

In general, the concerned parents of the anxious child have usually already tried juggling with diet and/or toilet training as well as the developing ego in an attempt to relieve the abdominal discomfort. It is most important to inform and educate the parents and child in detail about the pathogenesis of constipation and to establish a coherent long-term treatment plan.

- A diet that is balanced with fruits, vegetables and plenty of water is conducive to keeping constipation at bay. Excessive sugar, refined flour and cow's milk can often be the underlying factors in chronic constipation.

- A milk-free diet may help (especially in lactose intolerance).

- Enough **exercise** is important, as are **regular toilet visits** without psychological pressure. Small awards for the child when she has been successful can be of help too.

- Simple massaging using relaxing oils such as German camomile in a base of massage oil on the soles of the feet can be very helpful, as can rubbing the tummy.

- Constipation is often aggravated by tension or stress related issues. Parents can often help by being aware of stressful situations and helping the child to be at ease.

Allopathic medical treatment

An initial evacuation may be required in patients with severe constipation: hard fecal masses are disimpacted manually, after which time enemas are used. Then paraffin oil is used as a lubricant until the stool becomes soft. Paraffin oil needs to be given in high doses and should be administered for about 4 to 6 weeks. The treatment then switches to lactulose for about 4 weeks, before being phased out gradually.

Painful rhagades are treated with soothing skin-care products.

Fresh fruit that is slightly overripe is often sufficient in children with constipation that is not severe, especially the fruit that is in season. Constipation in very young babies can often be alleviated by water with milk sugar (lactose). The effect of lactose is different in each case and the treatment is difficult to control.

Osteopathic treatment

Osteopathic treatment of chronic constipation should include all aspects of the CNS, ANS and the musculoskeletal system that are associated with the function of the GI tract. All restrictions leading to a reduced flow of nervous information, arterial or venous blood and lymph, as well as mucus in the organs themselves, must be considered.

As mentioned before, the GI tract is an emotional brain, and as such it is very sensitive and does not take kindly to being directly poked, prodded and pushed. It is already overburdened with greater than the normal volume of retained fecal matter with its toxins and therefore it wishes to be treated with respect and empathy. Therefore, any treatments methods employed to relieve constipation must be slow and gentle. Sudden, springing manipulations especially of the spine should be avoided. Functional or low velocity techniques work very well, especially in neonates; some gentle articulatory procedures are helpful in the older child. Quite often, treatment remote to the abdomen will often be enough to achieve the desired result. If there are still areas of impaction or sagging of the colon that remain, lifting the gut and bringing it to a still point is enough to increase the vitality of the bowel to perform its function. As with many gut conditions, it is beneficial to treat the gut from the lumen outwards, but only when the rest of the body has reached a comfortable state of integration.

The gut is very sensitive and therefore it is important to not over-treat. For severe chronic constipation, little and often treatment is useful in the 1st week. Thereafter a couple of weekly sessions are followed by 3–4 weekly until a regular habit has evolved.

Prognosis

Where the constipation is due to organic pathology, surgical intervention is necessary. This should then be followed up by osteopathy to enable the body to recover from the operation and assimilate the surgical procedures.

Where the constipation is functional, if left untreated it often becomes self-perpetuating and more severe with progression of time, especially when there is an emotional contribution. In the long term, bouts of so-called diarrhea present intermittently with constipation, thereby becoming a 'an irritable syndrome'. The diarrhea is questionable as the loose material may just be the fluid contents of the diet finding their way out ahead of the solid components!

Osteopathy is of enormous benefit with excellent prognosis. However, this must also be maintained by correct bowel habits and dietetic advice as suggested above, under Treatment.

GASTRO-ESOPHAGEAL REFLUX

Tajinder K. Deoora

Definition

Because the gut of the newborn and small baby is immature, it is quite normal for young babies (especially in the first week of life) to spit up small amounts of milk after a feed. This occurs especially whilst burping or from being moved into different positions or when the baby is fed lying down instead of being upright.

However, sometimes the newborn and very young babies will have a tendency to persistent fussiness or vomiting after a feed or even between feeds. This spitting up of milk can also present as a wet burp, and the infant takes ages to settle. The wet burping and post-feeding vomiting or regurgitation is due to the gastro-esophageal reflux (GER), which occurs when the acidic contents of the stomach move back up into the esophagus (reflux), and out of the mouth.

Usually the child does not have a problem with thriving and the symptoms disappear when the child is usually in an upright position; that is, when she learns to sit and walk.

Pathogenesis

The developmental relationships of the esophagus and the stomach in relation to the diaphragm can have a bearing on the function of the stomach after feeding. Whether the lower esophageal sphincter lies above or below the diaphragm plays a part in contributing to the GER.

The commonest cause is a defect in the mechanism responsible for closing the lower esophageal sphincter (LOS), resulting in an ineffective anti-reflux barrier. In this setting the LOS forms a pressure barrier between the stomach and esophagus. In normal circumstances the pressure in the LOS – which is higher than that in the stomach – ensures that the stomach contents do not reflux back into the esophagus.

Transient reflexive relaxation of the LOS takes place only during the act of swallowing. However, if LOS tone is too low, the stomach contents are able to reflux back into the esophagus due to the negative pressure in the thorax. Therefore, as a response to the acid in the esophagus, salivation is stimulated and this reduces the pH and protects the mucosa.

However, if reflux persists over a longer period of time, the aggressive gastric juice (HCl) damages the esophageal mucosa and reflux esophagitis ensues. This condition leads to chronic blood loss, narrowing due to scarring, and chest pain, with the result that the child refuses food and consequently fails to thrive. If the stomach contents reach the trachea, lungs or nose, the infant will suffer from episodes of suffocation or apnea, and aspiration pneumonia may result.

Normal physiological pressure is lower in premature and newborn babies than in older infants. If in addition there is momentary relaxation of the LOS and a brief absence of esophageal peristalsis, reflux may develop.

A further mechanism contributing to GER in children concerns the relationship between raised pressure in the stomach and the transient reduction in tone in the LOS and diaphragm. Preterm babies and infants seem to have delayed gastric emptying, leading to abdominal distension. As a result, gastric pressure is elevated compared with the esophagus, and in that situation, when the LOS relaxes, reflux ensues.

When there is insufficient elongation of the esophagus relative to the development of the neck and thorax, a congenital hiatus hernia may occur. This means an upward displacement of the stomach through the esophageal hiatus of the diaphragm into the thorax.

Reflux may occur as a secondary phenomenon in disorders of gastric emptying, e.g. pyloric stenosis (see Pyloric hypertrophy, below), or in CNS lesions (e.g. cerebral palsy).

Any restriction to the passage of the vagus nerve at the jugular foramen (between the occiput and the petrous temporal) can affect the tone of the esophagus and result in symptoms of reflux.

Signs and symptoms and differential diagnosis

An infant with GER usually spits up and vomits after a feed; this may continue for over an hour after the feed. The wet burps or spits may be associated with hiccups and these are worse during burping and with change of positions; that is, in the lying position. This can be reduced with feeding in the upright position. The affected infant will push away and refuse feeds, in spite of being hungry. The infant is inconsolable and cries suddenly and constantly, she may even present with signs that indicate stomach discomfort or colic. Sleeping is difficult and there may be poor weight gain. The vomiting/spitting may continue past the first year of life, when most children have grown out of it. Colic is often misdiagnosed in conditions of reflux (see Ch.11, Irritable infants and colic). It is thought that recurrent otitis (see p.283), pharyngitis or laryngeal edema may also be caused by GER.

In severe forms the most prominent aspect of the clinical picture may be failure to thrive or the patient's history features recurrent episodes of (aspiration) pneumonia and asthma-like bronchitis.

Other, less common additional signs may be gagging or choking, hoarseness, frequent sore throats or respiratory problems (such as bronchitis, pneumonia, wheezing, or coughing) and bad breath. With an older child, the reflux may be aggravated by certain foods, such as sweets and fried or fatty foods.

The presence of blood or hematin in vomited matter is indicative of esophagitis.

Differential diagnosis

The differential diagnosis must consider all other conditions that are associated with vomiting.

Pyloric stenosis (see Pyloric hypertrophy, below) can present as vomiting, although this is of a projectile nature. That of reflux is not this forceful. There is often a firm palpable area of tension in the abdominal wall at the upper right quadrant overlying the site of stenosis. Weight gain may be more severely affected than in reflux, which may or may not affect weight gain.

In stenosis or atresia of the duodenum, there is a delay in vomiting after the feeds. As the milk has had time to reach the stomach, the contents are curdled milk or partially digested food. There is often an associated poor gain in weight.

Diagnosis

Conventional diagnosis

The best and most sensitive test is the 24-hour probe study, which monitors the acid levels in the esophagus. Consistently high acid levels indicate the refluxing of stomach acid.

The presence of esophagitis is demonstrated by esophageal endoscopy and biopsy.

Ultrasonography can be used to assess hernia width and observe reflux episodes.

The most common test used to diagnose GER is a barium swallow X-Ray of the upper GI tract, but this is easier to do with an older child. It displays whether the esophagus is irritated or if there are any physical abnormalities in the upper digestive tract; the study may show barium refluxing from the stomach into the esophagus. This test unfortunately only shows a picture of the moment so that a reflux is not necessarily discovered.

Osteopathic diagnosis

The mechanical 'position' of the organs and their place within the thorax, the abdomen and the pelvis should be evaluated. This means not only concentrating on the GI tract but getting an impression of the body as a whole.

Additionally, possible restrictions of the cranial base and the course of the vagus nerve should be examined. The diaphragm is also assessed.

Treatment

Very young babies tend to be guzzlers, so will often down milk as well as air very quickly, thus distending the stomach and consequently raising the gastric pressure. Since the peristaltic wave patterns may not yet have been established in the esophagus, reflux is likely. Babies should be fed in a vertical position and burped frequently but not too forcefully. After meals, the baby should be kept in a seated position or held upright. Meal size may have to be reduced and the feeding frequency increased so the stomach is less distended; and for the older child spicy, fatty, and acidic foods (like citrus fruits) should be avoided.

Whether the baby is breast or formula fed seems to have no bearing on GER. Breast milk, however, is emptied more quickly from the stomach than is formula milk and this may indirectly affect GER through the effects on distension. It seems that slightly thickening the baby's formula or breast milk with rice cereal may cause less reflux due to altered gastric emptying time.

Conventional treatment of GER

The doctor may also prescribe antacids to reduce the incidence of reflux.

If medical treatment alone is not successful and the child is failing to thrive, owing to complications of reflux, a surgical procedure called 'fundoplication' may be an option. A valve is created at the top of the stomach by wrapping a portion of the stomach around the esophagus. However, this is not without side effects, such as the sensation of gagging during meals and feeling full more quickly. In addition, the child may have great difficulty in burping or vomiting.

Osteopathic treatment

The upward displacement of the proximal stomach above the diaphragm is only a part of the story of GER. The esophagus pierces the diaphragm behind the 7th left costal cartilage, at the esophageal hiatus, where it is circled by fleshy fibres of the right crus at the level of the 10th thoracic vertebra to join the stomach just below. The fibres of the right crus appear to act as a sphincter for the cardiac end of the stomach and prevent its contents from returning to the esophagus.

The lower esophageal sphincter is a physiological one also known as the gastric or cardiac sphincter. It is supplied by the vagus nerve, which has the effect of relaxing the sphincter, and the sympathetic nerve which causes contraction. The vagus nerve also affects gastric emptying time as well as the tone of the abdominal muscles.

Since the esophagus and its nerve supply pass through the diaphragm, any interruption or restriction that affects the respiratory function and overall balance is a predisposing factor to GER. Therefore, it is important to release all the attachments of the diaphragm at the lower thoracic and upper lumbar areas, as well as the presence of any torsion strains within the diaphragm. In particular, the right crura should have a balanced tone, as should the thoracolumbar fascia.

In addition, the journey of the esophagus begins at the pharynx and extends to the stomach. It therefore has cervical, thoracic and abdominal portions. Through its course, the esophagus has four constrictions; at its origin in the neck, at the aortic arch in the superior mediastinum, at the tracheal bifurcation and where it passes through the diaphragm. These constrictions should be free of any restrictions from its related structures; therefore all the portions need to be assessed.

Most babies with reflux are agitated due to the discomfort of feeding. This may be in addition to the already altered tone of the ANS, both systemically and locally in the GI tract. The vagus and the sympathetic nerves influence the lower esophageal sphincter, stomach pressure and the tone of the abdominal wall. Therefore, any osteopathic treatment protocol should include balancing the ANS, both locally and systemically.

Prognosis

Most babies outgrow the condition by the time they are a year old and it is uncommon for a child to have GER after the age of 2 years. However, if there is a neurological or developmental disorder such as cerebral palsy, then there is greater risk of GER and the child may even experience more severe symptoms.

Osteopathic treatment is successful, especially if the ANS is balanced accordingly. Treatment should be given as soon as possible because feeding problems often lead to stress between mother and child and tend to become a behavioral pattern that is difficult to release after it has existed for a while.

NERVOUS (FUNCTIONAL) STOMACH ACHE

Tajinder K. Deoora

Definition

As mentioned in the introduction, babies and young children will predominantly complain of pain in the stomach area regardless of the fact that it may originate from somewhere else. For this reason, a thorough history and examination must be performed before pinpointing the cause to the GI tract, especially when considering a nervous stomach.

Etiology and pathogenesis

When a child is anxious, or when there is a change within the family/social environment that the child is having difficulty in adjusting to, she may exhibit symptoms of abdominal discomfort such as constipation, diarrhea, bloating or altered appetite. Often the child suffers from pressure in the family or at school. I do not to believe that a child will make up symptoms for no apparent reason. There is always a cause and this must be sought, no matter how insignificant it is in the bigger scheme of things. It is real enough for the child and therefore needs to be dealt with. Only when other pathophysiological reasons for GI tract disturbance have been eliminated should a diagnosis of nervous stomach ache be made.

Autonomic nervous system

The ANS plays an enormous role in the origin of nervous stomach ache. Regarding the effects of the ANS on the viscera as mentioned in the text above, a disturbance of the ANS can lead to any possible reaction of the GI tract. Symptoms from diarrhea to cramps and change of the mucosa can arise. As the ANS reacts to psychological stress, psychosomatic reactions are often seen in osteopathic practices.

One of the contributing agents to the responses of the GI tract to any number of situations is that great bundle of autonomic nerves, the solar plexus. It is the primordial, even instinctive method of communication for feelings such as distrust, fear, elation, sorrow, excitement, anxiety and joy. It communicates with the bundles of nerves from the various abdominal organs and their blood vessels to become the center point for signals.

The solar plexus radiates nerves to and from the walls of the chest, the diaphragm, the organs of the abdomen: liver, spleen, stomach, intestines, mesentery, the testes and ovaries, the kidneys and adrenal glands. Because of its incredibly wide distribution, the solar plexus orchestrates the balance between the effects of emotions and the normal function of organs. Emotions are also relayed into physical symptoms at the level of the hypothalamus and the limbic system. When considering a stomach problem due to nervous origins, the extent of radial distribution of the solar plexus plays a huge role in somatovisceral and psychosomatic, psychovisceral reflexes, both locally and at the craniosacral regions. Therefore the implication of the hypothalamus and cranial base, as well as the influence of the lower thoracic and upper lumbar region and the diaphragm, are essential components in any osteopathic treatment protocol.

Mechanical

During delivery, especially if it is complicated by ventouse or forceps intervention, or emergency caesarean, there is degree of axial spinal compression. This axial compression may result in a lack of space within the thoracic and abdominal cavities for the GI tract and other abdominal contents. Also there may be some residual inertia present within the abdominal and thoracic organs that the unmolding pro-cesses after the birth have not been able to resolve. This has the effect of creating tensions and torsions within the mesentery and GI tract so that their function is altered.

A short umbilicus or a cord round the neck at birth may also result in an umbilical tension that can be the fulcrum for reduced function and residual aching in the stomach. Quite often, the mother will deliver her child in the same manner that she was delivered; for example as a breech, or with a cord wrapped round the neck if the mother had a cord wrapped round the neck. One has to search the answers by sensitive and careful questioning of the mother. The treatment of the child is then administered by including the mother within the fulcrum of the treatment.

Signs and symptoms

The hallmark symptom is abdominal pain, possibly associated with stomach cramps. These usually occur in the area surrounding the umbilicus; the further removed they are from that region, the more likely the etiology is to be organic. The pain occurs mainly in the mornings and is unrelated to meals; nocturnal pain attacks are very rare. The pattern of physical development is normal. Nausea and vomiting may also be present as accompanying symptoms.

Often the nervous stomach ache alternates with headaches. Here the ANS also has an influence on the lumen of the arteries and can cause headache if the blood supply to the head decreases due to an orthosympathetic reaction to external influences.

Differential diagnosis

Organic causes of chronic and recurring stomach ache are not limited to particular times of the day and may also waken the patient at night. They are felt at locations away from the umbilicus and may be associated with loss of appetite, vomiting, fever, irregular bowel habit and weight loss. The pattern of physical development may be disturbed.

Differential diagnostic considerations should include the following possibilities: constipation, carbohydrate malabsorption, infections, post-enteritic malabsorption syndrome, peptic gastrointestinal disorders, allergic food intolerances, coeliac disease, Crohn's disease, ulcerative colitis, gallstones, pancreatitis, urolithiasis, partial obstruction of the small intestine, familial Mediterranean fever, porphyria, Meulengracht's disease.

Diagnosis

It is of importance to the osteopath to carefully listen to the description of the ailments. Stomach ache cropping up when the child is in school or before exams or when visiting a parent that lives apart from the child may give us a hint as to whether there is a psychological cause.

It is also important to look at the interaction between parents and children to see if the cause may lie in their relationship or the parents' expectations of the child.

Allopathic medical diagnosis

Clinical laboratory tests are generally inconclusive here and therefore they should be used to a limited extent only. Abdominal ultrasonography provides information concerning changes in the size and texture of organs, space-occupying lesions, positional anomalies of organs, concretions, and thickening of the intestinal wall.

Otherwise specific diagnostic procedures should be followed, depending on the suspected underlying disease (see above, Differential diagnosis).

Osteopathic treatment

It is advisable to perform a full osteopathic examination with special consideration of the ANS and possible retaining shock-patterns.

Treatment

The main issue is to calm the parents and convince them that the child is not suffering from a severe illness. Problematic situations such as conflicts and pressure should be discussed and solved if possible.

Conventional treatment

Conventional treatment is not necessary. It may be useful for a child psychiatrist to see the child too.

Osteopathic treatment

The solar plexus supplies a large area and plays an important part in somatovisceral, psychosomatic and psychovisceral reflexes as well as having influence locally and on the craniosacral system. Therefore osteopathic treatment should consider the pituitary gland and the cranial base, also the lower thoracic spine, the upper lumbar spine and the diaphragm.

It may be useful to include the mother in the treatment fulcrum. This can be done by placing one hand on the child and the other on the mother.

Prognosis

Once you have recognized the pattern in the tissues you can treat the stress patterns caused (e.g. by birth) and help the child to develop a better function. This allows the child to function from an optimal physiologic fulcrum.

PYLORIC HYPERTROPHY

Clive Hayden

Definition

In hypertrophic pyloric stenosis (pyloric hypertrophy) there is hypertrophy of the sphincter muscle, causing a narrowing of the pyloric orifice. Food can therefore no longer pass into the duodenum, instead accumulating in the stomach, which ultimately leads to projectile vomiting.

The condition affects boys four times more frequently than girls and usually develops in the first 2 to 15 weeks of life.

Etiology and pathophysiology

The etiology is unclear. However, genetic disposition is indicated by the fact that the disease is usually more common in families. Children with blood groups O and B are affected most often.

In congenital pyloric hypertrophy, there is a thickening of the walls of the muscles of the pyloric canal. This results in a marked tightening, or stenosis, of the pylorus, and food is unable to pass on to the duodenum. The child's abdomen becomes more and more bloated, and is suddenly emptied as he or she vomits explosively.

Pyloric stenosis is associated with a disturbance of the nitric oxide synthesis in the solar (coeliac) plexus. It is thought that nitric oxide plays a major role in muscle relaxation.

Clinical signs and differential diagnosis

If a baby suddenly starts to vomit large amounts of food forcefully, and if the tendency to do so increases, it is usually a symptom of pyloric stenosis. The food contains no bile. The baby is usually restless and has a serious facial expression (often with a wrinkled brow).

This may be followed by dehydration, weight loss and pseudo constipation (the stools look like rabbit pellets).

Differential diagnosis

Other diagnoses to consider are gastro-esophogeal reflux (see earlier section), adrenogenital syndrome with salt loss, raised intracranial pressure, gastroenteritis, pyelonephritis, annular pancreas, duodenal stenosis, peptic ulcer of the duodenum or stomach, an allergy to the protein in cow's milk, and congenital metabolic defects.

Diagnosis

Occasionally peristaltic waves can be recognized periumbilically from left to right following feeding. The pylorus can often be felt as an olive-shaped lump through the abdomen while feeding or after vomiting.

Allopathic medical diagnosis

Laboratory tests will show hypochloremia, hyponatremia and hypokalemia as well as metabolic alkalosis.

Sonography shows a thickened pylorus and an elongated pyloric canal.

Osteopathic examination

As well as the mechanical 'position' of the organs and their situation within the thorax, the abdomen and the pelvis need to be examined thoroughly, in conjunction with the usual examination of the child from the feet to the cranium. The practitioner should not focus solely on the GI tract, but should obtain a complete picture of the body. Palpation of the abdomen often reveals areas of increased tension in the upper abdomen.

Treatment
Allopathic medical treatment

The first step is to correct the acid-base balance and replace lost fluid.

A conservative treatment approach may be made with i.v. atropine derivatives and many (12–24) small meals. Although this is time-consuming, it can lead to spontaneous involution of the pyloric hypertrophy.

The treatment of choice is therefore surgical pylorotomy after Weber-Ramstedt, in which the pyloric muscle is separated as far as the mucosa.

Osteopathy

In some cases the pyloric spasm is variable; in other words, the baby does not vomit after every meal. It may then follow that the vagus nerve is compromized around the jugular foramen, and the cause of the pyloric stenosis may be treated osteopathically.

If a pylorotomy is performed, the scar should be treated osteopathically after surgery.

Prognosis

After slow postoperative feeding, babies soon recover. Osteopaths do not often see pyloric stenosis. Children in whom this condition is diagnosed have usually already undergone surgery. From the osteopathic aspect, the cranial compression, which may still be present, should be treated.

Bibliography

Behrman R E, Kliegman R M: Nelson essentials of pediatrics. 4th edn. Saunders, New York/London 2002

Moore K L, Persaud T V N: The developing human: clinically oriented embryology. 6th edn. Saunders, Philadelphia 1998.

Pathology involving the ear, nose and throat is commonly encountered in pediatric patients. The various clinical conditions often occur concurrently or one may carry over into another. Chronic infections of the pharynx, for example, may lead to hyperplasia of the adenoids (pharyngeal tonsils), and the resultant obstruction of the pharyngeal orifice of the auditory tube often gives rise to glue ear, or to recurrent otitis.

Allopathic medical therapy embraces pharmacological management and supportive measures, such as saline inhalation or irrigation, decongestant nasal drops, and autoinflation with the Otovent system, through to surgical intervention. Antibiotic administration may be necessary where the situation is extremely acute; however, frequent antibiotic administration is associated with adverse drug reactions (see Ch.10, Effect of nutrition on the immune system). Surgical procedures also expose the child to anesthesia-related stress and, as illustrated by the frequent insertion of grommets to ventilate the middle ear, may resolve the problem only for a time. Such interventions should be a last resort. The milieu within which the typical ear, nose and throat (ENT) diseases of childhood occur is highly amenable to modification by osteopathic treatment. Many chronic ENT conditions can be improved in this way. In high-grade acute infection, however, concomitant allopathic pharmacological or homeopathic treatment is indicated in most cases unless the opportunity exists for the child to receive regular osteopathic treatment.

The nose is normally the portal of entry for inhaled air and is ideally equipped as an organ of filtration and defence. However, many children are mouth-breathers and are exposed to frequent infections as a result. In most cases mouth-breathing is due to a local or general loss of muscle tone or to obstructed nasal breathing – and in each case all these situations can be positively influenced with the help of osteopathy.

If the organs of the ear, nose and throat are to function properly, their structures, and especially their mucosa, need to have a good blood supply and efficient lymphatic drainage. It may be necessary to treat cranial and facial asymmetries in order to ensure this.

GROWTH AND DEVELOPMENT OF THE NEUROCRANIUM AND VISCEROCRANIUM

Cranial growth

Certain features typical of cranial shape in the neonate can already be identified at first glance. Large bright eyes, high intelligent-looking forehead, rounded cheeks, tiny nose with a flat nasal bridge and a small mouth. Overall, the proportions appear to be short and broad. The maxillae and mandible are small, and the eyes are relatively far apart. These and many other features of the neonatal cranium undergo extensive changes as the years unfold. The neurocranium (cranial vault) grows very rapidly during the first year of life. The growth of the viscerocranium (the bones of the face) occurs at a much slower rate. At birth the neurocranium has attained 25% of its final size; this increases to 50% by the age of 6 months and to 75% by the 2nd year of life. By the 10th year the neurocranium has attained 95% of its final size, whereas the viscerocranium has attained only 65% (Fig. 13.1).

Factors influencing growth

The shape and architecture of a bone are the result both of hereditary factors and of the mechanical stresses to which it has been and still is exposed. Genetic factors play a role only

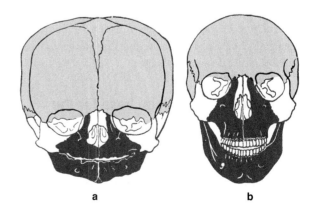

a   b

Figure 13.1 Growth-related change in cranial proportions (the maxillae and mandible are shown in black). **a:** Neonatal cranium. **b:** Adult cranium.
With permission, Benninghoff, Goerttler: Lehrbuch der Anatomie des Menschen, volume 1. 10th edn. Urban & Schwarzenberg, 1968

initially in that they determine the size, shape and approximate growth of the bone.

Every cranium and every face is an individual composition. If every regional structure and its corresponding counterpart in the other half of the cranium increase in size to an equal extent, the result is balanced growth between the two. Shape, structure and function are then in balance at every moment. An imbalance arises if a certain facial or cranial region and its contralateral counterpart grow to a differing extent and in different directions (Sperber 1989). This may be triggered by traumatic forces, such as by accidents and falls, or by the birth process (see Ch.5, Difficult delivery, onwards; Ch.8, Intraosseous strains). However, asymmetrical muscle traction also has a pronounced influence on growth as it unfolds.

The model of the functional matrix has been described over the past 20 years, chiefly by Moss (1989). According to this concept, all bone growth should be understood as a response to the functional relationships produced by all the soft tissues working in association with the particular bone in question. Consequently, the bone is not the sole determinant of the extent and direction of its own growth. This idea helps us to understand the many interactions that occur in the process of facial growth. The detailed mechanism by which functional mechanical forces produce deforming changes in bone structure has not yet been fully elucidated.

One theory, suggested by Moss (1989), postulates that biomechanical stress is mediated by piezoelectric currents produced by bioelectrical factors. When it undergoes deformation, bone behaves like a crystal. It generates a tiny electrical current. Bone-producing cells (osteoblasts) and bone-resorbing cells (osteoclasts), as well as their matrix, respond by building up bone in areas with a negative charge and conversely by resorbing bone in areas with a positive charge. These bioelectrical stress potentials are perhaps responsible for the adaptation or more extensive compensatory modification of bone structure in response to new functional requirements. A change in bone loading in the form of mechanical stress influences local calcium metabolism.

Importance of the cranial base for the growth of the viscerocranium

The development of the viscerocranium is in a dependent relationship to the growth and development of the neurocranium, in particular of the cranial base. With the conversion of mesenchyme into cartilaginous tissue, the formation of the cranial base commences around day 40 in utero. The ossification of the cranial base takes place between weeks 10 and 20 (Fig. 13.2). The development and growth of the nasal cavity form part of this overall process.

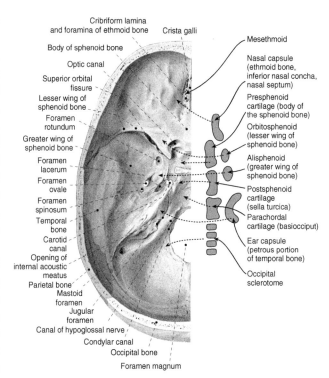

Figure 13.2 Development of the cranial base (viewed from above). With permission, Henriette Rintelen, Velbert

The increasing size of the cranial base results from the interplay of two factors: first, the growth of cartilaginous tissue between the bones, and second, the expansive forces that have their origin in the growing brain. As a result of the interstitial growth of the cartilaginous areas at the synchondroses, contiguous bones are pushed apart, and the bones increase in size due to appositional growth at the suture margins.

The greatest contribution to the development of the cranial base is made by the postnatal growth of the sphenobasilar synchondrosis (SBS), which is preserved as a growth zone into early adulthood.

The spatial development of the nasal cavity occurs in parallel with the growth of the cranial base. The extended growth period enables the maxillae to enlarge continuously in a posterior direction. All the cranial and facial structures located anterior to the middle cranial fossa will develop anteriorly, depending on the expansion of this structure, which forms the central part of the cranial base. Via the growth pressure of the cartilaginous part of the nasal septum the growth of all facial structures is directed inferiorly and anteriorly, and this creates an enlarged space in the nasal cavity. Development of a nasal cavity of normal size is strongly dependent on good cranial base development. Compressive or asymmetrical cranial base patterns may appreciably interfere with the development of the nasal cavity. One of the repercussions of inadequate spatial development may be permanent mouth-breathing due to narrowing of the nasal cavity. Early osteopathic treatment of the cranial base therefore has a very good effect on the shape and spatial development of the nasal cavity and on the function of its mucosa. Treatment should commence just 3 to 5 weeks after birth. In my experience, this timing is ideal for influencing the development of these structures.

Auditory tube

In order to understand the pathophysiology of otitis media and of glue ear (chronic seromucinous otitis) (see later sections in this chapter), it is important to have a precise overview of the anatomy and physiology of the auditory tube.

Embryological development

The auditory tube develops from the first pharyngeal pouch, an outpouching from the pharyngeal gut. This derives from the cranial segment of the foregut and corresponds to the pharyngeal segment of the gastrointestinal tract. Already at this stage there is a close functional relationship with the visceral system, and this is important for an understanding of the pathophysiology and its treatment along osteopathic lines. Both regions are of endodermal origin (Langmann 1989).

Functional anatomy

Topographically, the auditory tube commences at the anterior wall of the tympanic cavity with the tympanic orifice; it then descends slightly in an anteromedial direction and emerges into the nasal part of the pharynx through a wide opening known as the pharyngeal orifice.

Anatomically, the auditory tube consists for one third of its length of a bony part that is still within the temporal bone, and for two thirds of its length of a cartilaginous part that is suspended like a hammock at the cranial base. This part is not a closed tube, but rather a cartilaginous groove, the superior margin of which is bent into a hook shape, while being wide open laterally (Fig. 13.3). The lateral boundaries of the cartilaginous part of the auditory tube are formed by the tensor veli palatini and the belly of the levator veli palatini muscles. The junction of these two muscles is also the narrowest part of the auditory tube (the isthmus). This is located in the vicinity of the external cranial base, inferior to the sphenopetrosal suture.

Mucosal and muscle innervation

The mucosa of the auditory tube is a continuation of that in the pharynx and is also referred to as respiratory mucosa. Its sensory innervation is supplied by the tympanic nerve, a branch of the glossopharyngeal nerve. Although the tympanic nerve also carries parasympathetic fibres from the superior

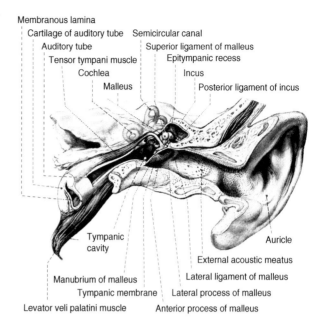

Figure 13.3 Topography of the auditory tube. With permission, Benninghoff, Goerttler: Lehrbuch der Anatomie des Menschen, volume 2. 8th edn. Urban & Schwarzenberg, 1967

ganglion of the glossopharyngeal nerve, these have no influence on the auditory tube mucosa. Because the production of secretions and their absorption are continuous phenomena, only one component of the autonomic nervous system is required. The production of secretions by goblet cells occurs under the control of the sympathetic nerve fibres, which come from the stellate ganglion and which use the internal carotid artery to gain intracranial access. The cilia receive autonomic innervation via the pterygopalatine ganglion.

The muscles of the auditory tube are innervated as follows:

- **tensor veli palatini:** by the lesser palatine nerve from the pterygopalatine ganglion and by a branch of the mandibular nerve; it is thus supplied by two different nerves
- **levator veli palatini:** by the chorda tympani, a branch of the facial nerve
- **tensor tympani:** by a branch of the mandibular nerve.

Vascular supply

Arterial blood is supplied by the anterior tympanic, posterior tympanic and superior tympanic arteries. All three arise from the external carotid artery and reach the middle ear by separate routes.

The tympanic veins carry blood to various venous networks, including the pterygoid plexus and the pharyngeal plexus. Communications may also exist with the sinuses of the dura mater.

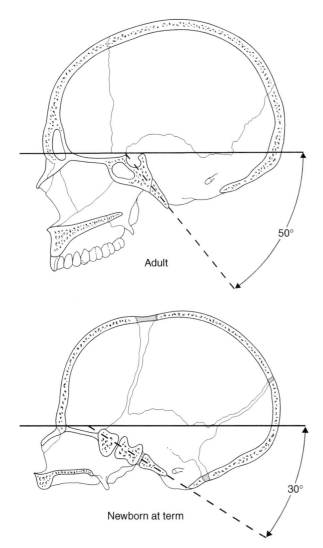

Figure 13.4 Change in the angle of the cranial base. With permission, Jane E. Carreiro, Biddeford; courtesy of the Willard and Carreiro Collection

Lymphatic drainage

A dense network of lymph vessels surrounds the auditory tube. Lymphatic fluid from the middle ear region flows to the deep parotid lymph nodes, which drain into the right and left venous angles via the deep anterior cervical lymph nodes, the inferior deep lateral cervical lymph nodes, the right and left subclavian trunks and the right and left jugular trunks. These venous angles are located between the first rib and the clavicle.

Change in orientation of the auditory tube

In the neonate the auditory tube is oriented more horizontally than in the adult (Fig. 13.4). As the neurocranium and viscerocranium grow, this orientation is subject to continuous change. Factors such as the expansive growth of the cranial base, the horizontal widening of the cranial base in the

region of the petrous portion of the temporal bone, and the increasing vertical orientation of the face due to the inferiorly directed growth of the nasal septum contribute appreciably to this, as does the enlargement of the pharyngeal space and the growth of the mandible anteriorly and inferiorly. As a result, the orientation of the auditory tube shifts from a horizontal to an anterior declined plane.

This orientational shift promotes a more efficient drainage from the middle ear and explains why otitis media or glue ear occur less commonly after the age of 6 years.

In the fetus the opening of the auditory tube in the pharyngeal wall is below the hard palate, at birth it is level with the hard palate, and in the adult it is well above the hard palate.

Physiology of the auditory tube

The auditory tube has several important functions, namely to:

- regulate **pressure equalization** between the middle ear and the atmosphere – something that is important for sound conduction
- serve as a **reflux barrier** to secretions and bacteria from the nasopharynx, and thus from the gastrointestinal tract, into the middle ear
- ensure the **drainage** of fluids formed in the middle ear.

In normal auditory tube function a balanced relationship exists between the forces which keep the tube closed and those which open it (Ingelstedt et al 1967). Under normal circumstances the auditory tube is kept closed by the following factors (Feldmann 1973):

- the elastic tension of the auditory tube cartilage
- the surface tension of the mucus film covering the mucosa
- the pressure exerted by the peritubal tissue
- certain configurations of pressure and suction effects.

According to research conducted by Rich (1920), Bluestone et al (1975), Cantekin et al (1979) and Honjo et al (1981), the auditory tube is opened by the direct traction of tensor veli palatini. The muscles are subconsciously contracted during swallowing and yawning and cause brief lateral opening (Huang et al 1997).

If passive closure is to occur after active opening, the cartilage tissue must possess a degree of elasticity in order to return to its original state under the influence of its inherent tension. For this to happen, according to evidence presented by Matsune et al (1992), the cartilage matrix of the auditory tube must show a certain maturity, which is in turn dependent on the concentration of elastin. The maturation of cartilage matrix is well advanced by the age of 6 years. The tendency for functional disorders of the auditory tube to develop therefore also declines steadily from the age of 6 years.

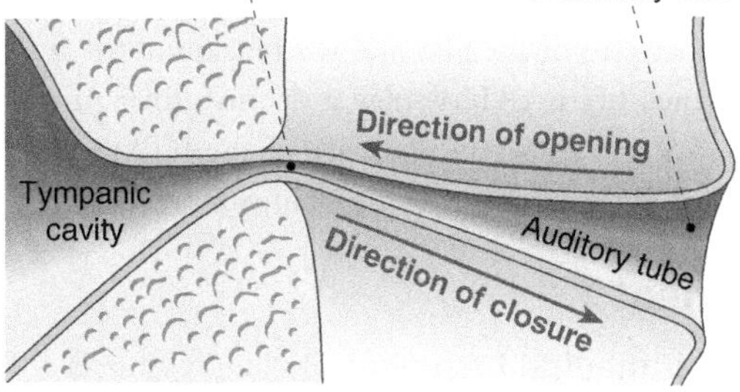

Isthmus of auditory tube   Pharyngeal orifice of auditory tube

Direction of opening

Tympanic cavity

Auditory tube

Direction of closure

Figure 13.5 Direction of auditory tube closure and opening. With permission, Henriette Rintelen, Velber

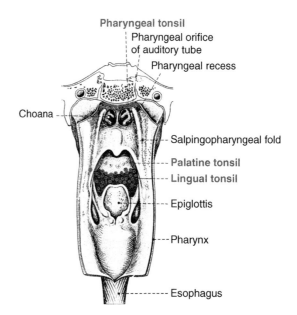

Figure 13.6 Topography of the pharyngeal, palatine and lingual tonsils, which together form the ring of lymphoid tissue in the pharynx.
With permission, Benninghoff, Goerttler: Lehrbuch der Anatomie des Menschen, volume 2. 8th edn. Urban & Schwarzenberg, 1967

Owing to the surface tension of the mucus film, the walls of the auditory tube adhere to each other. The more viscous this mucus, the more difficult it is for the tube to open. Closure by the surface tension of the mucus film is strongest at the isthmus and weakest at the pharyngeal orifice of the tube. Simultaneously, muscle traction to open the tube is weakest at the isthmus and strongest at the pharyngeal orifice. This combination of forces means that active opening of the auditory tube runs from the pharyngeal orifice to the isthmus and releases the mucus film in this direction rather like a zip fastener (Fig. 13.5). Conversely, closure of the auditory tube starts at the isthmus and travels from there towards the pharyngeal orifice (Flisberg 1963).

Pathophysiology of the auditory tube

The maturity of the cartilaginous part of the auditory tube depends on the elastin concentration. Where the elastin concentration in the cartilaginous part is too high, the tensor veli palatini cannot open the auditory tube even when muscle tone is normal because the cartilage tissue is unable to resist the muscle tonus. Instead of opening, the tube becomes elongated in response to muscle contraction and undergoes deformation, possibly resulting in auditory tube obstruction – a finding also referred to as the floppy tube phenomenon. The consequence is inadequate ventilation of the middle ear with an increase in negative pressure and in the resultant build-up of effusion.

In adults the auditory tube cartilage becomes increasingly firm. In this context the cartilage tissue of the medial wall is able to resist the traction exerted by the muscle, while the lateral wall yields. This mechanism is responsible for the open tube phenomenon.

ADENOIDS
Definition

Adenoids (adenoid vegetation) is the term used to describe hyperplasia of the pharyngeal tonsils (Fig. 13.6) and of the

ring of lymphoid tissue in the pharynx (Waldeyer's tonsillar ring). Marked enlargement may even cause obstruction of the nasopharynx.

Etiology and pathogenesis

In childhood especially, the ring of lymphoid tissue in the pharynx is one of the important zones in the body for the development of immunity. Humoral antibodies (immunoglobulins) are synthesized in the pharyngeal tonsils and T- as well as B-lymphocytes are immunologically determined. Chronic and recurrent infections in the pharynx may lead to hyperplasia (an abnormal increase) of lymphoid tissue in the pharyngeal tonsils.

The ring of lymphoid tissue in the pharynx becomes inflamed, for example, owing to inefficient mouth closure, constant irritation by environmental antigens, or pH shifts towards hyperacidity. Especially in gastro-esophageal reflux, hydrogen ions ascend constantly and cause tissue hyperacidity.

Moderate hyperplasia of lymphoid tissue in the nasopharyngeal space in childhood need not be accorded any pathological value initially because it occurs in virtually all children in the course of immunological activity. A marked increase in size occurs between the ages of 1 and 3 years; regression of lymphoid tissue is to be expected at about the age of 10 to 12 years. This moderate increase in pharyngeal tonsil size is attributable to hormonal and hereditary factors, and especially to continuous contact with an ever-changing spectrum of pathogens in childhood. Current knowledge indicates that it is not only the abnormal increase in the size of adenoid tissue that is important, but also its function as a bacterial reservoir, which leads to re-infection (Gates et al 1988).

Pharyngeal tonsil growth is entirely variable. It may be regarded as a personalized response of the individual as immunocompetence develops. Consequently, pharyngeal tonsil enlargement is only considered pathological and treated if signs of illness are also present.

Clinical signs and symptoms

The nasopharynx may become partially or completely blocked due to adenoidal hyperplasia, such that nasal breathing is prevented and the patient breathes with mouth open (mouth-breathing). Speech may become nasal or thickened, and snoring and restless sleep are more common. In extreme cases obstructive apnea may be encountered, especially at night. Affected children suffer from chronic tiredness.

Recurrent infections, such as constant colds or sinusitis, may ensue as a result of mouth-breathing. Originating from inflammation of the nasopharynx, auditory tube obstruction may produce otitis media or glue ear, which in turn may lead to hearing loss.

Diagnosis

The lymph nodes in the angle of the mandible and neck are commonly swollen.

Allopathic medical diagnosis

On laryngoscopy the pharyngeal tonsils appear enlarged and may show reddening; they may obstruct the entire nasopharynx. A mucopurulent track may be visible on the posterior wall of the pharynx.

Osteopathic examination

The patient's face appears swollen and the mouth tends to be slightly open, with the tongue displaced forwards between the maxillae and the mandible. The entire viscerocranium usually looks disproportionately small compared with the neurocranium.

This impression is often confirmed on palpation. Physiologically, a balanced expression of the involuntary mechanism is to be expected; that is, one can observe in the bones of the face intraosseous motion, external and internal rotation in the paired and flexion and extension in the unpaired structures. Frequently, however, the bones are found to be so inelastic that expression of the involuntary mechanism is hardly in evidence, if at all. For a diagnosis it is essential to establish precisely which of the facial bones is having this disruptive effect. In this context too it is certain that the patterns of the SBS and the tension of the reciprocal tension membrane (RTM) play a decisive role. Any pattern of the SBS or a tension imbalance of the RTM inhibits the expression of the involuntary mechanism in the face.

Treatment
Allopathic medical treatment

Diet, change of climate (North Sea, Baltic Sea) and cortisone nasal sprays are recommended as conservative therapy. If symptoms do not clear up despite such treatment, and if auditory impairment or recurrent glue ear occur, then adenoidectomy is advisable. Nevertheless, even with this operation, adenoid tissue often grows back in children under 4 years of age.

Osteopathic treatment

One objective of osteopathic treatment is to bring about a local and general improvement in the child's immune system. Another objective is to minimize the consequences of adenoidal hyperplasia.

This can be achieved, for example, by seeking to optimize posture and mouth closure. For example, the patient's shoulders are often in elevation and protraction, with the cervical spine in extension. In this position consistent mouth closure is rendered difficult. Moreover, unilateral and bilateral atlanto-occipital joint dysfunctions or strain patterns of the cranial base may be limiting the development of the pharyngeal space. The tension of the muscles of the soft palate is then altered in such a way that the tongue does not find its resting mid-position with the mouth closed, and the mouth has to be kept open. Where the maxilla is in internal rotation dysfunction, the tongue can also only find a mid-position with the mouth slightly open.

Stabilization of the tongue depends on guidance by muscles and the interplay of their bony attachments. Thus the tongue has connection with the temporal bone via the styloglossus muscle; the genioglossus muscle is attached to the mandible, and the hyoglossus muscle is connected to the hyoid bone. The palatine aponeurosis, a fibrous sheet underlying the anterior part of the soft palate, has insertion at the posterior margin of the hard palate, which is formed by the palatine bones (Fig. 13.7). Laterally, the two pterygoid processes form bony supportive buttresses that are formed by the palatine bones and the pterygoid processes. Raised tissue resistance causes an increase in the general muscle tone of the body. More pronounced lumbar lordosis leads to increased internal rotation of the lower extremities. As a result of this posture

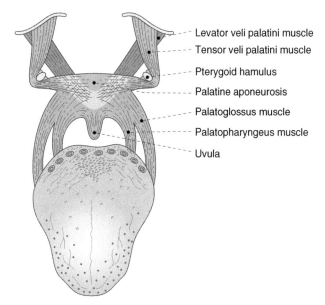

Levator veli palatini muscle
Tensor veli palatini muscle
Pterygoid hamulus
Palatine aponeurosis
Palatoglossus muscle
Palatopharyngeus muscle
Uvula

Figure 13.7 Muscles of the soft palate.
With permission, Henriette Rintelen, Velbert

the entire motor system appears to be flaccid and rather devoid of tension.

The development of the pharyngeal space is not only determined by local factors. The muscle connections from the scapula to the hyoid bone via the omohyoid muscle also act on the hyoid bone and hence indirectly the hyoglossus muscle, which has attachment with the tongue. In this anatomical situation, functional triangles can be recognized that must be in functional equilibrium if adequate mouth closure is to be achieved. The larger triangle comprises the scapula, mandible and temporal bone, and the lesser triangle is defined by the connections between the palatine bone, pterygoid process and hyoid bone.

All the facts cited here illustrate that the interplay between the various structures is highly complex. In my experience, the following treatment approach can be recommended: as a first step, all the diaphragms should be balanced in themselves as well as in relation to each other because they are interconnected in functional terms. This includes the cerebellar tentorium, floor of the mouth, thoracic inlet, abdominal diaphragm, urogenital diaphragm and plantar aponeurosis. As the peripheral resistances steadily decline, the involuntary motion out of the midline begins to permeate the organism more easily, more evenly and in a way that reaches all tissues. If tissue resistance persists in a circumscribed region, this also needs to be treated locally. These resistances may be encountered in the parietal, visceral or cranial region. Depending on region and the age of the patient, the appropriate treatment principle should be adapted to the dysfunction. Balanced tension states and an expression of the involuntary mechanism

that effectively pervades all tissues are prerequisites for tissue unfolding and spatial development.

Prognosis

Normal mouth closure can be expected after four to six treatment sessions. Over this period it is possible to reduce tissue resistances that adversely affect all basic functions, such as perfusion, innervation and the immune system. On the support of the immune system, see p.291.

OTITIS MEDIA

Definition

Acute otitis media is a serous or purulent inflammation of the middle ear that is extremely painful in most cases.

Etiology and pathogenesis

In general, otitis media is the consequence of a nasopharyngeal infection that ascends along the auditory tube. The pathogens responsible may be bacteria, such as pneumococci, *Hemophilus influenzae*, streptococci or *Pseudomonas* spp, as well as viruses. An allergic constitution and environmental factors, as well as a familial predisposition, may also be causally involved (Linder et al 1996). General weakness of the immune system is also commonly a factor.

Swelling of the auditory tube mucosa leads to insufficient opening of the tube with a resultant disturbance of ventilation and drainage in the middle ear and mastoid. The secretions formed as a result of inflammation are unable to drain away. Owing to the increased negative pressure in the middle ear, the fluid in the peritubal tissue is sucked inwards. This leads to increased tissue resistance that can no longer be compensated for by inadequate muscle traction as it seeks to open the auditory tube. The increase in negative pressure in the middle ear, compared to external pressure, brings about a change in the sound-conducting function of the tympanic membrane. As a result, auditory capacity may be reduced.

Tasker et al (2002) have demonstrated that in otitis media, the pepsin content in gastric juice is 1000 times higher than that in serum in 83% of children studied. The conclusion suggests itself that gastric reflux disease may be a further cause of otitis media because the increased acid concentration in the vicinity of the respiratory mucosa destroys the surface immunity. Neuralgic ear pain may also be triggered by gastro-esophageal reflux because the acid may irritate the vagus nerve and the mucosa of the oropharynx. For diseases of the ear, nose and throat, therefore, it may also be important to take account of all factors contributing to the anti-reflux barrier, such as the abdominal diaphragm.

Clinical signs and symptoms

In older children throbbing or stabbing ear pain is reported, which, however, disappears in most cases following perforation. Fever and headache are also common.

In infants and preschool children the picture is dominated by uncharacteristic symptoms, such as feeding weakness, refusal of food, restlessness, crying, fidgeting with the ear, vomiting and diarrhea.

Complications

Acute and/or chronic otitis media may involve the neighboring mastoid and lead to mastoiditis. About 2 weeks after the start of otitis media (i.e. in the recovery phase), tender redness and swelling develop behind the ear. The ear may also protrude.

Perforation in acute mastoiditis may lead to meningitis.

Diagnosis

The cervical lymph nodes are usually swollen. The tragus is exquisitely tender.

Allopathic medical diagnosis

Otoscopy (see p.143) reveals reddening of the tympanic membrane, initially often only at the margins. The light reflex is absent. In the case of purulent otitis media there is bulging of the tympanic membrane, and pus is discharged after perforation.

In chronic disorders a hearing test and auditory tube function test are recommended. Where mastoiditis is suspected, X-ray examination or MRI will confirm the diagnosis.

Osteopathic examination

It is recommended that the osteopathic examination begin with an assessment of respiration. Is the patient breathing preferentially through the mouth? What is the impression created by the face? In relation to overall cranial shape, does the face tend to look narrow and small? What space is taken up by the nasal cavity, and can it be ventilated adequately? These initial observations may already provide a clue as to whether the prerequisites are in place for the efficient drainage of the middle ear.

Good mouth closure is necessary for normal salivation. If saliva is formed in adequate quantities it stimulates the act of swallowing. In the course of each act of swallowing the auditory tube is opened for a period of milliseconds. Naturally, the mouth can only be closed if nasal breathing is assured. In my experience, the impression gained by visual inspection is in most cases confirmed during palpation with the help of involuntary motion.

What is the expression of the inhalation and exhalation phase of the involuntary mechanism in the region of the cranial base and the face? According to Sutherland, we should think particularly in terms of strain patterns of the cranial base. Because of asymmetry in this area the origin and attachment of the tensor veli palatini and levator veli palatini muscles may be altered. The effectiveness of these muscles may suffer as a result, their tensile forces are diminished and the forces that normally keep the auditory tube closed cannot be overcome. If the temporal bones are found unilaterally or bilaterally to be in a pattern of exhalation/internal rotation, the soft tissues beneath the cranial base in particular will be compressed. This compression may manifest itself at the junction of the two named muscles. Precisely at this location, which is found in the vicinity of the sphenopetrosal suture and is termed the isthmus, the lumen of the auditory tube is at its narrowest.

The petrous portion of the temporal bone and the basilar part of the occipital bone articulate with each other via a type of tongue and groove mechanism. This tiny articulation is of major mechanical importance (Sutherland 2004). If the occipital bone is subjected to torsion on its anterior-to-posterior axis, it becomes elevated on one side and lowered on the other. The elevated side of the occipital bone brings the petrous portion and hence the temporal bone into internal rotation. On the other side the temporal bone behaves in an opposite manner and undergoes torsion into external rotation. The sphenoid bone is also involved in this torsion pattern. On account of its motion during the inhalation and exhalation phase, the pterygoid process of the sphenoid bone usually holds the tensor veli palatini muscle under tension. Before the muscle attaches to the soft palate it travels round the pterygoid process, which it utilizes as a kind of pulley. Therefore, when palpating the involuntary motion in this region, we pay special attention as to whether the tiny posterolateral movement of the pterygoid process occurs during the inhalation phase.

Traumatic forces, such as a fall on to the face, may compress the palatine bone via the maxilla, and thus appreciably interfere with the movement of the pterygoid process. Where there is possible compression between the pterygoid process and the palatine bone, the pterygoid process is unable to glide either laterally or anteroposteriorly. As a result, not only does muscular tension control become ineffective, but also the filling pressure of the veins in the peritubal tissue is increased. According to Feldmann (1973), this is one of the factors responsible for the constant closure of the auditory tube. Because they are highly elastic, veins have a high capacity for receiving blood.

Among other mechanisms, the venous drainage of the auditory tube and its mucosa takes place directly via the pterygoid plexus, which is located as a venous plexus between the temporalis, medial pterygoid and lateral pterygoid muscles and drains into the external jugular vein. Traumatic dysfunctions of the mandible or possible strains of the cranial base may influence the tension of the medial pterygoid muscle to such a degree that the pterygoid plexus becomes compressed. Hypertonus of the medial pterygoid muscle can be detected in older children by observing TMJ movements during opening and closure of the mouth. If there is an imbalance of muscle tone, the mandible deviates towards the side of the contracted muscle. The possible consequences are congestion and increased filling pressure in the peritubal tissue, which also has repercussions on venous filling in the mucosa. If pressures are not equalized due to failure of auditory tube opening, this results in negative pressure in the middle ear which additionally causes blood to be sucked into the vessels and prevents outflow.

Sutherland (2004) repeatedly referred to the importance of free movement between the palatine bone and the pterygoid process. An attentive watch is therefore kept to establish whether the articulating surfaces between the pyramidal processes and the pterygoid plates are able to glide anteriorly and posteriorly. It is essential to have this special mechanism in mind because the sphenopalatine ganglion is located in the sphenopalatine notch. This ganglion sends out the lesser palatine nerve, which carries efferent motor fibres for the tensor veli palatini muscle. Further innervation is provided via the mandibular nerve, which also carries efferent motor fibres for the tensor veli palatini and tensor tympani muscles. Given its course, compression at the sphenopetrosal suture could lead to a disturbance of innervation. Because the etiology of otitis media and glue ear may be extremely varied, it should also be remembered that functional disorders do not only arise locally but may also emanate from other regions.

Treatment
Allopathic medical treatment

Bacterial infections of the middle ear are treated with antibiotics. The success rate of antibiotic administration is reported to be 14–23% (Rosenfeld 1992). For pain management paracetamol may be given. Decongestant nasal drops are used to restore ventilation to the middle ear via the auditory tube. Where there is considerable tympanic bulging, very severe pain or lack of treatment success (after 48–72 hours), tympanocentesis is performed to relieve pressure and to obtain material for pathogen identification. The pus can drain through the incision made. This acute measure affords protection against spread of inflammation. Where there have been multiple recurrences of tympanic effusion with auditory impairment, treatment takes the form of tympanocentesis and possibly grommet insertion and/or adenoidectomy (Scholz et al 1995).

It should be noted that otitis media in infants up to the age of 6 months is more commonly associated with complications such as mastoiditis and meningitis. Intravenous antibiotic therapy is indicated in principle and close daily clinical monitoring is recommended.

Osteopathic treatment

Acute otitis media has a tendency to recur if treatment is limited to symptomatic measures only (e.g. antibiotics). Fundamental improvement of the terrain can be achieved with osteopathic treatment, one goal of which is to improve the mechanics of drainage from the middle ear and to modify any constitutional allergic factors that may be present. A good treatment outcome can be achieved in chronic recurring otitis media and in glue ear (see next section). Osteopathic treatment alone is often not sufficient in acute otitis media. In most cases simultaneous homeopathic treatment or antibiotic therapy is necessary until the acute stage has passed.

The appropriate local treatment will emerge from the sum total of osteopathic observations and examinations. In my own experience, a sitting position for the child during treatment has a positive effect on auditory tube opening. In any case, preschool children – especially if they are suffering from disorders involving the ear – are usually not happy to lie down for treatment. A treatment approach to positively influence the opening of the auditory tube has already been described by Sutherland (2004) and Magoun (1976). This approach only becomes fully effective if existing dysfunctions of the temporal bones, SBS strain patterns or tension imbalances in the RTM have already been treated and are in the best possible balance. A specific supportive technique to ventilate the auditory tube and hence drain the middle ear can be implemented after such dysfunctions have balanced.

In their investigations Feldmann (1977) and Thullen (1979) pointed out that the auditory tube has a tendency to close when the patient is lying down and to open when the patient is upright. The hydrostatic pressure acting on the mucosa and on the peritubal tissue tends to hold the auditory tube closed in the supine position. The upright position supports the drainage of transudate as far as the tympanic orifice. From that point on, ciliary activity continues to transport the transudate (Rundcrantz 1969). Consequently, it may be beneficial to treat the child in the seated or semi-supine position.

The basic ideas and mechanism of action of the following approach, to be performed with the child in the upright or seated position, are consistent with the principles described by Sutherland and Magoun.

Active drainage of the middle ear

Sit the child on the treatment table, the head- and back-support sections of which are set at approximately 90°. This preset position permits an upright posture in which the child can lean comfortably against the treatment table without the need for secondary tension.

Stand behind the child and place your hands in such a way that they are adapted to the upright position of his head. Position your ring and little fingers on both sides so that they are in contact with the mastoid process. Bring the tips of your thumbs together and place them over the glabella (Fig. 13.8). Your index and middle fingers have no special function. Place them lightly against the patient's head on the right and left side.

With your ring and little finger now induce a combined movement, involving gentle medial pressure on the mastoid processes bilaterally and posterior traction to bring the temporal bones into external rotation. While holding this position with your fingers, use your apposed thumb tips to perform rhythmic compressions and decompressions, in a type of pumping motion directed posteriorly over the glabella. Gently, steadily and rhythmically perform the pumping action 10 times. At the end allow the temporal bones to find their way back again into their normal motion pattern. If necessary, you may deliver light pressure medially and anteriorly on the mastoid bones bilaterally to support the temporal bones into internal rotation. Finally, check the normal expression of external and internal rotation of the temporal bones to ensure that they have returned to their normal motion pattern.

The effect of this approach can be explained as follows: the temporal bones move into external rotation due to the medial and posterior motion induced via the apex of

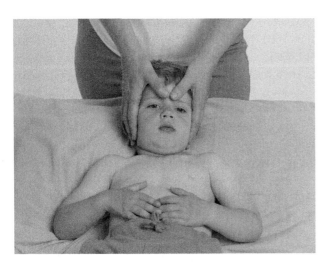

Figure 13.8 Active drainage of the middle ear. With permission, Karsten Franke, Hamburg

the mastoid processes. This acts to stretch and straighten the auditory tube. By means of the pumping motion induced over the glabella, motion is transmitted to the pharyngeal part of the auditory tube via the ethmoid and sphenoid bones. If this part of the auditory tube moves posteriorly, the tension of the tube is neutralized. In this process the auditory tube assumes a kind of sagging position. Consequently, the pumping motion has an alternately stretching and then relaxing effect on the cartilaginous part, which opens and closes the auditory tube. In this way the fluid build-up in the middle ear can be mobilized and drained.

Prognosis

Definite normalization of middle ear physiology is often seen after 2 to 4 osteopathic treatment sessions. If no positive result is recorded after the first series of treatments, the possibility of an allergic constitution should also be considered.

In the supportive treatment of the immune system, efforts should then be made to identify as far as possible all dietary substances consumed to which the body may be showing an allergic reaction. In the event of repeated recurrences, an allergy test should be performed. Exposure to environmental toxins and electrosmog should also be taken into account. However, immune function may also be impaired by endogenous factors, such as inadequate elimination of metabolic end-products by the liver or kidneys, congestion in the lymphatic system, inadequate thymus activity or general tissue acidosis. A series of about five to ten treatments is usually necessary to bring about a fundamental improvement in the functional anatomy of the cranium.

GLUE EAR (CHRONIC SEROMUCINOUS OTITIS)

Definition

Glue ear (chronic seromucinous otitis, otitis media with effusion) is said to be present in patients without signs of acute inflammation whose condition is characterized merely by increased accumulation of fluid in the middle ear which drains poorly if at all. Glue ear is encountered in both acute and chronic forms.

Etiology and pathogenesis

The acute form of glue ear is generally caused by nasopharyngeal infections. This leads to obstruction of the pharyngeal opening of the auditory tube with subsequent disturbance of middle ear ventilation. If the middle ear is not ventilated, complete pressure equalization cannot be achieved and negative pressure develops in the middle ear. If a negative pressure of -153 Pa is reached then ciliary activity, and hence the transport of fluid in the middle ear, are clearly impaired (Takahashi et al 1992).

Persistent negative pressure in the middle ear causes the tympanic membrane to retract. The mucosa of the auditory tube reacts initially by swelling and later by forming a transudate. The transudate further reduces the air volume of the middle ear, with the elastic gas now being replaced by fluid which cannot be compressed or expanded (Feldmann 1973). If this condition persists for longer than 3 months, the still relatively fluid effusion becomes increasingly viscous and sticky, hence the name: 'glue ear'.

The chronic form is caused by allergies that produce swelling of the auditory tube or by adenoidal hyperplasia.

Clinical signs and symptoms

The child first draws attention to himself because of hearing loss. Often the patient does not experience any pain or else the pain is very intermittent. Differentiation from otitis media is not always particularly straightforward.

Diagnosis

Allopathic medical diagnosis

Otoscopy reveals a retracted tympanic membrane that is intact but may also be bulging; however, its mobility is always poor. Air-fluid levels and bubbles may possibly be visible.

Osteopathic examination

As for otitis media (see p.284).

Treatment

Allopathic medical treatment

Where appropriate, treatment for the underlying disease should be implemented. If needed, decongestant nasal drops and analgesics such as paracetamol are administered.

In children with first-time glue ear and an unexceptional history of ear problems, autoinflation of the middle ear with the Otovent system is recommended. In this process air pressure is briefly delivered in order to open the auditory tube, thus enabling the pressure to equalize. However, it is inadvisable to use this system for long-term therapy because of the risk of over-inflating the tympanic membrane (Linder et al 1996).

In chronic disease courses tympanocentesis may be performed, with grommet insertion.

Osteopathic treatment

This corresponds largely to that described for recurrent otitis media (see p.285).

Prognosis

Even where chronic glue ear is present, a definite improvement in middle ear physiology can be achieved after four to six treatments. Children with a tendency to recurrences should be treated before the start of the colds season. This also includes supportive treatment for the immune system.

SINUSITIS

Definition

Acute inflammation of the paranasal sinuses is a commonly encountered infection in childhood. In most cases it occurs following a viral infection of the upper respiratory tract.

Where persistent or allergic inflammation is present in the area of the respiratory mucosa, chronic sinusitis may develop.

Etiology and pathogenesis

Pharyngeal tonsil enlargement is not infrequently the cause of sinusitis (Becker et al 1989). The pathogenesis is often but not invariably characterized by secondary bacterial infection.

Development of the paranasal sinuses

At birth the ethmoidal air cells are already present. The development of the inner chamber system continues into the 2nd year of life. Infection may already occur during the child's 1st year.

The maxillary sinus (paired) is also already present at birth, but it is only a small slit. From the 5th year of life onwards it can be detected on X-ray examination and it develops into its final shape and size by pre-puberty. This coincides with the time of eruption of the permanent teeth. Infections occur mostly after a child reaches 4 years old but in younger children they cannot always be reliably diagnosed radiologically.

Development of the frontal sinus (paired) begins in the 6th year and is dependent on the union of the metopic suture. The frontal sinus only attains its final shape and size during puberty. Infections in this region usually do not occur until a child is at least 10 years old. The sphenoidal sinus (paired) also starts to develop in the child's 6th year and this process continues into early adulthood.

The entire paranasal sinus system communicates via ostia with the meatuses of the nasal cavity.

Factors influencing the development of the paranasal sinuses

At birth the face is relatively small by comparison with the neurocranium. This is because of the need to save space to ease labor and because dentition has not yet occurred.

Traumatic compressive forces during the intrauterine period or acting on the neonate at the time of birth may result in alterations to the shape of the cranium. Usually these changes self-correct spontaneously during the postnatal period; however, if these asymmetries persist, they may interfere with or restrict the involuntary mechanism in such a way that the growth forces emanating from the cranial base are only inadequately transmitted from the neurocranium to the facial structures. The viscerocranium thus remains smaller and in particular the mid-facial region around the maxillae and nasopharyngeal space develops inadequately. This is very often a key factor when children with sinusitis are brought for osteopathic treatment. On inspection, the mid-facial region often has a swollen appearance. Breathing often takes place almost exclusively through the mouth.

Mucosal function

The inhaled air is pre-warmed, moistened and thus purified by a dense network of muscular veins in the mucosa which function rather in the same way as a central heating radiator. The cilia also have a cleansing function because they remove fluids and substance particles from the sinuses.

The mucosa of the sinuses is abundant in lymph vessels and lymphocytes which have a protective function. Goblet cells produce mucus as well as a secretion possessing antibacterial and – to a small extent – antiviral activity. The cilia can only fulfil their task if this mucosal secretion is of the correct viscosity. In this process the colloidal secretion film is continuously moved like a large conveyor belt from the sinus ostia towards the choanae.

Optimal mucosal function depends on its innervation, perfusion, pH and spatial development. However, chronic inflammation, regardless of whether it is of bacterial or viral origin, and medication with antihistamines cause this mucosal secretion to thicken. The net result is a reduction in ciliary motion and an attendant delay in mucociliary clearance. The composition of the mucosal film may be altered by all the factors listed above. In particular, tissue hyperacidity enables antigens to spread more easily. If the mid-facial region is compressed, as mentioned above, stasis results and the secretions formed by the nasal mucosa cannot drain away.

Sutherland's 'pump mechanism'

According to Sutherland (2004), the sinuses are dynamized and drained with the help of involuntary motion, which acts as a kind of pump mechanism. Not only does the global expression of the involuntary motion act as a mobilizing pump in the cranium, but local, particularly dynamic pump systems, also exist. The 'plumber's best friend' (Sutherland), a 'suction plunger', operates in various positions to improve mobility and hence drainage. Thus, according to Sutherland, a pumping motion dynamizes the maxillary sinus via the zygomatic bone, the sphenoidal sinus via the vomer, the frontal sinus via the perpendicular plate of the ethmoid bone, and the ethmoidal air cells via the crista galli. Any resistance detected between the connecting soft tissues and sutures of the facial bones may disturb the function of the paranasal sinuses and their mucosa. Excessive intracranial or extracranial membrane tensions, strain patterns of the cranial base or viscerocranial dysfunctions may also be responsible for such disturbances.

The following example is intended to describe the viscerocranial relationship more precisely: where gastric tone is lost, the tension is transmitted via the esophagus as far as the cranial base. This tension prevents normal transmission of the involuntary mechanism to the region of the nasal cavity and restricts the function of the pump mechanism.

Clinical signs and symptoms

Where sinusitis occurs as a consequence of recurrent colds, symptoms such as irritating cough or chronic runny nose will be more or less prominent. According to Palitzsch (1990), symptoms such as anorexia and failure to thrive may also be encountered.

Pain on percussion or tenderness over the corresponding sinus may be present where there is inflammation of the ethmoidal air cells or of the frontal sinus. Local redness may also be visible. Where the maxillary sinus is involved, children may also complain of toothache. Pain behind the eye may be indicative of frontal sinus, ethmoidal air cell or sphenoidal sinus involvement. The pain may become worse when the patient's head is tilted forwards.

Complications

In infants meningitis may very easily develop from ethmoidal sinusitis.

Diagnosis
Allopathic medical diagnosis

The suspected presence of sinusitis can be clarified by ultrasound or X-ray examination.

Osteopathic examination

As described for adenoids (see earlier section).

Treatment
Allopathic medical treatment

Allopathic medicine advocates treatment with antibiotics for febrile, purulent sinusitis. This recommendation is supported by results from a randomized controlled study in 136 children from the early 1980s. At that time amoxicillin and amoxicillin/clavulanic acid displayed a statistically significant advantage in terms of efficacy compared with placebo. Now, more than 20 years later, these results have been called into question by a placebo-controlled study in children with acute sinusitis: the cure rates for amoxicillin, amoxicillin/clavulanic acid and placebo were similar at around 80% (Garbutt et al 2001).

Decongestant nasal drops (especially in infants), irradiation with red light, local heat application and saline inhalations are also recommended.

Osteopathic treatment

The increasing spatial development of the nasal cavity and its paranasal sinuses in infants and preschool children is dependent on the growth forces of the cranial base. The involuntary mechanism with its slow rhythmic pattern of inhalation/flexion/external rotation and exhalation/extension/internal rotation supports the spatial formation of the tissues. This elementary rhythmic force coordinates dynamic mass movement. Its direction of flow is the expression of the metabolic activity that forms the basis for growth, development and function. Consequently, treatment must ensure firstly that generous spatial development can occur so as to guarantee optimal tissue function, and secondly that general mobility supports the effective drainage of the entire region.

In my experience it can be helpful here to liken the anatomical relationship between the cranial base and viscerocranium to a decorative mobile. The anterior part of the cranial base is formed by the sphenoid bone, which is in direct or indirect contact with most of the bones of the face. The cranial base and the sphenoid bone in particular occupy a kind of key position in the transmission of forces to the viscerocranium. The guiding threads of the mobile are the falces of the reciprocal tension membrane (RTM). If these are restricted then the sphenoid, frontal and temporal bones are restricted in their motion. In consequence, the expression of the involuntary mechanism in the face is reduced.

At the ethmoid bone the falx cerebri is very intimately attached to the crista galli. At this point, at the junction of the falx cerebri and the crista galli, the mobility and flexibility of the RTM form the basis for the physiological transmission of growth forces to the upper face. If this articulation is restricted, the vertical development of the face may be held back.

According to Sutherland, a restriction between the sphenoidal spine and the ethmoid bone may also be responsible for the failure of force transmission to the face. This tiny articulation transmits force to the midline bones of the upper face, to the frontal sinus and to the ethmoidal sinus. In the midline, beneath the crista galli, is located the perpendicular plate of the ethmoid, which in conjunction with the vomer forms the nasal septum. In my experience, the function of the midline bones is of major importance, especially for the drainage of the sphenoidal sinus.

Tissue quality and hence health can be decisively improved by osteopathic work on mechanical dysfunctions. Frequently, however, the patients also have to be tested for dietary intolerances and for environmental substance exposure. Stress, and familial and emotional strain may also sustain an allergic constitution. All these aspects need to be included in the treatment strategy.

Relevance of the sinus mucosa

Innervation

The autonomic nervous system regulates the perfusion, secretion and ciliary activity of the mucosa. This complex regulatory task is performed by the pterygopalatine ganglion, which is lodged in the pterygopalatine fossa. This small space may undergo impingement following compression of the palatine bone. Commonly, trauma to the maxilla is responsible for restricting the palatine bone and hence the surrounding soft tissues, and consequently for disturbing the balance of this autonomic regulation.

Parasympathetic fibres enhance secretion and have a vasodilator effect on the mucosa. These fibres derive from the facial nerve (intermedius nerve), divide off from the main motor trunk of the facial nerve in the geniculate ganglion of the petrous portion of the temporal bone, and travel as the greater petrosal nerve via the hiatus of the canal of the greater petrosal nerve into the middle cranial fossa. Beneath the dura mater, the fibres run anterior and medial to the foramen lacerum, and then pierce this cartilaginous plate to attain the pterygopalatine fossa via the pterygoid canal. Here, in the pterygopalatine ganglion, the parasympathetic fibres are relayed from their preganglionic to their postganglionic neuron.

The sympathetic fibres originating from C8 to T2 have a vasoconstrictor effect and inhibit secretion. In the superior cervical ganglion they are relayed to their postganglionic neuron and, together with the internal carotid artery, they gain access to the cranial cavity. From the point of entry into the cranial cavity, fibres divide off as the deep petrosal nerve. In their further course the sympathetic fibres pass through the foramen lacerum and then travel through the pterygoid canal to reach the pterygopalatine ganglion. The sensory fibres originating from the trigeminal ganglion travel via the maxillary nerve through the foramen rotundum to the pterygopalatine ganglion. These fibres are responsible for the perception of pain, pressure and temperature.

As with the nasal cavity, the sensory nerve supply for the paranasal sinus mucosa is derived from the first and second divisions of the trigeminal nerve.

The frontal sinus and the ethmoidal air cells derive their parasympathetic fibres from the oculomotor nerve via the ciliary ganglion. In the case of the sphenoidal sinus all the fibre types mentioned meet in the pterygopalatine ganglion. This small relay center has the very wide-ranging task of regulating all the different mucosal functions. If motility between the palatine bone and the pterygoid process is established during treatment, then the pterygopalatine ganglion can swing back and forth with the motion of the involuntary mechanism (Sutherland 2004). Regulation may stimulate increased tear secretion from the lacrimal gland. The tear fluid draining via the lacrimal canal into the nasal cavity exerts a disinfectant effect on the mucosa there.

Venous drainage

The structure of the mucosa of the nasal cavity reveals a large number of venous plexuses. Owing to their extremely variable filling with venous blood, they regulate filling pressure and hence mucosal thickness. The functionally useful cross-section of the internal nasal cavity and of the paranasal sinus outlets is determined as a result.

If there are disturbances of venous return, the space available for ventilation becomes smaller. Nasal breathing becomes more difficult due to the increased respiratory resistance, which may also lead to increased respiratory resistance in the lungs.

The transverse venous drainage pathway carries the blood via the ophthalmic vein to the cavernous sinus and thence via the superior petrosal sinus to the sigmoid sinus and into the internal jugular vein. The inferior petrosal sinus, which occupies a small groove above the petrobasilar suture, feeds directly into the internal jugular vein. From this it is clear that the direction of drainage via the venous network runs posteriorly.

The functioning of the drainage system of the venous cerebral vessels depends on the reciprocal tension membrane and the bony-membranous covering of the cranium. By treating existing strain patterns in the cranium it is sometimes possible to bring venous wall tone into balance. In this context it is primarily important to help balance existing strain patterns of the spheno-basilar synchondrosis and the reciprocal tension membrane. The veins then increase their uptake capacity and this helps to reduce mucosal swelling. As a secondary phenomenon, the respiratory resistance of pulmonary tissue can thus also be improved.

Extracranial factors important for treatment of the sinuses

Apart from the functions already described and their possible disturbance, this account should also include factors that help to determine the function of this region but are located outside the cranium. Negative pressure in the thorax increases with every inspiratory diaphragm contraction. At the same time the oropharyngeal muscles contract in order to keep the upper respiratory tract open against the negative pressure in the thorax. The attachments of the oropharyngeal muscles are located at the cranial base which, due to its stability, possesses a kind of lever function in keeping the upper respiratory tract open. The cranial base therefore needs also to be flexible and able to adapt to patterns in all directions. Treatment of all the diaphragms may also be necessary to rectify any pressure imbalance that might be present.

The occipital bone and the atlas together form the atlanto-occipital joint. Dysfunctions involving this articulation may alter the tension of the oropharyngeal muscles and disrupt the muscular stability that keeps the pharyngeal space open. Dysfunctions in this area can be resolved very gently with the aid of Sutherland's peripheral techniques involving the principle of balanced ligamentous tension (see p.183).

Similarly, ascending tension from the abdominal cavity may reach and adversely affect the nasal cavity via the esophagus or via the unbroken fascial continuity that extends as far as the cranial base. The entire gastrointestinal system is connected to the cranial base via the esophagus and pharynx. When thoraco-abdominal pressure equilibrium is lost, the diaphragm will seek to compensate for the pressure imbalance. However it achieves this compensation, the question is raised as to whether it can sustain its function as an anti-reflux barrier. If the gastro-esophageal junction is unable to close properly, stomach acid can ascend via the esophagus and disrupt mucosal functions in the mouth, nose and ears. In order to normalize the closing function of the gastro-esophageal junction, it is important to include all components that contribute to this closure mechanism. This means normalizing the tension of the stomach and liver, and the function of the abdominal diaphragm and its crura. These are difficult to palpate directly but their tonus can be normalized indirectly by treating the 12th ribs and the arcuate ligaments, as described by Sutherland (2004) (see p.192). In ptosis of the small intestine, tension is transmitted to the right crus of the diaphragm via the ligament of Treitz. It then normally responds with an increase in tension in order to stabilize the small intestine. A lowered kidney or a urinary transport disturbance in the renal pelvis can also be compensated for by increasing the tonus of the crura of the diaphragm. Aside from such mechanical factors, the neurovegetative control of the gastro-esophageal junction should also be included in the assessment and treatment. The hypothalamus and the region of the fourth ventricle may be relevant in this respect. Potential irritation of the sympathetic and parasympathetic fibres may be located in the region of the jugular foramen, the occipito-atlantoaxial complex, the superior thoracic aperture and in the territory of T5. All these regions should be examined and, where appropriate, treated.

Prognosis

A marked improvement in nasal mucosal function can usually be achieved by a series of four to six treatments. This also includes supportive treatment of the immune system. Frequently, patients have to be tested for dietary intolerances and for environmental substance exposure. Stress, and familial as well as other emotional strain may also sustain an allergic constitution. Once all components have been included, the body finds a sound basis for recovery. This applies especially in the allergic form of sinusitis.

OSTEOPATHIC TREATMENT OF THE LYMPH SYSTEM IN ENT DISEASES

The development and maturation of immunocompetence is a learning process of the immune system; the immune system involves the whole organism and reflects an increasingly developing 'memory'. As memory cells the B-lymphocytes are responsible for the development and maintenance of immunity. In this endeavour they are supported by cooperating populations of T-lymphocytes (Heine 1997).

In order for the organism to be able to draw on its memory, it passes through various phases of the cell-mediated immune process. Initially, a histiocyte palisade is formed around the site of antigen invasion. Biochemically, this initial defence process is set in motion by a range of tissue hormones, for example prostaglandins, leukotrienes and interferons. This is immediately followed by the microphage phase, which is also still a local reaction. The subsequent macrophage phase is associated with the active involvement of the whole organism. To overcome an infection, the lymphocytes need to become active in the final phase. If the phases of the immune defence process are hindered, chronification is difficult to avoid in the long term.

According to Pischinger (1998), monocyte factor is necessary to trigger the macrophage phase. This factor is found ubiquitously in the intercellular substance of the tissue matrix. A deficiency of this unsaturated fatty acid or its inactivity means that the macrophage phase is insufficiently pronounced and activation of the overall immune defences of the organism is hindered. Frequently, this occurs due to suppression of common colds because the organism is incapable of breaking through this inhibition of its defences. According to investigations conducted by Pischinger (1998), one prerequisite for overcoming blockade of the immune defences is the presence of monocyte and lymphocyte factor. The lymphocyte factor is found in lymph node fluid. As a result of the liberation of lymphocyte factor from the lymph nodes, B- and T-lymphocytes are activated and cross over into the circulating blood.

In my experience, the lymphatic techniques of Sutherland are very well suited for activating lymphatic flow, eliminating tissue stasis and thus supporting the release of lymphocytes. Depending on region, either vibration or agitation is performed until resonance and a palpable suction effect are produced in the tissue.

In addition to the relief of lymphatic stasis, the organism must also be supported to bring about the excretion of metabolic toxins and of cells and their toxic constituents. In order to ensure this process, the spleen, liver and heart must be in a functional equilibrium with each other and undergo treatment, as necessary. By its pulsatile force and its electrical frequency field, the heart stimulates the thymus, which drives forward the maturation of lymphocytes, especially in childhood. All the factors cited here contribute to supporting the immune system.

Bibliography

Becker R: Life in motion. Stillness Press, Portland, Ore. 1997

Becker W, Naumann H, Pfaltz C: Hals-Nasen-Ohrenheilkunde. 4th edn. Thieme, Stuttgart 1989

Bluestone C, Cantekin E, Berry Q: Certain effects of adenoidectomy on eustachian tube ventilatory function. Laryngoscope 85, 1975: 113–127

Cantekin E, Doyle W, Reichert T, Phillips D, Bluestone C: Dilatation of the eustachian tube by electrical stimulation of the mandibular nerve. Annals of Otology Rhinology Laryngology 88: 1979

Feldmann H: Physiologie und Pathophysiologie der Mittelohrventilation. Z Laryng Rhinol 52: 1973

Feldmann H: Physiologie und Pathophysiologie von Tube und Mittelohr. In: Beck C: Papers delivered at the symposium 'Physiologie und Pathophysiologie von Tube und Mittelohr.' Univ.-HNO-Klinik Freiburg 1977

Flisberg K: Clinical assessment of tubal function. Acta Otolaryngologica 188, 1963

Garbutt J M, Goldstein M, Gellman E et al: A randomized, placebo-controlled trial of antimicrobial treatment for children with clinically diagnosed acute sinusitis. Pediatrics 107, 2001: 619–625

Gates G, Avery C, Prihoda T: Effect of adenoidectomy upon children with chronic glue ear. Laryngoscope 98, 1988: 58–63

Heine H: Lehrbuch der biologischen Medizin. 2nd edn. Hippokrates, Stuttgart 1997

Honjo I, Okazaki N, Kumazawa T: Experimental study of the eustachian tube function with regard to its related muscles. Acta Otolaryngologica 91, 1981

Huang M, Lee S, Rajendran K: A fresh cadaveric study of paratubal muscles. Journal of Plastic and Reconstructive Surgery 100, 1997

Illing S, Claßen M: Klinikleitfaden Pädiatrie. 6th edn. Urban & Fischer, Munich/Jena 2003

Ingelstedt S, Ivarsson A, Jonson A: Mechanics of the human middle ear: pressure regulation in aviation and diving, a nontraumatic method. Acta Otolaryngologica 228, 1967

Langmann J: Medizinische Embryologie. 8th edn. Thieme, Stuttgart 1989

Linder T, Funke G, Schmid S, Nadal D: Die akute Otitis media und der Tubenmittelohrkatarrh: Ein Überblick über die Pathogenese und Empfehlungen zur Therapie. Z Schweiz Med Wochenschr 126, 1996

Magoun H: Osteopathy in the cranial field. 3rd edn. Journal Printing, Kirksville, Mo. 1976

Matsune S, Sando I, Takahashi H: Elastin at the hinge portion of the eustachian tube cartilage in specimens from normal subjects and those with cleft palate. Annals of Otology Rhinology Laryngology 101, 1992

Moss. In: Sperber GH: Embryologie des Kopfes. 4th edn. Quintessenz, Berlin 1989

Palitzsch D: Pädiatrie. Kinderheilkunde für Studenten und Ärzte. 3rd edn. Enke 1990

Pischinger A: Lehrbuch der Grundregulation. 9th edn. Haug, Heidelberg 1998

Rich A: Physiological study of eustachian tube and its related muscles. Bull Johns Hopkins Hosp 31, 1920

Rosenfeld R, Post J: Meta-analysis of antibiotics for the treatment of otitis media with effusion. Otolaryngology Head and Neck Surgery 106, 1992

Rundcrantz H: Posture and eustachian tube function. Acta Otolaryngologica 68, 1969

Scholz B: Handbuch 1995. Deutsche Gesellschaft für pädiatrische Infektiologie e.V. (DGPI). Futuramed, Munich 1995

Sperber GH: Embryologie des Kopfes. 4th edn. Quintessenz, Berlin 1989

Sutherland W: Das große Sutherland-Kompendium. Jolandos, Pähl 2004

Takahashi H, Honjo I, Hayashi M, Futjita A: Clearance function of eustachian tube and negative middle ear pressure. Annals of Otology Rhinology Laryngology 101, 1992

Tasker A, Detter P, Panetti M, Koufmann J, Birchall J, Pearson J: Reflux of gastric juice and glue ear in children. Lancet 359(9305), 2002: 493

Thullen A: Prüfung von Tubenfunktion und Paukendruck. In: Berende, Link, Zöllner (eds): Hals-Nasen-Ohrenheilkunde; Praxis und Klinik, vol. 5: Ohr 1. Thieme, Stuttgart 1979

EMBRYOLOGY AND ANATOMY

Development

During the 4th week in utero, the lower part of the respiratory system begins to develop. From the primitive pharynx, a groove called the laryngotracheal groove develops. This later deepens and forms a laryngotracheal diverticulum, which lies ventral to the primitive pharynx. The lining of the diverticulum is of endodermic origin and it is surrounded by splanchnic mesenchyme (Fig. 14.1a). The distal end enlarges to form a primitive lung bud.

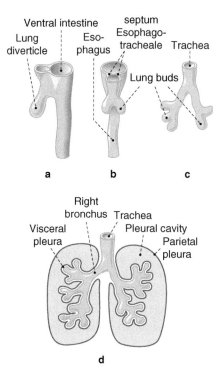

Figure 14.1 The development of the lung. **a:** Formation of the lung diverticle at 3 weeks on the ventral wall of the ventral intestine. **b:** The septum esophagotracheale separates the trachea and esophagus at 4 weeks. The lung diverticle forms 2 sacks, the lung buds. **c:** At 5 weeks the lung buds divide into 3 main bronchia for 3 lobes of the lung on the right, and on the left. **d:** This is followed by further dichotomous divisions of the main bronchia. The entire lung is surrounded by pleura. With permission, Henriette Rintelen, Velbert

A partition or septum develops on the 32nd day, separating the laryngotracheal diverticulum from the pharynx. This is known as the tracheoesophageal septum (Fig. 14.1b), which divides the foregut into a laryngotracheal tube on the ventral side (which in turn will develop into the larynx, trachea, bronchi and lungs) and the esophagus on the dorsal side.

If this septum is incomplete or defective during this early stage of development, a tracheoesophageal fistula (TEF) will ensue (Fig. 14.2). There are a variety of types of TEF, often associated with an esophageal atresia, but in all cases, there is communication between the trachea and esophagus at birth. This leads to regurgitation of feeds after birth and/or gastric reflux, which can enter the lungs and lead to pneumonia if not detected. It is associated with polyhydramnios in pregnancy because the fetus is unable to swallow the amniotic fluid, which would normally pass through the digestive system where a percentage would be absorbed. The detection of polyhydramnios is therefore important by the osteopath treating the pregnant woman, if it has not already been picked up by the obstetric team. Postnatally the infant has foamy secretion in her mouth and nose. When the infant tries to drink for the first time this may lead to aspiration and then to pneumonia. Ultrasound scanning can then be used to detect the fistula, and early surgery may be performed postnatally to prevent serious complications.

In the case of oligohydramnios, on the other hand, there may be compression to the thorax and therefore of the lungs. If this is the case, it can interfere with normal alveolar development, leading to a variable degree of pulmonary hypoplasia.

The distal end of the lungbuds grow caudad quickly and thereby form the trachea.

By the end of the 4th week in utero, the endodermal lung bud divides into two bronchial buds (Fig. 14.1b, c). During the 5th week, these buds enlarge and form the right and left bronchi and grow lateral and caudad into the pleural cavities so that they are covered by pleura from the beginning (Fig. 14.1d).

During weeks 5–17 in utero, all major parts of the lower respiratory system are formed in structure but gas exchange is still not possible. This means that respiration is not possible and a baby born at this stage cannot survive.

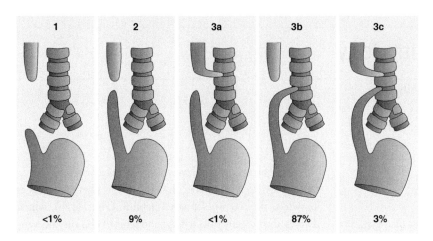

Figure 14.2 Different types of tracheo-esophageal fistula according to Vogt. TEF is seen in type 3 a–c.
With permission, Stange, Borrosch: Pädiatrie in Frage und Antwort. 3rd edn. Urban & Fischer, Munich/Jena, 2006

During weeks 16–25 in utero, the lumen of the bronchi and bronchioles become larger and highly vascular. The respiratory bronchioles give rise to terminal sacs or primitive alveoli, which become thin-walled. This makes some respiratory effort possible and means that a fetus born towards the end of this period may survive, given intensive care.

Between week 24 in utero and birth, the terminal sacs continue to grow. The epithelial lining grows thinner and thinner and allows the surrounding capillaries to grow into them. The epithelial cells have a secretory function and the type II pneumocytes begin to secrete surfactant. This counteracts surface tension and then at birth facilitates expansion of the alveoli. After 26 weeks gestation, the fetus has a chance of survival although surfactant is not really produced adequately until 32 weeks in utero. The presence of adequate surfactant and the development of the pulmonary vasculature are together essential for the survival of premature infants.

During the latter weeks of pregnancy, and right up until the child is approximately 8 years old, the immature alveoli continue to develop.

They increase in number and in size until, at this age, the full complement of adult alveoli are present.

Surfactant deficiency

As we have seen, the absence of surfactant makes it impossible for the alveoli to fill with air, and if gas exchange cannot take place the infant cannot survive. A primary surfactant deficiency is found in 50–80% of premature infants younger than 28 weeks or with a weight at birth of less than 1000 g. A secondary surfactant deficiency may occur through cardiovascular shock, hypoxia, acidosis, severe bacterial infections or aspiration of meconium. If, however, some surfactant is present and the premature infant survives, there is still a strong risk of a respiratory distress syndrome. Many of the immature alveoli may still be filled with fluid and will not have fully inflated.

This fluid is said to have the appearance of a 'glassy' or 'hyaline' membrane, often the condition being referred to as 'hyaline membrane disease'. This is a common and serious condition in the newborn, especially if already compromized from all the complications of prematurity. The infant's breathing quickly becomes labored and rapid. It is possible that periods of severe asphyxia in utero may lead to a lack of adequate perfusion to the alveoli. This would cause impairment to the type II pneumocytes which are responsible for surfactant secretion.

These infants need intensive care in hospital with surfactant substitution, artificial respiration and fluid substitution. However, if, as osteopaths, we are allowed to treat the baby in the incubator, we can help greatly to encourage adequate circulation to the lung fields, aid drainage via the lymphatics and encourage neurotrophic flow via the vagus and sympathetic nerve supply.

The thorax – structure and function

In order to be able to treat the many dysfunctional conditions of the respiratory system in children, we need to have a clear picture and knowledge of the thorax. We need to be able to visualize instantly the 'workings' of the thorax, encasing the lungs. We will look here at the bony and membranous attachments and the passage of the relevant nerves and circulatory vessels, which are all involved in normal pulmonary function.

Bony connection

We recognize instantly the importance of free mobility along the thoracic spine itself, especially T1–T6. We must remember, however, to include the unimpeded mobility of the lumbar spine because of the attachment of the diaphragmatic crurae at the levels of L1/2/3. The sacrum needs to have free mobility between the ilia in order to aid normal reciprocal tension within all other horizontal diaphragms. Full rib mobility

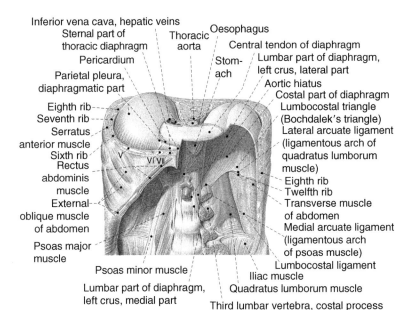

Inferior vena cava, hepatic veins
Sternal part of thoracic diaphragm
Thoracic aorta
Oesophagus
Central tendon of diaphragm
Pericardium
Stom-ach
Lumbar part of diaphragm, left crus, lateral part
Parietal pleura, diaphragmatic part
Aortic hiatus
Eighth rib
Costal part of diaphragm
Seventh rib
Lumbocostal triangle (Bochdalek's triangle)
Serratus anterior muscle
Lateral arcuate ligament (ligamentous arch of quadratus lumborum muscle)
Sixth rib
Rectus abdominis muscle
Eighth rib
Twelfth rib
External oblique muscle of abdomen
Transverse muscle of abdomen
Medial arcuate ligament (ligamentous arch of psoas muscle)
Psoas major muscle
Psoas minor muscle
Lumbocostal ligament
Iliac muscle
Lumbar part of diaphragm, left crus, medial part
Quadratus lumborum muscle
Third lumbar vertebra, costal process

Figure 14.3 Construction and position of the diaphragm (from front).
With permission, S botta:At las der Anatomie des Menschen. Publisher:R. Put za nd R. Pabst, 2 $t edn. E sevier/U rban & Fischer, Munich/ na, 20

is obviously essential, not only because the ribs form the entire lateral cage, underneath which the lungs can express their mobility in normal breathing, but also because of the importance of the autonomic nerves, the thoracic ganglia, which are situated along the rib heads.

The clavicles, scapulae and sternum need free mobility because of their direct and indirect connections to the whole ribcage via their fascial attachments. The clavicles are closely related to the first ribs and brachial plexus. The sternum lies anterior to the mediastinal lymphatic chain and posterior to the manubrium lies the thymus gland, which is responsible for a large part of the immune function, especially in young children. The scapulae are connected to the cranial base via their strong muscle attachments as well as all the direct attachments to the ribs and spine.

The upper cervical spine must not hold any bony restrictions as these would create tension deep within the cervical muscles, and therefore in the entire cervical fascia running from the cranial base to the mediastinum, via the sternomastoid muscle.

The temporal and occipital mobility is paramount due to the passage of the vagus nerve through the jugular foramen. These bilateral foraminae are formed by the articulations of the petrous portions of the temporals with the condyles of the occiput.

Membranous connections

It is on this level that I have personally found the greatest amount of strain affecting full pulmonary function. It is clear that all pulmonary lobes need the freedom in full expression of mobility to achieve normal inhalation and exhalation. It is, after all, this full excursion of the lungs that leads to adequate oxygenation of all the organs and cells of the body.

If these individual lobes are 'held' in position by the fascial bags within which they are enclosed, then their inherent mobility is impeded. I have found this restriction of full breath to have one of the most 'crippling' effects on the whole person. These effects are on every level: physical, emotional, mental and spiritual.

In order for one to be able to inhale and exhale fully, the membranous or fascial structures connected to the pleurae must have freedom of movement and optimum balance. I will not go into the anatomical detail of all the small and specific membranous connections but want to draw your attention instead to the far-reaching indirect fascial connections throughout the entire body, which have relevence to pleural mobility and balance.

I want you to think of connections from the parietal pleura medially to the mediastinal fascia. Then think of the connections inferiorly to the diaphragm and via the crurae, which blend with the anterior longitudinal ligamentous sleeve of the spine to attach to the sacrum. Laterally, the medial and lateral arcuate ligaments (Fig. 14.3) create a ceiling over the massive bellies of the psoas major and quadratus lumborum respectively. The 12th ribs lie in close association with these important ligaments and are a valuable tool for the osteopath in releasing tension in this entire area of the body. Restrictions and torsions in this area can cause serious impediment to arterial, venous and lymphatic flow. Superiorly, visualize the connections from the apices of the lungs; that is, the suprapleural membrane (Sibson's fascia) as it travels via the thoracic inlet and all the associated deep cervical fascias, leading superiorly to the cranial base via the pharyngobasilar fascia. In the early embryonic development, this whole fascial connection was apparent as the membrane called the pleuropericardial sac, suspended from the cranial base.

When you keep this entire fascial continuum in mind, it is easy to understand how a membranous strain at any point can affect either the bony structure, the mobility of the lungs themselves and/or the pathway of the nerves and circulatory vessels to and from the lungs. Treatment will therefore always include the release of this fascial continuum.

Circulation and lymphatic drainage

It is essential to check and ensure unimpeded circulation and drainage to and from the thorax and lung fields. Here again, we look at the thoracic inlet with its close relationship to major vessels, at the clavicles and the deep cervical fascia.

Then we turn our attention to the thoracic diaphragm (see Fig. 14.3) and the passage of the aorta, inferior vena cava and the cisterna chyli.

In almost every case of respiratory dysfunction that I have treated, I have found some degree of restriction in the movement of the diaphragm. It is easy to see how tension or torsional strains of the diaphragm can clamp down on these vessels, leading to backlog and extra strain on the heart, which in turn leads to congestion and stasis of the pulmonary system. I will deal with the diaphragm in greater detail later.

Innervation

The parasympathetic supply is via the vagus and its exit from the cranium via the jugular foraminae. The vagus originates in the floor of the 4th ventricle and we can understand the importance of checking and treating the cranial base in the case of any pulmonary dysfunction.

Sympathetic nerve supply is derived from T1–T6 via the thoracic chain ganglia. I will discuss the importance of inhibiting and balancing the autonomic nervous system (ANS) via the rib heads in this area when I describe individual cases later.

The diaphragm

(See Fig. 14.3)

I would like to discuss the thoracic diaphragm separately although it has already been mentioned. Its function and connections to all vital organs and vessels is of the utmost importance, not only to normal lung physiology but also to the normal function of the total being. A.T. Still wrote, 'By me you live and by me you die' as he spoke about the diaphragm. He also taught his students the 'parable of the goat and the boulder'. This is a wonderful simulation of the passage of arterial blood through the diaphragm:

The goat is running down a mountain path but is stopped by the presence of a large boulder right in the middle of the path. He backs up and tries to run and push the boulder ever harder, but each time it will not shift. The harder he tries to butt the obstructing boulder, the more he is flung backwards in the air.

So it is with the valves of the heart and the arterial blood (the goat) flowing along the aorta (the pathway). If there is great tension in the crurae of the diaphragm (the boulder), the blood cannot flow adequately through and is pushed back towards the heart, which tries harder and harder to get more pressure behind it. Eventually, if the diaphragmatic tension is not released, the backlog of blood to the heart builds up, the blood pressure increases and a congestive state ensues. Now you can imagine the effects on the pulmonary circulation and congestion in the lungs and then think about oxygenation of organs and tissues of the entire body. The parable also demonstrates the importance of arterial flow.

Now let us look at the passage of the inferior vena cava and the lymphatic channels. Diaphragmatic tension will again impede the free flow of venous return and lymph from all parts of the body below this level. Think of the congestion created in the lower extremities and pelvic organs leading to varicosities and/or edema of the lower extremities, vulval varicosities and hemorrhoids. These will not usually be common symptoms in children but pelvic congestion will certainly add to the dysmenorrhoea in teenagers or to the more generalized low backache experienced by older children and adolescents. It will also affect venous return and balance in the intestine in conditions such as chronic constipation in children of all ages. The cysterna chyli must have a free passage in order for lymph to drain upwards into the mediastinal lymphatic channels through the thoracic duct and into the left subclavian vein. Remember the passage of the esophagus and the effect on the cardiac sphincter leading into the stomach. I'm sure you have all treated many babies with gastric reflux due to the imbalance in the area of this sphincter caused by diaphragmatic tension.

Then we turn our attention to all the vital organs in close association with the diaphragm. Lying on this horizontal platform are the lungs themselves and the heart. Suspended from it are the liver and gallbladder, the stomach, the spleen. Visualize the fascial connections to the adrenal glands and kidneys. Think of the colonic flexures, hepatic and splenic, tucked up into the recesses at the lateral aspects of the diaphragm. All of these organs are constantly in need of the inherent massaging movement of the thoracic diaphragm, allowing each one to swing, rotate and 'breathe' in its own range of inherent motility for the optimal functioning of that organ. This is just a brief overview of how important the diaphragm is and how its balance and freedom of motion is essential in any condition affecting the lungs.

THE FIRST BREATH

As a midwife for many years, I always had great interest in the first gasp of the newborn infant. This may well have been for two reasons. First, because of the medical significance of this initial breath in initiating and stimulating the alveolar function of gas exchange, crucial to the infant's survival. Secondly, it was a moment of great relief for myself, the attending midwife (who could then release her own 'held breath'!!), signifying that all was well.

This first breath fascinated me, along with all the other 'miracles' involved in pregnancy and birth. I was amazed by the miracle of conception and the embryological development of the whole being, by the automatic physiological changes that take place in the fetus from life in utero, where the fetus is dependent on her mother and placenta, to life after birth, when she becomes a physiologically and emotionally independent human being for the first time.

Physiological changes associated with the first breath

We have already discussed some of the events and changes that take place in order to stimulate the initiation of the first breath. We know that primitive amoebic-like movements of the respiratory system occur from the start in utero. We have discussed the role of surfactant, a phospholipid and protein, which is secreted into the alveolar space. We saw how it decreases the surface tension between the walls of the alveoli, enabling the alveoli to inflate fully with the first gasp of air drawn into the lungs at birth.

Prior to this first breath the tiny alveolar sacs are filled with fluid. As air is drawn in and the alveoli inflate, this fluid is expelled and absorbed into the pulmonary vasculature and the lymphatics. Fluid is also dispersed from the lungs via the nose and mouth, from the pressure on the thorax during the final stage at the birthing process.

It is thought that many factors are involved in the initiation of the first gasp. We have seen above that the tactile, visual and auditory stimuli experienced at the time of birth encourage inhalation of the secondary respiratory mechanism.

The change of position of the fetal head during the final stages of the birthing process is also most probably involved. The fetal head is usually held in anatomical flexion during the first stage of labor. During the second stage, as we know, it goes through a phase of rotation and then is born by extension over the maternal symphysis pubis. This anatomical extension of the fetal head, as submitted by Dr. Viola Frymann, DO, leads to relative external rotation at the sphenobasilar synchondrosis. 'This is the mechanism of inhalation of the primary respiratory mechanism. Almost immediately the infant draws its first breath' (Frymann 1998). She writes, 'The postural change induced by delivery carries the respiratory mechanism into a position of inhalation and this in turn stimulates the inhalation center in the floor of the fourth ventricle. The secondary mechanism is thus initiated into its rhythmic, cyclic activity.'

A certain amount of circulating catecholamines in the fetus at the time of delivery are also said to be necessary, to aid the quality of the vigorous first breath. This will almost always be the case as even a perfectly normal labor and delivery is a stressful situation for the mother and the baby. The presence of glucocorticoids stimulates the production of surfactant. They also help in the absorption of the alveolar sac fluid at birth, which in turn allows for full inflation of the lungs to occur. Another important role of these circulating catecholamines is that they provide a 'state of alertness' in the baby at the time of delivery. This is essential because the infant needs energy and strength to respond promptly to the stimuli at birth and to have the ability to take the deep respiratory inhalation necessary for the first breath.

Ineffective first breath

In some cases, the baby will attempt her first gasp while the torso is still in the birth canal and only the head is delivered. From my midwifery experience I can confirm that this occurred quite often, especially in cases of shoulder dystocia. It also occurred if the umbilical cord was wrapped tightly around the baby's neck several times, necessitating clamping and cutting of the cord at that stage, before the body was born. In these cases, there is a longer period of time between delivery of the head and the rest of the body. The head is exposed to the cooler air and the light and sounds from the delivery room. This leads to tactile, visual and auditory stimuli, which encourage the in-drawing of breath. Clearly the effects of this 'premature' first breath can lead to inadequate inflation of some of the alveoli due to thoracic compression. We will discuss this presentation and osteopathic treatment later.

Think now of the babies whose mothers have been sedated with pethidine during labor. This drug has powerful analgesic and sedative properties. If given to the mother at an inappropriate time; that is, a short time before the actual birth (second stage) or if the drug has been repeated through the first stage of labor, the sedative effect on the fetus is seen in a drowsy, lethargic baby, not able to make that full respiratory effort necessary to inflate the alveoli fully. This can also be the case if a labor has been very prolonged and both mother and baby are unduly exhausted.

These children are later prone to recurrent chest infections and you will find that there is nearly always the imprint of that inadequate first breath which manifests physically with medial compression of the thorax. This may be found posteriorly at the costovertebral junctions or anteriorly at the costochondral junctions. The sternum often gives the impression of being sucked in and the lung fields may have the feeling of 'underinflation'. The fulcrum is deep within the mediastinum or lungs.

The first breath and its association with shock

We have just discussed 'ineffectual' first breath, which leads to the feeling of 'underinflated' lung fields. Now we will look at another type of first breath and its association with shock.

It is my experience, in very many cases of children whom I have treated, that there is a strong element of shock held in the thorax. In certain instances there has been a reason for this finding in the history; for example the severe trauma of a road traffic accident (RTA), a significant fall or a major emotional fright, leading to a state of shock. However, in many cases, when there was no history whatsoever to explain this shock imprinted in the child's thorax, I questioned and concluded that this shock was experienced at the time of the first breath. The birth histories confirmed my hypothesis. Often it is due to a precipitate delivery, usually the second stage of labor, though the first stage can also be very rapid. The baby is literally pushed or almost 'falls out' (as mothers often describe it) within seconds to a few minutes. There has been no time for a gentle molding of the vault bones in these cases. This rapid transition from life in utero to the outer environment is usually a total shock to both mother and baby. The baby takes a huge sudden gasp of air associated with a shock to the whole system and it feels subsequently to the osteopath's fingers as if that shock has remained imprinted in the tissue memory of the lungs.

Mostly I find this 'first-breath shock' in the center or superior third of the sternum, although occasionally it seems to be present through the entire mediastinum.

Other reasons for 'first-breath shock' may be a traumatic instrumental delivery, either an elective or emergency caesarean section or any other abrupt trauma at the time of the first gasp.

Let us consider the consequences of this shock in the infant and growing child. As with the 'ineffectual first breath' discussed earlier, these children will also be more prone to recurrent chest infections and congestion due to the associated restriction of the structural thorax. The lungs in this case however, feel 'overinflated'. It feels as if the lungs within the ribcage are ready to burst. You will find that, physically, the thorax appears 'full' and feels hard and compressed at the

junctions of the ribs. The sternum feels hard and generally the shocked tissues seem to push you away. The fulcrum may be quite far off the body.

Reaction types of the lung

Whether there is a feeling of 'underinflated' or 'overinflated' lung fields, I have found that these children can present in one of two ways. This is, of course, not black and white and in some cases the symptoms and signs may be mixed.

Type I – the 'underinflated' first breath

This is associated with the 'ineffectual' first breath leading to the underinflated lung feel (see p.297).

Clinical signs and symptoms

This is the child who presents with recurrent infections of the upper and lower respiratory tract (i.e. ear, nose, throat and chest infections). The immune system is often weak and this may be because of the long term and frequent use of antibiotics and/or inhalers.

The appetite is usually very poor and the child looks thin, pale and may be small for her age. Her diet consists of carbohydrates and refined sugar foods, which in turn leads to further exhaustion of the immune system and often chronic candidiasis.

Emotionally, this child is the timid type and is very often a victim of bullying in school. She may feel 'different' and isolated and prefer to play imaginary games alone or be more comfortable in the presence of adults, where she may feel more secure and understood.

There is also a history of lethargy and these children are hypersensitive to foods, drugs and their environment, leading to varying degrees of skin allergies and eczemas.

There is often a reactive hypoglycemia as the pancreas and whole digestive system is dysfunctional.

Diagnosis

The osteopath will find the underinflated feel of the lung fields. There will be medial compression of the anterior thorax and mediastinum and the entire involuntary mechanism may be held in internal rotation. The hips and feet will also show this internal rotation on a structural level. The hard feel to the sternum, especially the manubrium, impedes the inherent mobility and therefore physiological function of the thymus, a large part of the immune system in the infant and young child. The tense diaphragm is clamped down on the adrenals, coeliac plexus and spleen, leading to a further compromised immune system.

Osteopathic treatment

In the type I child, the osteopath will need to meet the compression in the anterior thorax. The fulcrum will be hidden deeply in the mediastinum. I usually find in this case that a more localized contact is necessary, around the area of the manubrium or central sternum. Sitting on the right side of your patient, you may place the distal parts of your three middle fingers on this area as a sensory hand and the tips of your fingers of the other hand on top, as a motor hand (Fig. 14.4). Make sure you have a good fulcrum, for example your elbows on the couch, as you will need to have a direct contact with your patient. Match the compression, acknowledging the underinflated and 'timid' feel of the tissues under your hands. You will quickly feel the shock, which builds to a crescendo and is then released. The child will usually take a very deep breath or an infant may cry and then quickly fall into a deep state of relaxation. You will see the relief in the whole countenance as if the child has taken a proper full in-breath for the first time. The child's color usually improves instantly and the parents invariably remark upon this.

In each case the first breath shock must be released before any of the other structures/organs will be able to change.

Type II- the 'overinflated' first breath

This is associated with the sudden shock of the first in-breath at birth, leading to the overinflated lung feel.

Clinical signs and symptoms

This child often presents with chest symptoms which have been labelled as asthma. She may not have any actual physical chest problems but may be brought to the osteopath with a history of being hyperactive and destructive. This child is highly stimulus bound, in a state of constant alert. In school, her concentration is very poor because each time there is a visual, auditory or tactile stimulus, the child will immediately be drawn towards it, distracting her attention from the teacher. The parents report that she is always on the go and cannot sit still for any length of time. She therefore uses up all her energy and this can lead to exhaustion when a project is finished. She may be quite a perfectionist.

Emotionally, this child's moods swing from being hyperexcitable to depressed states.

Diagnosis

The osteopath will find a 'full' thorax, like a suit of armour, with the mechanism held in external rotation. The tension in the diaphragm affects the associated organs, as before, and there will also be hyperfacilitation of the autonomic nervous system, along the thoracic chain ganglia at the rib heads, at the coeliac plexus and the adrenals.

Osteopathic treatment

In each case the first breath shock must be released before any of the other structures or organs will be able to change.

In the type II child, the osteopath will need to give great space and respect to the full thorax which feels ready to burst. In this case, I believe that it is more beneficial to place my two whole hands on the anterior thorax (Fig. 14.5). The upper hand is placed across the thoracic inlet, covering the clavicles, manubruim and upper ribs. The second hand is placed at right angles to the first, along the length of the sternum.

As you 'watch' and 'listen' very carefully to the tissues under your hands, acknowledging the overinflated, stimulus-bound feel of the first breath, you will often be pushed off the body wall. This may literally be a physical backing off of your hands or it may be that you take your intention away.

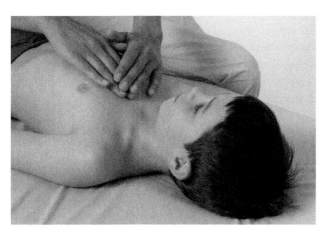

Figure 14.4 Treatment of a type 1 child with an underinflated lung and an ineffective first breath.
With permission, Karsten Frank , Hamburg

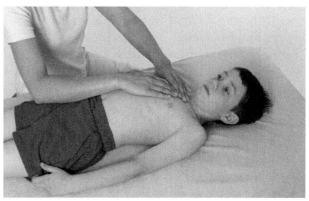

Figure 14.5 Treatment of first breath type II child.
With permission, Karsten Frank , Hamburg

In this case, the osteopath needs to give as much space as is necessary to the child and her communicating tissues until you will feel the shock releasing. As in type I, a long, deep breath may follow, leading to a state of deep relaxation, or often a fit of laughing in the older child for no apparent reason. There is again a sense of great relief over the child's whole countenance and demeanour as if it has let that first held in-breath out for the first time.

In both cases of the child having released the first breath the osteopath continues to treat/release all the other compromized organs, structures and tissues associated with this first breath.

The changes that follow over the subsequent weeks are profound and the emotional relief as well as all the improvements in physical symptomatology are truly wonderful to observe. These children not only become empowered and self-confident but also feel safe to give and receive love and affection as the fourth chakra region (the heart center and lungs) is opened up and in a state of balance for the first time in their lives. The parents will report these changes but you will also witness them for yourself.

THE LUNGS AND EMOTIONS

Now let us look at the lungs and the association with emotions. I consider the heart and lungs very much like a horse and carriage (i.e. you can't have one without the other!). Structurally, they descended from the developing forebrain, suspended from the pleuropericardial membrane and came to rest on the transverse septum, later to become the central tendon of the diaphragm (see Fig. 14.3). All these structures are totally interrelated and interdependent upon each other.

In my experience, I have felt many emotions held in the tissues of the lungs. The main emotion is that of grief, and when this is the case I usually palpate it in the right lung field. When there is sadness held in the tissues, I tend to feel it more in the heart center, retrosternally or spread generally within both lungs. If it is fear, then I feel this emotion more inferiorly towards the lower lobes of the lungs, through the diaphragm to the kidneys.

Let us examine the emotional effect of diaphragmatic tension, considering that the heart and lungs are resting on and relying on diaphragmatic motion.

Immediately our attention is drawn to the clamping down on the coeliac plexus. It is the recurring feeling of having been 'kicked in the guts'. It leads to an imbalance over time of the autonomic nervous system, usually with hyperfacilitation of the sympathetics in this area. This is a state of 'fight or flight'. It is a child on constant alert. We see them every day in our practices and the parents wonder why the child is lacking in confidence and self esteem. These are consequences

of dysfunction of this 3rd chakra area of the body. They may throw tantrums at all ages from toddlers to teenagers and they complain of intermittent nausea and 'tummy aches' when presented with a challenging or new situation. Great fear can be held in this entire area and you will 'feel' it in the tissues, in the kidneys, through the coeliac plexus tucked beneath the diaphragm and into the lung fields.

It is essential for us as osteopaths to find and release these 'emotional holding' patterns in the treatment of children (see Ch.9, Diagnosing and treating emotional factors). It will enable them to 'let go' of such patterns, thus allowing them to move forward in their healing journey.

CROUP OR LARYNGOTRACHEOBRONCHITIS

Definition

Any obstructive condition of the larynx or trachea, characterized by a hoarse, barking cough and difficult breathing is known as croup. It is usually due to a viral infection and occurs most often in autumn.

Etiology and pathophysiology

Croup is an infection of the upper trachea and larynx usually caused by parainfluenza viruses. It is often precipitated by a cold. It has been proved that environmental factors are also of importance, even if only to a small degree. Owing to the infection, an obstruction of the upper airways occurs with a sudden onset of breathing difficulty due to swelling of the mucosa and inspiratory stridor caused by turbulent air passage.

Clinical signs and symptoms

The child has a barking cough which usually gets worse at night due to parasympathetic activity, is hoarse, and inspiratory stridor is to be heard. She has difficulty breathing, is restless and tachycardia can sometimes be noticed. The child may also have fever. Anxiety worsens the situation. Intercostal and subcostal recession may be palpated. In severe cases dyspnea, cyanosis, impaired consciousness and muscular hypotony may occur.

Diagnosis

The diagnosis is found according to the clinical signs.

Allopathic diagnosis

It is important to differentiate between epiglottitis and croup. It is of great importance that this differentiation is made as soon as possible as epiglottitis can be life-threatening. In case of doubt and the possibility of epiglottitis, the doctor can inspect the pharynx under anesthesia and be ready to intubate. This is necessary since a reflectory cardiac arrest and apnea can occur. The virus causing epiglottitis is usually hemophilus influenza type B and leads to a very sore throat, swelling of the lymph nodes of the throat and swelling of the epiglottis and often dyspnea.

Osteopathic examination

In addition to case-history taking and general examination (see p.180; Ch.8, An osteopathic approach to the newborn and infant) an inspection of the thorax should be conducted. Please keep the following points in mind:

- skin color
- intercostal recessions
- deformities of the thorax
- symmetry of the thorax and the diaphragm
- breathing: are there problems breathing in or out? Are the secondary respiratory muscles used as support? Does the child use abdominal breathing or thoracic breathing? What is the breathing frequency?

Afterwards palpate:

- tension around the thoracic inlet and the anterior throat area
- mobility of the ribs against the thoracic spine and the sternum and their movement with respiration
- position and mobility of the thoracic spine
- mobility of the lobes of the lung during respiration
- symmetry of the thoracic diaphragm, torsion, tension and quality of movement during respiration
- involuntary movement of the lung
- quality of blood supply and drainage of lung tissue
- shock in the lung tissue (see p.298) that may be felt in the lung tissue and along the sympathetic chain.

Treatment

General treatment

The first and most important thing to do is to calm the child. Cold air can help (open the window) or inhalation of steam; for example filling the bathtub with hot water and keeping the child in the bathroom until breathing gets easier.

Allopathic treatment

If this is insufficient, inhalation with epinephrine (adrenalin) may be necessary. In severe cases cortisol (i.v. or rectal) is given and occasionally intubation is necessary.

Osteopathic treatment

This is similar to the treatment given in bronchitis (see p.306). The ANS should be balanced and the lymphatic flow enhanced to deal with the infection. Any restrictions to the fascia of the throat and the thoracic inlet should be dealt with as mentioned on p.299.

Prognosis

Croup is a condition that usually occurs in infants and small children from 1 to 7 years of age. It often appears at the end of a respiratory infection and another attack on the night following the first attack is common. Osteopathic treatment to improve the immune system is helpful and prevents croup attacks.

PNEUMONIA

Young children who have been suffering from chronic lower respiratory tract infections and who are unable to clear secretions may be at a higher risk of bronchopneumonia. Any existing chronic illness in a young child, leading to a weakened immune system, may also render the child more prone to this condition.

Definition

Pneumonia is the name given to inflammation of lung tissue. This is classically of three types: bronchial, interstitial and lobar. The infection may be caused by a variety of microorganisms. The condition may occur in healthy individuals or in the immunosuppressed.

Bronchopneumonia

This type of pneumonia is the most common and is seen more in the very young, very old or immunosuppressed patients. The infection is widespread, often involving both lungs.

Lobar pneumonia

Here the infection is limited by the segments of the lung and is therefore restricted to one lobe only. The symptoms are acute.

Interstitial pneumonia

This type of pneumonia is characterized by diffuse or local damages of the alveolar septa. The bronchioles are not affected here as is the case with bronchopneumonia. Other symptoms are congestion of the lung tissues, where edema, exudation from the alveoli, development of hyaline membranes, emphysema and hyperplasia of the alveolar epithelial layers can be found.

Etiology and pathophysiology

The cause of the infection may be:

- **Primary pneumonia (caused by infection):** viruses, pneumococcus (lobar pneumonia), *Streptococcus pneumoniae*, staphylococcus, *Hemophilus influenzae*, mycoplasma, pseudomonas, chlamydia, fungi, *Pneumocystis carinii*.

- **Secondary pneumonia (symptomatic):** caused by other illnesses: aspiration, artificial respiration, cystic fibrosis, asthma, bronchiectasis, heart valve problems, AIDS, immunopathy, Down syndrome.

- **Non-infectious pneumonia:** not caused by infectious organisms: allergies, rheumatoid arthritis, autoimmune diseases, aspiration or other toxic substances.

The infection leads to inflammatory cells and exudate, which may be within the alveoli, terminal bronchioles and/or air spaces. The untreated inflammation can lead to consolidation of the lung parenchyma.

Toddlers who suffer from chronic infections of the respiratory tract and are not able to cough up the phlegm are at higher risk of developing bronchopneumonia. Any other chronic disease which weakens the immune system can make the child susceptible to bronchopneumonia. Prior to the advent of penicillin, the mortality rate in this type of pneumonia was high and those who recovered were often left with permanent lung damage.

Clinical signs and symptoms

The symptoms in bronchopneumonia are less acute and more diverse than in acute lobar pneumonia. In the beginning you will find a dry cough which becomes more productive later on. The pyrexia is usually milder and there are more symptoms of general malaise. Later there will be breathlessness and pleuritic chest pain.

The child with a lobar pneumonia presents with severe cough, high fever, pleuritic chest pain and dyspnea. In very young children, this may present as grunting, flaring of the nostrils, shallow, rapid breathing and occasionally intercostal recession. The child will have a very flushed face and will appear very ill. Young children often complain of tummy ache and have to vomit.

Diagnosis

Clinical chest examination will show dullness to percussion and crackling on auscultation over the affected lung.

Percussion will also show congestion of the lung and an extensive lobar pneumonia may show a dull percussion. The distribution of sound (see p.115) is increased in lobar pneumonia and decreased in effusion of the lung.

Allopathic diagnosis

Bloodtests are necessary to diagnose pneumonia. The leucocytes are increased and/or the lymphocytes; the ESR and the CRP are usually increased. Only if the pneumonia is very severe is it necessary to analyse the blood gas and test for organisms and bacteria in the blood and sputum. If antibiotics have already been prescribed this may confuse the results of the blood tests.

X-ray shows shadows of consolidation over various lobes of the lungs.

Osteopathic examination

As for croup; see p.301.

Treatment
Allopathic treatment

Children presenting with the above symptoms are usually hospitalized. As the child is very ill, antibiotic cover is usually given prior to or on admission to hospital, and therefore later blood culture results can be misleading.

Cough medicines are only used to ameliorate a severe, painful cough to prevent congestion of the lung. The positive effect of secretion-dissolving medicine has not been proven.

As the child's condition will not be improving and she will be generally very unwell, hospital investigations are usually necessary. Antibiotic treatment is given, even though viral pneumonia may be diagnosed later. The route of administration will depend on how ill the child is and any known predisposing conditions.

Fluid balance is carefully monitored, as the child may be dehydrated. If the fever is very high and the pleuritic chest pain severe, antipyrexial and analgesic drugs may be given to support the child. Oxygen may be administered if dyspnea is causing distress.

Bronchopneumonia can lead to lung abscess or empyema. It can also spread to the pericardium, but the main complication that I have seen is of chronic, recurring inflammation in the form of chest infections due to fibrosis of the affected lung tissue.

Osteopathic treatment

In my experience, I have not been presented with a case of acute pneumonia, although quite often a child will present with subacute respiratory systems similar to the picture given above. I have, however, treated many children subsequent to both lobar and bronchopneumonia who had already been treated conventionally in hospital. I encourage the parents in such cases to bring the child for osteopathic treatment as soon as she has been discharged from hospital. As the treatment of each case has been very specific due to the predisposing causes, age of the child, and so on, for this condition I will describe the osteopathic approach which can be used to treat the acute symptoms and the after-effects of pneumonia.

You may decide to treat a child who presents with the symptoms outlined above before you refer the patient for conventional treatment. This of course will depend on how ill the child is. It may also be possible to treat daily while the child is hospitalized, if this is allowed in your area. In the acute picture, your aim will be:

- to free up all the surrounding structures of the lung or lungs affected; i.e. on the bony, muscular and fascial levels
- to ensure lymphatic drainage: this is obviously of the utmost importance as free passage of toxins is paramount so that the offending inflammation can disperse through the fine lymphatic and venous channels
- to approach the 'wounded' lung tissue itself
- to then use IVM to bring balance to the entire mechanism in order to enhance immune function and the child's inherent ability to heal herself.

This may sound like a lot of work or a very long treatment on an ill child. I assure you that all the above aims can be brought together easily and very effectively in a short and gentle fashion and with great compassion for the ill child in your hands.

The structures involved in the acute picture will be:

- the thoracic spine, especially from T6–L1/2/3, C3/4/5
- the ribs in the area of lung affected, but also
- rib 1 and rib 12 (to ensure adequate drainage through the cysterna chyli and the thoracic inlet)
- the clavicles
- the sternum.

In releasing the above structures, you will have dealt also with the nerves supplying the affected lung, whether phrenic or the sympathetic chain ganglia. You will also have dealt with the attached and associated muscles, whether paraspinal, intercostal or the secondary muscles of respiration.

The major horizontal muscle of the body now needs special attention; that is, the diaphragm.

Releasing the diaphragm and 12th ribs will free up the medial arcuate ligaments, in turn improving arterial, venous and lymphatic drainage, as well as further encouraging fuller expansion of the whole thoracic cage and freedom and space for the affected lung. You will already have indirectly released the anterior cervical fascia, though you may need to address this more specifically if necessary. From prior release of the sternum and clavicles, you have mobilized the fascial continuum through the mediastinum right up to its attachment to the cranial base, thus stimulating the function of the thoracic duct and thymus gland.

At this stage, having released and encouraged fuller excursion of the thoracic cage and enhanced better arterial, venous, lymphatic and nerve supply to and from the affected lung, you have prepared the body to receive the outpouring of infected exudate and indeed 'shock' from the sick lung. When speaking of pneumonia, Still (1986) writes: 'in changes of atmospheric conditions, the lungs receive shocks which wound or disturb the natural harmony of lung-action by irritating the nerve-terminals as they appear in the mucous membrane of the lungs'.

To release the consolidation in the lung field, you can hold the affected area depending on the site needing treatment, either anteriorly, posteriorly or anteroposteriorly (a/p) (Fig. 14.6). I almost always treat small children with this condition, using an a/p contact, while they sit on my lap. You can feel the sick, congested and 'loaded' or 'heavy' part and you will sense the need to gently lift or just wait for the lobe to release from its pleuritic envelope and regain its freer, inherent motility. You will almost always feel the release of shock to some degree, depending on the severity of the case.

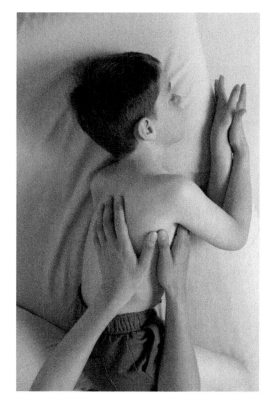

Figure 14.6 Release of a consolidation in the lung field. With permission, Karsten Frank, Hamburg

You have now reached the final step of engaging the entire IVM, preferably at the cranium, and allowing balance and rhythm to reinstate. This in turn leads to the calming and balancing of CNS and ANS activity and allows the neuroendocrine and immune systems to function to the best of their ability for the healing process of pneumonia in this child.

In children who have had bronchopneumonia and are now suffering from more chronic and recurrent chest infections due to fibrosis, the above treatment approach is still appropriate. In these children, I would also discuss diet and encourage a regular form of exercise. I would also demonstrate a diaphragmatic breathing exercise to be carried out with the supervision of a parent in the older child.

Prognosis

Treatment with the appropriate organism-sensitive antibiotic is good and a previously healthy child should make a full recovery.

Osteopathy is highly beneficial in the treatment of pneumonia, in conjunction with the appropriate allopathic treatment. As mentioned earlier, it would be wonderful if osteopaths in all areas were allowed to treat the children during the acute phase in hospital as this would greatly influence and speed their recovery. However, if this is not possible, osteopathic treatment is still highly recommended as soon as possible after the infection, where prevention of chronic lobar dysfunction due to fibrosis is possible.

BRONCHIOLITIS
Definition

This is an acute viral infection of the lower respiratory tract. It affects infants and toddlers under the age of 24 months. The children have an increased need for oxygen, and present with tachypnea, dyspnea and labored breathing.

Etiology and pathophysiology

Bronchiolitis is usually associated with the respiratory syncytial virus (RSV) though other viruses may be found. Recurrent episodes may lead to fibrosis and a long term overinflation picture and it is unclear whether there is a relationship between bronchiolitis in infancy and subsequent asthma or recurrent lower respiratory infections in older children and adults.

Clinical signs and symptoms

The illness usually begins with a common cold. The symptoms are of coughing associated with feeding difficulties. Breathing becomes labored. Usually only slight fever is present.

Intercostal retractions may be seen, as well as tachypnea with nasal flaring and sometimes cyanosis and crackling. Breathing can become very shallow – the more it does the greater the danger for the child.

Control via monitor is vital due to danger of apnea and sudden death.

Diagnosis

The symptoms such as labored breathing lead to the diagnosis. The breathing is shallow, the more shallow, the more dangerous to the child. Auscultation shows crackling and wheezing, prolonged expiration sounds are heard.

Allopathic diagnosis

X-rays show 'overinflation' of part of a lung and in serious cases may show lung consolidation or collapse. Tests of blood gases may show an increase in CO_2.

Osteopathic examination

As for croup, See p.301.

Treatment
Allopathic treatment

Infants hospitalized are usually nursed in an oxygen enriched environment. If the breathing difficulty is exacerbated by attempts to feed, nasogastric tube feeding may be necessary – or infusion in the short term for very ill babies – to guarantee enough fluid intake. Antibiotics should not be necessary unless the condition is superimposed by a bacterial infection.

In some cases intubation and artificial respiration are necessary as the labored breathing can tire children easily.

Control via monitor is vital due to danger of apnea and sudden death.

Osteopathic treatment

> **Case history**
> Michael, aged 13 months, was brought by his parents with a history of recurrent bronchiolitis. The worst episodes occurred when he was 6 weeks and 3 months old and he was hospitalized each time. Although bronchiolitis was diagnosed each time, he was given antibiotics, prednisolone and nebulized. He was then given a preventative inhaler to be used twice daily at home. More recently he had also suffered from ear infections and nasal congestion.
>
> Michael was the third of three boys in his family. His birth history was uneventful apart from a very fast second stage of labor. On examination, Michael was a very contented and

happy little boy and all his development milestones were excellent. I found a very sluggish and weakened expression of involuntary motion and immune system. He had restrictions through the right mid and upper ribs anteriorly. The main focus however was of a significant intraosseous strain of the occipital squama, with the right side grossly flattened in relation to the left side. The left occipitomastoid suture was also restricted and both temporals were held in external rotation. There was a discrepancy of the flexion and extension phases of IVM expression between the vault, viscerocranium and cranial base.

Michael's first treatment was mainly involved in releasing the right ribs at the costochondral junctions and some release of the cranial base. I suggested a change from cow's to goat's milk.

At his second appointment, Michael's parents reported that he had had a runny nose, thick and yellow since the first session. He had also had an episode of coughing for which he had been given another course of antibiotics. He was drinking goat's milk happily. During this and a subsequent three treatments, the focus of release was at the cranium, as the thorax and ribs had maintained wonderful mobility since the first session.

The main focus of dysfunction was the discrepancy of IVM expression between the vault and cranial base. The vault was in the extreme extension phase and the cranial base, including the temporals, was in the extreme flexion phase.

Michael responded beautifully to balanced membranous tension (BMT) release and balancing of his whole reciprocal tension membrane system through the ribcage and diaphragm. At each visit his parents reported 'wonderful improvements', with no symptoms and no need for an inhaler.

When I saw him for a 6 monthly check up he had continued to maintain all the changes that he had made during his first four treatments. I arranged to see Michael every 6 months so that any imbalances caused by growth spurts, falls or emotional traumas could be treated and integrated.

Case summary

In Michael's case, although he had been diagnosed with viral bronchiolitis on a couple of occasions, it was clear that he was now prone to recurrent respiratory infections. Each time he was offered antibiotics and other medications which, over time, were dampening his immune system. At this young age, this could easily be picked up on palpation, with the sluggish and weak amplitude of the IVM expression.

In this case the thorax and ribs seemed only compensatory and the focus of osteopathic treatment was in the cranium. There, the disturbed RTM was affecting the venous sinus drainage through the entire cranium, leading to stasis and lack of drainage. This in turn was leading to ear infections and nasal congestion. The disturbed RTM to the thorax and mediastinum was holding the anterior ribs, and in Michael's case I suggest that he had an already compromized, overinflated lung field due to his rapid first breath.

Prognosis

This disease is self limiting and usually resolves after 4 to7 days. Complications can appear by secondary bacterial infections or insufficient breathing, making artificial respiration necessary.

Osteopaths can obviously play an important role in treating infants as soon as possible after an episode of bronchiolitis. It is essential that we treat all the underlying somatic dysfunctions, in turn preventing recurrent infections and the likelihood of permanent damage to the lungs due to fibrosis.

BRONCHITIS
Definition

Acute bronchitis is an inflammation of mucous membranes of the bronchial tubes. A large number of such cases will be brought to the osteopath with symptoms of recurrent chest infections. This inflammation is seen mostly in autumn and winter.

The classical definition of chronic bronchitis is a productive cough lasting for 3 months at least twice in 2 years. This type of bronchitis is usually seen in the older child and adult.

More common in younger children is obstructive bronchitis.

Etiology and pathophysiology

Acute bronchitis is usually caused by infectious agents, such as bacteria or viruses and mycosis. It may also be caused by physical or chemical agents – dusts, allergens, strong fumes, and those from chemical cleaning compounds, or tobacco smoke. Acute bronchitis may follow the common cold or other viral infections in the upper respiratory tract. It may also occur in children with chronic sinusitis, allergies, or those with enlarged tonsils and adenoids. It is usually a mild condition although pneumonia is a complication that can follow.

In children obstructive bronchitis is often due to a viral infection, seldom allergic in origin and often amplified by stress and exertion.

Clinical signs and symptoms

In the earlier stages of acute bronchitis, children may experience a dry, non-productive cough, which progresses later to an abundant mucus-filled cough. Younger children may have some vomiting or gagging with the cough. The symptoms of bronchitis usually last 7 to 14 days, but may also persist for 3 to 4 weeks.

Children with a chronic bronchitis have a productive cough in the mornings. The mucus is yellow to green. Pyrexia is found in the early stages but disappears after a couple of days.

The symptoms in obstructive bronchitis are similar (as mentioned above) but may include: spasm of the bronchi, dry cough with expiratory dyspnea, rhonchus, wheezing, tachypnea, prolonged expiration and tummy ache.

Differential diagnosis

It is important to differentiate between pneumonia, asthma, aspiration of objects, bronchiolitis and cystic fibrosis.

If the case history is not clear and there is sudden onset of the illness, without having signs of infection (e.g. a runny nose), aspiration of an object is probable.

Diagnosis

Allopathic diagnosis

Acute bronchitis is easily diagnosed solely on the history and physical examination of the child. Crackling can be heard over the lung field on auscultation and the throat may be inflamed and red. Further examination is not necessary.

A chronic cough as seen in chronic bronchitis has to be examined further for differential diagnosis. Blood tests, chest X-rays, pulse oximetry, sputum cultures and lung tests are helpful.

In a child with spastic bronchitis, wheezing and crackling can be heard over the lung field on auscultation.

Osteopathic examination

As for croup, See p.301.

Treatment

Allopathic treatment

The treatment for acute bronchitis is to ameliorate the pain, increase fluid intake, lower the fever, and breathing exercises are given to mobilize the mucus. Inhalation with sodium chloride is possible. Cough mixtures and secretolytics do not help.

The treatment for chronic bronchitis is according to the underlying disease. It is most important to banish cigarette smoke in the environment, and allergens. Medicines to mobilize the mucus are only of questionable help. Usually antibiotics are given, but it is best that they are prescribed according to a culture of the mucus.

Most of the treatment in spastic bronchitis is supportive of the symptoms the child has, and may include: calming the child, increasing fluid intake, cool mist humidifier, and bronchodilator therapy in combination with parasympatholytics. In severe cases theophyllin or cortisol is given. Cough medicine is not useful.

Antihistamines are avoided, in most cases, because they dry up the secretions and can make the cough worse. A continuing therapy with steroids is common in recurrent obstructive bronchitis.

In many cases, antibiotic treatment is not necessary to treat acute and obstructive bronchitis, since most of the infections are caused by viruses. Should there be danger of bronchopneumonia, antibiotics are indicated.

Osteopathic treatment

These cases are regularly seen in the osteopathic practice, often with symptoms of recurrent infection of the respiratory tract.

Case history

Laura, aged 6 years, was brought by her parents after having suffering from recurrent chest infections since she was 2½ years old. One such infection led to pneumonia when she was 5, for which she was in hospital for 5 days. She had also been in hospital at 9 months old when she had an apneac attack. She had glandular fever when she was 3 years of age. Over the years, she had been prescribed courses of antibiotics and various inhalers for chest infections almost every winter month of her young life.

Laura was the eldest of three children. She was induced at 42 weeks gestation because of post maturity and her weight was slightly light at 7 lbs. Although the first stage of labor was average, the second stage was very prolonged. After 2 hours of pushing, a high rotational forceps delivery was carried out.

At our first consultation, I observed Laura to be a complex little character, quite fidgety and constantly answering questions with a joke or a totally opposite response to what one might expect. It was very obvious to me from the beginning that she was not happy in her body, was acting in a 'babyish' manner and had an extremely close bond to her mother, which the latter described as 'unhealthy'. Laura was very underweight and pale and her appetite was extremely poor. She never ate breakfast and had to be fed mashed vegetables at dinner. She craved milk and all refined sugar foods, including spoonfuls of actual refined sugar.

On examination, I found a very disturbed posture of the whole body with marked kyphosis and strain across the cervicodorsal area. There was a side shift of the head on neck and a 'rigid' feel to the entire spine. There was significant vertebral restriction from T4–T6 and T7–T10. There was hypertonus of the diaphragm and the posterior cervical muscles. I found a medial compression of the mediastinum and compression of the right occipital condyle. My first treatment involved not only much osteopathic release and balancing of the whole body but a long discussion with Laura's parents regarding her diet.

I tested Laura for various typically offending foods and found that milk and sugar completely weakened her system. I therefore strongly advised that all sugar and milk be excluded from her diet if at all possible until the next appointment 2 weeks later. I also suggested a natural herbal immune system enhancer, probiotic supplementation and regular swimming.

As treatments continued, Laura improved gradually but slowly. Although the strain patterns in her body released and improved, she found it extremely difficult to avoid her sugar foods and had been found in a cupboard eating sugar lumps. The immune system and IVM expression was weak and slow to respond. However, with persistence of treatments on my part and continuing to cut down on sugar on her part, improvements eventually did occur.

After six treatments, Laura was eating a healthy breakfast cereal (without sugar!), drinking lots of water and her general appetite was much better. She had experienced a cough on two occasions in all that time but had never needed antibiotic or other medication. The main focus of disturbance was the medial compression of the mediastinum and the occipital condylar compression, both of which are not now evident.

A year after I first met her, Laura was looking much better, was gaining weight and had not suffered from any further chest infections. However, because her system was so exhausted and low, I knew that I needed to continue working with her every few months for a while until she became stronger.

Case summary

Laura's case is interesting in that there was evidence of a traumatic forceps delivery with a poor first breath and medial compression of the mediastinum. However, these strain patterns released quite quickly and it was her addictive personality that seemed to be more the focus of her chronic condition than any physical element. She found it very difficult to 'let go' of things; for example the womb (induced for postmaturity and prolonged labor). Other examples were the bond with her mother and her craving for sugar. Following osteopathic treatment and releasing her physical body, and by Laura altering her diet, she was better able to accept and feel more comfortable in her own body. She eventually felt more confident and independent and has 'let go' a lot from her mother. Her sugar diet was exacerbating the chronically lowered immune system caused by the vicious cycle of chest infections and antibiotics. It has been wonderful to witness the changes she is making, and the rapid growth of her mind, body and spirit.

Prognosis

Most often this condition is not too severe and is usually self-limiting but pneumonia as a complication is possible.

Bronchitis can be influenced by osteopathy. In acute bronchitis few treatments are necessary to help the child cope with the infection and improve breathing and lung function. However, in cases of recurrent bronchitis it is important to see the child for a longer period of time in order to strengthen the immune system and to treat old restricting conditions. A special diet avoiding milk protein is also helpful.

BRONCHIAL ASTHMA

Definition

Bronchial asthma is characterized by strong reactions to inhalation stimuli causing bouts of bronchospasm, with obstruction of the respiratory tract caused by hyperreactivity of the tissues and an inflammation that leads to symptoms of dyspnea.

Etiology and pathophysiology

The occurrence of asthma is most probably genetic. There are two independent factors, the bronchial hyperreactivity and the allergic disposition (allergic reaction type 1) which lead to this condition and they can amplify each other.

The obstruction of the respiratory tract is caused by

- production of too much viscous mucus
- mucosal edema due to increased blood flow, edema and infiltration of inflammatory secretion
- bronchospasms (spasm of the smooth bronchial muscles).

Asthma triggers may be viral respiratory infections, allergens (pollen, mites, animal fur, food), exertion, psychological stress, and non-specific irritants. Usually the family has a history of asthma or other allergies.

Asthma patients tend to have high palates, corresponding with an extension pattern of the cranium. The ANS is often facilitated.

Clincial signs and symptoms

The child has a combination of symptoms: a dry cough, usually worse at night, wheezing, chest tightness and difficulty in breathing, tummy ache, anxiety, cyanosis, expiratory dyspnea, prolonged expiration. In chronic cases of obstruction the posture of the child may have adapted to her condition, causing deformation of the thorax and shortening of the pectoralis muscles.

Differential diagnosis

As differential diagnosis, keep in mind bronchiolitis, bronchitis, aspiration of objects, pneumonia, cystic fibrosis, bronchial obstruction due to other causatives (lymphnodules, vascular), gastro-esophageal reflux.

Diagnosis

To distinguish asthma from other lung disorders, physicians rely on a combination of medical history, physical examination, and laboratory tests. During auscultation, expiratory wheezing can be heard and the breathing may be shallow during a strong attack. This is an alarm signal showing a change for the worse.

Allopathic diagnosis

The basic diagnosis includes: spirometry, peak flow monitoring, chest X-rays (to check for deformities and local disturbances), blood tests (eosinophils, alpha-antitrypsin), allergy tests (pricktest, IgE test in the serum), sweat tests.

Osteopathic examination

As for croup, See p.301.

Treatment

Allopathic treatment

The aim of the treatment is to avoid asthma attacks and to enable normal physical and psychological development as well as normal lung function. Therefore it is necessary to treat infections and to normalize the hypersensitivity of the bronchi. Furthermore, it is important to avoid obstruction of the respiratory tract by abolishing the causative factors and to reduce medication.

The non-medical therapy includes: seating the child in an upright position so that she can use the secondary respiratory muscles, avoidance of allergens, keeping the child calm, abolishing smoke in the environment, breathing therapy and breathing exercises.

The aim of medical intervention is to eliminate bronchial obstruction and infection. Inhalation of bronchodilators (beta-mimetic drugs) and corticosteroids (theophylline) and antihistamines (if an allergic disposition is present) are given. Antibiotics are seldom necessary. Sedatives are to be avoided as they depress breathing; also beta blockers as they increase obstruction.

If an allergy is present a hyposensitivity therapy may be useful.

Osteopathic treatment

Asthma is a common condition in young children and cases will very often be brought for osteopathic treatment.

In my practice, the majority of children who have been 'labelled' as asthmatics are on a combination of corticosteroid and bronchodilator inhalers long term, even though the children may not have had any symptoms for more than a year.

Case history

Fred, aged 9 years, presented with 'asthma'. He had been medically diagnosed at 2½ years old. Since then he had been hospitalized five or six times. He had been taking both preventative and bronchodilating inhalers over these years and had been given courses of antibiotics and prednisolone on many occasions.

Fred became very wheezy when the seasons changed and was affected by cat hair, dust, pollen and the air in aeroplanes. His symptoms were of a wheezy cough that repeatedly developed into chest infections.

Fred was a very quiet but sociable boy. He had no problems with schoolwork. An interesting part of his history was that he was the first born of two boys and his parents had been trying to conceive for 10 years. His mother reported having felt 'totally stressed and worried' during the entire pregnancy and during Fred's 1st year of life.

Although the onset of his labor was spontaneous at 41 weeks gestation and his weight was average, his mother could not explain why he had been rushed out of the delivery room after birth. She managed to breast feed for 1 week only, and then gave up as she and the baby were so stressed. He had a caput succedaneum at birth and had slight jaundice. One aunt had a history of eczema.

On examination, I found that Fred's whole body was compromized, possibly due to an extended head in utero, leading to a ventouse delivery. His whole posture was grossly disturbed with a functional scoliosis, unlevel scapulae and posterior superior ilisc spines (PSISs) and a significant side-bending of his head. His upper to mid-thoracic spine was significantly kyphosed.

Interestingly, on further examination, I found that his ANS and CNS were hyperfacilitated, which could have been due to the high adrenal setting from his mother in utero and/or exacerbated by his long term use of sympathomimetic drugs.

My treatment plan consisted firstly of releasing all layers of chronic postural compensations. I advised on diet, excluding orange drinks and dairy, which he had been taking, and suggested alternatives. His anxious mother was reassured.

After the first treatment, his postural alignment was almost perfect. He was a happy and well-loved child and therefore had the ability to make changes quickly and easily with treatment. He had taken all the dietary advice. It became apparent at the second treatment that the primary focus was at Fred's disturbed head-neck relationship, where there was a strong structural extension pattern at the occipito-atlantal joint (probably due to an extended head in utero).

On the third treatment, the cervical spine was much improved and the focus now lay at the left parietal where I found a traumatic fulcrum of trauma and traction on a membranous level, possibly as a result of the ventouse extraction. The shock which was released was immense and I had to work to integrate the CNS, in this case the occipital lobe with the left hemisphere. The following month Fred returned and his mother reported a 'great improvement' on all levels. She said he had not suffered any episodes of wheezing since the first treatment, though he had coughed for a few days after each session. He was much happier in himself and was enjoying PE (physical exercise) in school for the first time in his life.

During the following two monthly sessions, Fred continued to change. His confidence improved immensely and his mother reported that, academically and socially, his school life had become so much easier.

I treated Fred again, 9 months after his initial consultation, and both he and his mother were really happy and well. He had no further wheezing, coughs or chest infections. His balanced posture was being maintained very well. There was no evidence of any strain pattern and his involuntary mechanism was vibrant and relaxed. He had discontinued all inhalers with the consent of his general medical practitioner. I asked to see Fred again 3 months later.

Case summary

Fred may well have had an extrinsic asthma but, osteopathically, it was obvious that his body was significantly compromised due to stress during the pregnancy and possibly an extended head in utero, which led to a traumatic ventouse delivery. He then suffered all the compensatory effects of that primary trauma over the following 9 years. It is easy for us as osteopaths to understand how our findings led to his symptoms of coughing, wheezing and chest infections. The main foci in his case were disturbances in his atlanto-occipital junction, leading to a structural extension pattern, which was disturbing vagal function to his lungs. The ANS/CNS facilitation was also disturbing autonomic distribution to the respiratory system. The shock which was retained in the dural membranes from the trauma of the ventouse was affecting the whole RTM.

Prognosis

As the case history demonstrates, asthma does respond well to osteopathic treatment, especially if nutritional aspects are included. The importance of cooperation with the medical practitioner must be emphasized, particularly when medication is supposed to be reduced or discontinued.

Bibliography

Carreiro J: An osteopathic approach to children, Elsevier, Edinburgh 2003

Frymann V: The collected papers of Viola M. Frymann, DO. American Academy of Osteopathy, Mich. 1998

Goldbloom R: Pediatric clinical skills. 2nd edn. Churchill Livingstone, New York 1997

Moore K: The developing human. Clinically oriented embryology. 4th edn. Saunders, Philadelphia 1988

Rowley N: Basic clinical science. Describing a rose with a ruler. Hodder and Stoughton, London 1991

Still A T: The philosophy and mechanical principles of osteopathy. Osteopathic Enterprise, Kansas City, Mo. 1986

Sutherland W G: Teachings in the science of osteopathy. Rudra press, Portland, Ore. 1990

Giles Cleghorn, Eva Moeckel

COMMON ORTHOPEDIC CONDITIONS

Giles Cleghorn

Babies and young children are often presented on account of asymmetries of the head (plagiocephaly), the neck (torticollis) and the body (such as scoliosis), each of which is dealt with in further detail in this chapter. In small children these asymmetries may cause immediate symptoms, but not invariably. However, asymmetries of any kind predispose the child to the development of other postural abnormalities or scoliosis with its known damaging effects. As a general rule, osteopathic treatment can be beneficial here, and guard the child from late sequelae.

Less common orthopedic disorders of early childhood which we encounter in practice, and which we will look at more closely in this chapter, include craniosynostosis and hip dysplasia. Treatment of these is indeed more difficult, but in many cases osteopathy will improve both the general health of the child and bring about positive changes in the tissues of the problematical area.

Older children are often presented because of malposition of the spine, pelvis, knee or feet. At this time, these deviations from the normal position are often, although not always, asymptomatic, but if left untreated can lead in many cases to muscular pain and premature osteoarthrosis. Osteopathic treatments are successfully used to treat functional disturbances of the spine, but they can also be of help in pathological conditions.

Osteopaths are often also asked to treat children with disorders of the lower extremities. Properly functioning legs are a prerequisite for normal walking, running, hopping and jumping. More demanding movements are required for dancing, gymnastic exercises or sporting activities. If the function of the legs is limited, the body is robbed of many opportunities. Many conditions of the lower extremities are functional in nature and usually one must then advise against surgical correction. When one treats the legs, the body's proprioceptive system is also addressed. The feet, the interosseous membrane of the lower leg and the lumbar fascia deserve especial mention here as they are particularly rich in proprioceptors. Normalization of these tissues usually reduces atypical feedback mechanisms, which

could worsen any functional disorder of the lower extremities still further. Children normally walk, hop and run a great deal; if the locomotor system is in equilibrium, they have a balanced sensory input, which is important for the appropriate linkage and integration of the developing sensory and motor systems. These considerations of course also apply to movements of the upper extremities and of the torso.

Worried parents often ask us to examine their children's feet because of a 'pigeon-toed' gait (see Genu varum, Genu valgum, below) or flat feet. This perceived 'deformity' is often purely physiological in origin, therefore age-appropriate for the developmental stage of the legs and/or feet, and does not require treatment. In some cases, however, examination will uncover delayed development of the normal axial changes of the legs, or in the development of the plantar arches. Osteopathic treatment can be especially helpful in functional problems. Early and consistent treatment can then prevent the child developing structural deformities during growth. But even in pathological conditions, osteopathic treatments can often considerably lessen deformity.

Children with disorders such as Perthes disease, slipped capital femoral epiphysis or juvenile rheumatoid arthritis are less often brought to an osteopathic practice but we will also deal with these in this chapter. Treatment in such a case is not easy; osteopathy will probably be only a part of a more comprehensive plan of treatment. As it may well happen, however, that an osteopath is asked to participate in the treatment of such a disorder, these conditions are also discussed in this chapter.

I would like to stress at this point that in all cases of pathology we should always work together with orthopedic consultants and doctors. I never take on an orthopedic case without the knowledge that the child is also under a consultant's care and constant review. With pathology, osteopathy can be seen as an adjunct to the child's overall treatment and care. It can, nevertheless, be a vital part of the total care package. It may help in securing great changes and improvement in health which I feel would not be achieved without our osteopathic care and skills.

In my osteopathic practice, my experience is that two therapeutic approaches are particularly useful for children with orthopedic conditions: intraosseous work (see Ch.8, Intraosseous strains) and treatment of the blood vessels.

Intraosseous treatment

In order to decompress an intraosseous lesion pattern, one must 'place oneself inside' the interior of the bone; that is, inside the bone marrow and the bone matrix. To achieve this it may be helpful to bring to mind how the bone has come into being.

The principle for this type of treatment is: the lighter the touch, the deeper the contact. Hold the bone quite gently, like a bird alighting on a small twig. If you work forcefully, the bone will probably guard itself to protect itself from you. With children, it is generally possible to obtain a decompression of the bone by being very gentle. The lesion will resolve spontaneously. In some cases, however, a greater expenditure of effort is required, appropriate to the tissue tension in the relevant case.

Treatment of the blood vessels

For Dr. Still, treatment of the blood vessels was a special concern (1910). One of his favourite mottoes was: 'The rule of the artery is supreme.' Osteopathic treatment of the blood vessels is one way to improve blood supply. It can definitely benefit many orthopedic conditions.

Blood vessels are large muscular structures with an enormous vital potential. They are no more difficult to palpate than the pituitary through the bony cranium. During palpation, one has only to concentrate consciously on the blood vessel and to turn one's attention away from other structures. Practise feeling for the major arteries in the legs. Practise palpation of the heart and then attempt to palpate the blood in the heart. This hot, rich and vital fluid is as easy to feel as cerebrospinal fluid.

PLAGIOCEPHALY

Giles Cleghorn

Definition

Babies with plagiocephaly are quite often brought to the practice of an osteopath who does cranial work. In plagiocephaly the two sides of the cranium visibly differ from each other and the cranium is often completely asymmetrical, with flattened or bulging areas. The name plagiocephaly comes from the Greek and means 'crooked head' (from *plagios* = crooked and *kephale* = head).

Etiology and pathogenesis

In some cases, plagiocephaly is caused by the strong molding forces of an asymmetric uterus. If, for instance, the mother suffers from a big myoma this may mold the child's head as he grows in utero. A deformation of the child's head can also ensue from a difficult labor, especially if delivery is with the aid of ventouse or forceps. A marked asymmetry may occur especially when the child's ability to self-correct his cranium is restricted (see Ch.5, Difficult delivery). A normal birth does not, to my knowledge, result in plagiocephaly.

In premature births the risk of deformity to the child's head increases because the bones will be still very soft and malleable at the time of birth. Also, premature babies may develop plagiocephaly postnatally, from not having their position alternated enough – if they lie too long in one position and their still very malleable heads are not adequately supported by cushions. As premature babies are usually moved as little as possible, especially in intensive care, the head often stays in the same position for far too long.

Another cause, which is also usually connected with the intrauterine position, or the birth of the baby, is torticollis (see p.316). Craniosynostosis can also cause plagiocephaly (see p.315).

A mild plagiocephaly can also often arise with the advised supine position, which is intended to minimize the risk of sudden infant death. Here, a typical flattening of the occiput is found.

Rarely, rickets can produce plagiocephaly, as it can also soften the cranial bones. Genetic causes have also been discussed as an etiological component.

Clinical signs and symptoms

Inspection of the head shows that part of the cranial vault is very much flattened whereas another part has an unusual bulge. The cranium may show the typical 'parallelogram head', an asymmetric head shape, which owes its name to the observation that it resembles a parallelogram when viewed from above (Fig. 15.1). The position of the eyes and ears can differ greatly from one side to another.

In craniosynostosis, you might find a protuberance of the affected cranial suture or abnormal hair growth. Plagiocephaly can quite often also be found in older children with idiopathic scoliosis. The plagiocephaly may possibly have been a cause of this form of scoliosis.

Diagnosis

Diagnostic procedures include inspection and palpation of the cranial bones with reference to their position, and palpation of the cranial sutures and fontanelles.

Slow head growth, a continual increase of the plagiocephaly and delayed development, whether alone or in combination,

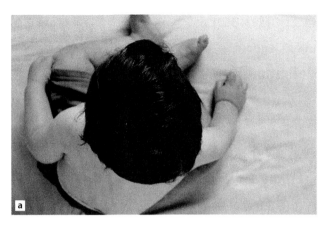

Figure 15.1 Baby with plagiocephaly. **a:** View of the head from above. **b:** View of the head from the side. **c:** Frontal view of the head. **d:** Helmet therapy.
With permission, Karsten Franke, Hamburg

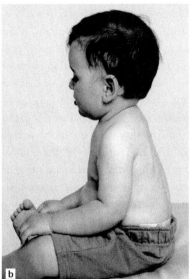
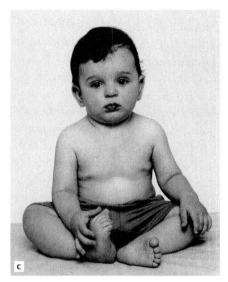
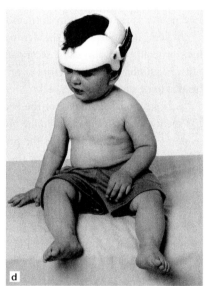

can point to craniosynostosis (Carreiro 2004). To rule out craniosynostosis or torticollis, a careful examination of the head, cranial sutures, neck and especially the sternocleidomastoid muscle is needed.

Allopathic diagnostic procedures

If craniosynostosis is suspected, X-rays ultrasound and CCT are the usual diagnostic tools.

Osteopathic examination

Apart from the above mentioned examination, osteopathic diagnostic examination also includes palpation of the head with the aid of involuntary motion. Special attention is paid here to intraosseous restrictions and strain patterns of the cranial base. All functional associations which emerge from the diagnostic findings relating to the rest of the body are of course also taken into account.

Treatment

Allopathic medical treatment

Helmet therapy has been increasingly offered for some time (see Fig. 15.1d). As with osteopathic treatment, the results of this treatment are best if it is started before the age of 6 months and applied within the first 12 months of life. Especially in extreme cases of plagiocephaly, a combination of helmet therapy and osteopathy may be useful.

Osteopathic treatment

The type of osteopathic treatment, its intensity and success depends to a large extent on the cause in each case.

Primary plagiocephaly

Intrauterine molding and extreme forces in labor, as in an especially lengthy birth, above all if it was ended with forceps or ventouse, are usually the cause of a primary plagiocephaly. The fluid field may be disturbed by the difficult labor, and distortions frequently occur at the cranial base. For an appropriate treatment of the cranium see Ch.8, Principles of osteopathic treatment.

Secondary plagiocephaly

This is a secondary cranial asymmetry which has other underlying causes. It generally develops more slowly and therefore often does not appear for some weeks or months. Here, the causative factors must always be treated and eliminated as far as possible. For instance, one reason could be a lesion of C1 fixing the head in a unilateral rotation and thus leading to a corresponding malformation of the head.

Problems in the region of the sternocleidomastoid muscle, like torticollis, can also cause secondary plagiocephaly; they must be eliminated if the treatment of the asymmetry of the head is to be successful.

With positional flattening of the occiput, when the baby has spent too much time in a supine position, it is important to point out to the parents that the prone position does not only promote the development of the arm and leg muscles but also completes the shaping of the occipital bone through the increased use of the erector spinae muscles in the prone position.

If craniosynostosis has been diagnosed, cranial osteopathic treatment may help improve malleability within the bone.

Prognosis

The prognosis depends on several factors; above all, however, on the severity of the pathological change, the cause and the time treatment begins. The earlier the child is treated the better are the results, and they are best if one can treat the child as early as the first months of life. Regular and frequent treatment is often necessary, especially if it is suspected that the change in head shape is caused by the position in utero.

In mild or moderate cases a satisfactory resolution can be expected with osteopathic treatment. The course of the treatment may last between 12 and 18 months. After that I recommend 6-monthly check-ups until the situation has stabilized. At every visit the whole spine must be examined to rule out a secondary scoliosis, even if the cranial problem has improved already.

In severe cases the cranial asymmetry might persist long-term. The developing face, however, distracts considerably from this disorder, because we look at people's eyes and not at the shape of their heads. At the very least, this asymmetry will cease to look unsightly once hair growth increases.

CRANIOSYNOSTOSIS
Giles Cleghorn
Definition

Craniosynostosis is the premature closure of the cranial sutures and fontanelles, leading to abnormal head shapes, depending on the site affected. It is found in about 1:2000–3000 babies.

Etiology and pathogenesis

Genetic causes seem to play an important role in some types of craniosynostosis; for example, if craniosynostosis is found as part of a syndrome. However, as part of a syndrome it is, at 1:25,000–100,000 births, very much less common. Most genetic forms are dominant; in other words, an affected person has a 50% chance of passing this predisposition to his or her children.

One of the external (non-genetic) causes is said to be compression of the child's cranium in utero, as can easily occur in multiple pregnancies or if the mother has a uterine myoma.

Carreiro (2004) regards strain patterns in the cranial base as causative, leading to abnormal mechanical stretching forces on the vault. In her opinion, the premature ossification of the sutures arises from these powerful stretching forces, not from a compression in the region of the suture.

Certain diseases, such as hyperthyroidism, thalassemia or sickle cell anemia, are associated with an increased risk of craniosynostosis.

Clinical signs and symptoms

From a medical viewpoint, the main concern is that a premature fusion of the cranial sutures will not allow sufficient space for the growing brain, because the growth of the cranial bones occurs chiefly in the region of the cartilaginous sutures. The result can be an increase in intracranial pressure with grave neurological consequences.

The most obvious clinical finding is a change in the shape of the head (Fig. 15.2). Normally, it is the growth of the brain that determines the shape of the head. The bony cranium grows by the enlargement of the individual bones which grow peripherally (i.e. to the side of the sutures). Growth takes place at an angle of 90° to the direction of the suture. If a suture has fused prematurely this growth is no longer possible.

Therefore, the premature fusion of, for instance, the sagittal suture will prevent the widthways growth of the cranium. As the growing brain demands space, however, the cranium grows into a longish, narrow shape, which is termed scaphocephaly (boat-shaped cranium or long, narrow cranium), as the vault

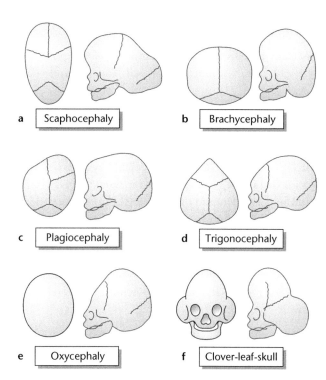

Figure 15.2 Skull shapes in craniosynostosis. **a:** Scaphocephaly in synostosis of the sagittal suture. **b:** Brachycephaly in bilateral synostosis of the coronal sutures. **c:** Plagiocephaly in unilateral synostosis of the coronal suture. **d:** Trigonocephaly in synostosis of the frontal suture. **e:** Oxycephaly (turret skull) in multiple synostoses of the sutures. **f:** Clover-leaf skull in premature synostosis of all the sutures.
With permission, Henriette Rintelen, Velbert

tapers towards the vertex in a wedge shape. The forehead is relatively prominent. A premature closure of the sagittal suture is the most common, occurring in about 55% of cases. Boys are three times more commonly affected by this than girls.

The second most common, at about 20%, is a synostosis of the coronal suture, which prevents cranial growth lengthwise. The cranium therefore has to grow widthways and a brachycephaly occurs (short or broad head). Bilateral coronal suture synostosis is more common in Crouzon and Apert syndromes.

Other cranial shapes arise if only part of a suture fuses prematurely; this can be a cause of an asymmetrical cranial shape, plagiocephaly.

Premature fusion of the lambdoid suture is rarer. If, however, the lambdoid suture fuses on one side, the cranium will seem flattened on that side, whereas the other side will be prominent. With bilateral synostosis of the lambdoid suture, the head seems short and broad.

Premature closure of the frontal suture often leads to a wedge-shaped elevation. Looking at the head from above, the anterior region of the head seems triangular. This is why

it is called trigonocephaly (triangular head). It is often associated with general developmental disorders caused by genetic conditions.

Premature ossification of all cranial sutures leads to a cloverleaf cranium, which is associated with markedly elevated increases in intracranial pressure.

Diagnosis

With any cranial asymmetry, and especially if a premature fusion of the sutures is suspected, the sutures are carefully palpated to feel for any ridge-like thickenings and to ascertain the size of the fontanelles. The head circumference is measured at regular intervals (see p.103) to see whether head growth is lagging behind.

Allopathic diagnostic procedures

If a craniosynostosis is suspected, X-rays are done to ascertain precisely where the sutures have fused prematurely; and a CCT is carried out to rule out brain abnormalities.

Osteopathic examination

Palpation with the aid of involuntary motion often reveals marked local intraosseous lesions or generalized global compression patterns. If craniosynostosis is suspected, the child will be referred to a specialist for further investigations (CCT, X-rays) to find out the extent of the prematurely fused sutures. The extent of the premature fusion determines whether osteopathic treatment is given first or whether an operation is necessary.

Treatment
Allopathic medical treatment

With mild craniosynostosis, it is usual to wait and observe the growth of the head. If the craniosynostosis is associated with plagiocephaly, helmet therapy may be suggested.

If craniosynostosis is marked, and especially if there is a risk of elevated pressure on the brain, an operation is usually done in the 1st year of life. The ossified sutures are removed, retaining the dura mater, and the cranial bones remodelled.

Osteopathic treatment

In milder forms of craniosynostosis, where no operation is needed, osteopathic treatment may be very useful. First, the body as a whole is treated, to optimize the expression of health.

On the cranium, one works both on the head as a whole (lesions of the reciprocal tension membrane, of the vault and of the cranial base are treated) and also on the affected suture. Even though the cranial base is often a problem zone, the pathological suture must be treated directly. I also like to support the de-molding of the bones by using shaping techniques (see p.166). You could do this, for example, with the parietal bones by placing your fingertips around the parietal eminence and encouraging the bones to expand. As you do this, it is useful to imagine the bones as a living calcium phosphate matrix enveloped in fascia. In this way you come into contact with that part of the bone which is plastic and not solid. This fascial envelope of the bones, the periosteum, is continuous with the intrasutural tissue; through this work with the fascia one therefore has direct access to the sutures, which can be modified through this.

Such an approach to treatment makes sense in a milder form of craniosynostosis, but can also be used even in a severe form after the operation. Here, in my experience, it is appropriate to wait 2 to 3 months after the operation until the area has healed, and then to treat the remaining strain patterns of the reciprocal tension membrane, the vault and base.

To be on the safe side, I would not treat exclusively osteopathically if the area of the premature sutural fusion is large or bilateral. In such a case an operation is normally the best solution.

During the cycle of treatment one must in every case document cranial growth (this can of course be done by the pediatrician) and watch carefully to see whether the child develops normally.

Prognosis

Frequent and regular treatment over a fairly long period of time is often appropriate. If one can restore function and mobility in the region of the premature sutural fusion, a favorable change in the shape of the head follows. How far this remodelling goes, however, can be very variable.

TORTICOLLIS

Giles Cleghorn

Definition

Muscular torticollis (muscular wry neck) is a widespread fixed malposition of the head, which I often see and treat in small patients. It leads to an inclination towards the affected side and a rotation of the head towards the other side. Plagiocephaly and a faulty development of the cervical spine or viscerocranium may ensue.

If the torticollis is caused by a spasm or contracture without pathological changes in the muscle tissue it is termed a functional torticollis.

Etiology and pathogenesis

Muscular torticollis arises from a shortening of the connective tissue in the sternocleidomastoid muscle. The causes may be:

- genetic factors, which lead to this malformation.
- injuries to the muscle from stretching, strain or rupture of the belly of the muscle with hematoma formation and subsequent scarring. These generally originate from a difficult labor, if, for instance, the child's head moved forward well in the birth canal but the shoulders were stuck (the opposing forces of the emerging head and the wedged shoulders may then lead to a muscular rupture) or from the pulling in a birth finished with the help of forceps or ventouse.
- a prolonged intrauterine forced posture of the head and neck, in which the scalene musculature may also be involved (Carreiro 2004).

Clinical signs and symptoms

In mild cases of torticollis the affected child prefers to turn his head in one direction but can also turn it in the other.

In more severe cases the child shows the typical head posture and cannot turn his head in both directions; the mobility of the cervical spine is restricted. In babies, nursing at the breast in the direction in which the child does not like to turn his head can be more difficult. In addition, a C-shaped curvature of the body may also be present.

In older children, in whom this condition has been present for a longer time, adaptive asymmetries have often already developed in the cranium and body, such as a scoliosis of the viscerocranium, the cervical or the whole spine.

Sometimes a swelling about the size of a cherry is palpable in the distal sternocleidomastoid muscle from the 2nd week of life; later on the muscle is thick and stringy both on inspection and palpation.

Differential diagnosis

The differential diagnoses to be considered are:

- an acute wry neck, which is produced by a lesion in the cervical spine. In adolescents this can also occur as psychogenic torticollis with emotional stress. This is probably attributable to a normally well-compensated dysfunctional area in the cervical spine. If there is increased tension in the region of the mediastinum or the diaphragm (for example for an emotional reason), the cervical spine decompensates.
- bony malformations, such as found in Klippel-Feil syndrome (congenital fusion of two cervical vertebrae), Sprengel

deformity (congenital elevation/upward displacement of the scapula), atlas assimilation or a unilateral cervical rib.

- ocular causes, such as a unilateral paresis of the superior oblique muscle and consequent squinting to avoid seeing double.
- otogenic causes.
- secondary to an infection of the nasopharyngeal space.
- a benign tumor in the muscle.

Diagnosis

First inspect the face, cranium, neck and the whole body posture. Then observe the spontaneous, active movements. How far does the child move his head in each direction? With babies, ask the mother to sit down first on one side and then on the other side of the table and speak to her child.

This is followed by palpation of the sternocleidomastoid and scalene muscles and passive movement tests of all neck muscles.

In functional torticollis the muscle is in spasm, but the belly of the muscle shows no abnormalities. Usually, the head can be turned in both directions by gentle passive movement.

In torticollis due to muscle rupture one can palpate a hardening in the belly of the muscle which stems from a hematoma. In the first weeks after birth one can feel something hard and gel-like in the area of the injury. The ability to rotate to the side opposite the injury is severely restricted.

If a tumor is the cause of torticollis, you can palpate a hard nodule. On passive movement towards the opposite side you will come across great resistance. If a nodule is palpated, the patient must be referred to a specialist.

Allopathic diagnostic procedures

To rule out a Klippel-Feil syndrome or a Sprengel deformity, a detailed investigation, ultrasound and X-rays are required.

Treatment
Allopathic medical treatment

In functional torticollis and torticollis caused by a hematoma the advice is to position the baby so that he looks at an uninteresting wall in his preferred position and therefore has an incentive to turn actively in the direction of the optical and acoustic stimuli. Physiotherapy is recommended.

If conservative treatment is unsuccessful, or if the deformity progresses despite treatment, an operation is advised, if possible at 12 months: a caudal sternoclavicular tenotomy of the sternocleidomastoid muscle followed by plaster cast in overcorrection.

If the torticollis originated from a tumor, the tumor is removed surgically.

Osteopathic treatment

It is important to treat this disorder as early as possible. If there is no improvement soon, the wry neck can lead to the development of plagiocephaly or functional restrictions of the cervical spine. The diagnosis determines the type of osteopathic treatment.

Functional torticollis

Functional torticollis is treated by addressing present lesions, particularly in the cranial vault and base, in the neck, the upper thorax including the ribs and the scapulae, and of course everything else that is relevant. I like to direct the forces of treatment on to the accessory nerve and the other nerves supplying the neck muscles. As functional torticollis can also originate from molding in utero, where the adaptive malposition of the head and neck may last for quite a while, a global approach to treatment is needed. The problem is that the muscle deforms the cranium by constant traction, so that opposing forces can act even as the treatment is working. If the muscle itself has not been injured, a complete restoration of its function is possible. The emphasis of treatment is on breaking down the neuromuscular reflexes which are causing the wry neck.

In functional torticollis, especially, it is a good thing if the parents can get the child to look in the affected direction as often as possible. This counteracts the tendency to turn the head away from the affected side.

Torticollis caused by muscular tear

If a muscular tear is the cause of the torticollis, we are confronted by a problem of quite a different nature. The muscular forces will here again tend to deform the cranium. As, however, the muscle is weakened by this acute injury, cranial deformation will not occur at all if the child is treated soon after the injury. A hematoma which has not been completely absorbed can lead to scarring. In this case, fluid drive techniques (see p.185) along the muscle and regular osteopathic treatment (starting twice weekly, later once weekly) are recommended, until the situation has normalized. Hematomas are sometimes very difficult to treat. To support the process of the blood being absorbed, I therefore sometimes like to use homeopathic or herbal remedies.

Alongside the local treatment procedures mentioned, the entire body must of course be treated, so as to keep the risk of adaptive changes in posture as low as possible.

Torticollis due to tumor formation

After surgery the scar tissue may be treated osteopathically.

Prognosis

The treatment of functional torticollis is relatively uncomplicated. I personally would nevertheless recommend several months of treatment for the child, to make quite sure that all the factors which have caused this condition have indeed been completely eliminated. The torticollis should have resolved completely after the treatment has been completed. As soon as that is the case, I recommend the parents to come with the child for a check-up every 3 to 6 months in the first year after the treatment, so that one can be certain that the situation has stabilized.

In torticollis due to muscle rupture osteopathic treatment can be used as a supportive measure to treat scarring and strictures within the muscle. Treatment success can however not be guaranteed. Complete restoration is not always possible, but osteopathic treatment will help the belly of the muscle to regain as much elasticity as possible. With some luck and complete re-absorption of the blood residues only a minimal functional impairment will remain.

SCOLIOSIS

Giles Cleghorn

Definition

Scoliosis is defined as a lateral curvature of the spine in the frontal plane.

A functional scoliosis can be corrected fully, or at least to a great extent, by active muscular effort, for instance by bending forward, or by elimination of the cause, unless it has been present for so long that structural changes have already followed. So a functional scoliosis is usually reversible and shows no vertebral rotation.

A structural scoliosis is a permanent deformity, which cannot be corrected actively or passively. It involves a rotation of the vertebral bodies with the ribs following this movement: at the convex side of the curvature the vertebral bodies are rotated forwards and protrude, while on the concave side the opposite is the case.

Etiology and pathogenesis

Functional scoliosis

There often seem to be no obvious, visible underlying structural anomalies in functional scoliosis.

The causes of a functional scoliosis may be:

- poor posture.
- compensatory processes in static problems, such as a pelvic tilt, different leg length, abductor or adductor contracture of a hip joint or ptosis.
- a forced posture due to pain, as in sciatica.

Infantile scoliosis is congenital or develops in the 1st year of life. There are no structural changes in the spine. It is probably the consequence of a dissonance in neuromotor development in the fetal period with unilateral contracture of the muscles of the trunk. Often it is associated with plagiocephaly, a torticollis without shortening of the sternocleidomastoid muscle and occasionally with club foot, hip dysplasia, congenital heart defects or a developmental disorder which affects postural function.

Structural scoliosis

In only about 10% of all structural scolioses is there a known cause. These include:

- Congenital scoliosis – caused by congenital skeletal malformations of individual vertebrae, larger parts of the spine or of the ribs, e.g. hemivertebrae, wedge vertebrae, absence of segmentation, schisis, fusion of several vertebrae or rib defects.
- Myopathic scoliosis – the result of muscular disorders or defects such as myasthenia gravis, muscular dystrophy or arthrogryposis.
- Neuropathic scoliosis – as a consequence of a weakened, imbalanced musculoskeletal system due to neurological disorders, such as neuropathy, a flaccid paralysis as after poliomyelitis, after viral myelitis, meningomyelocele, spinal muscular atrophy, syringomyelia or spinal tumors. With cerebral palsy scoliosis often develops, as a result of paralysis of spinal or other muscles (see Ch.16).

In the most common idiopathic scoliosis (approx. 90%) the cause often remains unknown. Possible causes which have been discussed among osteopaths are the sequelae of birth trauma or accidents. I personally am not sure whether these events are really always the reason for an idiopathic scoliosis. There is of course a temptation to see the cause of pathology in things we believe we understand. And usually osteopaths who work in the cranial field tend to be of the opinion that they know about birth trauma and accidents. In some cases it is certainly right to consider a trauma as a possible cause of scoliosis, while in other cases it is in my opinion impossible to speculate about causes. Carreiro (2004) suspects a connection between idiopathic scoliosis, vestibular dysfunctions and abnormal postural reflexes, such as the righting reflex or proprioceptive reactions.

'The degree of spinal curvature appears to correlate with the amount of equilibrium disturbance.' According to Carreiro, however, 'the nature of the relationship is unclear'; in other words, it is not clear which is cause and which is effect. Three forms are distinguished: infantile, juvenile and adolescent idiopathic scoliosis (characteristics see Table15.1).

Clinical signs and symptoms

Most idiopathic scolioses are discovered by chance at the age of 10–12 years and only seldom does the patient have any symptoms.

Scoliosis with a lateral curvature of up to 10°, which is detectable on X-ray as a slight bend, can be termed mild. There is only a slight rotation within the body and no deformity of the ribcage. The patient is mostly pain-free.

Severe scoliosis can cause a deformity of the whole body, but especially of the ribcage. The function of the internal organs can be considerably restricted. Among the possible serious consequences is a restricted vital capacity with shortness of breath and pulmonary heart disease.

The possible late sequelae of scoliosis – backache and pain in the cervical spine – are a matter for controversy among experts. Whereas some research shows no relationship between scoliosis and backache, in others a direct relationship has been demonstrated.

Diagnosis

When taking the case history of adolescent and older girls, ask about the menarche, because spinal growth continues for another 2 years from the time of the menarche. Measure the body height at each diagnosis to detect an accelerated growth in height, which is important for treatment as far as progression is concerned.

When inspecting the standing child, check the level of the shoulders (for shoulder elevation), waist triangles (for asymmetry), the level of the pelvis (for tilt, level of gluteal folds), note any skin changes (e.g. neurofibromatosis) and whether the spine is perpendicular (plumb line falling from the spinous process of C7, which ends in scoliosis not at the anal cleft but next to it).

Then the child is asked to sit down on the treatment couch. If the abnormal lateral inclination disappears, this points to a functional scoliosis, which is secondary to a difference in leg lengths. If the scoliosis persists while sitting, the child is asked to do a forward bending test, in which he clasps his hands behind his neck in order to keep the shoulder girdle as balanced and stabilized as possible, and then bends forward (Fig. 15.3). In a small child it is sometimes necessary to guide the movement somewhat. If the scoliosis disappears during the forward bending, this indicates good

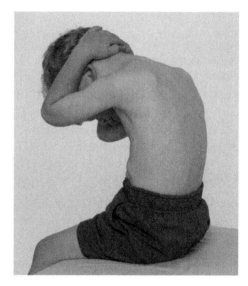

Figure 15.3 Forward-bending test for scoliosis, in a sitting position. In this, a structural scoliosis will persist, and a rib hump and lumbar protuberance might be discernible.
With permission, Karsten Frank, Hamburg

Table 15.1 Characteristics of idiopathic types of scoliosis

Type	Age	Sex ratio	Form	Incidence	Progression
Infantile	0–3 years	Mostly boys	Left convex, thoracic	Rare (2–3%), often additional malformations	90% severe progression
Juvenile	4–9 years	Mostly girls	Right convex, thoracic but also lumbar	Rare (10–15%)	70% severe progression
Adolescent	≥10 years	Mostly girls	Right convex, thoracic	Common (approx. 85%)	10% severe progression

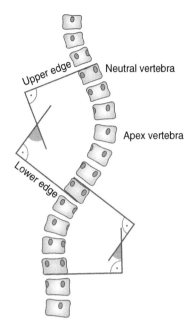

Upper edge

Neutral vertebra

Apex vertebra

Lower edge

Figure 15.4 Ð finition of the Cobb angle of scoliosis with above apex and below apex.
With permission, Henriette Rintelen, Velbert

mobility and a postural and functional origin. If the scoliosis persists, or if a rib hump or a lumbar bulge appears, this points to a structural scoliosis. One often finds a scoliosis with both functional and structural components.

Allopathic diagnostic procedures

Anteroposterior X-rays are made of the entire spine in a standing position. In scoliosis, the description covers:

- Side – right-convex, left-convex
- Level of the apex vertebra – thoracic, thoracolumbar, lumbar, thoracic and lumbar
- Shape of curvature – C-shaped, S-shaped, double curve
- Sagittal profile – lordosis, kyphosis.

Ascertaining the angle of scoliosis (degree of deviation from the axis) is done by the Cobb method of measurement (Fig. 15.4): a parallel line is drawn in relation to the superior surface (upper edge) of the superior neutral vertebra (this being the most strongly inclined towards the horizontal and the least wedge-shaped) and to the inferior surface (lower edge) of the inferior neutral vertebra. The angle at the intersection of these two lines is the angle of scoliosis (Cobb angle). The apex vertebra is the vertebral body with the most lateral wedge-shaped deformity.

The larger the Cobb angle, the more severe the scoliosis. Curvatures below 25° are graded as mild, up to 40° as moderate and over 40° as severe scoliosis. An annual radiological examination gives information about the progression of the scoliotic change. It also helps document the success of treatment.

The method presented here is only one of many for evaluating the degree of severity of a scoliosis. Which method is used may vary from country to country and is also basically irrelevant. The decisive thing is that the same procedure should be used each time for comparative X-rays. Studies show that the assessment of X-rays is to some degree subjective. As a child's spine must be monitored regularly for several years, the most reliable results are obtained if the angle of scoliosis is always ascertained by the same physician (Carreiro 2004).

In order to assess the rate of growth, the stage of ossification of the iliac apophysis can be evaluated. Ossification begins laterally at the iliac apophysis and its timing coincides with the pubertal growth spurt. When the apophyses are completely closed growth is complete.

Treatment

Allopathic medical treatment

The aims of treatment are:

- to arrest a proven progression
- correct the existing curvature
- maintain the result of correction and thus prevent long term consequences.

Outpatient checks are made every 6 to 12 months, during puberty every 3 months. The available modes of treatment are: physiotherapy, bracing and surgery.

With a lumbar scoliotic angle of up to 15° or a thoracic angle of up to 20° (after completion of growth up to 40°), physiotherapy is recommended to strengthen the muscles, improve posture and improve lung function. Nevertheless, this often cannot halt the progression of scoliosis.

With a lumbar scoliosis angle of 15–35°, thoracic of 20–50° or if there is rapid deterioration, a brace is supplied with adjunctive physiotherapy. It is scientifically proven that bracing can slow the progress of deterioration, but only in rare cases is a reduction in the angle of scoliosis achieved. Parents and children must be supported in the process of deciding for or against bracing. Bracing is indeed unpleasant but certainly less drastic than an operation. Boston, Cheneau and Milwaukee corrective braces are used.

If the lumbar scoliosis angle is greater than 35° and in a thoracic angle greater than 50° surgery is indicated, because research has shown that these scolioses cannot be arrested in any other way. The action of gravity on the postural muscles is so great that the curvature deteriorates very quickly. Here, an operation can stabilize the curvature and prevent further structural damage and deterioration. There are numerous procedures available which all have the aim of correcting and stabilizing the curved spine. This is done with metal implants. They are classified as ventral compressing and de-rotating (Dwyer, Zielke), purely dorsal (Harrington, Luque, Cotrel-Dubousset) and combined procedures. Unfortunately, complications such as chronic back pain are not rare.

Osteopathic treatment

Treating scoliosis is not always easy. It is important to examine and treat the patient without any preconceived ideas. One must learn to listen to what the body says and needs. On this topic, Becker says (1997): 'There are always three factors to consider every time a patient enters your office: the patient's ideas and beliefs of what he considers his problem to be; the physician's concepts of what he considers the patient's problem to be; and finally, what the anatomical-physiological wholeness of the patient's body knows the problem to be.' All patients, regardless of the type of scoliosis, need a treatment which is adapted to their individual needs. Both types of scoliosis, functional and structural, show a number of points in common. In both cases, the axial skeleton, that is pelvis, spine, ribs and the cranium as a whole, must be brought back to correct functioning, oriented towards the midline.

Not infrequently one finds the sphenobasilar synchondrosis (SBS) in an extension phase, so that movement in the flexion phase is greatly reduced. It seems compressed; in some cases both the base and vault of the cranium are affected by the scoliosis. The sacrum and iliac bones can also be restricted in their function. Often the iliac bones are in an extension situation and appear to be rotated inwardly, while the sacrum is pulled cranially and is suspended between the iliac bones with its base tipped anteriorly and its apex posteriorly (Fig. 15.5). The hip joints are also frequently rotated inwards, causing the knee to rotate into a knock-kneed position.

It is important to look to the anterior body wall in treatment. One may find relevant osteopathic lesions at the anterior end of the ribs at the sternum and manubrium. Diagnosis of this area followed by treatment to reduce existing distortions in the ventral region of the rib cage is worthwhile. Sometimes the abdominal muscles and their attachments to the pubic bone must also be treated to normalize muscular activity in the umbilical region. The umbilicus may be a possible starting-point for an osteopathic approach because it can give clear indications of stress patterns and strains in the abdominal cavity, through its close attachment to the network of fascial tissues in the anterior abdominal region.

One may also find a segmental disturbance as the cause of both structural and functional scoliosis. A focal lesion may occur during embryogenesis, disturbing a developmental

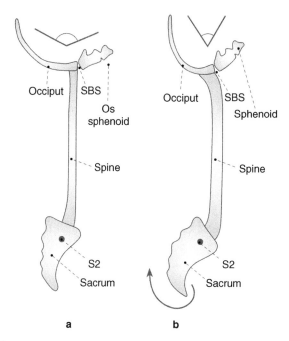

Figure 15.5 a: Normal spine and base of skull. **b:** Possible dysfunction of the base of the skull and the os sacrum in scoliosis. With permission, Henriette Rintelen, Velbert

segment. All three germinal layers (endoderm, ectoderm and mesoderm) may be more or less seriously affected, ranging from an obvious pathological lesion to a more functional disturbance (osteopathic lesion). Such changes in the germinal layers may be sensed by the hands of an skilled osteopath once the child is born. In a structural scoliosis there are often, apart from the changes at the spine such as malformed vertebrae, associated skin lesions such as hyperpigmentation and hair tufts, and organ malformation such as ventral septal defects. This shows that usually all three germinal embryonic layers are affected.

In functional scoliosis, though there are no obvious pathological changes of the spine, osteopathic lesions may be detected on osteopathic palpation in all three germinal layers. Osteopathic treatment may then remedy such focal lesions in the deeper layers associated with the segment, which sometimes hold the key for unravelling the musculoskeletal component of the scoliosis.

For that reason, in my experience, it makes sense to evaluate quite precisely all three germinal layers as part of the osteopathic examination and treatment of scoliosis. The vertebrae and associated tissues which belong to such an affected embryological segment often show viscerosomatic or somatovisceral lesions. Also the associated support structures around organs, such as the pericardium. or other support structures (e.g. the falciform ligament) may be found to be involved.

Rib lesions or dysfunction may also be present, and other tissues such as the spinal ligaments may be affected.

The intervertebral disc material can also suffer lesions, and osteopathic work focusing on disc and notochord is often useful.

Typical of structural scoliosis is the lasting character of the problem. The spine feels like a solid bamboo stick. It can resist change with the utmost obstinacy. In severe structural scoliosis, bracing and surgery are often the only means of choice to stabilize the curvature. However, before these procedures are carried out, the condition is often still observed, investigated and given conservative treatment. If intensive osteopathic treatment can bring about an improvement in the condition, a less drastic intervention may be possible. Perhaps the operation can be postponed to a later date and a brace worn instead. Osteopathic treatment has the potential to preserve the condition of a C- or S-shaped curvature from deterioration. A scoliotic change in the spine is in my opinion one of the conditions in which structural manipulations (high velocity thrust, HVT) are appropriate after a certain age, as the fixation of the spine can be very severe. Both a functional and a structural scoliosis may profit from manipulative procedures.

The role of osteopathy in surgically corrected scoliosis

After an operation the treatment of shock occupies prime position within the framework of osteopathic treatment. Shock may make itself noticed in the form of oscillations or vibrations, which occur in a cycle of about 40 times per minute in the body fluids. In my experience it feels like an effervescence, like air bubbles in carbonated water. If you have well-developed palpatory abilities, you may sense that the shock is sited in the sympathetic nerve fibres and is intensified by hormonal secretions from the adrenal cortex. Once discovered, it is easy to treat and disappears (on the treatment of shock see p.208; the treatment described there for premature babies can also be applied to older children). Without help shock may persist in the system for years, where it slowly 'burns in' and causes complete exhaustion at a deep neuronal level. In a renewed situation of shock this can prevent the person affected reacting appropriately, which is extremely dangerous to the entire organism. Selye (1984) was the first to describe this phenomenon in his book *The stress of life*. Several treatments might be necessary to remove shock completely from the tissues. The value of this therapeutic procedure must not be underestimated. It supports the healing process by increasing the rate of epinephrine catabolism in the body, and reduces the risk of a sympathetic reflex dystrophy.

Functional and cranial work according to the principles of Sutherland on scars and traumatized areas supports a further process of healing. Gentle fluid drives in the areas strengthened with metal and bone grafts help the body to overcome the effects of these foreign bodies.

Later, regular treatment at 6- to 12-monthly intervals helps to maintain the inner balance and adaptation of the body to the operation; growth will then be as symmetrical as possible. I never give up but always return to my programme of treatment in order to maintain the body's health and integrity. An improvement in the state of health is always possible, even after a radical intervention like an operation. Perhaps the key to good health lies in the spine's ability to continue to function even if perfect symmetry is not possible. A good fluid exchange and optimum elasticity of the tissues are the most important factors.

Case report

A woman patient, now 35 years old, was diagnosed with idiopathic scoliosis at the age of 12 years, with a scoliotic angle of 20°. I treated her osteopathically for severe backache. To put it more precisely, I performed a fascial 'unwinding' of the entire body fascia. After only two treatments her spine was perfectly straight. Three years later the patient attended on account of a strain in the region of the sacroiliac joint. However, the scoliosis had not recurred. This case is certainly exceptional but shows what potential lies in our work.

Prognosis

The prognosis depends on the progression. As long as the child grows a deterioration is possible. Prognosis is more severe:

- if the child is very young at the onset
- the higher the curvature lies
- the greater the curvature.

Normally scoliosis stabilizes after puberty. In some cases, however, the condition deteriorates by about 1° per year, if this process cannot be halted by treatment.

In children and adolescents with a mild curvature of 10–15°, I have seen the scoliosis disappear quite often; mostly after about 3 months and 6 to 10 treatments. With curvatures of 15–40° and more, one battles for years against the effects of growth and gravity. At first a treatment interval of a week or a fortnight is recommended; later treatment once a month is sufficient. During growth, or after illnesses or shock it is necessary to give treatment at shorter intervals in order to stabilize the curvatures, because these factors as a general rule cause the angle of scoliosis to deteriorate.

Osteopathic treatment normally strengthens the child's health considerably, lessens the curvature of the spine and improves its functionality. There are cases where scoliosis completely disappears with osteopathic treatment.

DISORDERS OF MATURATION OF THE HIP, HIP DYSPLASIA AND DISLOCATION, AND SUBLUXATION OF THE HIP

Giles Cleghorn

Definition

A disorder of maturation of the hip is a disturbance of ossification in the cartilaginous acetabulum and leads to hip dysplasia (Fig. 15.6) with a steeply sloping and shallow acetabulum, which is protracted cranially. As a result, part of the acetabular roof over the head of the femur is missing. Hip dysplasia is generally associated with coxa valga, an abnormally steep rising femoral neck (see later in this chapter), and also lax ligaments.

In subluxation of the hip (Fig. 15.6) the femoral head is sited on the acetabular rim, but does not quite leave the acetabulum. The margin of the acetabulum and its convexity are deformed and protracted. Mostly, the femoral head slips back into the acetabulum if the hip joint is brought into flexion and abduction and subluxates on extension and adduction of the hip joint. In dislocation of the hip (see Fig. 15.6) the femoral head comes out of the dysplastic acetabulum completely but still lies within the stretched joint capsule. At

birth only the dysplasia is present which is the prerequisite for the dislocation; the actual dislocation, however, mostly takes place post-partum.

Congenital/developmental hip dysplasia is quite common. It can be unilateral or bilateral (Jäger/Wirth 1986).

Etiology and pathogenesis

Following factors play a part:

- Genetic – consistent sex ratio, 6:1 girls to boys: increased familial and geographic incidence, bilateral in about 40% of cases.
- Hormonal – post-partum hormonal imbalance with consequently weak ligaments.
- Mechanical – lack of space in utero, e.g. higher incidence with breech births (because of the extreme flexion of the femur), in oligohydramnios or twin births.

If hip dysplasia remains undiagnosed and untreated, or if the treatment is not effective, the consequence is a femoral head which is no longer centered within the acetabulum; there will be not enough stimulus for further development of the hip joint; there will be changes in the acetabulum, femoral head, joint capsule and muscles; and, long-term, a secondary osteoarthrosis of the hip may develop because of the incongruence of the joint surfaces.

Clinical signs and symptoms

In neonates and infants, asymmetries of the folds in the upper thigh, the buttocks, the groin and adductors can be a clue. From the 2nd month of life reduced abduction may show, owing to the increased tension in the adductors with off-center hips (normal abduction in neonates is 80–90°, from the 2nd month 65°, definitely pathological is reduced abduction of 45° or less). A shortening of leg length or discrepancy in leg length becomes visible if the knees are at different heights on flexion at right-angles (warning: not with bilateral dislocation). The affected leg lies in increased external rotation and its lack of movement is striking. When the child begins to walk he shows a limping gait; if the pathology is bilateral, a type of waddling gait.

In the UK ultrasound screening of neonates viewed to be at risk of DDH may occur as part of the health screening at the age 6 weeks. This helps prevent some hip dysplasias and subluxations from going undiagnosed.

Differential diagnosis

A paralytic dislocation should be considered; for example associated with cerebral palsy, meningomyelocele, after poliomyelitis, a subluxation caused by coxitis or a dislocation detectable right from birth, as in congenital arthrogryposis multiplex.

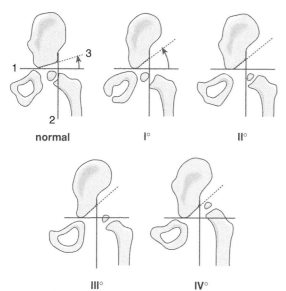

Figure 15.6 Degree of severity of hip dysplasia. 1 = Hilgenreiner line:horizontal through the Y-joint;2 = Ombrédanne line:perpendicular from the edge of the acetabulum to the Hilgenreiner line. 3 = tangents to the acetabular roof to ascertain the angle of the acetabular roof. I°:Femoral head still within the lower inner quadrant, but smaller epiphyseal nucleus and acetabular roof is shorter and has a steeper slope, a sign of hip dysplasia. II°: Progressive lateralization and decentering of the femoral head. III°:Subluxation, the lateralized femoral head rises cranially above the Hilgenreiner line. IV°:Complete dislocation.
With permission, Henriette Rintelen, Velbert

Diagnosis

During case history taking, ask about abnormalities during pregnancy and labor (breech birth, caesarean section, premature birth), hip disorders in the family and other anom-alies in the child (club foot, metatarsus adductus, torticollis, spinal deformity).

The Ortolani sign, a palpable and audible click, is the most important sign of instability in subluxation or dislocation of the femoral head and is sometimes detectable only in the first days of life (procedure see p.125, Fig. 7.10).

Allopathic diagnostic procedures

Ultrasound examination assesses bone and cartilage morphology.

X-rays are seldom needed for early diagnosis. However, it is recommended to monitor treatment. In osteopathic treatment of a subluxation of the hip, X-ray monitoring is reasonable only after 9 to 12 weeks of treatment. Before this time the ossification process has not proceeded far enough for the joint to be evaluated. With the aid of X-rays the development of the joint can be exactly documented (see Fig. 15.6).

Osteopathic examination

In rare cases hip dysplasia or subluxation remains undiagnosed or inadequately treated. At the age of 2 years or older the affected person may show the following characteristics in a:

- unilateral subluxation – lumbar scoliosis with contracture of the quadratus lumborum muscle and a palpable mass in the upper region of the acetabulum
- bilateral subluxation – palpable mass in the upper region of the acetabulum or above, no scoliosis, no crawling, late walking or walking absolutely impossible.

A late diagnosis is quite devastating. From the point of view of allopathic medicine, an operation is the only treatment of choice. That means opening the joint capsule, partial reconstruction of the acetabulum and/or adjustment of the angle of inclination of the femoral neck. An early-onset osteoarthrosis of the hip, usually necessitating an artificial hip replacement as early as 20 years old, is unfortunately, almost invariably the consequence.

Treatment
Allopathic medical treatment

The aim is reposition and retention, with centering of the femoral head in the acetabulum for later maturation and formation of a normal acetabulum. This necessitates flexion and a position of abduction at the hip. The younger the child, the less needs to be done; and the earlier treatment begins, the better the prognosis.

Depending on the severity of the malposition, the affected child wears an abduction brace to obtain abduction at the hip joints; this allows flexion and kicking movements but prevents extension. This considerably restricts the freedom of movement of the legs. The duration of treatment varies from 6 to 8 weeks to up to 6 months. If the hip is very unstable, a plaster cast or splints are used. If this treatment is given early, it normally proves highly effective. However, neither abduction braces nor plaster cast can correct the causative asymmetrical pattern in the hip joints.

In dislocation the femoral head is gently and slowly repositioned into the acetabulum. Suitable reposition procedures include a Pavlik harness and (overhead) extension procedures. The subsequent treatment consists of splints, abduction braces, and bandages or plaster casts.

If a dislocated hip cannot be adjusted by a closed procedure, or if there is a pseudarthrosis with the iliac bone, an operation is indicated. Depending on the extent of the acetabular dysplasia, various pelvic osteotomies and corrective osteotomies are appropriate to correct the malposition.

Osteopathic treatment

During osteopathic palpation (see pp.125, 180) one usually feels that the body is still trying to cope with a strain. It is important to treat exactly this underlying strain, even if the hip dysplasia has been successfully treated by allopathic medicine, as this persisting asymmetrical pattern opposes the unrestricted function and full health of the body.

The secret of success almost invariably lies in the treatment of the three parts of the acetabulum and of the femoral head, with the aid of the capitis femoris ligament as a vector to restore the normal orientation and function of the hip joint. Through an intraosseous treatment of the iliac, the ischial and pubic bones, a reorganization of the acetabulum takes place (for a detailed description of this treatment see p.189). The shear force pattern through the cartilaginous part of the joint is reduced and the blood supply improved. The use of a fluid drive or similar techniques in the same direction as the ligament of head of femur may also contribute to a re-positioning of the femoral head.

A spasm or contracture of the psoas major must also be released in some circumstances. Mostly, the psoas major, together with the other muscles of the hip, tries to splint the dislocated or subluxated hip with the aid of a typical protective spasm, in order to keep the bone immobile while it grows together. Even when the underlying condition has changed, a chronic contracture can remain and may not be able to release itself on its own.

As every child displays his or her own individual pattern of dysfunction, more procedures are of course needed besides this, adapted to needs in the relevant case.

Prognosis

With early diagnosis and treatment, healing generally takes place without negative consequences. The danger of necrosis of the femoral head with poor prognosis is remote with adequate treatment.

In cases of subluxation, the prospects of an osteopathic treatment succeeding are really pretty good; but the patient must nevertheless be clinically monitored by an orthopedic consultant at regular intervals. Osteopathic treatment should be part of the child's overall care and treatment. The acetabulum can improve its orientation and the femoral head can and will return to its position on its own. In the early phase the treatment should be given at weekly intervals; after a few months, only once a month. Regular monitoring to the onset of adolescence would be ideal. Growth spurts, injuries and illnesses can cause disturbances in the body, necessitating a few cycles of treatment from time to time. If there is a true dislocation, osteopathy cannot, on its own and without other measures, enable the femoral head to return to its position.

COXA VARA

Giles Cleghorn

Definition

In coxa vara the angle between femoral neck and shaft is reduced (Fig. 15.7), with shortening and thickening of the femoral neck. In extreme cases this leads to deformity of the femur, looking like a shepherd's crook (Fig. 15.8). The angle between the neck and shaft of the femur is normally about 150° in neonates and 125–130° in adults. Coxa vara can be unilateral or bilateral.

Etiology and pathogenesis

There are three distinct forms; the term used for each depends on the causation:

- If it is present right from birth, it is termed congenital coxa vara (primary form); this pre-natal defect may have been induced by teratogens (see Ch.4, Influences in pre-natal experience).

- If bending of the femur occurs with defective ossification of the femoral neck under the influence of muscular traction and stress and there is a hypoplastic growth of the epiphyseal joint cartilage, the term used is infantile coxa vara (secondary form).

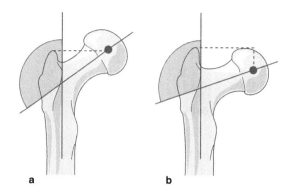

Figure 15.7 Variation in the angle between femoral neck and shaft. **a:** Normal angle of neck and shaft. Center of femoral head and tip of trochanter are at the same level. **b:** Coxa vara with a neck-shaft angle ⩽20°. The tip of the trochanter stands higher than the center of the femoral head.
With permission, Henriette Rintelen, Velbert

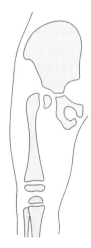

Figure 15.8 Congenital coxa vara with a vertical epihyseal growth cartilage at the femoral head.
With permission, Henriette Rintelen, Velbert

- Symptomatic coxa vara. This arises from systemic disorders of the skeleton, mostly as stress deformity, e.g. in rickets, Perthes disease, slipped capital femoral epiphysis, osteomalacia, chondrodystrophy (achondroplasia, see Ch.17), tumors, osteomyelitis or hip fractures.

Clinical signs and symptoms

Unilateral coxa vara is manifested as a high-standing greater trochanter and a shortening of leg length on the affected side. If the child is already walking, he will probably limp; the Trendelenburg sign is positive; the ability of the hip to abduct reduced. In addition, the affected hip shows an increased internal rotation.

In a bilateral coxa vara there is a forward-tilted pelvis and also a lumbar lordosis. The typical manifestation of this disorder is a waddling gait.

Diagnosis

Allopathic diagnostic procedures

The X-ray (general view of the pelvis) gives information about the severity of the disorder and shows a reduced angle between the femoral neck and shaft, spotted or streaked zones of lucency in the femoral neck, a widened and steeply rising epiphyseal joint, and, in adolescents, a deformation of the femoral end of the hip joint.

Osteopathic examination

Besides a local examination of the hip joint, this also includes a complete evaluation of the musculoskeletal system, and also of other systems, to ascertain how the child is compensating for this pathology and how the expression of health in the body can best be supported.

On local examination, besides palpation of the various tissues and testing of active and passive range of movement, an evaluation with the help of expression of primary respiration is helpful.

Treatment

Allopathic medical treatment

In infants with only slight varus deformity a conservative treatment may be tried (observation with possibility of spontaneous correction; if necessary an orthosis). In general an intertrochanteric valgus-producing osteotomy is done as early as possible. Physiotherapy is recommended.

Osteopathic treatment

In small children the bones can still be molded with the aid of intraosseous fluid drives and molding techniques. I like to treat the whole body and not just the lower extremities. The spinal axis and the anterior body wall should be evaluated in detail.

The three parts of the hip bone and the femoral head must be treated and the position of the femoral head with reference to its relative internal or external rotation reorganized. The leg must be evaluated in its entirety and treated as far down as the plantar aponeurosis (see p.187).

If a disorder such as osteomyelitis or Perthes disease is present, this should be treated as a priority. The aim is to assist normal immune function, for example by techniques to support lymphatic circulation. In children from 8 years of age a CV4 can be used at the occiput; in small children

this should be done from the sacrum. Also, care should be taken to ensure a good arterial circulation, as this is often impaired in many cases. If there is an infection, a fulcrum must be found for this bodily activity and this should be worked with.

Prognosis

The severity of the disorder in the individual case and the precipitating factors determine the prospects for healing. Osteopathic treatment is helpful in many cases. It may take several months, sometimes even years, before a real change sets in. Until then, recovery proceeds in small steps. I expect some kind of progress to show itself within the first three treatments. The entire process of recovery can, however, require 10 to 30 treatments. I personally only give up if the tissue has not changed at all and it is obvious to me that I can do nothing further with osteopathy. If I succeed in improving the femoral neck-shaft angle by at least 50%, in my eyes this is enough to make the treatment worthwhile.

COXA VALGA

Giles Cleghorn

Definition

This is where there is an abnormally steep angle of inclination of the femoral neck, with an angle between the neck and shaft of 140° in adults, and ⩾155° in a 2-year-old child (Fig. 15.9). The angle between the neck and shaft of the femur decreases physiologically in the course of growth. Coxa valga is frequently bilateral.

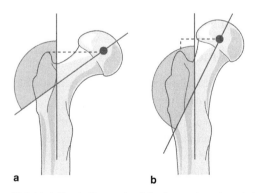

Figure 15.9 Variation in the angle of the femoral neck and shaft. **a:** Normal angle of neck and shaft, center of femoral head and tip of trochanter are at the same level. **b:** Coxa valga with neck-shaft angle ⩾140°. The tip of the trochanter stands lower than the center of the femoral head.
With permission, Henriette Rintelen, Velbert

Etiology and pathogenesis

A congenital coxa valga is termed a constitutional coxa valga of unknown etiology. A genetic predisposition is possible, because there seems to be a higher incidence of this disorder in some families. Mostly it is well compensated and then remains asymptomatic. In rare cases there will be a tendency to secondary arthrosis.

Various pathological processes may underlie an acquired secondary coxa valga, such as muscle imbalance in flaccid or spastic paralysis, caused for example by cerebral palsy, myopathy, or meningomyelocele. Mostly the coxa valga is then bilateral; in hemiplegia, however, a unilateral malposition is possible. A unilateral coxa valga may be due to damage to the epiphysis at the femoral neck or greater trochanter; for example from an injury, inflammation (osteomyelitis) or a tumor. Even a poorly healed fracture in this region can lead to the development of a unilateral coxa valga. Over the course of time the problems and symptoms become more and more pressing, as more and more demands are made on the body's adaptive mechanisms. The unilateral secondary form of coxa valga, above all, often leads to a secondary arthrosis of the hip later on.

Clinical signs and symptoms

In a bilateral coxa valga the child has often been asymptomatic for a long time or even never had any problems. In some circumstances he or she becomes tired more quickly when walking and standing and has groin pain dependent on weight bearing. In some cases hip abduction is limited or the Trendelenburg sign positive.

In secondary coxa valga the symptoms of the underlying disorder are more evident. Abduction on the affected side might be restricted, or the Trendelenburg sign positive.

A coxa valga is often combined with an increased femoral antetorsion (see next section).

Diagnosis

Allopathic diagnostic procedures

An X-ray (general view of the pelvis) confirms the diagnosis.

Osteopathic examination

Besides a local examination of the hip joint, this also includes a complete evaluation of the musculoskeletal and other body systems. The aim here is to find out how the child compensates in this pathology, how the biomechanical forces are distributed in the body and how the expression of health in the body can best be supported.

With the local examination, besides palpation of the various tissues and testing of the range of active and passive movement, an evaluation with the help of the expression of primary respiration is also informative.

Treatment

Allopathic medical treatment

A chance finding of an isolated congenital coxa valga normally requires no treatment, as in most cases there are no symptoms and later consequences in the form of arthrosis are not expected. Should arthrosis nevertheless occur, an operation to reduce the angle between the femoral neck and shaft, repositioning the femoral head (intertrochanteric varus-producing osteotomy) may be considered.

In secondary coxa valga the causative systemic disorder is treated, as far as is appropriate and possible. Surgical correction may be considered.

Physiotherapy is strongly recommended with hip muscle insufficiency (Trendelenburg sign positive).

Osteopathic treatment

The approach to treatment is the same as for coxa vara, above.

Prognosis

The femur of an adult is a very pliable bone. It is said that this bone can be bent by many degrees before breaking. How this may be with children's bones I do not know, but I suspect that the potential for flexion must be several times greater. The structure of this bone is in a permanent state of remodelling. Against this background one can imagine what transformations it undergoes in the course of a lifetime. Osteopathic treatment can support this process of reshaping and modelling. If an abnormal stress on the bone disappears by optimizing the distribution of biomechanical forces, there is certainly a possibility that the bone will find its own way back to its genetically predetermined norm. With secondary, constitutional problems, however, the decisive thing is how well the child reacts to the correction of the primary disorder.

FEMORAL ANTETORSION

Giles Cleghorn

Definition

There is an increased AT-angle (antetorsion angle), which describes the position of the femoral head and neck in relation to the shaft of the femur in the transverse plane (see Fig. 15.10). That means that the femoral head and femoral neck are inclined further forward than normal. This disorder is usually bilateral.

A decrease in the antetorsion angle is one of the physiological changes in the axes of the lower limb which occur in the course of normal growth. In children up to 2 years of age a femoral antetorsion is said to be present if the antetorsion angle is ⩾ 40°, in a 12-year-old ⩾ 30° and in an adult ⩾ 20° (Jäger and Wirth 1986).

Etiology and pathogenesis

A genetic predisposition is demonstrable. Normally, a femoral antetorsion develops when the normal physiological processes which cause the AT angle to change are slowed. A post-traumatic etiology is possible. In such a case the abnormal angle will usually normalize itself by the time the child stops growing. An anteverted hip is seen most often at the age of 2 to 4 years. The condition may deteriorate if the child usually sits between his lower legs (in a W position), when playing on the floor.

Clinical signs and symptoms

An intoeing gait ('pigeon-toed gait') is typical of femoral antetorsion; the child may easily trip over his or her own feet. It is pain-free and seems to have no problems with walking or running. Sometimes, however, affected children fall over more often and so walk with extreme caution, avoiding a more rapid gait. After weight bearing there might be pain in the hips and the area of the thighs.

Femoral antetorsion is often combined with a coxa valga (see previous section).

Differential diagnosis

To be considered are a pseudo femoral antetorsion in club foot or pes adductus, a torsion problem in the lower leg i.e. the

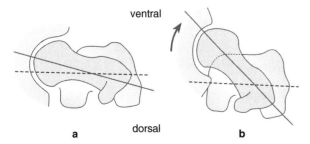

Figure 15.10 Variation in the antetorsion angle (AT angle). **a:** Normal antetorsion. **b:** Femoral antetorsion with increased AT angle. With permission, Henriette Rintelen, Velbert

tibia, movement disorders of cerebral origin, a post-traumatic rotation problem, or coxa valga with femoral antetorsion in congenital dislocation of the hip.

Diagnosis

A femoral antetorsion is usually detectable on inspection (leg axis, gait). When testing movement on both extended hips in the prone position, the internal rotation is increased (up to 90°) and the external rotation restricted.

Allopathic diagnostic procedures

This is done with the aid of X-rays.

Osteopathic examination

As with every osteopathic examination, a complete examination of the musculoskeletal system and other relevant areas is carried out.

Treatment
Allopathic medical treatment

The normal course is to wait to see whether the angle has reduced by itself at the end of growth. The parents are instructed to ensure that the child does not sit between his or her lower legs at play ('between-the-heels'), as this posture favours the internal rotation of the hips.

If the increased femoral antetorsion has not regressed sufficiently once growth is complete, and if the adolescent is suffering pain with weight bearing, surgical correction (intertrochanteric derotation osteotomy) is recommended. This is only seldom necessary.

Osteopathic treatment

Basically, the approach is the same as for coxa vara and coxa valga (see under coxa vara). An osteopathic treatment can usually contribute considerably to accelerating the normalization of the angle of femoral antetorsion.

Prognosis

If a significant change in the tissues has set in after one cycle of treatment and the system is stable, I recommend treating the child once a month. A complete recovery can be expected within 1 year. However, this may happen in a shorter period if the problem is due to poor posture only. It is advisable to work closely with the doctor in charge or a hospital for regular X-ray monitoring.

PERTHES DISEASE

Giles Cleghorn

Definition

This is spontaneous, acquired aseptic bony necrosis, of ischemic origin, of the epiphysis of the femoral head, frequently including the epiphyseal joint. First described by Perthes in 1910. This disorder usually occurs from the 3rd to 12th year, with a peak at the 5th to 6th year, lasts for 2 to 4 years, is bilateral in 10–20%, and has a boy-to-girl ratio of 4:1.

Etiology and pathogenesis

The cause is not clear. Congenital vascular anomalies at the proximal end of the femur and a hormonal dysregulation are discussed.

A circulatory impairment may lead to necrosis of the bone nucleus of the epiphysis in the femoral head. Remodelling processes follow, which can last for 2 to 4 years, with breakdown and rebuilding of the necrotic bone. During this time the epiphysis should bear less weight because of the risk of deformity. If the epiphyseal joint is involved, the result may be a significant impairment of growth.

With the onset of puberty, the blood supply routes to the epiphysis and metaphysis in the femur unite; until then the supply to the femoral head can be impeded a lot easier. Therefore at this point in time spontaneous healing frequently occurs.

Clinical signs and symptoms

As diagnosis by X-ray will only later be positive, it is important to pay attention to the early clinical signs. The child feels generally well, but may complain of pain on weight bearing in the hip, and also pain in the knees. After walking or playing for a longer time, there is an increasing (pain-related) limp, mostly unilateral but also bilateral. Many children tire quickly when walking, and are not able to walk far. Whereas older children may report mild pain in the hip and knee, smaller children can also complain of abdominal pain. The symptoms may be intermittent, and sometimes even disappear for weeks on end. Knee pain may therefore point to a primary serious hip disorder.

Differential diagnosis

Above all, one must rule out other forms of coxitis which are usually associated with fever and malaise. Consideration should be given to coxitis fugax, slipped head of femoral epiphysis (see p.330), tumors, rheumatic fever, septic arthritis, juvenile rheumatoid arthritis (see p.345) and hypothyroidism.

Diagnosis

With the pathology in its early stages, the testing of movement in the hip joint during an examination in the prone position will generally show a restricted abduction and internal rotation. The child may complain of pain at the extreme point of the range of movement.

At a more advanced stage the child suffers from an atrophy of the gluteal and femoral muscles. A flexion contracture may develop and lead to a shortening of leg length. The Trendelenburg sign may be positive.

If both sides are affected, the progression is often not simultaneous on both sides, so that an asymmetry may nevertheless be seen (Jäger and Wirth 1986).

Allopathic diagnostic procedures

X-rays (general view of the pelvis and axial film, Lauenstein method) confirm the diagnosis and make a prognosis possible, from the extent of the necrosis (Catteral stages, Salter-Thompson classification; Fig. 15.11). The Herring classification evaluates the involvement of the lateral pillar of the femoral head. Radiological risk signs, whose appearance means a poorer prognosis, are:

- foci of calcification lateral to the epiphysis
- lateralization (subluxation) of the femoral head

		a.p.	axial
Salter and Thompson, type A; ≤50% of the ossification center	**Catteral group 1** Only anterolateral sector affected		
	Catteral group 2 Approx. 50% of the epiphysis necrotic		
Salter und Thompson, Typ B; ≥50% of the ossification center	**Catteral group 3** Approx. 75% affected		
	Catteral group 4 Total necrosis (poor prognosis)		

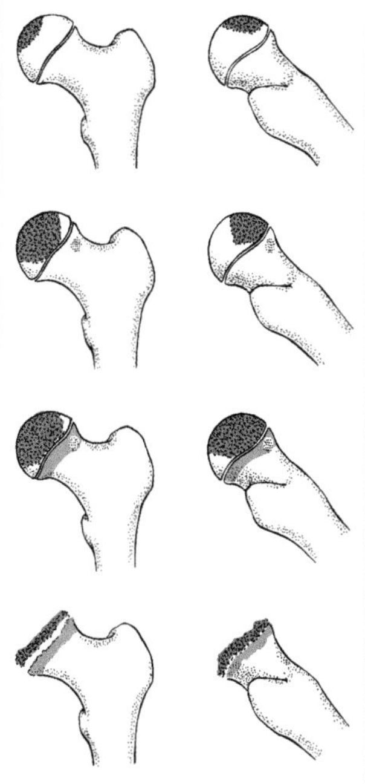

Figure 15.11 Classification of morbus perthes after Salter and Thompson and after Catteral.
With permission, Gerda Raichle, Ulm, in association with the series Klinik und Praxisleitfaden, Urban & Fischer Verlag

- metaphyseal involvement
- horizontal position of the epiphyseal plate
- hinge abduction.

In some cases, further diagnostic procedures are used:

- Ultrasound – to assess whether there is an effusion
- Magnetic resonance imaging (MRI) – for early diagnosis and to determine the extent of necrosis of the head
- Bone scintigram – in exceptional cases, for differential diagnosis.

Osteopathic examination

Local osteopathic examination includes palpation of the tissue and motion testing. Additional information is obtained from a precise evaluation of the hip area with the help of the expression of primary respiration. Often it becomes obvious that this region has suffered some trauma. The general osteopathic examination will also offer information about other areas that may contribute to preparing the ground for a necrotic disease in the hip region.

Treatment

Allopathic medical treatment

The aim of treatment is to rebuild the femoral head in a normal shape with the fullest possible roofing for the femoral head and good mobility of the hip joint.

Views differ about the 'right' therapeutic approach. In the early stages the treatment is mostly conservative (bed rest, analgesia). Otherwise, a functional treatment with physiotherapy is instituted; swimming is supportive; excessive weight bearing as in jumping is to be avoided. In isolated cases a short-term extension or orthosis treatment (Thomas splint) may be useful to take the load off the joint.

To improve the roofing of the femoral head, an operation (varus osteotomy or pelvic osteotomy) which improves centering in the acetabulum may be necessary.

Osteopathic treatment

The important thing – as always – is to take account of the child's individual condition. A local intraosseous osteopathic treatment of the bones and surrounding tissues supports both the circulation and the cellular fluid exchange. A fluid drive along the capitis femoris ligament can be useful, because the blood supply to the femoral head runs through the artery enclosed by this ligament.

The arteries supplying the region around the femoral head originate from the external and internal iliac arteries. Osteopathic lesioning may occur at any site in the arterial plexus above the femoral artery and in the circle of arteries that supply the soft tissues and bones in this area – the lateral and medial circumflex arteries. Such osteopathic lesions must also be treated. You might find that the osteopathic lesion extends into the aorta, so that the entire circulation is impaired. An improvement in venous drainage can also contribute to treatment, as this also promotes drainage from the arterioles. I remind you of Dr. Still's maxim: 'The rule of the artery is supreme.' This applies particularly when to treating a child with Perthes disease osteopathically.

Prognosis

If the pathology makes its appearance before the 7th year of life, the prospects for cure are normally better than when it appears later. The fundamental principle applies that the larger the affected area, the worse the prognosis. About 5% of all cases of coxarthrosis are attributable to Perthes disease, which is a very aggressive pathology. In my opinion it is very important to treat children with Perthes disease osteopathically, as one can definitely have a favourable effect on the severity of the disorder and thus avoid potential negative consequences later.

SLIPPED CAPITAL FEMORAL EPIPHYSIS

Giles Cleghorn

Definition

Slipped capital femoral epiphysis is an atraumatic disorder during (pre-)puberty, in which the epiphysis of the femoral head becomes detached from the femoral neck at the epiphyseal plate and slips (mostly posteriorly and inferiorly; Fig. 15.12).

There is a higher incidence of the pathology in some families. In boys it usually appears between the 12th and 16th year of life, in girls between the 10th and 14th year, and shows a boy-to-girl ratio of 2:1 to 3:1. In girls this disorder generally occurs before the onset of menstruation. In up to 80% both hips are affected (often with a latency period for the second hip of up to 18 months).

Slipped capital femoral epiphysis is a rare disorder which occurs in about three people out of 100,000. However, as in most cases it is associated with a secondary osteoarthrosis in later years, it should never remain untreated. The following forms occur:

- Chronic form (more frequent) – slow slippage or tilting of the capital femoral epiphysis over weeks and months
- Acute form (rare) – acute detachment of the capital femoral epiphysis.

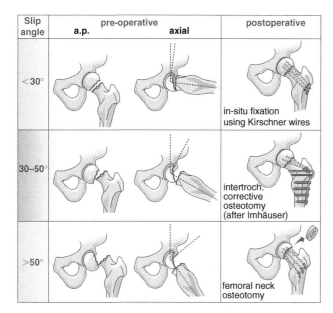

Slip angle	pre-operative a.p.	axial	postoperative
<30°			in-situ fixation using Kirschner wires
30–50°			intertroch. corrective osteotomy (after Imhäuser)
>50°			femoral neck osteotomy

Figure 15.12 Radiological representation of the epiphyseolosys capitis femoris and surgical therapy of the same.
With permission, Henriette Rintelen, Velbert, in association with the series Klinik und Praxisleitfaden, Urban & Fischer Verlag

Etiology and pathogenesis

The etiology is multifactorial. It is striking that overweight, excessive height and gonadal underdevelopment are often present at the same time, which suggests a possible hormonal dysregulation in the pre-pubertal growth spurt. The mechanical triggers under consideration are a reduced anteversion of the femoral neck and an increased load on the epiphyseal plate, whose anatomical location in any case already exposes it to heavy loads from shearing forces.

In the chronic form there is a gradual loosening of the epiphyseal plate without a known reason or trauma. The resulting deformity of the hip joint causes pain and leads to restriction of movement.

The slippage may stop at any stage but can also – for example, after an injury or as a result of the chronic process of detachment – suddenly convert to an acute slippage (acute form), where there is the risk of destruction of the epiphyseal vessels, which may then lead to necrosis of the femoral head.

The entire process generally lasts from 8 months to years. Only the end of the growth phase and the fusion of the epiphyseal plate can give an assurance that the process has indeed been halted. Until then the chronic form may become acute at any time.

Clinical signs and symptoms

There is often tall stature with obesity.

In the chronic form the symptoms are initially slight. Knee pain may be the first symptom, but also backache, groin or thigh pain. The adolescent tires quickly when walking or standing and begins to limp. The limp may be painless. The preferred position for the leg is in external rotation.

The acute form is associated with severe hip pain and a sudden inability to bear weight on the hip (inability to walk and stand). The leg is in external rotation.

Diagnosis

On testing movement, the striking features are an increased external rotation of the leg and a limited and in some circumstances painful internal rotation and abduction. In guided flexion of the externally rotated leg the hip deviates into forced abduction (positive Drehmann's sign).

Allopathic diagnostic procedures

X-rays (general view of the pelvis and Lauenstein's axial image) confirm the diagnosis. They show a widening of the epiphyseal plate, an apparent narrowing of the epiphysis and the tilting or angle of tilt of the epiphysis (see Fig. 15.12).

Osteopathic examination

The osteopathic examination is the same as the examination for other hip disorders, such as in Perthes disease, above.

Therapy
Allopathic medical therapy

Therapy is always surgical. The surgical procedure depends on the extent of the tilt (see Fig. 15.12). If the epiphyseal plate is still open, a prophylactic stabilization of the other hip is always undertaken.

In the acute form strict bed rest is necessary, and weight-bearing on that hip is prohibited. The operation will be performed as soon as possible.

Osteopathic treatment

The osteopathic treatment is an adjunct to surgical treatment of the hip joint. The basic principles of the therapeutic approach are similar to those for hip dysplasia (see p.323) and other hip disorders. However, as slipped capital femoral epiphysis does not appear until shortly before or at puberty, we are confronted with a body which has probably been exposed to considerable forces and stresses for many years.

We must examine and treat the child's whole body carefully, so as to minimize all the factors which negatively influence the child's health. As there is always a considerable risk of developing osteoarthrosis of the hip later (around age 40 or 50 years), the aim is to optimize the biomechanical forces so that potential negative consequences later are largely eliminated. Osteopathy will make a valuable contribution to the treatment of a surgically fixed femoral head.

Prognosis

The prognosis depends on the degree of the tilt. It is good with early diagnosis and correct surgical treatment. With angles of slippage ≥30° and the occurrence of necrosis of the femoral head, however, the early development of secondary osteoarthrosis of the hip is a threat.

In my opinion osteopathic treatment which normalizes the tissues and blood supply reduces the risk of coxarthrosis later, prepares the child's hip well for surgery and promotes postoperative recovery. A long-term study which could measure the efficacy of osteopathic treatment in reducing the risk of osteoarthrosis of the hip would be interesting here.

GENU VARUM

Giles Cleghorn

Definition

Unilateral or bilateral misalignment of the leg axis, in which the leg is bent outwards at the knee (bow leg; Fig. 15.13).

Etiology and pathogenesis

Bow legs are quite common in children. In the first months of life a mild form is physiological, and it corrects itself later.

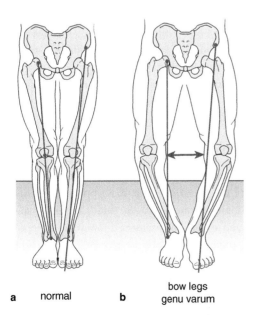

Figure 15.13 Leg alignment. **a:** Physiological leg alignment. **b:** Varus deviation.
With permission, Henriette Rintelen, Velbert

In just a few cases there is an underlying disorder. If the axis is not corrected, the deformity will increase from the raised pressure of weight-bearing; the ligaments may loosen as a result and degenerative changes are more likely (varus arthrosis of the knee).

Physiological genua vara

The leg axes change during the infant's development from a lying position to crawling and walking. A baby has physiological bow legs, with both the femur and the tibia contributing to this form. The legs assume a straight form little by little, and a genu varum is not termed pathological until after the 2nd year of life. A physiological genu valgum very often develops in the course of the 3rd year (knock-knees; see next section). At the age of 5 to 6 years the child's legs should have made the transition to a relatively straight leg form by themselves. Physiological changes in the leg axes in the course of childhood growth are:

- At birth the normal alignment of the knee is around 10–15° varus deviation.
- Neutral femur-tibia position during the 12th–14th month of life.
- Maximum valgus position of 10–15° at the age of 3–3½ years.
- Physiological valgus deviation in adulthood of 5–7°.

Pathological genu varum

Pathological genu varum is quite rare and occurs mostly secondary to another disorder. Causes of such a faulty leg alignment may be:

- unilateral – idiopathic, inflammations, tumours, paralyses, Blount's disease (see below), lesions of the epiphyseal plate, post-traumatic
- bilateral – metabolic disorders (rickets, phosphate diabetes), achondroplasia (see Ch.17), osteogenesis imperfecta.

Blount's disease is a deforming osteochondrosis of the medial tibial epiphysis. With early onset, both sides are generally affected; later onset (at the age of 6–12 years) it is mostly unilateral. Excess weight and early walking seem to be etiological factors. A secondary compensatory hypertrophy of the medial femoral condyle leads to the typical bow legs.

Bow legs occurring after the 2nd year of life are often attributable to biomechanical strain patterns, which stand in the way of correct physiological development of the leg axes. The body may for example not be able to self-correct local intraosseous strains which are the result of molding processes in utero or forces at birth.

In some cases the entire leg (that is, also including the foot and hip), is in a molding pattern in which the hip joint is in external rotation. The fibula may be pulled inferiorly in relation to its normal position with reference to the tibia.

Clinical signs and symptoms

Symptoms are rare. There is often a pes planovalgus, caused by compensatory processes.

Diagnosis

Inspection generally shows that both legs – seldom only one leg – are bowed. With children who are already walking a glance at the shoes is sufficient; heavy wear at the lateral areas of the shoes indicates the existing problem.

The leg axes are precisely measured, assessing the gap between the knee condyles and between the malleoli.

Testing of movement shows free motion of the joint; in the older child there is often an internal rotation of the tibia.

Allopathic diagnostic procedures

X-rays (films of the leg axes in a standing position) show the extent of the deformity, the site of the greatest axial deviation and the configuration of the epiphyseal plates. To avoid frequent radiography, progress is often monitored by making outline drawings on a large sheet of paper of the child's legs in a supine position, or by taking photographs.

To rule out rickets, the phosphate, alkaline phosphatase and calcium levels in the blood are measured.

Osteopathic examination

The child's entire body is carefully examined to ascertain which biomechanical strain patterns may influence the situation at the knee. Besides testing movement in all the joints of the lower extremities, a careful analysis is made of the intraosseous condition of the affected bones, with the help of the expression of primary respiration.

Therapy
Allopathic medical therapy

The aim is to prevent a later osteoarthrosis of the knee by correcting the physiological leg axis.

The classic medical approach is to wait and see how much the bow legs self-correct. In rickets especially, there is a great tendency to spontaneous correction. Raising the outer edge of the shoe or appropriate orthoses are recommended for correction. In case of excess weight, weight reduction may be helpful.

If a deformity does not tend to improve, surgical correction is advised (corrective osteotomy, temporary epiphysiodesis in the Blount procedure between the 10th and 13th year).

Osteopathic treatment

If there is no pathological cause, the axial deviation is often due to a molding process in utero or at birth. Although the advice is often given that the bowing will correct with growth, I have found that this is not always the case, and that the varus position can indeed persist into adulthood. It is impossible to predict in which person the bowing will self-correct with growth and in which it will not. I therefore always treat the condition. I have the impression that those in whom the condition might have self-corrected anyway respond very quickly to treatment. Other children, in whom it would probably not have corrected itself at all, respond less quickly to therapy and need very intensive treatment.

All the tissues in the leg area need support to find their way back to the normal state. An intraosseous decompression treatment for all the bones in the lower extremities, including the feet, is recommended.

The fascia must also be 'derotated.' This includes the interosseous membrane of the lower leg and the iliotibial tract.

Biomechanical strain patterns throughout the body which influence the leg are of course treated.

Another reason why osteopathic treatment is especially important in genu vara is that the child often has problems with walking because his biomechanics are disturbed. Children with tibial torsion do indeed trip and fall quite often, and so have difficulties not just with sport but also with perfectly ordinary activities. As mentioned earlier, a balanced and intensive use of the legs is crucial for sensory input, which drives forward the appropriate cross-linking and integration of the sensory and motor systems.

Prognosis

The prognosis depends on the cause, the extent and the progression of the misalignment in each case.

If the intraosseous strains in the child you are treating are concentrated principally in the tibial region, correction of the varus position is possible after only a few treatments. However, if the configurating effect was greater, and the entire leg has been involved, regular treatment can be required for more than 2 years to correct the existing strain pattern. Only treatment and regular monitoring will make it clear how refractory the problem is.

Bow-leggedness that persists beyond the 2nd year of life and which is attributable to a delayed development of the leg axes is very amenable to osteopathic treatment. In very rare cases there is an underlying pathological cause which makes complete normalization of the leg structures impossible; however, in such cases an improvement in the condition can often be achieved. With consistent osteopathic treatment of the mechanical axes an improvement in function sets in, which counteracts the development of osteoarthrosis of the knee in later years.

GENU VALGUM

Giles Cleghorn

Definition

A unilateral or bilateral axial misalignment of the leg, in which the leg is bent inwards (knock-knees; Fig. 15.14). If both legs are affected the knees are close together and the ankles are wide apart.

Etiology and pathogenesis

If the axis is not corrected, the deformity increases from the pressure of increased weight bearing; the ligaments will become more loose as a result and degenerative changes may ensue later on in life (valgus osteoarthrosis of the knee).

Physiological genua valga

The leg axes shift in the course of the child's growth. A physiological genu valgum very often develops in the course of the 3rd year of life. At the age of 5 to 6 years the child's

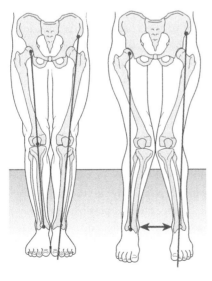

Figure 15.14 Leg alignment. **a:** Physiological leg alignment. **b:** Valgus deviation.
With permission, Henriette Rintelen, Velbert

legs should have made the transition to the normal adult leg form by themselves. Physiological changes in the leg axes in the course of a child's growth are:

- At birth, the normal alignment of the knee is 10–15° varus deviation
- Neutral femur-tibia position during the 12th–14th month of life
- Maximum valgus position of 10–15° at the age of 3–3½ years
- Physiological valgus deviation in adulthood of 5–7°.

Pathological genu valgum

Rarer causes of this leg misalignment may be:

- unilateral – idiopathic, inflammations, tumors, paralyses, Blount's disease (see p.332), epiphyseal lesions, coxa valga, adduction contracture of the hip, valgus position of the foot, post-traumatic, inhibition malformation (sometimes also accompanied by hip dysplasia).
- bilateral – metabolic disorders (rickets, phosphate diabetes), endocrine disturbances (pituitary, in Marfan syndrome).

Biochemical weight-bearing patterns and/or a connective tissue weakness are more often the reason why the physiological valgus position does not correct itself by 7 years of age.

Remember that the knee is not the only problem. The knee is a universal joint between hip and foot. As such it must compensate for strains coming both from above and from below, in motion and at rest. If the biomechanical forces are too great or not centered, the knee may not be able to compensate the strain and so shifts into a knock-kneed stance. Not infrequently, internally rotated hip joints are the triggers for a functional adaptation of this kind in the knees. The hips in their turn can be put under pressure by an inflexible sphenobasilar synchondrosis, especially if the pelvis and sacrum are also restricted by osteopathic lesions. This scenario is similar to that described for scoliosis (see p.318), except that here the hip-joints and knee are affected and not the spine.

Clinical signs and symptoms

Symptoms are rare. Often a pes planovalgus arises through compensatory mechanisms due to the usually weak muscle tone. The child has a tendency to malpositions of the patella and early degenerative changes in the patellar joint. Knee pain may be felt in the anterior part of the knee.

In some circumstances the child has developed a compensatory gait, in which the two legs are each swung rather more outwards to prevent the knees from meeting and rubbing against each other (circumduction gait). The child may therefore tire more quickly when walking or running, or try to avoid running fast.

A child with knock knees may also fall more frequently, and this can produce additional strains in the body and cranium and worsen the situation.

Diagnosis

Inspection generally shows that both legs – seldom only one leg – are knock-kneed. With children who are already walking, a glance at the shoes is sufficient: heavy wear at the medial areas of the shoes indicates the existing problem.

The leg axes are precisely measured by assessing the distance between the condyles and between the malleoli.

Allopathic diagnostic procedures

X-rays (films of the leg axes in a standing position) show the extent of the deformity, the site of the greatest axial deviation and the configuration of the epiphyseal plates. To avoid frequent radiography, progress is often monitored by making outline drawings of the child's legs on a large sheet of paper in a supine position, or by taking photographs.

To rule out rickets, the phosphate, alkaline phosphatase and calcium levels in the blood are measured.

Osteopathic examination

Osteopathic examination includes motion testing of all the joints of the lower extremity: feet, ankles, knees and hips. Additional information, especially relating to possible intraosseous restrictions, is obtained by observing the tissues of the lower extremities with the expression of primary respiration.

The child's entire body is carefully examined to ascertain which biomechanical strain patterns may influence the situation in the knee. By careful examination of the whole of the body's structures you may discover primary dysfunctions leading to compensatory genua valga.

Therapy

Allopathic medical therapy

The aim is to correct the physiological leg axis in order to prevent later osteoarthrosis of the knee.

The classical medical approach is to wait and see how much the bow legs self-correct. With rickets especially, there is a great tendency to spontaneous correction. Orthopedic support or appropriate orthoses are recommended for correction. In the case of excess weight, weight reduction can also be helpful.

If the deformity is not improving, surgical correction (corrective osteotomy, temporary epiphyseodesis by the Blount procedure between the 10th and the 13th year of life) is advised.

Osteopathic treatment

As a matter of principle I check all the body's structures; that is from the cranium and the SBS down to the foot. If there is a dysfunction of the spinal mechanics it must be treated first. In this case partial success is not enough, as even the smallest dysfunctions in the biomechanical system lead to restricted function in the entire body.

As soon as the vertebral axis is working well, which often means up to 6 months of hard work, I start to treat the hip joints. The hip position must be corrected; whether the problem is an increased internal rotation or external rotation does not matter. Frequently, one hip joint is also internally rotated and the other externally rotated (correction of the hip joint see pp.189, 211).

Up to this point I have often ignored the knee when giving treatment, because its dysfunction is caused by compensatory mechanisms. It is treated later when the correction of the bodily structures as a whole has already progressed further. An osteopathic lesion of the knee is much easier to treat later when the problems at the upper and lower end of the leg have already been eliminated. For that reason, after the spine and hips, I first treat and correct the mechanics of the feet. In my experience treatment of the entire foot is usually necessary. It is especially important to evaluate, and if necessary treat, the subtalar joint between the talus and calcaneus, as this often plays a quite special role in correct weight distribution. Often the navicular drifts medially and inferiorly in rotation, and the tarsal and metatarsal joints are greatly compressed (Fig. 15.15). This part of the treatment may last for up to 6 months and may need to be repeated frequently during the course of the growth of the child in order to obtain stability in the foot area. I recommend that the child wears

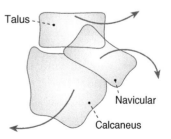

Figure 15.15 Rotation of the bone in the foot (right foot, from front). The os naviculare is rotated to medial and inferior. The talus is rotated to medial and superior, the calcaneus to lateral. With permission, Henriette Rintelen, Velbert

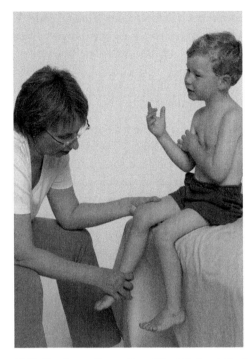

Figure 15.16 Passive motion testing of the tibia in relation to the femur.
With permission, Karsten Frank, Hamburg

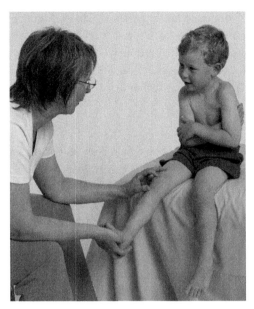

Figure 15.17 Test for patella tracking.
With permission, Karsten Frank, Hamburg

arch supports. These must be very stable in form and correctly adapted. While good therapeutic results may be obtained without these aids, in my experience the ligaments can adapt better to the new situation with the help of such support.

When treating the feet, the fibula and the interosseous membrane of the lower leg must also be addressed. Their correct alignment is very important because the entire neurovascular supply to the foot runs across the interosseous membrane. The fibula also has a close relationship to the knee. I check the degree of rotation of the tibia in relation to the femur (Fig. 15.16). For this, use one hand to stabilize the femur at the distal end and the other hand to clasp the tibia at the distal end to induce, first, an internal rotation and then an external rotation of the tibia. You also need to test the position of the patella (see Fig. 15.17).

As soon as the aforesaid mechanical disturbances have been removed, the knee generally self-corrects. Then the arch supports are no longer needed. In my experience it is better if they are no longer worn after self-correction. However, it is sometimes preferable to wait until the end of the growth phase before removing them because the arch supports stabilize and support the ligaments. This gives protection from an excessive biomechanical load in the growing body. Regular monitoring into late adolescence is important because treating the biomechanical structures in the child's body is a lengthy business. Sometimes it takes years to correct the disturbed pattern. Even

if the knock-knee is only unilateral and attributable to a pathological cause, osteopathic treatment can still be worthwhile and optimize the child's chances.

Prognosis

This depends on the cause in the individual case, and the extent and progression of the malposition.

Both in genua vara and in genua valga intensive osteopathic treatment can do much good. If the malposition has to be corrected surgically, try to postpone this intervention for a few months and meanwhile treat osteopathically. As neither knock-knees nor bow legs are life-threatening, an operation can usually be postponed without difficulty. You will be surprised at what you can achieve. Perhaps your treatment will make an operation unnecessary. However, if surgical correction is best for the child, 3 months of osteopathic treatment before the operation will make the tissues more flexible and make the work of the orthopedic specialist much easier.

OSGOOD-SCHLATTER DISEASE

Giles Cleghorn

Definition

Osgood-Schlatter disease is an aseptic necrosis (juvenile osteochondrosis) of the tibial apophysis. It most often appears during the major growth spurt in boys from 10 to 14 years of age who do a lot of sport, but girls, especially if athletic, may also be affected.

Etiology and pathogenesis

The cause is obscure. The precipitating event is said to be an imbalance between growth and development at the attachment of the patellar ligament to the tibial tuberosity, associated with increased traction on the patellar ligament from overuse in sport or other activities. A local disturbance in the process of ossification may lead to the tibial tuberosity developing a more prominent form.

An imbalance in the leg muscles often underlies this process, such as the muscles being too tense in the thigh ventrally or dorsally; or there is actually a faulty tension in the calf area. Mostly the quadriceps femoris muscle and its tendons are shortened. The excessive strain on the muscles may then produce microfractures in the fibrous cartilage where the patellar ligament attaches to the tibial tuberosity. Often the area where the patellar tendon attaches to the tuberosity is inflamed. However an avulsion, with aseptic necrosis of bone or cartilage fragments, occurs only rarely. Then the fragments lying below the patellar ligament are usually still palpable and cause a further local irritation.

Clinical signs and symptoms

As the aseptic necrosis of the bone mostly occurs at a very active phase in the child's life, it can cause considerable problems.

A notable feature is a swelling, tender to pressure, over the tibial tuberosity; on extension of the knee against resistance the pain is more severe. Pain in the region of the tibial tuberosity mostly occurs with activity such as walking, especially climbing stairs, and is worse with fast running or heavy strain. Sometimes those affected also complain of slight pain at rest.

Diagnosis

The site of origin and the nature of the pain are typical. Signs of local inflammation over the tibial tuberosity and tenderness to pressure on palpation are unequivocal indications. The pain is increased on extending the knee against resistance.

Allopathic diagnostic procedures

X-rays of the knee confirm the diagnosis; they show a fragmentation of the tibial apophysis. Not uncommonly a bony enlargement of the tibial head is detectable as a manifestation of a progressive healing reaction; sometimes also an avulsion of the tendon with a piece of dependent cartilage.

Osteopathic examination

In the general osteopathic examination special attention will be given to the distribution of muscular tensions in the leg region. An examination of the biomechanics of the entire body can indicate whether the overstrain of the quadriceps femoris muscle is really due solely to the increase in sporting activity, or whether this muscle also has to work harder than normal to compensate for a postural weakness.

Therapy
Allopathic medical therapy

As this disorder generally heals without problems, partial abstention from sports (especially jumping disciplines) and, if necessary, resting the knee are enough. A swollen knee is treated here by elevating the entire leg in an extended position. Here, a pillow should never lie under the knee, as this may cause venous thrombosis. The most effective is a slatted frame raised at the foot. Ice packs also relieve the symptoms. Place these on the knee for about 20 to 30 minutes every 3 to 4 hours for 2 or 3 days until the pain disappears. Anti-inflammatory creams may also be prescribed as an adjunct. Physiotherapy can also be helpful.

Surgical intervention to remove the avulsed fragments of bone is only very rarely needed. If done at all, then it should not be carried out until after the child's growth is completed.

Osteopathic treatment

When treating, it is important not to move the knee unnecessarily, so as not to set off any further inflammatory reactions. In my experience fluid drives and lateral fluctuations in the area of the epiphyseal plate work well. These will help the inflammatory reaction to subside.

In severe cases and with a tendon avulsion, fluid drives along the quadriceps femoris muscle can be helpful. As soon as the inflammation has gone down, the cause must be treated. In many cases there is a muscular imbalance in the leg, often a shortened quadriceps femoris tendon. For further therapeutic measures see the next section, Chondromalacia patellae.

Prognosis

Mostly, the disorder heals by itself without problems. However, this can last for about 6 to 24 months after the appearance of the first symptoms. An osteopathic treatment of the causes underlying the muscular imbalance considerably accelerates the healing process. The prominence of the tibial tuberosity may remain even after the symptoms have disappeared.

CHONDROMALACIA PATELLAE

Giles Cleghorn

Definition

Chondromalacia patellae is a softening of the cartilage on the posterior aspect of the patella, with varying degrees of severity. Adolescent girls and women are more often affected than boys and men.

Etiology and pathogenesis

The cause is multifactorial. It is probably precipitated by a discrepancy between the load and the ability to bear the load, an excessive or asymmetrical pressure from:

- muscular imbalance – which leads to an abnormal direction of force on the knee. The vastus lateralis and the vastus medialis muscles are often not balanced. The vastus lateralis may be more powerful than the vastus medialis and thus cause a lateral displacement of the patella when the quadriceps femoris muscle contracts and the knee is extended. This in turn leads to an excessive pressure on the lateral joint surface. If the patella is not correctly centered in the midline, it comes into contact with the femur in an abnormal fashion, which probably increases the 'softening' and destruction of the cartilage.

- bony abnormalities – variations in form of the patella, genua valga (knock knees). Any valgus position of the knee will usually intensify during a growth spurt, thus widening the angle between the thigh and the patellar tendon, so that every flexion of the knee increases the risk of a patellar dislocation. The pressure on the lateral joint surface of the patella is too great.

- ligamentous laxity.

- overuse (microtrauma).

- cartilage contusion (macrotrauma).

In teenagers there is a phase in which the articular cartilage of the patella has not yet been worn away, so that the condition is still reversible. This stage should correctly be termed 'anterior knee pain' or 'femoropatellar pain syndrome'.

In fact, in most teenagers the pain comes and goes for years until growth is complete. In most patients the pain vanishes completely after the end of the growth phase, while in others the pain intensifies over the years; the articular cartilage of the patella is destroyed and a true chondromalacia patellae develops. Osteopathic treatment can do much to prevent such a scenario.

Tall, knock-kneed teenagers, especially girls, with very taut vastus lateralis muscles are at increased risk of this disorder.

Clinical signs and symptoms

Affected teenagers mostly complain about bilateral spontaneous pain in the patellar area at or after long periods of knee flexion (e.g. sitting in a cinema), or when going downstairs or downhill. Not uncommonly the pain also radiates into the posterior aspect of the knee. The pain comes and goes. It intensifies with squatting, kneeling, climbing stairs or on changing from a sitting to a standing position.

On extending the leg, the persons affected often have the sensation that something is grinding inside the knee; they report that the knee gives way or that there are blocking phenomena.

Diagnosis

Many young people affected show a slight lateralization of the patella, which no longer lies in line with the femur (patellar subluxation). The knee may be tender to palpation and slightly swollen. On moving the joint a grating is usually palpable in the patella.

Testing passive movement of knee and patella

The movement of the tibia is palpated in relation to the femur, and that of the patella while the leg is being extended. The adolescent sits on the treatment couch and lets her legs dangle. Sit in front and place the middle finger, index finger and thumb of one hand on the femur, middle of the patella and tibial tuberosity of the flexed knee. On flexion these three points are normally in line. With your other hand now extend the knee and observe the movement of the patella (Fig. 15.17). Normally, the patella moves superiorly on extension and inferiorly on flexion. During extension the tibia also rotates externally, on account of the medial condyle of the femur being bigger and longer. As a result, the tibial tuberosity moves laterally in relation to the patella when the leg is extended.

A further passive movement test of the patella is to lay the outstretched leg on your thigh and to manually test the mobility of the patella, cranially, caudally, medially and laterally.

Active movement testing (patella tracking test)

If you suspect a femoropatellar pain syndrome, palpate the course of the patella (tracking) while the child actively extends the leg; that is, contracts the quadriceps femoris muscle. The test is positive if the patella moves laterally (Carreiro 2004). While extending the knee the patient may feel a grinding under the patella.

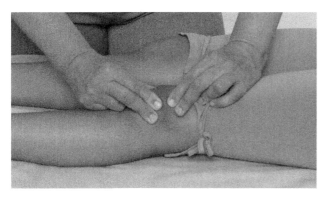

Figure 15.18 Patella compression test.
With permission, Karsten Frank, Hamburg

Patella compression test

The adolescent lies supine, with knees extended. Hold the patella caudally and ask the patient to tense her quadriceps femoris muscle. This can cause pain (*caution*: sometimes quite violent) (Fig. 15.18). If the patient cannot cooperate, you can also push the patella cranially and caudally and compress while doing so (McRae 1983).

Allopathic diagnostic procedures

The X-rays are normally unremarkable. A patellar deviation laterally or medially may indicate pathology. An axial film of the patella possibly shows variants in form, subluxations and signs of arthrosis in the femoropatellar articulation.

The affected anterior cartilaginous area is not visible on X-ray, but can be evaluated with an MRI.

Osteopathic examination

Besides the above-mentioned orthopedic examinations, a general osteopathic examination can give an indication of adaptive mechanisms in the biomechanics of the body, which may have led to imbalance in the muscular system (see Ch.7, Examination of the preschooler and schoolchild).

Therapy

Preventive measures in sporting activity

It is important to inform affected teenagers that warm-up exercises and stretching, especially of the quadriceps femoris and ischiocrural muscles, considerably reduce the risk of chondromalacia patellae. It is better to alternate various sporting activities; for example to alternate running, swimming and cycling.

Particularly susceptible adolescents should avoid squats, kneeling, and hill or mountain runs.

Allopathic medical therapy

The treatment is always conservative initially. Resting the knee and avoidance of long periods of sitting with the knees flexed, squatting and overuse from sport is recommended. Until the pain has fully subsided, the advice is to abstain from taking part in PE lessons or from strenuous activities. Anti-inflammatories (ointments, tablets) can also be helpful. Physiotherapy, above all, strengthening the quadriceps femoris and especially the weaker vastus medialis, stretching of the ischiocrural muscles and a patellar tendon stretching can bring relief.

Only after all the conservative options have been exhausted, and only on very strict indications, is surgery undertaken. The results are, however, quite often unsatisfactory.

Osteopathic treatment

Simple stretching of the patellar ligament has proved extremely effective. It makes no difference which technique you use for this. I personally prefer the patellar lift (see p.211). Normally the condition improves if the child is treated intensively, once weekly for a month. During this time the child should rest as much as possible. A simple patellar stretching, or soft-tissue massages, is also very effective.

Further treatment aims to regulate the existing muscular imbalance in the knee and also the precipitating factors.

Prognosis

The rate of spontaneous healing in adolescents is high. Both femoropatellar pain syndrome and chondromalacia patellae respond well to osteopathic treatment. In my experience the success rate is around 95%.

CONGENITAL CLUB FOOT

Eva Moeckel

Definition

Congenital club foot is a complex foot deformity, which cannot be passively corrected, with contractures of the joint capsules and tendon shortenings of varying degrees. The following components are present: pes equinus, inversion of the foot, adduction and supination of forefoot and hindfoot in relation to each other, and pes cavus (hollow foot) – hence the term pes equinovarus.

It is twice as common in boys and both feet are affected in 50% of cases. Congenital club foot is one of the most common congenital developmental disorders.

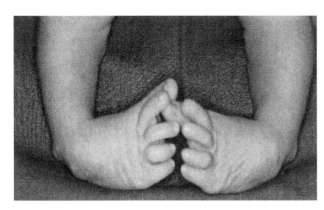

Figure 15.19 Congenital club feet in ventral and dorsal view. With permission, Rössler, Rü her:Or thopädie. 8 h edn. Urban & Fischer, München na, 20

Etiology and pathogenesis

Possible precipitating causes under discussion are chromosomal or embryonic defects; the embryonic skeletal anlage not developing further than an early developmental stage; and a mechanical impairment of foot development in the embryonic period. The functional equilibrium seems to be disturbed by a predominance of the supinator (tibialis anterior and posterior) and flexor muscles (triceps surae, toe flexors) and anomalies of the muscle attachments.

Errors in bone growth, contractures in the subtalar joint complex with tendon shortenings and deformities of numerous bones in the skeleton of the foot (e.g. talus, calcaneus) follow.

Club foot may also occur in neuromuscular disorders, such as spina bifida, cerebral palsy, muscular dystrophy, congenital arthrogryposis multiplex, and sacral dysgenesis.

Clinical signs and symptoms

The deformity is impossible to overlook. The typical components are unequivocally verifiable (Fig. 15.19); the examination is done in the supine position with the knee and hip at 90° flexion:

- pes equinovarus – contracted triceps surae muscle with the entire foot fixed in plantarflexion, the shortened Achilles tendon being palpable as a hard cord
- varus of the hindfoot
- adduction of the midfoot and forefoot
- supination of the entire foot
- pes cavus (hollow foot), with deepening of the longitudinal arch.

The calf usually shows signs of atrophy of the triceps surae muscle.

An investigation must always be made for other associated deformities or malformations, such as hip dysplasia, spina bifida occulta, congenital arthrogryposis multiplex and neurological defects.

Diagnosis

The clinical picture is sufficient for diagnosis. Only a harmless club foot posture, which can be fully corrected manually, can be differentiated from congenital club foot.

Allopathic diagnostic procedures

X-rays are suitable for monitoring development. They are not relevant before the 3rd month of life.

Osteopathic examination

Besides an evaluation of the entire body, the osteopathic examination will include a thorough examination of the lower leg and the foot. The practitioner tests the mobility of all the foot joints and, with the aid of primary respiration, the intraosseous situation in all the bones in the foot and lower leg.

Therapy
Allopathic medical therapy

The decisive thing is to start treatment immediately after birth and to continue with this consistently until growth is complete. The aims are correct anatomical axial relations, normal position and weight bearing of the foot, muscular balance and a freely mobile foot before walking begins.

A patient step-by-step manual correction is done and consolidated with a plaster cast which is frequently changed. Physiotherapy is given supportively. After the plaster casts splint treatment is used. First the adduction and varus position are eliminated and finally the pes equinus is carefully corrected.

If the result of conservative correction is inadequate, the remaining misalignments are treated surgically (arthrolysis, tendon lengthening, tendon transposition, osteotomy).

Osteopathic treatment

Osteopathic treatment should be given as an adjunct to orthopedic care. With good cooperation between orthopedic specialist and ourselves, it may be possible arrange to have the cast removed, give treatment that day, and then have the new cast put on, since the plaster cast needs to be frequently changed anyway. With splint treatment there is no difficulty in removing it for the treatment.

All the structures of the body, from the cranium and cranial base down to the foot are examined and, if necessary, treated in order to optimize the ability of the foot to self-correct. It is important to treat the relationship of tibia and fibula and especially the interosseous membrane of the lower leg (see p.187) to normalize as far as possible the muscular and fascial components of all the muscles which have their origin in this area. All the joints in the feet are treated using a balanced ligamentous tension approach (BLT; see p.183). It can be helpful here to have the embryonic central axis of the lower extremity at the edge of our consciousness without concentrating on it too much. We need to keep a special look-out for potential intraosseous lesions in this area. Often a good intraosseous change can be achieved by treatment using the BLT approach; however, it may also be necessary to work with fluid drives.

Prognosis

Lack of treatment or poor treatment leads to progressive deformity. With early treatment satisfactory results are obtained.

Adjunctive osteopathic treatment will in any case improve the prognosis. Thorough osteopathic treatment may even help to avoid operation. If surgery must be undertaken, the tissues will be more adaptable after previous osteopathic treatment.

The treatments should be given at least every 14 days, in some circumstances even every week, so as to exploit the window of opportunity of early development to the full. After about 6 months the intervals between the treatments can be lengthened.

INTOEING (METATARSUS ADDUCTUS)

Giles Cleghorn, Eva Moeckel

Normal intrauterine development of the feet

On the 27th to 28th day the lower limb bud appears, originating at the level of the lumbar and upper sacral segments. At the start of the 5th week the mesenchymal skeletal anlage appears, then at the end of the that week the first cartilage nuclei appear. At the end of the following week the entire skeleton of the extremities is laid down as cartilage. In the first days of the 7th week the anlagen grow ventrally. Towards the end of the embryonic period the legs rotate 90° medially, the extensors now being at the front. The arm buds rotate 90° laterally, the arm extensors now being at the back. In the 3rd month the fetus has his thighs in flexion, abduction and external rotation with the feet crossed over (Fig. 15.20).

The feet are in plantarflexion and adduction, the soles of the feet pointing towards the child's abdomen. As the fetus gradually develops, the thighs derotate inwards; the feet

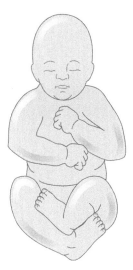

Figure 15.20 Fetus in the 3rd month. Thighs in flexion, abduction and external rotation with feet crossed over, the feet in plantarflexion and adduction, and pointing towards his own abdomen. With permission, Henriette Rintelen, Velbert

gradually rotate outwards and position themselves against the wall of the uterus. It is possible that this normal process is halted or delayed for some reason and the child is born with his feet in a plantarflexion and equinovarus position.

The normal newborn foot may still appear as it was positioned in utero: the forefoot is adducted in relation to the hindfoot, the sole of the foot is slightly supinated and the foot tends to be in plantarflexion. This physiological supination and adduction position, however, should disappear with kicking and be easy to correct passively.

Definition

Synonyms: Toeing-in, pigeon-toeing, metatarsus varus.

The forefoot is adducted and points inward; the metatarsal bones are angled medially. The outer edge of the foot is bent convexly, the arc of the convexity being greatest at the base of the fifth metatarsal bone. The hind foot is in a valgus position (Fig. 15.21).

Approximately 70% of cases of this disorder of the foot are in boys, and it is often bilateral.

Etiology and pathogenesis

Intoeing is commonly found in babies and children, from birth up to the age of 18 months. It is often accompanied by an internal rotation of the tibia. In neonates and babies this phenomenon is fairly normal. A metatarsus adductus which persists after this time, however, will hamper the child's walking. The child may fall over more often because of it.

The possible causes are a delayed derotation of the foot from its normal intrauterine position, or a persisting adaptation to

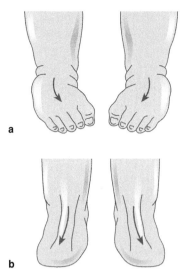

Figure 15.21 Metatarsus adductus (Intoeing). **a:** Ventral view **b:** Ðrsal view.
With permission, Henriette Rintelen, Velbert

the intrauterine lie, especially where conditions were quite cramped. In severe cases, an impaired development of the leg anlage may be the cause. The adduction position can also develop if the baby's preferred sleeping position is on his front.

Carreiro (2004) distinguishes three types, depending on the mobility of the forefoot.

- Type 1: Self-corrects on active movement (child kicking). Prognosis is good, the disorder self-corrects.

- Type 2: Can be corrected with passive movement (foot positioning). Prognosis is good.

- Type 3: Cannot be corrected even by passive movement. The most severe form.

In a severe case, the deformity tends to lie in the joint area between the cuneiform and metatarsal bones, or even rather more within the metatarsal bones, at their base. This is also the area in which intoeing is corrected surgically, by base wedge osteotomy.

Clinical signs and symptoms

The forefoot is in the adduction position. All the metatarsal bones, especially the first, are angled medially. The outer side of the foot has a convex curvature, with the inward curve being most marked at the base of the fifth metatarsal bone. The hindfoot is in the valgus position; the longitudinal arch of the foot is flattened.

With a severe deformity, painful calluses may appear on exposed sites from the pressure of shoes.

If the child can already walk he shows a more or less marked intoeing gait ('pigeon-toed gait').

Differential diagnosis

The differential diagnoses which we must consider are tibial torsion, functional malposition of the hip joint with increased internal rotation, club foot (in which the heel is in the varus position, see p.339) or femoral antetorsion (see p.327).

Diagnosis

Inspection clearly shows the clinical signs. Observe the baby to see whether he can compensate for the intoeing when kicking (active movement test). The following movement tests are useful:

- Stroke the lateral margin of the foot lightly. At this, the peroneal muscle contracts, and if the intoeing is only functional this will correct it (Type 1).

- If the intoeing has not corrected itself in this way, try to get the foot to assume the correct form passively. If this can be done, then it is a Type 2; if it is impossible, a Type 3.

- All the normal foot movement components are tested: plantarflexion, dorsiflexion, supination and pronation. No pes equinus position is found, and when the foot is dorsiflexed, there is no limitation as there is with club foot.

Allopathic diagnostic procedures

To confirm the diagnosis, X-rays can also be made. They show the adduction of the metatarsal bones, the first being inclined the most and the fifth the least.

Osteopathic examination

In a complete osteopathic examination (see Ch.7, Examination of the infant and toddler, Examination of the preschooler and schoolchild) particular attention is paid to the lower extremities. Here, besides the mobility of the foot, the position of the hip joint, knee, tibia and fibula are of special interest. In intoeing one will often find an external rotation of the femur with a compensatory internal rotation of the tibia. On examination with the aid of involuntary motion, pay attention to intraosseous restrictions in the feet, tibia and fibula, which may be a result of the position in utero.

Therapy
Allopathic medical therapy

Manual remedial work is done immediately after the birth. Mild form (Types 1 and 2) often self-correct. It may be enough if mother or father – following precise instructions – stimulates the lateral margin of the foot by stroking it. Antivarus shoes also may prove helpful.

Where there is resistance to therapy or Type 3, remedial plaster casts, and then splints and orthoses, are used.

Only rarely is a surgical correction needed (capsulotomy, serial metatarsal osteotomy).

Osteopathic treatment

In a Type 1 the self-correction can be supported by osteopathic treatment, and osteopathy is also useful in a Type 2. In a Type 3 osteopathic treatment will be used only as an adjunct to a remedial plaster cast.

In my experience it makes sense to examine the feet and leg axes of every baby brought to the practice and to judge whether the child's development is age-appropriate in this respect. If the normal development and changes in legs and feet lag behind, one can encourage the physiological developmental process with osteopathy. Much can be done even for severe deformities if they are discovered early enough. Sutherland's approach to the body as a whole (BLT) has proved very helpful both in normalizing the leg axes and for local foot treatment. For an exact description of this approach to treatment and for the relevant techniques see Ch.8 (An osteopathic approach to the newborn and infant). Intraosseous treatment of the foot may also be required. Often a good intraosseous change can be achieved by treatment with the BLT approach, but it can also be necessary to work with fluid drives, for instance.

Prognosis

The prognosis depends on the severity of the malposition. In Types 1 and 2 a full correction can be expected. Type 3 requires long-term treatment to obtain the best possible function of the foot. An early start to the treatment is always important.

FLAT FOOT (PES PLANUS)

Giles Cleghorn, Eva Moeckel

Definition

Congenital flat foot (talus verticalis or congenital pes planus, 'rocker-bottom foot') is a foot deformity with a vertical position of the talus, contracted valgus position of the heel, a high heel, abduction and pronation of the forefoot and flattening of the longitudinal arch of the foot.

Flat foot acquired in childhood (pes planus infantum) is a fairly common and mostly harmless condition of the foot in which the heel is in a valgus position (pes valgus) and the longitudinal arch of the foot is flattened (pes planus), and thus comes into contact with the floor. In some people the

arch of the foot never develops. Another component may also be present, a splay foot (pes transversus); the transverse arch of the foot is lowered, so that the heads of the metatarsal bones II–IV stand lower.

Etiology and pathogenesis

Congenital flat foot is probably hereditary, and in 50% of cases it is combined with other additional malformations. It is generally unilateral. Among the possible causes under discussion are: intrauterine lie, an inhibition malformation, neuropathies and muscular imbalances with a contraction of the triceps surae, peroneus and extensor muscle of the foot.

In babies and young children flat feet are normal, because the longitudinal arch of the foot has not yet developed. The longitudinal and transverse arches develop after the 1st year of life, when the child starts to walk. The longitudinal arch should be developed at the age of 3 years and the transverse arch at the age of 6 years. If the flat feet persist, this is regarded as a normal variant in most cases.

Flat foot acquired in childhood (pes planum infantum) develops when walking begins. The longitudinal arch of the foot does not develop properly or disappears again. The foot is nevertheless mobile; on standing the arch is not detectable, but if the child raises the big toe or stands on tiptoe the arch becomes visible. Hence pes planum infantum is also called mobile flat foot. In children with mobile flat feet the medial margin of the foot is often lowered. The toes point inward, so that the foot can be kept in balance.

Causes of flat foot acquired in childhood may be:

- Hypermobility of the joints. This is caused by weak ligaments and muscles. Predisposing factors are constant walking and standing on hard and smooth floors and also on paved streets. Typically, affected children show no interest in sport and have never had to walk long distances – especially not over rough terrain, which trains the foot muscles.

- Reduced flexibility. Here, one finds a shortened Achilles tendon, which contracts the muscles at the back of the leg and forces the foot into lowering its medial margin to compensate.

- A persistent medial tibial rotation. This may force the foot into a compensatory pronation, so that the foot points forward. According to Caillet (1987) about 10% of all 5-year-old children and 5% of all teenagers still have an internally rotated tibia.

- Excess weight.

- Genua valga or vara, which lead to compensatory flat foot.

- Flaccid and spastic paralyses.

A splay foot can develop from a flat foot. This is mostly a consequence of a compensatory supination of the forefoot, which overextends the transverse metatarsal ligament and the interosseous muscles. The heads of the metatarsal bones II–IV stand lower and must therefore bear a part of the body weight.

A synostosis in the region of the tarsal bones can also be the cause of painful flat foot in children. This is a fusion of two or more tarsal bones, which leads to a limitation of movement and often to the development of a flat foot.

Clinical signs and symptoms

In congenital flat foot the entire foot is rigid and cannot alter its shape on walking. Fluid movements are not possible. The longitudinal arch has a downward-pointing convex curvature, the feet are rotated externally on walking. In the early years the child is still asymptomatic but pain often begins in adolescence.

Flat foot acquired in childhood generally causes no symptoms in childhood. It is usually the worried parents who seek advice. However, with advancing age the feet may lose their mobility and pain can occur. Predisposing factors are tense foot muscles and long periods of standing ('adolescent flat foot'). If a mobile flat foot causes pain even in a young child there is usually another underlying problem, such as repeated ankle sprains or constricting footwear.

Splay feet are often painful, especially in walking and standing. The pain is caused by the lowered heads of metatarsal bones II–IV, which are not designed to bear weight.

Diagnosis

The gait will show up any paralyses if they are present.

Congenital flat foot is evident from the convexly curved sole of the foot, pronation of the heel and pronation and abduction of the forefoot. The entire foot is immobile. The longitudinal arch of the foot is not visible, even when the child stands on tiptoe.

In flat foot acquired in childhood the medial margin of the foot is lowered; the longitudinal arch of the foot is not visible. The navicular is lowered and the calcaneus stands in pronation. If the child stands on tiptoe the longitudinal arch reappears (flexible flat foot in contrast to the contracted congenital flat foot). Alternatively, you can get the child to raise his big toe while lying supine, and the arch of the foot will again appear. The hindfoot is often in the valgus position; the tibia can stand in internal rotation. The ankles are mobile, sometimes even hypermobile. The loss of the longitudinal arch and the intoeing gait greatly accelerates wear on the soles of the feet. If the shoes are placed side by side they will look as if they lean towards each other.

In splay foot there is an obvious spreading of the forefoot and a lowering of the transverse arch. The heads of the metatarsals are tender to pressure. Corns have usually formed on the sole of the foot at the level of the heads of the metatarsals.

Allopathic diagnostic procedures

In congenital flat foot an X-ray shows the axis of the talus almost as an extension of the tibia, the navicular being dorsally dislocated onto the head of the talus.

Radiography is only required for congenital flat foot or if there are symptoms in acquired flat feet. The hindfoot may then appear in the valgus position, the forefoot in abduction and pronation.

In splay foot the X-ray shows that metatarsal I deviates medially (the angle between metatarsals I and II is widened). The other metatarsals are splayed, the big toe frequently adducted (hallux valgus).

Osteopathic examination

A complete examination of the whole body (see Ch.7, Examination of the preschooler and schoolchild) can give important clues as to whether biomechanical factors are impairing the development of the arch of the foot.

Therapy
Allopathic medical therapy

Congenital flat foot is treated immediately after birth with corrective plaster casts. However, in many cases the position of the talus cannot be changed. In older children there is an option of surgical reposition of the talus and navicular; however, there is a risk that a talar necrosis will develop. Surgical subtalar arthrodesis after the end of the growth phase may also be considered.

Doctors usually treat mobile flat feet conservatively, by the careful choice of appropriate shoes, and, if there is pain, by prescribing arch supports. Walking barefoot and foot exercises to strengthen the flexor digitorum muscles will be helpful (gripping exercises for the toes, standing on tiptoe). In excess weight, weight reduction is recommended.

In a contracted flat foot the precipitating factors must be treated. If the cause is a synostosis in the tarsal region, the fusion of the affected bones can be eliminated surgically. In a more advanced stage or in older patients an osteotomy may be advised, with repositioning of the bones and also a fusion of the tarsals. In less severe cases supportive treatment with anti-inflammatories and splints or arch supports may be quite sufficient.

Osteopathic treatment

Flat feet are not always a pathological problem. Not every foot has to have a pronounced arch; a less marked arch can function well, whereas a very pronounced arch can be as stiff as a board. When examining the feet, mobility and elasticity are the deciding factors.

Correcting the plantar arch with the aid of osteopathy is a lengthy but straightforward undertaking if you bring the necessary patience to the task. Start with the cranium and the sphenobasilar synchondrosis (SBS), because a compression will be found here in many cases. Once a 10-year-old boy came to my practice because of chronic flat feet. I was of the opinion that his feet were normal, as were his legs and his pelvis. His SBS, on the other hand, was compressed. During treatment this pattern resolved; he stood up, and suddenly the arches of his feet were visible. We were all astonished. This case shows how the body as a whole has an effect on the individual parts.

It is important to treat the entire spine and the pelvis before starting work on the feet. The fibula, tibia and interosseous membrane of the legs are treated in order to balance out the foot muscles and their fascia, which have their attachments in this area, as far as possible. In the foot, turn your attention to the navicular bone first and foremost; this is often rotated medially. In order to restore the plantar arch, the navicular must be raised and rotated externally. One way of doing this is described on p.209 under the treatment of the transverse tarsal joint. All the foot joints must be mobile and correctly located. This is especially true of the subtalar joint. The plantar aponeurosis must also be normalized, because contractions in the foot depend to a considerable extent on the fascial components. Often, the bones are in odd positions, determined by the connective tissue. For this, I would like to suggest a lift for the plantar arch (see p.210).

Our feet love energetic treatment. The foot is so constructed that it can bear four times its own body weight during running and jumping. Consequently, in treatment we must truly reflect the fascial tissue of the foot and find the exact matching tone that is required.

Insoles can support the process of osteopathic treatment but should be abandoned once it is certain that the foot can again bear the body's weight independently.

Prognosis

Whether the flat foot is functional or pathological in nature is largely immaterial to the mode of approach in osteopathic treatment, because this is similar in both cases. However, it does make a difference to the prognosis. The more fixed and pathological the process is, the more long-term the planning for the treatment.

JUVENILE RHEUMATOID ARTHRITIS

Giles Cleghorn, Eva Moeckel

Definition

Synonym: Juvenile idiopathic arthritis (JIA).

Juvenile rheumatoid arthritis (JRA) is a rheumatic disorder of childhood and adolescence with an onset before the age of 16 years, which is associated with inflammations and stiffness of the joints, lasts more than 6 weeks, and for which no other cause can be found. Besides the joints, other organs may be affected. It can considerably impair the child's bone development. JRA can run a mild course with few problems but can also take a severe course with serious complications. Unlike chronic and incurable rheumatoid arthritis in adulthood, JRA may often heal spontaneously.

Girls are twice as commonly affected as boys.

Etiology and pathogenesis

Like rheumatoid arthritis in adulthood, JRA is an autoimmune disease in which the body's own immune system attacks the body's own healthy cells and tissues. However, the exact cause of JRA is not known. Some researchers suspect that in autoimmune diseases, like JRA, the lymphocytes lose their ability to protect certain parts of the body, such as cartilage, from the negative effects of bacteria or viruses. This releases messenger substances which can damage the body's own tissues as part of an inflammatory process.

There are probably many predisposing factors in JRA. It is likely that both genetic and environmental factors play a part. When a number of genes were being decoded, an HLA gene complex was discovered on chromosome 6, which is associated with JRA. If a child shows the specific HLA antigen type for JRA, which is called DR4, the risk of illness is increased. But even children without this antigen can have JRA. HLA antigen tests are therefore not an appropriate diagnostic method for existing disease or its possible later onset.

Clinical signs and symptoms

Even before the onset of joint symptoms, the children seem tired, weary and pale. The main symptom is an arthritis, which is not of traumatic origin, with swelling, effusion, painful limitation of movement and often hyperemia. Morning stiffness of the joints is typical but not regularly present. Knees, hands, fingers and feet are most commonly affected. The symptoms can fluctuate considerably from day to day, even in the course of a day. On some days the joint stiffness and pain are slight, while on other days so severe that the child can hardly move. Moreover, every child can feel the symptoms in a different way. Loss of appetite, poor weight gain and slow growth may also be present.

JRA is divided into 5 different subtypes (Table 15.2), which are distinguished from each other by the extent to which the joints are affected, the detection of specific antibodies, therapy, complications and prognosis.

- Polyarticular form without rheumatoid factor. Five or more joints are affected, mostly the smaller joints in the hands (especially metacarpophalangeal, proximal interphalangeal joints) and feet, but often also the large joints; never the lumbar spine. The joints are affected symmetrically. Fever can occur initially. Involvement of the hand can lead to an ulnar malposition, limiting the ability to write.

- Rheumatoid factor positive polyarthritis. Rapid cartilage erosion is possible. It is similar to adult rheumatoid arthritis. Rheumatic nodules appear.

- Early childhood oligoarthritis (type I oligoarthritis). Here, four joints or fewer, typically large joints such as the knee, ankle or wrist, are affected; conversely, fingers and toes are affected much less often. Half of this group will later develop a monoarticular arthritis. The joints are affected asymmetrically. In general the patients show a very mild course and recover fully. Patients with more than one joint affected may develop a polyarticular type of the disorder. Often a chronic iridocyclitis occurs, which, if inadequately treated or not at all, leads to lasting damage to the eye with later blindness (in up to 15%).

- Undifferentiated juvenile spondylarthropathy (previously type III oligoarthritis). This is associated with the HLA class I antigen B27. Psoriatic arthritis is classified under this: arthritis, psoriasis and two of the following criteria – dactylitis, nail abnormalities, dermatologically confirmed psoriasis in a first-degree relative. A transition to ankylosing spondylitis is possible.

- Still's disease. The systemic and most severe form of JRA. It is defined by the following symptoms:
  - arthritis, myalgia
  - intermittent high fever with rapidly spiking temperature ($>39°C$, for at least 2 weeks); the temperature generally rises late in the afternoon and becomes normal within the next few hours; the fever can be accompanied by chills; the child usually feels very ill; weeks or even months can elapse before the next bout of fever but seldom more than 6 months.

Table 15.2 Subtypes of juvenile rheumatoid arthritis

	Rheumatoid factor-negative polyarthritis	Rheumatoid factor-positive polyarthritis	Oligoarthritis of early childhood, Type I	Undifferentiated juvenile spondylarthropathy (previously Type II oligoarthritis)	Still's disease
Incidence	20–30%	5–10%	30–40%	15–30%	5–15%
Age at the onset of the illness	3	12	2	10	5
Sex distribution	More girls than boys	Predominantly girls	Predominantly girls	More boys than girls	Girls = boys
Rheumatoid factor	Negative	Positive	Negative	Negative	Negative
Antinuclear antibody (ANA)	Positive in 25%	Positive in 75%	Positive in 50%	Negative (except in psoriatic arthritis)	Negative
Association with human lymphocyte antigen	None	DR4	DR5, DR8	B27	None
Uveitis	Rarely	None	Up to 40%	Up to 25%	None
Joint prognosis	Doubtful	Poor	Good	Good	Doubtful to poor

– a mostly truncal, transient and confluent, fine rash that is visible only during the fever; this comes and goes over several days

– hepatosplenomegaly

– lymphadenopathy

– pericarditis, myocarditis, pleuritis

– abdominal pain

– anemia, leucocytosis (increased neutrophils), thrombocytosis, increased ESR.

Differential diagnosis

Differential diagnoses to be considered: septic arthritis, osteomyelitis, malignancies (leukemia, neuroblastoma), coxitis fugax, rheumatic fever, arthritis associated with an infection, collagenoses, 'growing pains'.

Diagnosis

The local findings are decisive: joint inflammations which have been present for at least 6 weeks. The joints are examined, with inspection, palpation, and testing of the range of motion of all joints.

Allopathic diagnostic procedures

Laboratory

As yet, there is no specific laboratory test to detect JRA. The following variables are investigated:

• Markers of inflammation: increased CRP and ESR, leucocytosis with left shift in Still's disease.

• Infective anemia, decreased serum iron, increased ferritin.

• Complement concentration decreased: may suggest an impaired immune system.

• Detection of antinuclear antibodies (ANA): may suggest oligoarthritis of early childhood, increased risk of chronic iridocyclitis.

• Rheumatoid factor (IgM): indicates rheumatoid factor-positive polyarthritis.

Arthrocentesis

Arthrocentesis (removal of joint fluid from the joint space) is used principally at the onset of the illness to rule out septic arthritis.

Imaging procedures

Ultrasound can detect joint effusion, tenosynovitis and soft tissue changes. X-rays are used at the start of the illness to rule out other disorders (e.g. osteomyelitis, tumor) and for documentation. The MRI scan can visualize all the joint structures and assess the extent of the inflammation.

Osteopathic examination

If a child is suspected of having JRA, the child is referred to appropriate specialists for investigation. However, commonly a child is brought to an osteopathic specialist when the diagnosis is already known. The osteopathic examination will therefore concentrate (see Ch.7, Examination of the preschooler and schoolchild) on finding indications as to how the child's immune system can be strengthened and his existing state of health optimized.

Therapy
Allopathic medical therapy

Resting the joint and pain-relieving medication are of fundamental importance. Putting stress on an inflamed joint can damage it permanently. For pain relief, non-steroidal anti-rheumatic agents and corticosteroids, in severe cases anti-rheumatic agents, such as methotrexate, can be given.

Cold packs may be used when there is active inflammation; after the inflammation has subsided, local heat therapy. Physiotherapy is intended to improve and maintain muscle and joint function. Daily active and passive exercises are important. Occupational therapy may be necessary to preserve independence in the activities of daily life.

A nutritional adviser checks the child's nutritional status. A nutritional plan can help ensure that the young patient, whose appetite may be impaired by the illness itself or by the medication given, has a balanced diet.

Because of the risk of blindness, close ophthalmological monitoring is mandatory, even if the joint symptoms have already disappeared.

Patient information programmes help reduce the frequency and severity of the outbreaks and prevent complications. The topics covered include sport and weight control, rest periods, and techniques of carrying and pulling heavy objects, using the large joints more, rather than the small joints. Psychological care is also important.

Osteopathic treatment

In the acute phase of the illness, CV4 treatments following the approach of Sutherland (2004) are very useful, in my experience. This method has a profound effect and produces a systemic change in the entire body. It may also modify the membrane permeability, so that leucocytes can penetrate into the tissues and reduce the cycle of inflammation. In both adults and children with rheumatoid arthritis it can take a very long time for the CV4 approach to show an effect. Although the treatment normally lasts only a few minutes, with these patients it may take up to 20 minutes. If the patient's state of health improves with regular treatment, the length of each session usually shortens. Under a CV4 treatment, prescribed medication works better. I have been able to achieve a full remission in many cases. Of course one never knows exactly whether the recovery is attributable to the osteopathic treatment, to the medication or to a spontaneous remission. However, studies seem to show that regular osteopathic treatment does much good. Here, a CV4 should never be carried out directly on the occiput of children less than 8 years of age, as a mainly mechanical application risks compressing this extremely fragile physiological area. An approach starting from the sacrum is better.

In non-acute phases, when the illness is temporarily quiescent, therapeutic approaches such as 'general osteopathic treatment' (GOT) or other methods can be useful in treating the affected joints.

Mobilization techniques such as GOT and manipulative methods of treatment with high velocity thrust (HVT) can, however, cause great damage to the joint in the acute phase of the illness and are in my opinion contraindicated in this period.

Prognosis

The course of JRA differs from one child to the next. The duration of treatment is indeterminate. Periods of remission and of flare-ups of the disease alternate. In some children the illness flares up once or twice, never to return. In other children, however, it continually recurs and never completely heals. After 20 years about 75% of cases are healed or have a low activity. The rest develop a severe disease in the joints, mainly in the rheumatoid factor-positive form. Early and consistent treatment is decisive in reducing the effects on the joints to a minimum.

The illness can severely restrict many areas of life for an active, growing young person (such as school, playing with friends and family, sport). It is important for the entire family to master the challenges associated with this illness. In asymptomatic phases the child should be encouraged in sport and other activities which keep the joints strong and flexible. Playing with other children is also important for the young patient's social development. There will always be times when the child cannot attend school. However, with appropriate support from the school most children with JRA can keep up. Many affected young people want to be like their peers, and feel isolated, imperfect and insecure. The pain and exhaustion caused by the disease are evident to everybody, but the anger and depression which grow out of the restrictions imposed by

the disease must be recognized. Regular osteopathic treatment seems to support a positive course.

FREQUENCY OF TREATMENT AND AFTERCARE
Giles Cleghorn
Frequency of treatment

Parents often ask about the frequency of treatment and the prognosis. The answer is not easy, because one never knows how each individual patient will react to the treatment. I have decided against dealing with this topic with reference to the different illnesses and have instead preferred to work out a few guidelines (not prescriptive rules) which may be of help to you.

For me, the following treatment schedule has proved useful. If I treat an acute infectious condition or a sudden trauma which has occurred only recently, then frequent, but not too invasive or intensive, treatments are appropriate. In acute infections it can be perfectly advisable to treat every couple of hours, after a traumatic event perhaps only once every couple of days. For example, the birth of a child can be a traumatic event for both the mother and the child. The intensity of the symptoms also determines the frequency of treatments to a certain extent. The more severe and painful the symptoms the more often must treatment be given. Babies and children in the acute phase of a disease must be treated more often because their immune system may be in crisis and need help to reach a crescendo and then find its way back to normality. As the symptoms of the illness regress the treatments can go deeper and the treatment interval increased.

Conversely, if one treats a child with a stable system but who has a bone disease, such frequent treatments do not make much sense because 3 to 5 weeks can go by before there is a change in the state of the bone. In such a period it remodels its trabeculae and the associated blood supply. Consider that a bone renews itself every 5 weeks; this is its tempo.

If the affected tissues are muscles at the reflex level, and the state of health is otherwise stable, the treatment can take effect more quickly. The blood supply also changes quickly, but as the nutrient supply to the affected tissues was deficient and the shortfall which has arisen must be made good, several days or weeks can easily go by until the tissues have renewed themselves at the cellular level – on this level the improvement in the condition is slower.

Accordingly, the type of tissue determines how long it is before one can expect a result and how often treatment must be given. In chronic disorders, overtreatment is more problematic than undertreatment. Remember that each system needs time to recover. Excessively short treatment intervals can lead to treating the reaction to treatment rather than the condition of the tissues.

We have to learn to recognize what input a system can tolerate and can only evaluate this by 'reading' the changes in the tissues during treatment. The first resonance in the tissues is often the only indication that a therapeutic process or healing is taking place. We often expect major changes to take place in the tissues, believing this to be better. But consider: a small change in the tissues can start the healing process like a snowball getting bigger and bigger as it rolls downward until a real 'health landslide' is let loose.

Follow-up treatment

'Follow-up' means a further treatment when the patient is actually asymptomatic and the tissues feel normal on palpation, or as normal as you think possible. The aim of follow-up is to ensure that the child's condition has remained stable and that growth and development have not disturbed the body's equilibrium. In answering the question about the follow-up interval, account must be taken of the child's age and development. Neonates should be seen again in 1 to 2 months, small children every 3 or 6 months, and 3- to 5-year-olds every 6 months. Between the 5th year of life and puberty an aftercare interval of 9 to 12 months is quite adequate if the health is otherwise stable.

In puberty itself, adolescents experience great growth spurts. Body and mind are transformed. In this time the changes caused by treatment may be greater than at other phases of life. Consequently, I would shorten the follow-up interval for adolescents to 3 to 6 months again if there are no symptoms and treat more frequently if there are any symptoms. I like to work very intensively with adolescents, as the changes in this period of life are tremendous and the success obtained in childhood lasts throughout adult life.

Bibliography

Becker R: Life in Motion. Rudra, Portland, Ore. 1997

Behrman R, Kliegman R: Nelson – essentials of pediatrics. Saunders, Philadelphia 1990

Breusch S, Mau H, Sabo D: Klinikleitfaden Orthopädie. 4th edn. Urban & Fischer, Munich/Jena 2002

Brooks W, Gross R: Genu varum in children – diagnosis and treatment. Journal of the American Academy of Orthopedic Surgeons 1995

Caillet R: Foot and ankle pain. 4th edn. Davis, Philadelphia 1987

Carreiro J: Pädiatrie aus osteopathischer Sicht. Elsevier, Munich/Jena 2004

Isogai K: Isogai dynamic therapy. Lattice, Tokyo 1982. Distributed Maruzen PO Box 5050 Tokyo International 100–31 Japan

Jäger M, Wirth C: Praxis der Orthopädie. Thieme, Stuttgart 1986

McRae R: Clinical orthopedic examination. 2nd edn. Churchill Livingstone, London 1983

Selye H: The stress of life. 2nd edn. McGraw Hill, New York 1984

Still A: Osteopathy, research and practice, Journal Printing Co, Kirksville, Mo. 1910, Reprint Eastland Press, Seattle, Wash. 1992

Sutherland W: Sutherland–Kompendium. Jolandos, Pähl 2004

Internet addresses

www.orthoteers.org.uk
www.ortho.hyperguides.com

ANATOMY AND PHYSIOLOGY OF THE BRAIN

William Goussel, Dina Guerassimiouk, Jens-Peter Markhoff

Brain stem

Reticular formation and ARAS

The brain stem (Fig. 16.1), which comprises the medulla oblongata, pons and mesencephalon (or midbrain), also contains a loosely interwoven net of nerve fibres known as the reticular formation. The development of this network structure is already evident in the cervical region of the spinal cord and it extends to include all three regions of the brain stem. The reticular formation consists of large and small nerve cell groupings that are varyingly interspersed between the fibre tracts and cannot be assigned either to the cranial nerves or to other groups of relay neurones. A number of cell groups of the reticular formation – the reticular nuclei – can be identified and these can be differentiated anatomically, depending on their location in the brain stem, but not functionally. The neurones in these groups send out ascending or descending axons and transmit many side branches to the cranial nerve nuclei and to the relay nuclei of the brain stem.

One crucial point to note is that the cells of the reticular formation receive input from all afferent signal systems. The function of the reticular formation here is determined not on the basis of which particular stimuli are received but by how many; in other words, the differentiation is quantitative rather than qualitative.

The reticular formation has an excitatory and an inhibitory component. These influence the cerebral cortex, brain stem nuclei and spinal cord to regulate tone and to control the level of activity. The excitatory, activating component, the arousal center, is also known as the ascending reticular activating system (ARAS). Via efferent connections with the thalamus the ARAS generally enhances the activity of the entire cerebral cortex, and this may be regarded as a prerequisite for alertness and effective perception.

The cranial nerve nuclei and the brain-stem centers governing vomiting, circulation and respiration will not be discussed in detail, although they supply the primary somatosensory and viscerosensory afferents for further processing and integration, and they project somatomotor and visceromotor efferents. They are important 'entry portals' through which conscious awareness gains access to the 'internal and external world'.

Substantia nigra

The substantia nigra is another important element that contributes to impulse processing: it is located in the brain stem and, as the largest nucleus complex in the midbrain, it constitutes an important motor center. In conjunction with the basal ganglia (see p.353) it regulates the modulation and control of coordinated movements. This center is especially significant for motor drive and the initiation of appropriate responses to sensory stimuli.

Nuclei in the tectum of the midbrain

Two important relay stations located in the tectal region (the corpora quadrigemina) also form part of the midbrain: these are the superior colliculi, which are responsible for optic reflexes and rapid ocular muscle movements, and the inferior

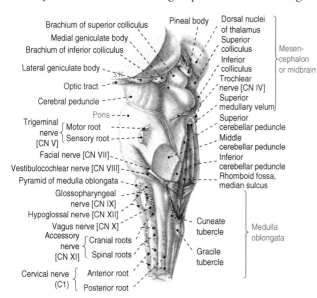

Figure 16.1 Structure of the brain stem (lateral view). With permission, Sobotta: Atlas der Anatomie des Menschen. Publisher: R. Putz and R. Pabst, 21st edn. Elsevier/Urban & Fischer, Munich/Jena, 2000

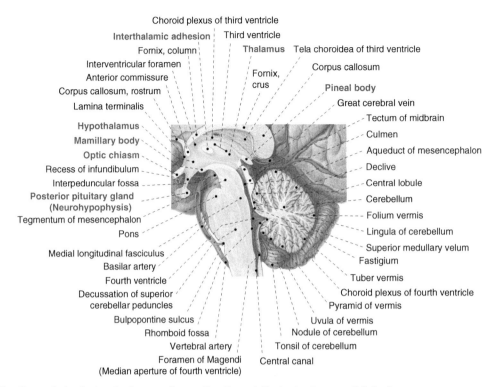

Choroid plexus of third ventricle
Interthalamic adhesion
Third ventricle
Fornix, column
Thalamus
Tela choroidea of third ventricle
Interventricular foramen
Corpus callosum
Anterior commissure
Fornix, crus
Corpus callosum, rostrum
Pineal body
Lamina terminalis
Great cerebral vein
Hypothalamus
Tectum of midbrain
Mamillary body
Culmen
Optic chiasm
Aqueduct of mesencephalon
Recess of infundibulum
Declive
Interpeduncular fossa
Central lobule
Posterior pituitary gland (Neurohypophysis)
Cerebellum
Tegmentum of mesencephalon
Folium vermis
Pons
Lingula of cerebellum
Medial longitudinal fasciculus
Superior medullary velum
Basilar artery
Fastigium
Fourth ventricle
Tuber vermis
Decussation of superior cerebellar peduncles
Choroid plexus of fourth ventricle
Pyramid of vermis
Bulpopontine sulcus
Uvula of vermis
Rhomboid fossa
Nodule of cerebellum
Vertebral artery
Tonsil of cerebellum
Foramen of Magendi (Median aperture of fourth ventricle)
Central canal

Figure 16.2 The diencephalon (color shading; median section through the brain stem, medial view). With permission, Sobotta: Atlas der Anatomie des Menschen. Publisher: R. Putz and R. Pabst, 21st edn. Elsevier/Urban & Fischer, Munich/Jena, 2000

colliculi, which form an important station on the auditory pathway where most of the auditory afferents are relayed and projected to the thalamus.

Cerebellum

The cerebellum is located behind the medulla oblongata and pons (Fig. 16.2) and forms the roof of the fourth ventricle. It is the highest and most important integration center for balance and the coordination of movements. Its function is to control and provide fine tuning for:

- aspects of posture and movement, including muscle tone
- motor aspects of gaze in terms of stabilizing on a target object
- targeted implementation of motor activity planned in the cerebrum
- motor aspects of speech.

Diencephalon

The diencephalon (see Fig. 16.2) has several subdivisions, the largest and most important of which is the thalamus, which forms the greater part of each lateral wall of the third ventricle. Almost all sensory projection pathways pass through the contralateral part of the thalamus before being projected onwards to the cerebral cortex in fibre tracts that travel via the internal capsule to the frontal, parietal, temporal and occipital lobes. For this reason the thalamus is also often referred to as the 'gateway to the cerebral cortex'.

In terms of its relationship to the cerebral cortex, two principal components of the thalamus can be differentiated on a functional basis:

- The specific thalamus, whose nuclei have qualitative specific connections with well-defined cortical areas; namely with the motor, premotor, sensory, visual and auditory regions and with the limbic system.
- The non-specific thalamus, whose nuclei are functionally part of the reticular formation and have connection with the cerebral cortex. However, this occurs in a fairly diffuse manner, resulting in arousal and wakefulness responses following stimulation of the ARAS of the reticular formation.

The most important function of the two thalamic components is impulse selection so as to prevent the cortex being overwhelmed with stimuli.

Another part of the diencephalon, located inferior to the two lobes of the thalamus, is the hypothalamus, which forms the floor of the third ventricle; with its nuclei it constitutes the

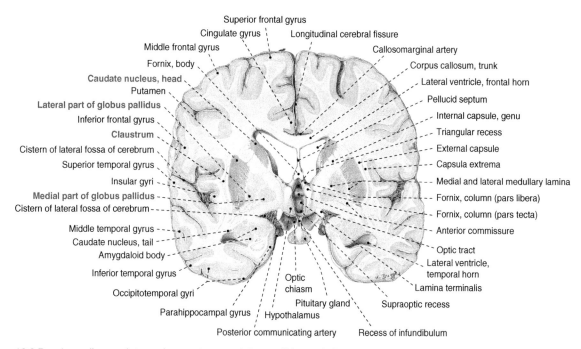

Figure 16.3 Basal ganglia: caudate nucleus, putamen, globus pallidus and claustrum.
With permission, Sobotta: Atlas der Anatomie des Menschen. Publisher: R. Putz and R. Pabst, 21st edn. Elsevier/Urban & Fischer, Munich/Jena, 2000

highest regulatory center in the autonomic and endocrine systems. The hypophysis or pituitary gland consists of an anterior lobe (the adenohypophysis) and a posterior lobe (the neurohypophysis) which in turn is still classed as part of the hypothalamus. Controlled by the anterior lobe, the previously described regulation of the endocrine system unfolds through the agency of appropriate releasing and release-inhibiting hormones.

Cerebrum (telencephalon)

The cerebrum, which in humans accounts for about 80% of the total brain mass, consists of two hemispheres interconnected by the corpus callosum, and the basal ganglia lying beneath them. In phylogenetic terms the striatum, paleocortex, archicortex and neocortex can be distinguished in the cerebrum.

Basal ganglia

The corpus striatum consists of the putamen and caudate nucleus as well as the lateral and medial globus pallidus and claustrum – all nuclei that are counted as belonging to the basal ganglia (Fig. 16.3). In functional terms, the subthalamic nucleus and the substantia nigra in the midbrain are also considered part of the basal ganglia.

All the basal ganglia share a key role in the central regulation of involuntary motor activity. Lesions in this area result in hypo- and hyperkinesias. Thus injury to the corpus striatum produces hyperkinetic syndromes, such as Huntington chorea. Injury to the substantia nigra is associated with hypokinetic syndromes, such as Parkinson syndrome.

Amygdala

The paleocortex – phylogenetically the oldest part of the cerebral hemisphere – accommodates the amygdala, with its distinct fibres connecting it with centers in the limbic system. The amygdala plays an important role in the emotional modulation of vegetative processes and in the regulation of behavior associated with fear and rage.

Limbic system

The archicortex is formed principally by the hippocampus, parahippocampal gyrus and parts of the cingulate gyrus. These areas are constituent parts of the limbic system (Fig. 16.4), which is largely classified as belonging to the temporal lobe and is composed of nuclei and cortical regions as follows:

- The hippocampus, situated at the medial wall of the inferior horn of the lateral ventricle. As a result of the rotational movement of the hemispheres during embryonic development the hippocampus acquires its characteristic curved shape. Beneath the corpus callosum – and forming

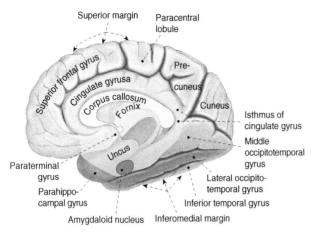

Figure 16.4 Limbic system (color shading) in the cerebral hemisphere (medial view).
With permission, Sobotta: Atlas der Anatomie des Menschen. Publisher: R. Putz and R. Pabst, 21st edn. Elsevier/Urban & Fischer, Munich/Jena, 2000

the roof of the third ventricle – it continues in the fibre structures of the fornix to terminate in:

- The mamillary bodies, which form part of the hypothalamus.
- The cingulate gyrus, which runs above the corpus callosum on the medial surface of the cerebral hemispheres and, together with the hippocampus, forms what might be termed the 'center' of the limbic system.
- The parahippocampal gyrus, which also forms part of the temporal lobe.
- The amygdala, which is located in the anterior region of the temporal lobe.
- The dentate gyrus, which is located further lateral to the parahippocampal gyrus.

The functions of the limbic system are diverse and may be defined primarily as being in the psycho-emotional and vegetative area. The hippocampus, for example, is very significant for learning processes and the associated development of memory (both short-term and long-term) as well as for motivational behavior and conscious appreciation. Similarly, it plays a key role in the pathogenesis of epilepsy. The cingulate gyrus affects many autonomic functions and plays a special role in psychomotor and locomotor drive.

The limbic system exerts a pronounced effect on emotional and vegetative functions (circulatory regulation, hormone secretion, immune system activity) and thus modulates motivation, drive, sexual behavior as well as emotional modalities (joy, rage, calm, despair, etc.). However, it should also be emphasized that the limbic system must not be viewed as the only cerebral location where these effects are manifested; many other areas can be equally influential.

Neocortex

In phylogenetic terms the neocortex is the most recent and therefore the most highly organized part of the cerebral cortex. The following functional distinctions may be made:

- Primary areas are principally sensory centers that receive their sensory afferents directly from the thalamus, examples being the auditory or visual pathways.
- Secondary areas are located, in most cases, adjacent to the primary areas and are responsible for the initial integrative processing of sensory information; i.e. some interpretation of sensory information already occurs there.
- Association areas neither receive primary sensory information nor are they classed as part of a particular primary area. Instead they have connections to numerous primary and secondary cortical areas. This results in circumscribed functional areas, as in the case of the motor speech center, which processes a large number of different afferents and projects them in its efferents.

Morphologically, the neocortex can be subdivided into four cerebral lobes.

Frontal lobe

The frontal lobe consists of four parts:

- The precentral gyrus (Fig. 16.5) is located immediately in front of the central sulcus and as the primary motor cortex it is the territory of origin for the greater part of the pyramidal tract. It is here in particular that fine motor movements of the contralateral half of the body are initiated.
- The premotor or supplementary motor cortex lies immediately anterior to the primary motor cortex, for which it performs a certain preparatory or programming function.
- The motor speech center (Broca's area) is responsible for the initiation of speech in terms of articulation and sentence structure. It is located only on one side, namely in the dominant – i.e. usually the left – hemisphere. A selective lesion of this center leads to motor aphasia with linguistic comprehension largely intact.
- Functionally higher-order psychological and intellectual processes are associated with the prefrontal cortex. A bilateral lesion in the territory of the frontal lobe may result in altered social behavior in the form of a diminished sense of social responsibility. Reduced self-criticism, inability to concentrate, poor movement programming and fine motor movement deficits are also encountered.

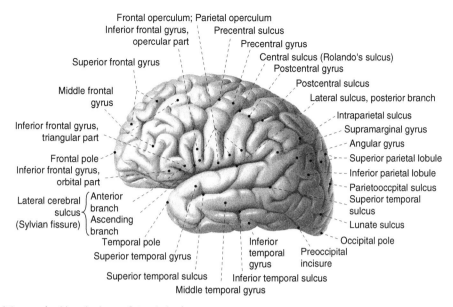

Figure 16.5 Gyri of the cerebral hemispheres (lateral view).
With permission, Sobotta: Atlas der Anatomie des Menschen. Publisher: R. Putz and R. Pabst, 21st edn. Elsevier/Urban & Fischer, Munich/Jena, 2000

Parietal lobe

The parietal lobe should also be considered part of the sensorimotor system. The postcentral gyrus (primary somatosensory cortex; see Fig. 16.5) is located behind the central sulcus and is the primary brain area on the somatosensory pathway where information relating to heat, temperature, pain, and fine or coarse touch are directly received. Owing to the somatotopic pattern of the gyrus, a lesion here produces loss of sensation in the corresponding sensory territory supplied.

The secondary somatosensory cortex lies directly behind the postcentral gyrus and is responsible for interpreting the information arriving from the primary somatosensory cortex. A lesion here is associated with tactile agnosia (i.e. objects touched can no longer be recognized.)

The angular gyrus (see Fig. 16.5) arches over the posterior end of the superior temporal sulcus. As the central relay station between the visual cortex and the sensory speech center (Wernicke's area) in the auditory association cortex, it is of major importance for reading and writing. Lesions in this area lead to an inability to read (alexia) and write (agraphia).

The posterior parietal lobe contains areas that play a crucial role in spatial perception, spatial orientation and development of personal body image. Right hemispheric lesions often lead to disorders of spatial orientation, while left hemispheric lesions usually result in apraxia.

Temporal lobe

The temporal lobe is the location of the neocortical manifestation of the auditory system. The auditory pathway (Fig. 16.6)

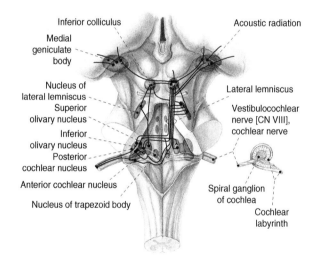

Figure 16.6 Auditory pathway.
With permission, Sobotta: Atlas der Anatomie des Menschen. Publisher: R. Putz and R. Pabst, 21st edn. Elsevier/Urban & Fischer, Munich/Jena, 2000

begins at the cochlear nuclei in the medulla oblongata: from there auditory impulses are transmitted sometimes ipsilaterally, sometimes contralaterally with relay stations in the inferior colliculi in the midbrain and in the medial geniculate body of the thalamus to the primary auditory cortex in the temporal lobe.

The primary auditory cortex is the zone where auditory impulses are first consciously perceived without being interpreted; that is, sounds or tones are consciously recognized but not perceived as language or music. A lesion of the primary auditory cortex does not result in deafness, but merely

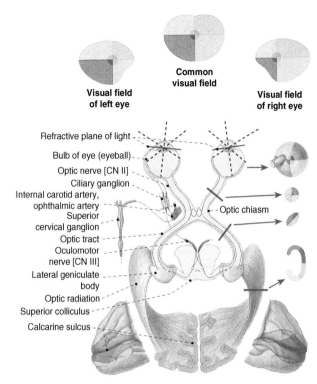

Figure 16.7 Visual pathway.
With permission, Sobotta: Atlas der Anatomie des Menschen. Publisher: R. Putz and R. Pabst, 21st edn. Elsevier/Urban & Fischer, Munich/Jena, 2000

in auditory impairment because the impulses from one inner ear terminate bilaterally in the temporal lobes.

The secondary auditory cortex, the most differentiated part of which is known as the sensory speech center (Wernicke's area), lies lateral to the primary auditory cortex. This is where the impulses arriving from the primary auditory cortex are interpreted: language is recognized as such and understood. The sensory speech center is developed in the dominant – usually left – hemisphere in each case. In right-handed individuals the auditory association cortex is located on the left side, and in left-handed individuals it may be on the right or left side. A lesion of the sensory speech center results in loss of linguistic comprehension, as well as a disorder of the individual's language formation capability (sensory aphasia).

Occipital lobe

The occipital lobe belongs to the visual system. The visual pathway (Fig. 16.7) begins in the retina and travels as the optic nerve (cranial nerve II) to the optic chiasm. Here the fibres of the nasal retinal halves decussate to the contralateral side. As the optic tract, the visual pathway continues to the lateral geniculate body of the thalamus, whence it continues as the optic radiation to the primary visual cortex in the occipital lobe.

In the primary visual cortex the visual impulses from the contralateral half of the visual field of both eyes are recorded without any interpretation of these impulses taking place. A lesion of this area of the brain results in blindness in the contralateral part of the visual field.

The secondary visual cortex is located radially around the primary visual cortex and is responsible for interpreting the visual impulses delivered by the primary visual cortex in the sense of assigning recognition to visual input. A lesion to the secondary visual cortex means that the individual affected is no longer able to process the visual input. The person is not blind and can see individual features. Instead the disorder means that these individual features cannot be assembled together to make whole images. For example, in optical agnosia the affected individual may mistake a telephone dial for a clock or fail to recognize his wife's face.

Functional anatomy

The following sections will describe a number of possible connections between cerebral functional impairment and osteopathic lesions. As with osteopathic treatment, it is not a matter here of listing 'if A, then B' causal relationships and patent remedies, which simply cannot exist given the individuality of each and every child, but of taking a didactic step closer to understanding the complexity of sensory disorders and their varied etiologies.

Hemodynamic aspects

The metabolic status and function of a tissue are both dependent on its supply by the blood vessels, which deliver and remove nutrients, metabolic products, oxygen, carbon dioxide, vitamins and electrolytes. If this hemodynamic equilibrium is disturbed, the result will be disorders of tissue homeostasis, possibly leading to functional impairment. These repercussions may occur at the level of blood glucose concentration, electrolytes, pH, neurotransmitters, and the immune system, etc. – all areas in which the sensory nerve tissue is particularly susceptible.

Arterial blood supply

(Fig. 16.8)

Still (1992) repeatedly maintained that from the osteopathic standpoint the arterial blood supply for every tissue is of central importance for function and self-healing. An osteopathic dysfunction in the sense of restricted tissue mobility can influence the arterial perfusion of a tissue via fascial and reflex pathways.

Given that the central nervous system (CNS) is equipped with terminal arteries and that in the event of a stenosis or

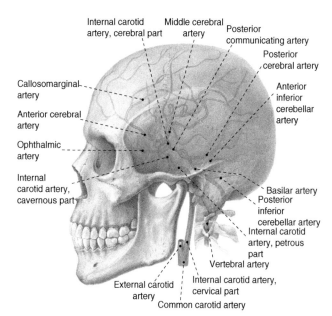

Figure 16.8 Course of vertebral artery and internal carotid artery. With permission, Sobotta: Atlas der Anatomie des Menschen. Publisher: R. Putz and R. Pabst, 21st edn. Elsevier/Urban & Fischer, Munich/Jena, 2000

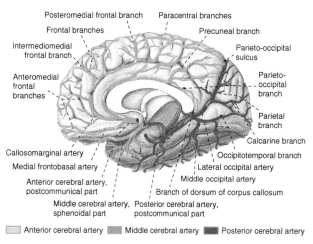

☐ Anterior cerebral artery ▦ Middle cerebral artery ■ Posterior cerebral artery

Figure 16.9 Territory supplied by the three major cerebral arteries, the anterior, middle and posterior cerebral arteries (medial view). With permission, Sobotta: Atlas der Anatomie des Menschen. Publisher: R. Putz and R. Pabst, 21st edn. Elsevier/Urban & Fischer, Munich/Jena, 2000

obliteration the existing anastomoses – including the arterial circle of Willis – can provide only inadequate compensatory perfusion, the potential problems associated with disorders of perfusion become even more significant. Osteopathic lesions relating to the territories supplied by cranial arteries and to the topographic location of certain brain areas involved in corresponding processing functions should therefore certainly be considered as possible causes of sensory disturbances. A number of examples will be given to indicate the location of individual lesions and their functional consequences for perfusion.

An osteopathic dysfunction in the region of the atlanto-occipital joints may impair physiological blood flow in one or both vertebral arteries. In the main these arteries supply the brain stem and cerebellum in the posterior cranial fossa. As a result, all the previously mentioned CNS structures important for impulse processing – the reticular formation, substantia nigra, colliculi of the midbrain and cerebellum – may be affected by circulatory disturbances.

Once the two vertebral arteries have united to form the basilar artery, there arises from the latter the (frequently double) posterior cerebral artery (Fig. 16.9), which essentially supplies the occipital lobe with the primary and secondary visual cortex, the caudal and basal part of the temporal lobe and the inner ear, as well as the midbrain and thalamus. Because the basilar artery and site of origin of the posterior cerebral artery are located on the clivus, intra- and interosseous lesions at the level of the occipital bone and

sphenoid body may have a disruptive influence on the arterial blood supply of these brain areas.

Where it passes through the cranial base in the region of the foramen lacerum, the paired internal carotid artery may also be vulnerable to dural tension and to lesions of the sphenoid and temporal bones.

After passage through the foramen lacerum and traversing the cavernous sinus, the internal carotid artery gives off the anterior cerebral artery, and itself continues in its larger terminal branch known as the middle cerebral artery. The branches of the middle cerebral artery (see Fig. 16.9) supply the corpus striatum, part of the globus pallidus and considerable areas of the frontal, parietal and temporal lobes. These locations are associated principally with the motor cortex, the motor and sensory speech centers and the angular gyrus, an important relay center between the optical system and language. Osteopathic lesions involving the sphenoid, frontal, temporal and parietal bones may exert a disruptive influence on these brain areas that have particular relevance for perception. The osteopath should pay special attention to the pterion, that region where the four above-mentioned cranial bones overlap and articulate with each other. Also worth emphasizing in this region is the sphenosquamous pivot point between the temporal and sphenoid bones; it is the site of least mobility above which the middle cerebral artery travels on its course.

After branching off from the internal carotid artery the anterior cerebral artery (see Fig. 16.9) travels above the optic chiasm into the longitudinal cerebral fissure and there extends as far as the end of the parietal lobe. Its supply territory is characterized by the medial parts of the frontal and parietal lobes; that is, it perfuses a major part of the prefrontal

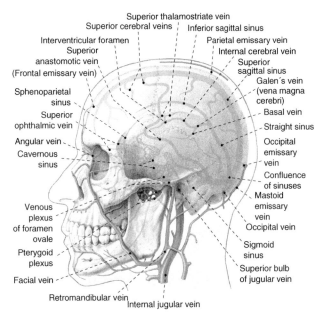

Superior thalamostriate vein
Superior cerebral veins
Inferior sagittal sinus
Interventricular foramen
Parietal emissary vein
Superior
anastomotic vein
Internal cerebral vein
(Frontal emissary vein)
Superior
sagittal sinus
Sphenoparietal
sinus
Galen´s vein
(vena magna
cerebri)
Superior
ophthalmic vein
Basal vein
Angular vein
Straight sinus
Cavernous
sinus
Occipital
emissary
vein
Confluence
of sinuses
Venous
plexus
of foramen
ovale
Mastoid
emissary
vein
Pterygoid
plexus
Occipital vein
Sigmoid
sinus
Facial vein
Superior bulb
of jugular vein
Retromandibular vein
Internal jugular vein

Figure 16.10 Schematic illustration of the dura mater sinuses and veins of the head.
With permission, Sobotta: Atlas der Anatomie des Menschen. Publisher: R. Putz and R. Pabst, 21st edn. Elsevier/Urban & Fischer, Munich/Jena, 2000

and premotor cortex and parts of the precentral and postcentral gyrus (somatotopic leg and foot region).

In terms of the vascular supply of the brain Kahle (1991) noted that the major cerebral vessels are without exception located at the surface of the brain. They send small arteries and arterioles vertically into the cerebral substance and these form subdivisions. Considering this, both intra- and interosseous (i.e. sutural) lesions affecting the tension of the cranial dura mater are potentially adverse factors for the arterial perfusion of certain areas of the brain.

Thus Magoun (1976) highlights the phenomenon – proven by many clinical studies conducted by Sutherland – that even mild sutural lesions have a reflex effect on neighboring nerve tissue and blood vessels.

Venous drainage

(Fig. 16.10)

Turning our attention to the venous part of the blood circulation, the aforementioned influences of sutural lesions on nearby blood vessels apply also naturally to the venous drainage system. Indeed, it is likely that this disruptive influence may be even more pronounced because veins have a less robust wall structure by comparison with arteries, indicating that the veins can be compressed more easily, particularly since the venous vascular system is a low-pressure system.

The venous blood from the neurocranium is collected in the cranial veins and transported to the intradural venous

sinuses, from where it is carried almost exclusively via the internal jugular vein to the superior vena cava. The cranial veins are subcategorized into superficial and deep veins.

The superficial cerebral veins collect blood from the cerebral cortex and from the underlying medullary layer and feed directly into the intradural sinuses. By contrast, the deep cerebral veins all conduct the blood first into the great cerebral vein, which in turn empties into the straight sinus. The drainage territory of the deep cerebral veins principally covers the subcortical cerebral structures and the diencephalon. At this point it is worth emphasizing again the importance of the thalamus, which is situated in the diencephalon and, as the 'gateway to the cerebral cortex', performs a kind of impulse selection of virtually all sensory afferents to prevent the cortex from being overwhelmed. This area appears to play a relatively pivotal role specifically in regard to sensory disorders.

Venous drainage from the brain stem also occurs via the great cerebral vein and directly into the inferior petrosal sinus and the transverse sinus. In the context of the present discussion, we should also recall the important place occupied by the reticular formation. The superior part of the cerebellum finally drains into the great cerebral vein and the straight sinus, and the inferior part into the superior petrosal sinus and the transverse sinus.

Sutherland (1990) draws attention to a phenomenon in the cranial field that is of immense functional importance from an osteopathic viewpoint. While the venous blood is received into veins with a typical morphological structure, it is then transmitted to the sinuses, which do not display the typical structure of veins but consist of duplicatures or folds of cranial dura mater. Sutherland characterizes them as 'large channels' for the venous blood. If we recall the osteopathic function of the reciprocal tension membrane (RTM), then the primary respiratory mechanism (PRM) may be regarded functionally as a type of 'suction pressure pump' for venous blood flow in the sinuses. Lesions of the RTM and associated sutures may directly impair venous drainage from the aforementioned brain areas and hence their function.

Sutherland (1990) emphasizes the importance of the PRM for venous blood flow in the neurocranium: the free mobility of the cranial bones is an important prerequisite for the unhindered flow of blood in the sinuses. The two parietal bones determine the quality of drainage for the superior sagittal sinus, and the occipital bone is important for the straight sinus and the confluence of sinuses. He went on to describe the transverse sinus, which is located on the inner surface of the occipital squama, as being particularly important. In that area Sutherland was unable to identify any compensatory capacity whatsoever for the venous blood flow. The inevitable repercussions of an occipital bone dysfunction in terms of circulatory stasis are therefore readily imaginable.

Also meriting mention is the region of the asterion, which represents a former fontanelle and on whose inner surface runs the transverse sinus, which empties into the sigmoid sinus. Here, free mobility of the parietal, occipital and temporal bones is a precondition for unhampered blood flow, with the temporal bones being of major importance also for the superior petrosal sinus and the inferior petrosal sinus (draining the cavernous sinus).

The cavernous sinus collects blood from the superior ophthalmic vein, the sphenoparietal sinus and the pituitary. It is of osteopathic relevance because the oculomotor, trochlear and abducent nerves pass in proximity to it. Hemodynamic disturbances at the level of the cavernous sinus in the form of impaired drainage may irritate these cranial nerves which are responsible for controlling eye movements. Coordination disorders of the eye, learning disorders due to ocular factors, as well as disturbances of balance may be a consequence of a pressure increase in the cavernous sinus.

The further drainage of venous blood from the neurocranium follows three main pathways. One leads from the cavernous sinus via the venous plexus of the foramen ovale to the pterygoid plexus or, depending on pressure factors, also via the orbits to the facial vein. This pathway may be disturbed by lesions involving the sphenoid bone and the pterygoid fossa and by lesions of the bones contributing to the orbits.

A small proportion of venous blood drains by a second pathway, via the basilar plexus epidurally through the foramen magnum into the internal vertebral venous plexuses within the spinal cord. The potential significance of lesions of the occipital bone, especially of intraosseous occipital lesions, for this venous drainage pathway is clearly apparent.

However, by far the greatest share of venous blood leaves the neurocranium by the third pathway, namely via the internal jugular vein. Consequently, the jugular foramen merits keen attention. Lesions in this area between the occipital and temporal bones may cause major disturbances of the circulation. This region may be affected in particular by birth trauma, occipito-atlanto-axial lesions, otitis media accompanied by mastoiditis, and other cranial trauma common in childhood.

Special attention should also be paid to the confluence of sinuses with its characteristic principal direction of flow: the superior sagittal sinus drains mainly via the right transverse sinus to the right jugular foramen, whereas blood from the straight sinus is drained mainly via the left transverse sinus and the left jugular foramen. This has significance in turn for the drainage of the great cerebral vein, which receives blood from the thalamus among other sources. A dysfunction in the region of the left jugular foramen may therefore have repercussions in terms of venous stasis and disturbed homeostasis extending as far as the diencephalon.

Unhindered circulation of the blood is enormously important for homeostasis in the neurocranium. Any changes to the internal environment may also involve nerve cell function and affect the production of neurotransmitters, resulting in disruption of intercellular communication in the CNS.

Cerebrospinal fluid

The cerebrospinal fluid (CSF) fills the central canal of the spinal cord and the ventricular system of the brain, and in the subarachnoid space it surrounds the brain and spinal cord like a fluid coat. In this way it protects the CNS against mechanical factors and compensates for hydrostatic pressure changes in the vascular system. In addition, the CSF fulfils a nutritive and drainage function for the brain and meninges.

Benninghoff (1994) considers the CSF system to be a modified lymph system for the CNS. The CSF contributes to the regulation of the biochemical environment in the CNS and performs immunological tasks, similar to the lymph in the rest of the body.

Benninghoff (1994) further observes that the CSF space communicates via the ventricular walls with the extracellular space of the brain. Thus the concentration of electrolytes in the CSF also corresponds to that in the extracellular space of the brain. Consequently, the chemical composition and fluctuations of the CSF are of prime importance for the function of the neurons and their intercellular communication.

Concerning CSF production, plexectomies performed in humans and monkeys (Benninghoff 1994) have shown that the choroid plexuses are not the only production sites for the CSF. Experimental investigation of this aspect has confirmed that 30% to >50% of CSF derives from sources other than the choroid plexuses, namely from the intercellular space of the brain. This functional aspect bears testimony to the communication and continuity of the body fluids. In the practice of osteopathy this body fluid continuity has great relevance that is reflected particularly in the drainage of CSF into the venous sinuses of the brain at the level of the arachnoid (Pacchionian) granulations.

Since important integrative brain centers are located immediately adjacent to the cerebral ventricles, the important role played by CSF fluctuations in sensory disorders is easy to appreciate. Most of the cranial nerve nuclei, the autonomic centers of the brain stem, the reticular formation and the cerebellum are grouped around the fourth ventricle. The thalamus, hypothalamus and pituitary surround the third ventricle and many basal ganglia and parts of the limbic system lie in immediate proximity to the lateral ventricles. The fluctuation of the CSF is therefore particularly important in terms of the osteopathic treatment of sensory disorders in children.

Sutherland (1990) points out that membranous restrictions impair both venous drainage and CSF fluctuation and therefore should be viewed as a significant factor in the causation of functional disorders of the CNS. The CSF system and CSF fluctuations depend functionally on the RTM and the circulation of the blood. Moreover, traumatic osseous lesions involving the neurocranium may compress the CSF cisterns and thus locally disturb the physiological fluctuations of the CSF. This in turn has an influence on neighbouring brain areas (Sutherland 1990).

Autonomic nervous system and CNS

The autonomic nervous system regulates those organ functions that are not under conscious volitional control. All its regulatory mechanisms promote homeostasis and help maintain the internal environment. Both parts of the autonomic nervous system, the sympathetic and the parasympathetic divisions, have a direct influence on the CNS. This affects both the regulation of perfusion as well as the flow of information from and into the periphery.

The sympathetic and parasympathetic divisions share a common control center in the diencephalon, the hypothalamus, which is under the influence of the cortex and the limbic system. In addition, there are also regulatory centers which are specifically assigned to one or other of the two divisions:

- Among the regulatory centers of the sympathetic system the superior cervical ganglion is especially relevant. It innervates the arteries of the head and thus regulates perfusion in the cranium. Fascial stress, in particular lesions of the upper cervical spine, may accordingly produce dysregulation of perfusion in the cranium and, depending on the innervation of the vessels, in circumscribed brain areas, thus in turn influencing neuronal processing activities. The regulatory centers in the spinal cord include all the ganglia of the sympathetic trunk with their anatomical and physiological connection to the lateral horns at the level of C8–L2. These modulate the function of the vascular system of the spinal cord and the internal organs so as to safeguard the homeostasis of the entire body.

- In the parasympathetic system the vagus nerve is important. It is estimated that it is made up of approx. 80% afferent fibres (Benninghoff 1994), a finding that underscores its importance in transmitting information from the periphery. The potential effect of this flood of information from the viscera on impulse processing in the CNS can be readily guessed. With regard to possible disruption due to osteopathic lesions, the spectrum in the visceral region is clearly diverse. The vagus nerve may also be subject to compressive forces and hemodynamic stress in other regions; e.g. in the cervical region with the upper thoracic aperture and in the jugular foramen.

- With reference to sensory perception and recognizing the fact that a child's visual perception should be regarded as an important precondition for harmonic development, another parasympathetic brainstem center is very important: the Edinger-Westphal nucleus of the oculomotor nerve in the mesencephalon ventral to the cerebral aqueduct regulates ocular accommodation and the pupillary reaction to entering light. Osteopathic lesions influencing CSF fluctuations or the circulation of the blood in the corresponding brain stem region may therefore be associated with problems of visual perception.

Fascial relationships

In embryological terms, the fascial system derives from the mesoderm. It constitutes an uninterrupted tissue unit and ensures the anatomical integrity of all the organs of the body. On account of their structural continuity, the fascias form a mechanical transmission system with twin functions: first, they enable and coordinate movements of the body, and secondly, they absorb and pass on forces from the outside, rather like a shock absorber. Trauma may therefore interfere with this fascial network and give rise to corresponding lesion chains (Paoletti 2001).

In this respect, as far as the neurocranium is concerned, there is a virtually inexhaustible variety of fascial relationships which includes both myofascial chains of the parietal system as well as viscerocranial connections.

Bibliography

Benninghoff A: Anatomie. Vol 2. Urban & Schwarzenberg, Munich/Vienna/Baltimore 1994

Kahle A: Taschenatlas der Anatomie - Nervensystem und Sinnesorgane. Vol 3. Thieme, Stuttgart/New York 1991

Klinke R, Silbernagl S: Lehrbuch der Physiologie. Thieme, Stuttgart/New York 1996

Magoun H I: Osteopathy in the cranial field. Journal Printing Company, Kirksville, Mo. 1976

Netter F H: Atlas der Anatomie des Menschen. Ciba-Geigy, Basel 1994

Paoletti S: Faszien. Urban & Fischer, Munich/Jena 2001

Silbernagl S, Despopoulos A: Taschenatlas der Physiologie. Thieme, Stuttgart/New York 1991

Still A T: Osteopathy- research & practice. Eastland Press, Seattle, Wash. 1992

Sutherland W G: Teachings in the science of osteopathy. Sutherland Cranial Teaching Foundation, Texas 1990

Trepel M: Neuroanatomie, Struktur und Funktion. 2nd edn. Urban & Fischer, Munich/Jena 1999

HYPOTONIA

Kok Weng Lim

Definition

Muscular hypotonia is defined as reduced tonus of the musculature with reduced resistance on passive motion testing of a joint. It is important to distinguish between peripheral muscular or motor-end plate weakness of the musculature and a centrally caused hypotonic musculature.

Weak infants are always hypotonic, but hypotonia may exist without weakness. A new born with muscular hypotonia is also called a 'floppy infant'.

Etiology and pathophysiology

Hypotonia in children is a common clinical problem, but it is important to bear in mind that the majority of floppy babies do not have a persistent neuromuscular disorder and may have benign neonatal/congenital hypotonia with a favorable outcome.

The classification of hypotonia is anatomical; it may be central in origin, or originate from the spinal cord, the peripheral nerves, the neuromuscular junction or the muscles themselves.

Central hypotonia

It is very important to recognize babies who are floppy but not weak, as muscular weakness is uncommon in central hypotonia. It only occurs in the acute stages or in infants with severe central nervous system malformations. Central hypotonia is the commonest cause of floppiness in babies and can be classified as follows:

- Primary central hypotonia due to:
  - **Chromosomal disorders:** e.g. **Down syndrome** and **Prader-Willi syndrome**. Children with Down syndrome (see Ch.17) will generally have good antigravity movements in the limbs, despite being floppy.
  - **Inborn errors of metabolism:** e.g. acid maltase deficiency, Zellweger syndrome. Afflicted term babies are born healthy, with normal tone and strength, and then become floppy after 12–24 hours. Such babies should have oral feeds withheld while a screening metabolic work-up is completed. They rarely present with hypotonia as the sole feature; commonly there are associated dysmorphic features and multiple malformations. The presentation varies, reflecting the energy deficiency or toxic states of acute or chronic CNS involvement; one sees hypotonia and seizures associated with the biochemical abnormalities. Metabolic disorders such as galactosemia may also present with hypotonia. But in such cases there are usually other features such as vomiting, hypoglycemia and an obvious depression of the level of consciousness. All these are potentially treatable conditions and should always be considered.
  - **Cerebral palsy:** babies are often hypotonic in the neonatal period; spasticity emerges several months later. Frequently, excessive tone occurs in specific regions while other areas remain hypotonic (see p.371).
  - **Brain malformations, brain dysgenesis:** e.g. lissencephalia, or aplasia of the cerebellum.
  - Benign congenital hypotonia
- Secondary central hypotonia due to:
  - **Anesthesia, drugs:** maternal medication such as diazepam or clomethiazole may affect the baby's muscle tone, also benzodiazepines, barbiturates and opiates, and anesthesia in a caesarean section.
  - **Meningitis, encephalitis, sepsis:** an otherwise normal baby who is unwell with respiratory problems or sepsis may be floppy. Indeed a baby who is floppy at birth is often considered septic until proven otherwise.
  - Respiratory distress
  - Hypoglycemia
  - **Trauma:** contusion, compression, bleeds.

Disorders of the spinal cord: spinal muscular atrophies

Birth injuries to the cervical spine and cord may result in hypotonia. But there are also a group of clinical syndromes arising as a result of genetically determined anterior horn cell degeneration: spinal muscular atrophy (SMA). The commonest form of SMA presents with limb girdle weakness; but other patterns of weakness are also found, such as scapuloperoneal SMA, and distal SMA with distal weakness of the upper limb predominating.

Even more rarely occurring spinal cord diseases presenting as hypotonia in infancy include syringomyelia and other forms of spinal dysraphism. Clues may be the finding of a hemangioma or tuft of hair in the midline over the spine, or a scoliosis. A history of bladder or bowel dysfunction may be obtained. On examination the presence of a mixed deep tendon reflex pattern and absent abdominal reflexes may be clues, and anal tone may be reduced.

SMA Type 1 (Werdnig-Hoffmann disease)

This is the most severe form of limb girdle SMA. The infant is often considered normal in the neonatal period. But in the first few months symptoms appear: striking proximal weakness (usually the legs are more affected than the arms), absent deep tendon reflexes, poor or lack of control of the head, atrophy of the intercostal muscles with tachypnea, fasciculations of the tongue, tremor of the hands, delayed motor milestones and floppiness. The weakness may appear quite suddenly in a previously normal baby. The baby typically lies in a 'frog' posture with the legs abducted, shoulders internally rotated and the elbows flexed. The face and external ocular muscles are mostly unaffected. Bulbar involvement often results in feeding difficulties. All affected children have onset of weakness before 6 months and 95% die of respiratory failure before 18 months.

SMA Type 2 and 3

SMA 2 has an onset before 18 months and affected children live longer. Type 3 has an onset after 18 months. They may be considered together as chronic SMA.

Typical symptoms are limb girdle weakness and depressed or absent tendon reflexes. Usually patients present with some degree of atrophy of the thigh musculature. The affected child may have a fine action tremor of the limbs. The severity may vary from children with only a mild disability to children who will never walk. The degree of weakness may progress but often remains essentially static, with growth spurts leading to an apparent deterioration. Parents cannot often be given a clear prognosis because of the variability of the condition. The most important aim in management of these children is to prevent the development of complications such as contractures and scoliosis.

Disorders of a peripheral nerve

Local palsies secondary to trauma are easily recognized. A generalized peripheral neuropathy is very rare in neonates.

Inherited axonal or demyelinating neuropathies are also very uncommon, but merit consideration in the assessment of the floppy infant with absent deep tendon reflexes. These include the Dejerine-Sottas syndrome (DSS) and congenital hypomyelination (CH) syndrome.

DSS is either congenital or of early childhood onset. There is a virtual absence of myelin on nerve biopsy and very low nerve conduction velocity. CH is of greater severity than DSS. The affected infants show severe hypotonia, weakness and respiratory and feeding difficulties.

Disorders of the neuromuscular junction
Transient neonatal myasthenia

Transient neonatal myasthenia occurs in one in seven children born to mothers with myasthenia gravis. The disease is caused by the passage of anti-acetylcholine receptor antibodies across the placenta. These babies may have feeding and respiratory difficulties and a progressively weakening cry. Maternal history and examination is of the utmost importance in the diagnosis. They respond to anticholinesterase drugs and improve after a few weeks.

Congenital myasthenia gravis

Congenital myasthenia gravis is a rare, genetically determined condition usually involving absence of a subunit of the acetylcholine receptor. There is usually a myopathic face, ptosis, generalized weakness and fluctuation of muscle strength, hypotonia and respiratory and feeding difficulties. They often present in later infancy and are only rarely encountered in the neonatal period.

Infantile botulism

Infantile botulism may mimic these myasthenic syndromes, but large, poorly reactive pupils should give the clue. It usually occurs within 6 weeks to 1 year after birth, usually where infants have been fed honey contaminated with spores of *Clostridium botulinum*. The first symptom is usually constipation but later listlessness, ptosis, facial weakness, decreased eye movements, feeding difficulties and progression to respiratory failure may occur.

Muscle disease
Congenital myotonic dystrophy

This should be suspected in a term neonate who is extremely floppy, with an immobile face and a tented, triangular, myopathic mouth. Affected children often require respiratory support and/or tube feeding. Often polyhydramnios may be detected in the pregnancy because of the fetus's swallowing difficulties in utero. The baby frequently has postural limb deformities like a clubfoot. Surviving children often have learning difficulties. The characteristic myotonia does not manifest until 8 to 10 years of age. In older children with myotonic dystrophy there may be delayed relaxation after muscular contraction, such as delayed relaxation after shaking hands.

Older children and adults present with a mild limb girdle weakness with specific involvement of the anterior neck muscles. Myotonic dystrophy is really a multisystem disease. There are abnormalities of gut mobility, which may produce dysphagia, small bowel bacterial overgrowth or abnormal anal sphincter tone. CNS involvement produces somnolence and fatigue, in addition to learning difficulties. Cardiomyopathy, arrhythmia and problems of the cardiac conducting system may occur. Endocrine problems such as diabetes mellitus, testicular atrophy and gynecological disorders are frequently seen in adulthood.

Congenital muscular dystrophy

Congenital muscular dystrophies are genetically caused myopathies with progressive muscular degeneration and atrophy. Babies born with this condition have poor muscle tone, severe weakness and limb contractures. Respiratory difficulties are not present in most cases. This is the single most commonly recognized underlying disorder in children with arthrogryposis. Some children may improve and gradually attain independent mobility.

Subgroups are recognized such as Fukuyama muscular dystrophy. This dystrophy is associated with microcephaly, myopia, global delay and seizures. The affected infant becomes progressively weaker through childhood and is usually unable to walk by 10 years of age.

Muscle-eye-brain disease presents with severe neonatal hypotonia, mental retardation and visual failure. Retinal degeneration with optic atrophy and a pale retina are typical.

Congenital (nondystrophic) myopathies

Congenital nondystrophic myopathies are myopathies with characteristic histological or electro-optic changes or metabolic defects. The types of congenital myopathy that are recognized include: central core, nemaline, myotubular, multicore and congenital myopathy with fibre type disproportion.

Infants present with hypotonia/flabby muscles and weakness which may also affect the face resulting in a lack of facial movement (in nemaline myopathy). Other signs are joint contractures and reduced tendon reflexes, along with other abnormalities such as micrognathia, open bite and a high arched palate leading to weakness of sucking and swallowing and consequent feeding difficulties. They may also have respiratory problems and often have learning difficulties later.

Clinical signs and symptoms

Hypotonia in the newborn ('floppy infant') usually presents after birth or may be identified in early life with reduced spontaneous movement, lack of control of the head, weak crying and weakness when suckling. The mother may have noticed little movement of her child in utero.

The majority of floppy infants, however, do not suffer from a persistent neuromuscular disorder but have benign neonatal/congenital hypotonia with a favourable outcome. Benign neonatal hypotonia is characterized by floppiness with normal strength. There may be a high familial incidence, and significant joint laxity is often a clinical feature.

It is important to note that the term benign congenital hypotonia is no longer considered to be a specific diagnostic entity as many patients with this diagnosis initially may well have a neuromuscular disorder with a well-defined structural or biochemical basis on further investigation.

Muscular hypotonia is associated with hypersalivation, an open mouth, a prominent head lag in pull-to-sit with traction from the arms, and the infant appears to 'slip through' on vertical suspension. Affected children also have a low-pitched cry or progressively weaker cry.

Clues to a central nervous system etiology include:

- significant dysmorphology
- abnormal size and shape of the head
- a disproportionately small body with normal head size
- seizures
- stridor
- brisk tendon reflexes
- axial hypotonia in excess of limb hypotonia.

Clues to a peripheral disorder include:

- facial weakness
- tongue fasciculations
- reduced or absent tendon reflexes.

Unusual skin creases extending over the pectoralis muscle from the axilla or additional thigh creases below the buttocks may signal underlying muscle atrophy. Truncal muscular atrophy will reveal bony prominences over spinous processes and ribs. Muscle bulk is of course related to the overall state of nutrition.

Arthrogryposis can be a feature of both central and peripheral disorders. A history of progressive weakness and hypotonia suggest a degenerative condition of either the central or peripheral nervous system.

The increased understanding of the genetic basis underlying some forms of hypotonia, the gene mutations that are involved and the current availability of DNA-based diagnostic tests have made the diagnosis of disorders such as Prader-Willi syndrome, congenital myotonic dystrophy and spinal muscular atrophy more straightforward. However, the differential diagnosis of hypotonia remains complex and the list of disorders that can be considered in the differential diagnosis of hypotonia grows ever longer.

Diagnosis
Case history taking

The history is a very important aspect in the clinical evaluation of the floppy infant or child as so many of the disorders involving hypotonia are heritable.

Family history

There may be a relevant family history. Ask about any history of neuromuscular problems in either parent or in the family in general. In congenital myotonic dystrophy, the mother is often mildly affected and may be unaware of the disease in herself. Ask if she has difficulty with hand grip; for example opening bottles or jars.

It is important to enquire about the age of walking and relative athletic ability in school for each family member. The diagnostic power of a negative observation (i.e. no family history) is diminished when the family is limited in size, without at-risk individuals (e.g. no at-risk males in a suspected X-linked disorder), or when the family is unavailable for examination. Note that for very rare diseases or for known recessive disorders, such as spinal muscular atrophy, the family history is usually benign.

Previous miscarriages and early neonatal deaths of siblings may indicate a genetic basis as in congenital muscular dystrophy or myotonic dystrophy. Miscarriages should be specifically asked for as parents do not always volunteer this information spontaneously.

Prenatal risk factors

An assessment of the prenatal, perinatal and postnatal risk factors is crucial. Look for a history of drug, medicine or alcohol exposure during pregnancy as they can act as CNS toxins.

Enquire about infections during pregnancy, especially systemic 'flu-like' illnesses. Infections such as congenital toxoplasmosis, rubella, cytomegalovirus and herpes (TORCH) infections are now recognized as a cause of widespread cerebral damage which can present in the newborn as hypotonia.

Also significant are maternal diseases such as diabetes and epilepsy. Other prenatal factors that should be enquired for include reduced fetal movements, especially when reported by an experienced mother. This may often be the first sign of hypotonia. The presence of polyhydramnios may be the result of disordered fetal swallowing, either from brain or motor unit dysfunction. Note that abnormal fetal presentation may reflect poor fetal movement or immobility, which may be due to poor muscle tone or simply a short umbilical cord.

Perinatal risk factors

A history of perinatal birth trauma that may suggest the possibility of cerebral damage includes delivery complications and persistently low Apgar scores. Floppiness at birth may sometimes be diagnosed in retrospect by an unusual pattern of the Apgar-score with low scores for tone, reflexes and respiratory effort more than for color. Severe complications of delivery, though rare, may be associated with cervical spinal cord injury.

Postnatal history

Was hypotonia noticed at, or soon after birth? A baby who is floppy at birth is often considered septic until proven otherwise. Term babies who are born healthy with normal tone and strength and then become floppy after 12 to 24 hours may have inborn errors of metabolism.

A newborn with brain dysfunction, either acute or long-standing, may have a number of important features. Enquire about the early signs of CNS impairment, such as altered levels of consciousness, seizures, feeding difficulties, abnormal breathing patterns, abnormalities of early primitive reflexes, and unusual posturing. These may last for under 24 hours if mildly neurologically compromised, and beyond if moderately or severely compromised; for example by hypoxia or ischemia.

The course of the floppiness after the newborn period can be revealing. Hypotonia due to CNS causes does not worsen with time. However, even if static, it may become increasingly apparent when compared with the tone in healthy children. Most infants with static brain disorders and floppiness will slowly develop increased tone, eventually becoming spastic. A static or slowly improving floppiness is possible with both central or peripheral causes of hypotonia. Worsening of the hypotonia may suggest degenerative disease of the CNS, the motor unit or both.

A history of delayed motor milestones is often the main or presenting complaint. Delayed social, fine motor or language milestones suggest a central etiology. If the child is weak, this itself may contribute to the developmental delay.

Clinical examination

General observation

Observe for dysmorphic features in the face and cranium as these may suggest a syndrome involving hypotonia. Also, abnormalities of head size (whether too large or too small) or cranial deformities are consistent with brain maldevelopment. Lack of facial expression may be seen in hypotonic infants. A high arched palate is often noted in infants with metabolic disorders (acid maltase/ Pompe disease). The presence of fasciculations, for example on the tongue, suggest anterior horn cell involvement and denervation. Other features to look for include lipodystrophy and inverted nipples (congenital disorders of glycosylation).

Eyes

Examination of the eyes may reveal ptosis, weakness of the orbital muscles (myasthenic syndromes), cataracts and pigmented retinas (peroxisomal disorders) and lens dislocation (metabolic disorders).

Limbs and joints

Examination of the limbs and joints may show fixed positioning and limitation of joint mobility: arthrogryposis that involves both proximal and distal joints. This is due to severe weakness in early fetal development, which immobilizes joints leading to contractures. This feature is encountered in both neurogenic and myopathic disorders. Such infants may be hampered more by the joint restrictions than by weakness or hypotonia.

Search for mild proximal joint contractures as they are common in floppy infants and can be corrected by passive stretching.

Hypermobility is the finding of increased joint range of motion, frequently seen both with weakness and hypotonia.

Visceral organs

Also important is the examination of the heart, liver and spleen. Enlargement of these organs may alert you to the possibility of storage disorders: for example glycogen storage disease. Renal cysts are characteristic of peroxisomal disorders.

Neurological examination

A neurological examination should be performed in order to ascertain if the hypotonia is a central ('floppy'/hypotonic) or peripheral (muscle weakness) problem. Many children with a peripheral disorder involving nerve, muscle, or the neuromuscular junction will be weak as well as floppy. Some children, although not all, with severe CNS involvement, particularly if in the acute stages, may also be weak as well as hypotonic.

Muscle tone simply refers to the least resistance that an alert but not overstimulated infant generates while opposing passive movement. The assessment of muscular resistance is subjective and must be related to the state of arousal. Tone can alter considerably in relation to feeds and sleep state and repeated examinations are required to confirm physical signs. Note that tone increases with gestational age and is high in term babies. Their limbs lie flexed and adducted, while preterm infants adopt an extended posture. Passive tone matures from below upwards.

Muscular weakness is determined by asessing the maximum muscle power that can be generated. Assessment of full muscle power requires maximal effort on the patient's part. Hence the crying baby offers the best information. Note should be made of any regional differences in muscle power. When muscular atrophy is present, it is useful to compare the muscle power to bulk. Weak infants are always hypotonic, but hypotonia may exist without weakness.

Muscle power is best assessed by studying the baby's spontaneous movements and looking at antigravity movements and posture in the limbs. The antigravity movements are reduced in the weak as well as hypotonic infant.

In infants and children attempts should be made to document the maximal functional abilities, such as the heaviest toy that can be picked up, the height of reaching above the head, or the degree of truncal tilt possible before head support is lost.

The distribution of the weakness should be noted. Comparisons should be made between the tone of the left and right sides and arms versus legs, versus trunk and neck. Axial weakness is often a feature of central hypotonia. A combination of weakness in the antigravity limb muscles, reduced or absent tendon reflexes, or facial weakness or tongue fasciculation suggest a neuromuscular disorder. Signs such as axial weakness and the relative preservation of limb muscle power with hypotonia and brisk tendon reflexes or abnormal eye movements, seizures and stridor suggest a central origin.

Certain classical patterns of weakness are important: acute infantile spinal muscular atrophy (Werdnig-Hoffmann disease) classically spares muscles of the face, diaphragm and pelvic sphincters. The various myasthenic syndromes in infants frequently affect the bulbar and eye muscles. Most myopathies tend to affect proximal limb muscle function more than fine distal movements of fingers and toes.

Excessive fatigability is rarely an isolated feature of floppy infants. Excessive fatigue implies progressive failure at the neuromuscular junction. It is the most difficult to demonstrate because it requires the infant to sustain maximum effort. However, fatigue can be deduced from an infant who is unable to breastfeed despite a strong urge to feed, good swallowing, and an initially powerful suck. Bulbar fatigue, accompanied by fixed weakness of eye movement and ptosis, suggest infant myasthenia.

The absence or relative strength of deep tendon reflexes should be assessed. In normal infants, reflexes can readily be elicited from the biceps, knees and ankles; other reflexes may not be as responsive. The floppy child with increased deep tendon reflexes almost certainly has a central dysfunction, in contrast to diminished reflexes with muscle disease. Absent reflexes out of proportion to minimal weakness may suggest either a neuropathy or central disease.

The posture of the infant may betray hypotonia. The floppy infant usually lies in a 'frog-leg' posture. This is a posture of full abduction and external rotation of the legs as well as flaccid extension of the arms. There is prominent head lag in pull-to-sit with traction from the arms. The infant appears to 'slip through' on vertical suspension, and on ventral suspension, the infant hangs limply.

The degree of alertness may be an important clue too: infants with neuromuscular diseases are often alert, compared to the depression of consciousness seen in infants with CNS involvement.

A clear distinction may, however, not always be possible. For example, arthrogryposis may be a feature of both central and peripheral hypotonia. Features may also overlap in certain conditions affecting both the CNS and peripheral nerves, such as the group of muscle-eye-brain disorders.

Parents

Examination of the parents, especially the mother, is essential. In many autosomal dominant conditions, disease expression is highly variable. Therefore a complete family history requires personal examination of the family. In suspected congenital myotonic dystrophy a the mother should be checked for signs of myotonic dystrophy, such as eyelid closure weakness and grip myotonia. She may have wasting of the temporalis muscles and an inability to open her hand quickly and completely after maximum grip, particularly the thumb. Another sign is percussion myotonia of the tongue or thenar eminence. Fatigability of the eyelids, when the mother gazes up for a while, or of the arms when maintained outstretched forward for 4 minutes, suggests myasthenia gravis.

Familial joint hypermobility is a common cause of infantile hypotonia and examination of the parents may reveal this.

Allopathic diagnostic procedures

Laboratory examinations include a full blood count, blood sugar levels, signs of infection, electrolytes, thyroid hormones, screening for viruses (if prenatal infection is suspected), selective metabolic screening, testing of CSF and genetic screening.

Nerve conduction tests, an electromyogram (EMG) or a muscle biopsy may be carried out (for example in congenital myopathies where one can find morphological abnormalities, variation in size and number of fibre types and/or presence of inclusions on electron microscopy).

Treatment

Delayed motor milestones are often the chief presenting complaint. This must be taken seriously, using all the available treatment approaches right at the outset rather than adopting a wait-and-see approach.

Truncal weakness should be addressed by encouraging the parents to place the infant prone and to ventrally suspend the infant for increasing periods in order to develop axial tone and strength. Exercises should be prescribed in the older child with muscle weakness or joint laxity.

Allopathic medical treatment

This may vary, depending on the cause of the hypotonia.

Osteopathic treatment

Osteopathic treament should be aimed at releasing any joint restrictions and muscle contractures wherever present. Scoliosis should be treated when present.

Peripheral and spinal joint restrictions can be approached using techniques such as joint stretching, joint articulation and balanced ligamentous technique (BLT), and muscle contractions can be released by using techniques such as muscle inhibition and muscle energy techniques (MET).

Case study

Lillian, a 5-month-old infant, presented with developmental delay involving nearly all the motor milestones, and she had slight difficulties with sucking and feeding.

The pregnancy was apparently normal; however, she suffered from anoxia at birth as the umbilical cord was wrapped around her neck. Directly after her birth she had to be resuscitated and was placed in the special care baby unit for a few weeks. Lillian was initially tube fed.

A developmental examination revealed that she had an asymmetrical tonic neck reflex and the grasp reflex was still present. She had no rooting reflex. On prone suspension, Lillian was just beginning to lift her head slightly but not her lower extremities: she appeared 'floppy'. There was head lag on pull-to-sit. There was some attempt at rolling from the supine position. When placed prone, she was able to lift her head to face forwards, but not her chest. She was able to grasp and reach for objects. She was able to smile. There was response to visual stimuli but the right eye did not abduct.

A neurological examination revealed decreased tone, normal muscle bulk, no fasciculations, normal or slightly elevated reflexes and axial weakness with no limb weakness. These findings suggested a central origin to the hypotonia, and the anoxia at birth may have been a contributory factor.

Osteopathic examination revealed a pronounced right lateral strain at the cranium. There was an overriding coronal suture with a pronounced ridging of the coronal suture and a palpatory sense of anteroposterior compression at the cranium. This suggested either molding in-utero or compression as a result of the forces of birth. There was also a palpatory sense that the infant had not taken her first breaths adequately, and this was suggested too by the rapid and shallow breathing and the case history. The incomplete first breath was felt as a lack of expansion of all the tissues of her body, particularly the CNS. There was a sense of venous congestion within the cranium, and this could perhaps have contributed to the neurological picture.

Treatment was carried out at 2 to 4 weekly intervals. The aim was to stimulate the first breath by matching the tone of the diaphragm, seeking a field of neutral that encompassed the diaphragm, the umbilicus and the ligamentum teres (derived from the fetal umbilical vein), to allow for full diaphragmatic excursion. The improved longitudinal fluctuation of the cerebrospinal fluid would allow the intracranial membranes to shift the strain pattern in the cranium, and therefore allow the CNS to express its inherent motility freely. The free movement of the fluids, membranes, bones and CNS would allow for better venous drainage of the cranium and the brain, and therefore better vascular perfusion. After four treatments, Lillian's parents noticed that the rate of her motor development was beginning to improve markedly. She was now able to roll, prop herself on straight arms prone, flex her knees and hips under her while prone, and transfer objects from hand to hand. It may be that some cases of benign congenital hypotonia may indeed have in part a mechanical-physiological basis, as this case appears to illustrate.

Regular further treatment throughout growth was necessary to support her body through its growth spurts. With children like Lillian it is also important to institute age-appropriate trunk- and limb-strengthening exercises.

Prognosis

Of course, the prognosis always depends on the cause of the hypotonia. For example, metabolic causes can readily be corrected when identified.

Osteopathic treatment is aimed not so much at the poor muscle tone itself as at the effects of this symptom and other associated symptoms on the musculoskeletal system. In cases of weakness the aim is to maintain or develop muscle strength; in cases of delay exercises should be given to stimulate development. It is important to reduce contractures by exercises and stretching and to address joint problems such as laxity or scoliosis to prevent or reduce complications in the future. The ultimate aim is to enable the child to develop as fully as possible in spite of the limitations of muscle tone. The ideal treatment regime is almost always long term: during the entire childhood period, and beyond if possible.

Bibliography

Bear L M: Early identification of infants at risk for developmental disabilities. Pediatric Clinics of North Am 51, 2004: 685–701

Gesell, A: The first five years of life. Methuen, London 1950

Singer T et al: Cognitive and motor outcomes of cocaine-exposed infants. Journal of the American Medical Association 287(15), 2002: 1952–60

DEVELOPMENTAL DELAY

Kok Weng Lim

Early recognition of infants at risk for developmental delay or disability is a challenge. Children are usually checked by a pediatric doctor at regular intervals. If regular osteopathic check-ups are performed throughout infancy and childhood, osteopaths are also well placed to observe any deviation from the normal. Early identification of developmental delay, particularly in the first year of life, is of the utmost importance, as early referral and treatment is the objective.

Definition

We speak about developmental delay if a child does not reach important developmental milestones in the motor, cognition, speech or psychosocial area within a reasonable range of their peers (see p.86). Charts of developmental milestones in these domains are largely based on Gesell's (1950) work.

It is difficult to differentiate between infants or children who are merely lagging behind with their developmental skills and those who are truly handicapped in some way. The former category of children would normally achieve the usual milestones in the course of time, whereas the same cannot be said for the latter. They will not achieve developmental milestones without specific help, if at all.

It is traditional to describe child development in terms of fine and gross motor skills, language, cognition, and social and emotional skills. However, all these domains overlap and should be looked upon as an integrated whole and as one continuous, cascading process. Skills may require the maturation of two or more of these areas. One example for this is perceiving shapes and being able to reproduce/draw them.

Etiology and pathophysiology

Developmental delay can stem from a myriad primary causes. The contribution of genetic inheritance is important and twin studies have suggested that up to 80% of the variance in intelligence in a population can be attributed to genetic transmission. Causative genetic pathologies could be Down syndrome (see Ch.17), fragile X syndrome, Rett syndrome, Prader-Willi syndrome or Angelman syndrome. Also metabolic, endocrinological (e.g. hypothyroidism) and neuromuscular disorders, or dysplasia of the brain may be the cause. Defects of special senses most commonly affect vision and hearing and can result in a severe restriction of the information a child receives. Thus a child with severe visual impairment may show delay in all areas of development.

Secondary causes of developmental delay may be:

- Prenatal – e.g. lack of oxygen, minimal cerebral dysfunction due to placental insufficiency, infections (TORCH), multiple gestation, illegal drug use, prescription medication, alcohol and smoking (see Ch.4, Influences in prenatal experience).

- Perinatal – e.g. fetal distress, lack of oxygen, asphyxia, bleeding, hypoglycemia, cerebral palsy.

- Postnatal – e.g. any chronic medical condition, infection (meningitis, encephalitis), deprivation, intoxication, trauma, environmental factors, psychosocial factors (e.g. altering the child's opportunity to learn by limiting or encouraging her exploration).

It is not always easy to pinpoint a definite etiology, but often a picture of the causative factors appears as we take the case history. More information may later emerge with osteopathic examination.

Risk category for developmental delay

The following factors are well known for increasing the risk of developmental delay (Bear, 2004).

High risk for developmental delay

- Birth weight less than 1250 g
- 30 weeks' gestation or less
- Intraventricular hemorrhage, periventricular leucomalacia
- Severe perinatal asphyxia
- Severe neurological problems
- Bronchopulmonary dysplasia that requires home oxygen
- Complex congenital, cyanotic heart disease
- Abnormal neurological examination at discharge following birth
- Significant feeding problems, requirement of gavage feeding
- Intracranial pathology – congenital or acquired
- Extracorporeal membrane oxygenation
- Diaphragmatic hernia
- Persistent pulmonary hypertension of the newborn and required inhaled nitric oxide/oscillatory ventilator

- Significant circulatory failure
- Congenital viral infection (HIV, TORCH)
- Prolonged or persistent hypoglycemia
- Multiple, major congenital anomalies and genetic disorders.

Moderate risk

- Birth weight of 1250–1500 g
- Prolonged ventilation and high-frequency ventilation
- Surgical: cloacal anomalies, gastroschisis, omphalocele
- Tracheotomy
- Metabolic disorders.

Clinical signs and symptoms

A circumscribed developmental delay shows in individual areas; for example motor or speech development. One or more abilities are delayed.

A global developmental delay and mental retardation show as reduced intelligence. This appears especially as delayed development, or little development, of age-specific abilities or a below average ability to learn.

Diagnosis
Case history

Reviewing a child's history of developmental milestone achievements enables detection of deviations from the normal. It must be noted that parents may be unreliable in their recall of when milestones were passed. Major milestones such as sitting or walking may perhaps be reliably recalled. But it is also important to ascertain whether the child has always had a problem or if there has been regression or loss of skills. A developmental assessment should therefore be undertaken regularly over a period of time. Therefore, it is very important to see a child regularly for osteopathic examination and treatment during the period of growth and development.

Any chronic medical condition can contribute to developmental delay, so the child's general health must be enquired after and explored. The family history is especially important and enquiries must be made about parents, siblings, aunts, uncles and cousins. In boys with learning disability a history of affected males on the mother's side must be sought.

Pre and perinatal history

This is of the utmost importance in order to assess risk factors that may have an impact on the child's functioning later. Prematurity, low or high birth weight, low Apgar scores, lack of prenatal care before the birth, high-risk pregnancies and increasing maternal age are all risk factors. Enquire about the health of the mother. Maternal conditions such as excessive maternal weight gain, diabetes, lupus, seizure disorders and other chronic diseases may be relevant. Of particular importance are placental insufficiency, infection, multiple gestation, illegal drug use, prescription medication, alcohol and smoking. Cocaine-exposed infants have significant cognitive deficits and a doubling of the rate of developmental delay during the first 2 years of life (Singer et al 2002).

The length of the labor and any complications of labor should be noted. Caesarean section or instrumentation may not in itself place a baby at risk, but the reason for the intervention might be important.

Always enquire about infection or signs of fetal distress during the delivery. A dropping heart rate, the passage of meconium or meconium aspiration may all suggest fetal hypoxia and distress. A low Apgar score may suggest but is not synonymous with asphyxia. The Apgar score was developed as a tool primarily to assess the condition of the infant at birth. Medications, congenital anomalies, gestational age and acute events can all also influence the Apgar score, not just oxygen deprivation and metabolic acidosis from fetal hypercarbia.

Factors affecting development

Both psychosocial/environmental and biological factors are relevant in assessing developmental delay.

When faced with a child showing a delayed or abnormal pattern of development it is important to consider which of the following biological or social factors are contributing. More than one factor may be operating and they may interact. Treating or managing the developmentally delayed child also involves looking at the family dynamics. This is particularly relevant when there is a biological abnormality, because the family's ability to cope may be stretched in the face of the child's special needs. Enlisting parental cooperation is important; the child may need parental help and encouragement in performing specific exercises.

Family environment

Interestingly, it is people rather than physical elements that are the most important factors in the environment of the infant and child. Note that the parents' ability to cope depends on the family structure, features of pregnancy, labor and delivery and life experience. Children from deprived environments tend to show developmental delay, especially of language and social skills. Children continue to practice and develop skills if they are encouraged, or if the behavior

is reinforced. This feedback is important in the process of learning and if severely deprived of positive feedback during her first year, the child's ability to learn can be affected for the rest of her life.

Brain pathologies

A child's development may be affected by abnormalities of brain function from brain damage, or genetic factors affecting the maturation of certain brain functions. Disorders of movement whether due to the brain (cerebral palsy), spinal cord (paraplegia), nerves (spinal muscular atrophy) or muscles (dystrophy or myotonia) not only have a direct effect on motor skill acquisition but can also limit the child's sensory experience.

Freedom of movement

The child who cannot move independently or freely, owing to a motor disorder, or even from physical restraint and lack of physical stimulation, does not fully and accurately experience space and distance; this in turn limits further motor development.

Examination

Subtle physical clues should be searched for in a physical examination. These include abnormal or unusual postures and positioning, which may lead you to the site of pathology. Growth parameters should be checked – weight, height and head circumference – as growth retardation is significant. Head circumference provides a rough estimate of brain size. Conditions such as microcephaly and macrocephaly may indicate a brain pathology or abnormality.

Facial asymmetries or dysmorphisms may suggest delay as part of a syndrome. Any physical anomaly in terms of structure or mobility may be significant in the etiology of delay. Skin lesions, skin elasticity and hyper- or hypopigmentation may lead to a specific medical diagnosis.

A neurological examination that is performed at regular intervals is essential. Subtle changes in a neurological examination may be enormous significance in eventual development of the child.

With regard to sensory development, special attention should be paid to examining the hearing and vision of any developmentally delayed child or child with learning difficulties. For example hearing loss due to otitis media may be missed in children with delayed speech, even with passing the 8th month screening. Examination of the eyes for visual acuity, squints, papillary response to light, eye movements, tracking, and visual dominance using the cover test should be routinely performed. Visual impairment can affect all areas of development and alter the interpretation of data from other parts of the examination.

Interpretation of abnormal development

If on observation of the child's play and from results of tests performed we conclude that at least one skill is definitely delayed, a systematic approach should be adopted. Consider whether the delay is affecting all tasks equally or whether the child is lacking in some skill areas more than others.

Some tasks, such as drawing a shape, require sub-skills such as cognition, fine motor control and vision, one of which may be lacking. Therefore, it may be necessary to break down the assessment further to determine the relevant defect. Is there a specific learning difficulty, such as autism or dyspraxia, that would make a maturational delay or even a simple learning disability unlikely? What disorders present with the particular pattern of disability that affects this child? Look for other associated symptoms such as hyperactivity, inability to concentrate, mild tremor or low IQ.

When assessing delayed motor patterns, the first question is whether the motor pattern is abnormal. Does the child present, for example, with toe-walking or signs of spasticity? The other question is whether development in other non-motor areas is normal. This will help to determine if there is global developmental delay, maturational lag, motor disorder or a mixture of motor disorder and developmental delay.

In the case of a child with delayed speech, it is necessary to determine the following factors: what is the child's understanding of language, her hearing, her ability in non-language areas in terms of symbolic play and drawing? What are her social skills, quality of speech and articulation of the few words in her vocabulary? How is the overall pattern of development? When taking an exact family history, a genetic predisposition may become visible which is common in developmental language disorder. In this way the differential diagnosis of an expressive language disorder learning disability, dyspraxia or autism may be clearer.

A child with any disability often presents as a child with developmental delay. A full assessment should enable the clinician to discuss with parents and child the nature of the difficulties and the prognosis and management. Based on this, a treatment program can be planned that is appropriate to the child's needs. This may involve enlisting the social services and local council for specific help. A diagnostic summary includes:

- A profile of the child:
  - limitation of motor ability; e.g. through spasticity or dyspraxia
  - sensory limitations, particularly of hearing and vision

  - cognition and understanding
  - the extent of the child's abilities, and tasks for which aid is needed
  - emotional components and behavior: does the child suffer from, for example, hyperactivity or has she difficulty concentrating?
  - social abilities: e.g. does the child suffer from autism?
- An etiology, including the possibility of genetic implications
- The environment – parenting skills, neglect, family structure and circumstances, school, etc.

Allopathic diagnostic procedures

Apart from a thorough neurological examination, the following tests are performed:

- Tests to assess possible cognitive problems (IQ-testing)
- Electroencephalogram (EEG) when sleeping and awake: typical changes in certain syndromes, evidence of seizures
- Magnetic resonance imaging (MRI)
- Laboratory testing: thyroid hormones, liver enzymes, urinalysis, TORCH – serology, metabolic screening
- Chromosomal screening
- CSF screening: if neurodegenerative pathologies suspected.

Treatment
Allopathic medical treatment

This involves treatment for underlying conditions where possible. Physiotherapy is very useful, and can be provided at the same time as osteopathy.

Osteopathic treatment

In managing children with developmental delay, it is important to assess the entire family dynamics as well as the child. In a healthy but delayed child the emotional well-being of the child, which depends on the environment in which she grows, will also influence her desire to move, develop her own activities, and so on. The degree of parental stimulation and encouragement, and their willingness to devote time and energy towards improving their child's skills, determines also the approach that we, as osteopaths, take.

Where motor skills such as commando crawling, crawling on all fours, skipping and hopping are deficient, then patterning exercises may be useful. For example, positioning the child, and then getting the child to eventually position herself, initially in a homolateral pattern in the prone position and then a cross-lateral pattern, may help the child's nervous system to rediscover developmental skills that may have been missed along the way. These exercises require a degree of long-term commitment from the child and her carers.

Osteopathic treatment should be directed firstly towards the peripheral joints and muscles. Joint restrictions should be addressed, muscle contractures and muscle tone normalized. These children often have a degree of extensor tone and you must always check for this.

The tone of both pelvic and thoracic diaphragms should be assessed. The ribs may need to be freed of restrictions to allow the tone of the sympathetic nervous system to normalize via freeing the sympathetic chain on the rib heads. This is especially important because there is often a degree of autonomic dysregulation.

Freeing the periphery allows sensory input to the nervous system to be normalized. Correct unimpeded sensory feedback is of the utmost importance for these children.

Chronic concurrent medical conditions, such as recurrent otitis media resulting in hearing loss, hip dysplasia or recurrent infections, should be addressed.

Developmental delay should not be merely watched over time in order to see how the complete picture emerges but should be treated immediately using all possibilities at the outset. Advantage should be taken of the potential for change and of the plasticity of the brain in the earliest years. Developmental delay is a precursor for learning difficulties in the school-age child and therefore early diagnosis and intervention is of the utmost importance.

Prognosis

The prognosis depends of course on the cause of the delay. The effect of osteopathic treatment may be especially significant where there is mechanical, fascial/membranous or emotional strain or shock from the birth. Be aware of structural asymmetries, whether from intrauterine molding or from birth or postnatal trauma. Where structural factors predominate in the etiology, such as compressed condylar parts resulting in pincering or irritation of the brain stem, osteopathic treatment may be very effective. By addressing these mechanical factors and allowing better neurotrophic flow and vascular supply, the prognosis can be greatly improved in some cases of delay.

As children present with a changing anatomy and structure, monitoring of developmental milestones, neurological testing, and treatment of delay should be carried out throughout childhood. Once again it must be emphasized that early detection and prevention are the primary aims.

Bibliography

Bear L M: Early identification of infants at risk for developmental disabilities. Pediatric Clinics of North America 51, 2004: 685–701

Gesell A: The first five years of life. Methuen, London 1950

Singer T et al: Cognitive and motor outcomes of cocaine-exposed infants. Journal of the American Medical Association 287(15), 2002: 1952–1960

CEREBRAL PALSY

Kok Weng Lim

Definition

Cerebral palsy (CP) is a group of disorders of movement and postural control caused by a nonprogressive defect or lesion of the developing brain. It is not a specific syndrome. The following features are characteristic of this disorder:

- The defect in movement and posture may manifest as spasticity, dystonia, dyskinesia, ataxia or a mixture of these.

- It is caused by a non-progressive lesion of the immature, developing brain.

- Although it is a permanent disorder, the clinical picture changes as the brain matures throughout childhood.

- Other associated problems, such as cognitive impairment, learning disabilities, mental retardation, impairments in vision (squints, cortical blindness), hearing or speech, and seizures may also present in children with cerebral palsy, although definitions of cerebral palsy often emphasize the motor nature of the defect.

- Note that this definition of damage to the 'growing brain' implies that a static encephalopathy after 2 or 4 years of age can still be considered as CP. The prevalence of CP is approximately 1.0–2.3 per 1000 live births.

Classification

Cerebral palsy may be classified in various ways:

- Etiology – This may be genetic, or may be the result of a malformation, an infarction or a hypoxic-ischemic injury.

- Site of brain injury – whether cortical, subcortical or periventricular white matter, cerebellar, etc.

- Body distribution – monoplegia, diplegia, quadriplegia, etc.

- Physiological type – spastic, dystonic, dyskinetic (choreoathetoid), ataxic or mixed.

- Severity – mild, moderate or severe.

Etiology and pathophysiology

The risk of CP is strongly associated with gestational age. Prematurity is probably the major factor associated with brain damage in newborns (Wood et al 2000). The risk among very preterm children is approximately 1 in 20 survivors, whereas the risk is less than 1 per 1000 survivors in children born weighing more than 2500 g. However, term or near-term infants, although individually at relatively low risk, constitute the large majority of all births and therefore contribute to at least half of all CP cases. Impairment may range from major disability to cognitive, perceptual and behavioral problems that could interfere with school performance (McCarton et al 1997).

Intraventricular hemorrhage (IVH) occurs in up to 40% of infants born before 35 weeks or with a birth-weight below 1500 g (Paneth 1990). Approximately 5% of infants with IVH will develop cerebral palsy (Paneth & Kazam 1994).

Premature infants appear to be at a higher risk for cerebral white matter damage (periventricular leucomalacia). Depending on the degree, timing and duration of the anoxic event, term infants tend to exibit subcortical white matter damage, selective neuronal necrosis affecting the cerebral and/or cerebellar cortex, hippocampus and anterior horn cells of the spinal cord, parasagittal cerebral injury, or status marmoratus affecting the basal ganglia and thalamus.

All these injuries are the result of asphyxia leading to hypoxic-ischemic injury, resulting from various intrinsic developmental factors such as a loss of autoregulation, free radical damage, sensitivity of oligodendrocytes to anoxia during the proliferative stage, and immaturity of the vasculature, both venous and arterial.

Note that asphyxia during complications of labor and delivery is seldom measured directly; commonly it is inferred on the basis of signs in the fetus and newborn that are not etiologically specific. Few efforts are made to distinguish interruption of oxygen supply as an initiating pathologic condition, from hypoxia or ischemia occurring as downstream complications of other pathogenic processes. Ischemia may therefore only be the final trigger in the pathogenesis of CP. Not only is this distinction important for primary prevention, it can also be an important focus for osteopathic treatment. Other prenatal factors such as malformations, prenatal strokes and TORCH infections (congenital toxoplasmosis, rubella, cytomegalovirus, herpes) are important in approximately half of infants with CP of normal birth-weight (Grether and Nelson 1997).

Congenital anomalies are more frequently found in infants with CP compared to the normal population (Dite et al 1998). It is now realized that multiple causes may interact via excitotoxic, oxidative, or other converging pathophysiological pathways. A single factor, unless present to an overwhelming degree, may often be insufficient to produce cerebral damage, whereas two or three interacting pathogenic insults may overwhelm the natural ability of the body to cope and produce brain damage.

Chorioamnionitis (CA) is a bacterial infection involving the chorionic and amniotic membranes and the amniotic fluid. It is present in 0.5% to 10% of all pregnancies and is associated with 45% of pregnancies complicated by preterm labor (Watts et al 1992). The clinical diagnosis of CA is based on the following symptoms: maternal fever, maternal or fetal tachycardia, uterine tenderness, purulent vaginal discharge and leucocytosis. Mostly the diagnosis is confirmed by laboratory tests, with positive stains of amniotic fluid for organisms or leucocytes, and positive cultures or histopathologic examination of the placental membranes and umbilical cord. This infection develops primarily by bacteria found in the lower genital tract ascending into the amniotic cavity, where they may induce placental inflammation. The most common organisms are *Bacteroides* species (25%), group B streptococci (12%), other aerobic streptococci (13%), *Escherichia coli* (10%) and other Gram-negative rods (10%). Such infections may also be transplacental or may be introduced during invasive procedures. An intrauterine infection of the mother can lead to a fetal inflammatory response; a fetal inflammatory response is evident in 70% of amniotic fluid infections (Yoon et al 1997). It has been proposed that cytokines produced by the placenta and fetal immune system during the course of maternal infection are harmful to the developing brain of the unborn infant, producing white matter damage (Eschenbach 1997). Grether and Nelson (1997) noted that clinical diagnosis of infection of the uterus and its contents during pregnancy as well as histopathological evidence of placental infection were associated with increased risk of unexplained CP. It is important to bear in mind when assessing a case history that most cases of chorioamnionitis are subclinical. Probably many fetuses are exposed to such an infection for extended periods of time before they are delivered. It is possible that the severity of CP is related to the duration of exposure and intensity of the inflammatory response.

Infarction of the great arteries in the brain, especially of the middle cerebral artery, can lead to a spastic hemi- or quadriparesis. Since 1992 reports have linked strokes (and other cerebral lesions) and subsequent motor defects with antiphospholipid antibodies in the blood of the mother of the affected infant, or more recently, with the factor V Leiden mutation (Silver et al 1992). Antiphospholipid antibodies are associated with risk of stroke or cerebral venous thrombosis in older children or adults, and there is evidence to suggest that they are also related to the risk of cerebral injury in the fetus or neonate. Cerebral thrombosis or thromboembolism also has been reported with the factor V Leiden mutation, the most common known genetic thrombophilia. Alone, the Leiden mutation is associated with a relatively low level of risk, but with the addition of other genetic or acquired risk factors, the risk of strokes increases sharply. A variety of other abnormalities of coagulation may coexist in affected children, indicating that more than a single risk factor may often be required to result in CP.

Abnormalities of the placenta or its vasculature have also been reported in association with antiphospholipid antibodies (Sarafia and Parke 1997) and factor V Leiden mutation (Dizon-Townson et al 1997). Thromboses from the placenta may embolize to the fetal circulation, reaching the cerebral vasculature via the patent foramen ovale. Such emboli might explain why the right-sided congenital hemiparesis is more commonly found. In placentas examined for medico-legal purposes in children with CP, thrombotic lesions were the most commonly identified pathological condition (Kraus 1997).

For a small proportion of CP cases a genetic basis has been described (McHale et al 1999). The genetics of CP may also be related to coagulation factors described above or to genetic components of the inflammatory response.

Posture and mobility

It is often assumed that the problems of CP are caused by spasticity alone. This limits the treatment of children with CP. Cerebral palsy is really a comprehensive disorder of the development of movement, posture and muscle tone, including dystonia and reflex excitability (Lin et al 1994).

The ability to move and to manipulate objects is dependent upon the successful control of posture. The development of posture involves the coupling of sensory inputs with motor actions. Postural control requires the countering of gravitational forces, control of the relationships and the parts of the body, and the maintenance of balance. Initially the infant has minimal head and trunk control. Then she arrives at independent sitting, standing and walking via increasingly sophisticated interactions between these three variables. Posture control can be thought of as the coordination of stability and body orientation in space for the purpose of executing movement tasks (Shumway-Cook and Woollacott 1985).

Nearly all motor skills have an underlying stability component. Consider the skills needed for a baby in order to reach for a toy: the baby would need to control her stability by maintaining her trunk and head within the base of support of the pelvis in order to successfully reach out in the sitting position. Only then can the upper extremities be oriented appropriately to grasp an object.

Maturation theory or reflex model of development

Although it is generally agreed that the central nervous system plays a role in the control of posture, the specific control mechanisms are still the subject of debate. Traditional approaches focus on CNS maturation as the basis for postural development. More current theories take a broader perspective and suggest that it is the interaction of the many body systems, along with the environment and task related factors, that is important.

Studies using longitudinal observations to document the sequence of motor behaviors in infants and young children have shown that development occurs in a predictable sequence (McGraw 1932; Gesell 1946). For example, development occurs in predominantly cephalocaudal and proximal-distal directions. It can be observed that infants first acquire control of the structures of the head, such as the lips, mouth and eyes. This control then progresses in a caudal direction, with the trunk, legs and feet being the last structures brought under control. Within the extremities, mastery of proximal joints occurs first, followed by gradual control of the distal joints. This suggests that there is a built-in unfolding and neural organization of the CNS over time. As the nervous system matures, new behaviors are revealed.

Therefore it is the maturation of the CNS that determines the sequence and the order of the motor milestones. This is the basis of the maturation theory of development. It is also often called the reflex model of development as the emergence of increasingly mature postural reflexes and responses is dependent on the maturation of progressively higher CNS structures: from the brainstem, midbrain and cortex upwards.

This theory implies that the postures and movement patterns seen in young infants are controlled by primitive reflexes that are organized at the spinal cord and brainstem levels. The tendon jerk and asymmetrical tonic neck reflex are examples of reflexes controlled at these levels. As maturation of the CNS proceeds to the midbrain, righting reactions become apparent. Mature postural, balance and movement responses are seen with the eventual maturation of the cortex. Motor skills also progress from low levels of reflexive movement as expressed in general movements in infancy to voluntary skills controlled at cortical level.

Based on the reflex model, reflexes and responses seen at lower levels disappear as control is taken over by higher centers. The integration of lower level reflexive responses into more mature ones and the suppression exerted on lower levels by higher centers therefore explains the disappearance of primitive responses with maturation. According to the reflex model, low-level motor patterns persist only in conditions of CNS pathology, such as CP. Abnormal maturation of higher centers is thought to be responsible for the retention of primitive patterns in these cases. When higher CNS levels do not mature there is resultant lack of inhibition of the lower centers, allowing primitive patterns to dominate (Horak 1992).

Another assumption of the reflex model is that the development of equilibrium must always progress in the following order: supine, prone, sitting, all-fours and standing. If a child does not obtain stability in one posture, control of balance in subsequent positions cannot develop fully.

Dynamic systems model of posture control

Although the reflex model of motor development has been generally accepted and has formed the basis for some types of therapeutic intervention for CP, research in the past decade has shown up inadequacies in this model. A simple example: protective, 'primitive' reflexes can be present in the absence of CNS dysfunction, such as the flexor withdrawal reflex on stepping on a sharp object. Therefore some primitive reflexes do not just disappear as the reflex theory suggests.

Rather than just looking at development as a consequence of suppression of inhibition of reflexes, the systems model of motor control proposes that development arises as a result of the interaction of the many subsystems in the body in relation to the task and the environment. Motor behaviors therefore arise from the cooperation of the various domains of development, such as sensory, motor, cognitive and emotional. Dynamic systems approaches in therapy 'seeks to understand the overall behavior of the system, not dissecting it into parts, but by asking how and under what circumstances the parts cooperate to produce a whole pattern' (Thalen 1996).

Factors which determine the rate of development include:

- neuronal organization
- muscle strength and elasticity
- development of muscle synergies that maintain stability involving head, trunk and legs
- joint structures and range of movement
- sensory systems, such as the vision, vestibular and somatosensory systems and the central sensory processing systems
- motivation and arousal levels
- the task.

This systems model places the role of the CNS in the context of other bodily systems in motor development. None of the subsystems listed above, including the nervous system, has priority or prime importance. It is the interaction of all these factors that is important. The interaction of these factors with the task and the environment is a changing and flexible one, as new behaviors emerge as one or more of these factors reach maturation.

An example of this is the myelination of the visual pathways – the improvement in the visual acuity enables a 12 week old infant to view her hand clearly. This in turn allows the baby to watch her hand as she moves it about. This coupling of the eyes and the arm movement allows the infant to develop motor pathways for both the arm and hand. Movement of the hand in turn allows the infant to develop her visual acuity further. As the infant is able to raise her head, further development of visual acuity and convergence is possible, so that the infant is able to recognize her mother's face at this point. Thus the developing visual and motor skills allow development of cognitive ability. There is therefore an interplay between the sensory and motor and cognitive systems, mutually reinforcing their development.

Contrast this situation with an infant with cerebral palsy. Many children with CP do not see their hands enough, if at all. However, it is very important that infants play with their hands in this early period. In fact, it has been suggested that the normal infant is more interested in her hands than toys. This is important from a therapeutic point of view because although a child may have developed some feel for her hands in the early months of life, with not being able to see them much, she will not be able to couple the visual information with the information from the sensors in the joints and muscles. This may be bewildering for the child and is an impediment to developing motor skills.

The dynamic systems theory and brain organization

Sporns and Edleman (1993) proposed that the brain selects a group or a population of neurons for the control of any one particular movement. During brain development, patterns of synaptic connectivity are dependent on cell proliferation, cell differentiation and cell migration, the formation of a vast number of connections between neurons, cell death and synaptic pruning. Over time, as the infant explores and interacts with the environment, selection amongst these initial populations of cells is achieved by the strengthening of particular synapses. In learning a movement, the infant is selecting a population of neuronal cells to coordinate muscle synergies to achieve that movement.

The infant is learning to select groups of neurons to accomplish a given task from an interaction between the CNS and the environment. This emphasizes the importance of experience and exploration in neural organization. Therefore, though a process of exploration, interaction and selection, neuronal self-organization emerges in the brain. This is consistent with the dynamic systems theory of development where patterned behaviors arise from self-organization at all levels of the body. As the infant develops, a repertoire of related neurons, associated with particular categories of action is organized. There is a constant correlation of efferent information to afferent information required to modulate the motor output between these neuronal groups.

By these means neuronal groups are selectively carved out, linking motor, visual and somatosensory systems with higher centers. These neural mappings and activity are dynamic and not fixed and predetermined, even in adults. Experiments using electrophysiological mapping of cortical areas in monkeys have shown that when one or two digits in monkeys were amputated, the cortical representations of adjacent digits and palm expanded to include areas formerly reflecting activity in the amputated segments (Jenkins et al 1990). And when the monkeys practised a food retrieval task, the specific areas in the somatosensory cortex that represented the digits making tactile contact increased their area of representation. When the practice stopped, area boundaries shifted again.

Therefore, fundamental to both the dynamic systems theory and contemporary ideas on brain development is the concept not just of self-organization, but a dynamic process of motor behavior and brain organization. This is a flexible process, influenced by many inputs and is not predetermined. This growing evidence for brain plasticity in adults, as well as in early life, indicates the importance of experience and exploration in neural organization (Kaas 1991).

In practice, this means that all the domains of development must be taken into consideration in treating a child with CP, as they are interdependent. Constant repetition of movement patterns and exploration in performing motor tasks are essential in order to exploit the capacity of the brain to form new neural pathways or networks.

Role of the stretch reflex

Motor problems in CP are frequently attributed to spasticity alone, which arises as a consequence of damage to the CNS. These children with spastic cerebral palsy have hyperactive stretch reflexes.

The functional significance of spasticity in relation to functional ability may be considered as dubious because numerous studies have failed to show a correlation between the two. Also the role of the stretch reflex in posture control is questionable. A study by Nashner et al (1983) investigated the response of ankle plantar flexors in children with spastic diplegia and hemiplegia to sudden forward sway disturbances to their standing posture. Because these muscles were hyperactive

when the children were tested clinically, the expected response to these sudden postural disturbances was that the stretch reflex would be evoked. Instead the plantar flexors of these children showed a delayed response to the test. This seems to support the contention that the stretch reflex and therefore spasticity may not be the primary cause of functional disability in CP (O'Dwyer and Nelson 1988; Vaughn et al 1988).

Musculoskeletal constraints in cerebral palsy

Spasticity is the main neurological factor that contributes to muscle tone in CP. Other factors contributing to muscle tone in other situations include:

- myotonia, which is a slowness to relax due to intramuscular electrical discharges
- movement, either voluntary or involuntary
- elasticity, which is length dependent
- contracture, either short muscle or short tendon, or both.

Studies have shown that children with spastic CP show a reversal of the normal muscular sequencing patterns with unclear onset and offset of muscle activation (Sienko-Thomas et al 1996).

Positional deformity may arise from any of the factors detailed above, especially from muscle shortening in tonically spastic muscles as in hemiplegia. In some children there is secondary change in muscle proteins so that stiffness and resistance to movement occur without any electrical activity on the EMG, which means there is plastic change in muscle. These muscles show a relaxation over time (e.g. 20 seconds) and are easily confused with fixed contractures or tonic spasticity.

In particular, children with severe motor disorders, such as quadriplegic CP, who are not able to change their own position during a period of growth develop deformities due to immobility, growth and gravity. These include plagiocephaly, chest asymmetry, scoliosis, pelvic tilt and a 'windswept' posture of the lower limbs. Prevention or amelioration with osteopathic treatment is ideal in these cases, as surgical treatment is rarely successful or indeed indicated.

Early diagnosis is essential to prevent positional molding and windsweeping, which can occur by 6 months of age if the infant has been totally immobile.

Sensory disorders in cerebral palsy

The ability to couple visual and non-visual information is vital for developing and maintaining movement. Under normal circumstances, it is not possible to keep an eye on every moving part of the body all the time. It is necessary to feel how each part of the body, especially the limbs, are moving.

This ability to couple visual and non-visual information has been shown to be impaired in children with hemiparetic CP in various studies. Lee and others (1990) measured how accurately these children and normal children could locate three types of target with their hand when that hand was hidden from view. There was a visual target (the children could see it but their other hand was not involved), a felt target (the children could see neither hand but could feel their other hand on the target) and a seen and felt target (the children could see and feel their other hand on the target). The hemiparetic children performed less well than the normal children when localizing targets, both when using their affected and their unaffected hand.

Nashner et al (1983) found that children with different types of cerebral palsy, particularly ataxic CP, had more difficulty than normal controls in maintaining balance on a movable platform when deprived of visual or proprioceptive input. They speculated that these sensory deficits may be a result of delayed or disrupted development of sensory organization systems, along with abnormalities in peripheral sensory inputs.

Loss of two-point discrimination, texture sense, dysgraphesthesia (recognition of shapes traced on the hand) and astereognosis may be found in hemiplegic CP. Sensory abnormalities may be found on the normal side too. Such sensory defects occur in about 25% of cases.

Rejection of a limb and failure to learn volitional tasks have often been attributed to failure of sensory feedback. There is no doubt that children with chronic motor disorders may experience a disordered body image and, unlike normal children, will not get feedback from using the limb during the vital periods of parietal maturation in infancy by exploring their hands, objects, textures and so on.

Clinical signs and symptoms

Symptoms of the child depend very much on the severity of the motor nature of the defect, how much of the sensory systems is involved, and whether there is another neurological dysfunction present. Disorders of cognitive development are common, ranging from learning difficulties to mental handicap. Visual impairment may be present as well, more often than hearing disorders. Epilepsy is common as well, especially if lesions are in the cortex.

Early signs are changes in muscle tone like hypotonia, failure to open the hands, opisthotonus and persisting reflexes like the asymmetrical tonic neck reflex (ATNR). If only one side is affected, there is asymmetry and difference in muscle tone. Later on, paresis becomes more obvious as the child fails to move normally.

The motor system of the child may be affected as well by spasticity, dystonia, athetosis or ataxia, which may all be a factor in classification.

Spastic CP

In spasticity there is raised muscle tone, and often exaggerated tendon reflexes, a tendency for muscle shortening and contracture. Other signs of spasticity include: clonus, extensor flexor response (positive Babinski sign), distal weakness and loss of fine motor dexterity. There is also a predilection for the involvement of certain muscle groups: the anti-gravity muscles; that is, the flexors of the arms and extensors of the legs are predominantly affected. The arm tends to assume a flexed and pronated position with the fingers flexed across adducted thumbs and the leg an extended and adducted one, indicating that certain spinal neurons are reflexively more active than others.

If in spasticity the arm or leg is flexed very slowly, there may be little or no change in muscle tone. However if the muscle is briskly stretched, the limb moves freely for a short distance and then catches with increasing muscular resistance. This resistance melts away on further stretching; this is called clasp-knife phenomenon and is a typical feature of spasticity. Forms of spastic CP are:

- Spastic tetraplegia, in which both arms and legs are affected in the same way, and spastic diplegia, in which the legs are more affected than the arms. More than 60% of these children have a severe disorder of motor and cognitive development, about 50% develop epilepsy and about 10% have visual impairment or are even blind. Spastic diplegia is associated with preterm hypoxic-ischemic encephalopathy.

- Spastic hemiplegia, in which only one half of the body is affected. The motor disorder varies in severity, the arm is in a flexed position, the leg slightly extended, and occurs often after a vascular insult, such as an infarction of the median cerebral artery. It may be associated with epilepsy.

Dyskinetic CP

Is generalized and affects legs, arms, thorax, shoulder girdle and face. Activation and excitement lead to a virtual storm of movement. Cognitive abilities may be quite good. Often there is a spastic component. The dyskinetic movement disorder can be mostly choreoathetoid or mostly dystonic. Usually it is due to hypoxia or kernicterus (bilirubin encephalopathy).

Athetosis is the inability to sustain the fingers and toes, tongue, or any part of the body in one position. The maintained posture is interrupted by relatively slow, sinuous, purposeless movements that flow into one another. These movements may be indistinguishable from chorea, which are involuntary arrhythmic jerky movements, hence the term choreoathetosis.

Dystonia is a persistent attitude or posture in one or other of the extremes of athetoid movement. It may take the form of an overextension or overflexion of the hand, inversion of the foot, arching and twisting of the back or forceful closure of the eyes. Dystonia is therefore not very different in appearance from athetosis. The term dystonia is used especially to refer to any variability in muscle tone, but it can also mean fixed abnormalities of posture that may be the end result of certain diseases of the motor system; hence hemiplegic dystonia, or the dystonic phase of diplegia. The dystonic phase of diplegia is an extensor hypotonus which is maximal when lying supine or when suspended vertically under the armpits. This phase lasts till 7 or 8 months when it merges into the spastic phase before developing the characteristic spasticity confined to the legs.

Atactic CP

Here signs of cerebellar ataxia are most prominent. Ataxia is an incoordination of postural control and gait and of the skilled volitional movements which are involved in hand manipulation and speech. The cerebellum is involved in the coordination of movements, which means the judgement of the speed required, the amount of force and the distance to be moved, stabilization of the limb or trunk during the movement and gradual relaxation of antagonists during agonist movement.

The child may show truncal ataxia or volitional ataxia. The former is a disorder of posture (standing, turning), tone, locomotion (walking, crawling, swimming) and equilibrium (standing from lying, rolling, changing center of gravity by leaning over). The latter shows clinically as an intention tremor, dysmetria and past pointing, dysdiadochokinesia, explosive and staccato speech and a dysarthria. Nystagmus may be seen.

This form is especially seen after bleeds, trauma and hypoxia.

Differential diagnosis

The differential diagnosis should include: neuromuscular disorders, ataxia, myelopathy, dysgenesis of the brain, tumors of the brain, genetic syndromes and neurometabolic disorders.

Diagnosis

Diagnosing CP early can be difficult, as early neurological symptoms, especially motor symptoms, may change.

The diagnosis does not imply a specific prognosis. Efforts to diagnose CP that focus on specific causes do not address the motor symptoms central to CP.

The main aim of diagnosis is early detection, in order that effective early intervention may be instituted. A specific diagnosis, although desirable, is not as important as early detection in a clinical setting. Indeed the specificity of the diagnosis will improve as the child ages and the nature of the disability evolves.

Allopathic diagnostic procedures

To make sure CP is diagnosed correctly, dysgenesis of the brain, genetic, neuromuscular, neurodegenerative and neurometabolic disease is excluded via computed tomography (CT), MRI, EEG, nerve conduction tests, checking the metabolic status, lumbar puncture and serological tests (TORCH).

Developmental diagnosis assesses cognitive and speech development. Vision and hearing are tested, and often psychological tests will be done.

Osteopathic examination

An assessment of the risk factors that are known to be associated with CP in each infant is essential. This is because from an osteopathic point of view, an approximate knowledge of the likely risk factors that are involved, or better still a precise knowledge of the etiology, is essential in the treatment process. An appreciation and acknowledgement of the etiology underlying a case of CP, either via palpation or via a diagnostic work-up, form an important fulcrum in the process of getting a change in the quality or a shift in the potency of the tissues in a child with CP.

There are palpatory findings that are often associated with CP. If there has been a sudden anoxic episode, the consequent anoxic shock can be palpated in the infant's tissues. This may be a feeling of inertia and a lack of motility in the CNS, as well as in the whole body. One can learn to recognize an anoxic feel to the tissues in these infants.

Physiologically, anoxia suffered at birth results in the diving seal response. This is a sympathetic nervous system mediated response to oxygen deprivation which results in a slowing down of the heart rate and an increase the contractility of the heart, and diversion of blood from the periphery towards the central organs, such as the brain, heart and the adrenals. This sympathetic response can often be felt in the infant's tissues following a birth involving fetal distress. One can learn to recognize this particular quality to the tissues (see p.208).

Treatment

Allopathic medical treatment

It is important to start physiotherapy early. The aim is to reduce secondary complications like muscular atrophy and joint contractures. Usually approaches following Bobath and Vojta are used.

Orthopedic treatment with splints, walking-frame and wheelchairs can help with the achievement of mobility. Night time splinting is used as prophylactic treatment against contracture. Surgery to lengthen the Achilles tendon will be done if necessary.

Logopedics helps in learning to chew and swallow and works on speech disorders. Strabismus is corrected where necessary

With epilepsy, antiepileptic drugs may be given. In some cases spasticity can be improved by baclofen or vigabatrin. Local injections of botulinum toxin are also used in some cases.

Osteopathic treatment

The aim of osteopathic treatment is to improve muscle tone and reduce spasticity in order to maximize the function of the whole musculoskeletal system. This can involve fascial chain work on the limbs, paravertebral inhibition, stretching techniques and exercises, and mobilizing exercises to improve the range of motion of affected joints. Also, prevention of deformity is important to prevent later complications such as arthritis and pain. Osteopathic treatment may influence the physiology of the CNS, by working on the venous drainage of the cranium, and the motility of the CNS by addressing the bony and membranous envelopes of the CNS that may be limiting motility.

In managing children with spasticity, it is useful to bear in mind the systems perspective: posture control is brought about by the interaction of many subsystems within the context of the task and the environment. Dysfunctions in the motor system in CP do not result solely from the retention of primitive reflexes and muscle tone abnormalities. The interaction of maturing parallel systems within the context of the neurological problems must be considered.

This point is emphasized by studies in which children with spastic diplegia have undergone selective dorsal rhizotomy to normalize muscle tone. The aim of the procedure is to selectively destroy the primary afferent input into the cord, thereby lowering the primary afferent input to balance the lowered suprasegmental inhibitory input to the motoneuron pool. This is based on the hypothesis that spasticity arises from a loss of suprasegmental control at the cord level. The reduction of spasticity as a result of dorsal rhizotomy is

variable and studies reveal the return of spasticity in as little as a year following the procedure (Sienko et al 1994). The significant finding, however, is that these children are not able to control posture normally in the absence of spasticity after this procedure (Guilini 1991). This supports the systems view of posture control and research has been focused in recent years on the role of musculoskeletal constraints and sensorimotor abnormalities related to posture control in children with CP.

If there are additional strains or strain patterns in the musculoskeletal system of children with CP, the aberrant proprioceptive and nociceptive information resulting from these long-term distortions may affect all aspects of learning, not just motor. Spatial maps are constructed from somatosensory information that comes into the CNS from the whole body. Distortions of this sensory mapping can adversely affect the body's interaction with the spatial environment. Therefore consideration of joint strains and contractures in CP with regard to abnormal sensory input from the trunk and peripheral joints is essential in the osteopathic management of CP, as is a program of sensory stimulation.

Case study

Anne was 3 years old when she presented with congenital spastic quadriparesis with epileptic fits, feeding problems, developmental delay and cortical blindness. The pregnancy was uncomplicated and the presentation was normal with a quick first labor lasting 6 hours in total. However, she did not breathe on delivery and was ventilated for a week. Apgar scores were very low at 1 and at 5 minutes. She was tube-fed for 2 weeks following birth. She was medicated for her fits which began within the 1st week of birth.

On osteopathic palpatory examination, there was an inferior sacral drag with a finding of a bilaterally locked sacrum in its respiratory axis, affecting the tone of the entire reciprocal tension membrane and fascial system. There was an irritable quality to the membranous tissue. There was also a poor palpatory sense of the expression of the primary respiratory mechanism from the lack of the first breath that should ideally have been taken at birth with the first cry. Her problems might have been triggered by the anoxia during the birth, but as is so often the case in brain injury, the precise etiology was not clear and may well have been due to intrauterine or genetic factors acting in association or alone.

Treatment on the first visit was directed at releasing the sacral and membranous/fascial drag using a sacral hold with compression to the point of membranous balance. This allowed the release of the dural membranes and resulted in the normal longitudinal fluctuation of the cerebrospinal fluid, which enabled the brainstem and cerebral and cerebellar hemispheres to expand and express their inherent motility. During the treatment it was noticed that the flexor muscles of Anne's hands became less clenched, and her hands became progressively more open as the treatment progressed. Osteopathic treatment at monthly intervals over a period of years has helped to reduce her high muscle tone and therefore the joint contractures.

Prognosis

The osteopathic treatment of cerebral palsy is aimed at improving the quality of life. Musculoskeletal function should be maintained or improved and later complications prevented. The presentation of cerebral palsy changes with growth, and treatment has to be adjusted accordingly. Osteopathic treatment should be carried out long term as regression of symptoms is common during growth spurts and any plagiocephaly or scoliosis tend to worsen during these periods. Treatment should be continued into adulthood and exercises prescribed where appropriate.

Bibliography

Bax M: Terminology and classification of cerebral palsy. Developmental Medicine and Child Neurology. 6, 1964: 295–7

Dite G S et al: Antenatal and perinatal antecedents of moderate and severe spastic cerebral palsy. The Australian and New Zealand Journal of Obstetrics and Gynaecology. 38, 1998: 377–383

Dizon-Townson D S et al: Fetal carriers of the factor V Leiden mutation are prone to miscarriage and placental infarction. American Journal of Obstetrics and Gynecology 177, 1997: 402–406

Eschenbach D A: Amniotic fluid infection and cerebral palsy. Journal of the American Medical Association 278, 1997: 247–248

Gesell A: The ontogenesis of infant behavior. In: Carmichael L (ed). Manual of child psychology. Wiley, New York 1946, pp 335–345

Grether J K, Nelson K B: Maternal infection and cerebral palsy in infants of normal birth weight. Journal of the American Medical Association 278, 1997: 207–211

Guilini C: Dorsal rhizotomy for children with cerebral palsy: support for concepts of motor control. Physical Therapy 71, 1991: 248–259

Horak F: Motor control models underlying neurologic rehabilitation of posture inchildren. In: Forssberg H, Hirschfield H (eds): Movement disorders in children. Karger, Basel 1992, pp 21–32

Jenkins W M et al: Neocortical representational dynamics in adult primates: implications for neuropsychology. Neuropsychologia 28, 1990: 573–584

Kaas J H: Plasticity of sensory and motor maps in adult mammals. Annual Review of Neuroscience. 14, 1991: 137–167

Kraus F T: Cerebral palsy and thrombosis in placental vessels of the fetus: insights from litigation. Human Pathology 28, 1997: 246–248

Lee D N et al: Basic perceptuo-motor dysfunctions in cerebral palsy. In: Jeannerod M(ed) Attention and performance. XII: Motor representation and control. Erlbaum , Hillsdale, NJ 1990, pp 583–603

Lin J P, Brown J K, Walsh E G: Physiological maturation of muscles in childhood. Lancet 343, 1994: 1386–1389

McCarton C M et al: Results at age 8 years of early intervention for low-birth-weight premature infants. The Infant and Health Development Program. Journal of the American Medical Association 277, 1997: 126–132

McGraw M B: From reflex to muscular control in the assumption of an erect posture and ambulation in the human infant. Child Development 3, 1932: 291–297

McHale D P et al: A gene for autosomal recessive symmetrical spastic cerebral palsy maps to chromosome 2q24-25. American Journal of Human Genetics 64, 1999: 526–532

Nasher L et al: Stance posture control in selected groups of children with cerebral palsy: deficits in sensory organization and muscular coordination. Experimental Brain Research. 111, 1983: 877–899

O'Dwyer N J & Neilson P J: Voluntary muscle control in normal and athetoid dysarthric speakers. Brain 111, 1988: 877–899

Paneth N P-M J: The epidemiology of germinal matrix/paraventricular hemorrhage. In: Kiely M (ed.): Reproductive and perinatal epidemiology. CRC Press, Boca Raton 1990, pp 371–399

Paneth N R R, Kazam E: Brain damage in preterm infant. MacKeith Press, London 1994, pp 171–185

Sarafia C M, Parke A L: Placental pathology in systemic lupus erythematosus and phospholipid antibody syndrome. Rheumatic Disease Clinics of North America 23, 1997: 85–97

Shumway-Cook A, Woollacott M: The growth of stability: postural control from a developmental perspective. Journal of Motor Behavior. 17, 1985: 131–147

Sienko S et al: Does gait continue to improve two years following selective dorsal rhizotomy? Developmental Medicine and Child Neurology 36 [Supp 70], 1994: 20

Sienko-Thomas S et al: Simulated gait patterns: the resulting effects on gait parameters, dynamic electromyography, joint movements and physiological cost index. Gait and posture 4, 1996: 100–107

Silver R K et al: Fetal strokes associated with elevated maternal anticardiolipin antibodies. Obstetrics and Gynecology 80, 1992: 497–499

Sporns O, Edelman G M: Solving Berstein's problem – a proposal for the development of coordinated movement by selection. Child Development 64, 1993: 960–981

Thalen E: The improvising infant – learning about learning how to move. In: Merrens M R, Branningan G G (eds) The developmental psychologists – research adventures across the life span. McGraw Hill, New York 1996, pp 21–35

Vaughn C W et al: Motor control deficits of orofacial muscles in cerebral palsy. Journal of Neurology, Neurosurgery and Psychiatry 51, 1988: 534–539

Watts D H et al: The association of occult amniotic fluid infection with gestational age and neonatal outcome among women in preterm labor. Obstetrics and Gynecology 79, 1992: 351–357

Wood N S et al: Neurologic and developmental disability after extremely preterm birth. EPICure Study Group. New England Journal of Medicine 343, 2000: 378–384

Yoon B H et al: Experimentally induced intrauterine infection causes fetal brain white matter lesions, and cerebral palsy. American Journal of Obstetrics and Gynecology 177, 1997: 797–802

SENSORY INTEGRATION DISORDERS

William Goussel, Dina Guerassimiouk, Jens-Peter Markhoff

Sensation is the product of a set of highly complex processing activities during which information about our own body and the outside world is gathered, analyzed and interpreted.

In the biological sense, life is a continuous confrontation with sensory input from our external surroundings as well as from our own body. It is important that our reaction to this input is always precise and appropriate. In terms of its quality and quantity, this reaction is determined by personal phylogenetic and ontogenetic experience, by the individual's acquired knowledge and experience, by intuition which is the 'daughter of experience', and by cognitive skills. These enable the brain rapidly and flexibly to construct a variety of dynamic functional systems so that information of all types can be taken in, processed – understood, interpreted, organized and integrated – and translated into an appropriate reaction. Dynamic functional systems are momentary, time-limited networks linking different brain centers which are able to analyze particular information from several sources. The more rapidly a brain is able to construct a dynamic functional system and the greater the number of cooperating brain centers that can be combined to form a circuit, the more gifted and versatile this brain – and hence the person whose brain it is – may be considered to be. Accordingly, such a brain has a better capacity for sensory integration, a superior memory and increased capability for logical, abstract and analytical thought.

Definition

Sensory integration (SI)

In order to receive input from the world about us, we are equipped with sensory organs that enable us to smell, taste, see, hear and touch as well as providing us with information about the position of our body in relation to gravity and about the state of our muscles, joints and internal organs. Each individual input is rarely picked up by a single sensory organ working in isolation; instead sensation almost always involves the combined function of several sensory organs. For example, watching a bird in the sky does not merely involve optical information from the eyes; the head, neck and body also have to be moved, causing the brain to receive additional information from vestibular receptors and proprioceptors. These complex items of information have to be processed in the brain. However, on those occasions where just one sensory organ is involved in sensation (e.g. if we smell an orange without touching it or seeing it), the brain makes other information available from personal experience so as to yield a complete picture of the object.

In the broadest sense, all these processing activities working in concert may be defined as sensory integration (SI). SI can be represented as a sequential chain (Fig. 16.11).

Sensory integration disorder

A malfunction in one link of the chain depicted in Fig. 16.11 is termed a sensory integration disorder. This may be an obstacle to the general and/or partial learning process and general development. These disorders of sensation and sensory integration include specific learning difficulties such as dyslexia, dysgraphia or dyscalculia, as well as attention deficit hyperactivity disorder.

Back in the 1950s and 1960s Ayres (1979, 1984) attempted to formulate sensory integration processes and their disorders on the basis of knowledge available at the time. Her theory underwent further refinement by a number of successors (Doering 1990; Fisher et al 1998).

The foundation of this theory is formed by the basic processes involved in sensation and the processing of information from the world around us. Five areas of SI have been identified in which basic dysfunctions may occur:

- Processing of vestibular and proprioceptive sensory input resulting from postural-ocular movements

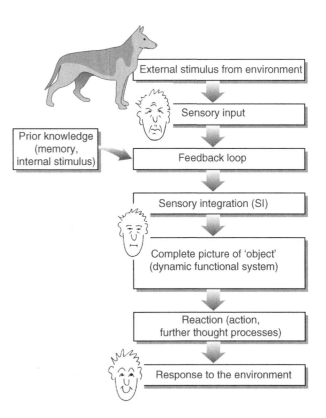

Figure 16.11 Processing activities involved in sensory integration. With permission, Henriette Rintelen, Velbert

- Somatosensory processing of tactile and proprioceptive information
- Bilateral integration and sequencing of vestibular-proprioceptive input at the level of the higher analytical brain areas, with involvement of additional motor centers
- Processing of tactile and vestibular-proprioceptive sensory input (somatopraxis)
- Sensory modulation of tactile, vestibular and proprioceptive sensory input involving the limbic system and the reticular formation.

Etiology and pathogenesis

A variety of prenatal, perinatal and postnatal factors have been discussed as possible causes of sensory integration disorders. These factors include:

- inadequate intrauterine supply of oxygen, vitamins and nutrients to the fetus due to an unfavourable maternal lifestyle
- chronic maternal illness during pregnancy; e.g. diabetes mellitus, bronchial asthma, valvular heart disease, etc.
- consumption of specific medicines by the mother during pregnancy; while many medicinal products do not necessarily lead to obvious deformity, they may be a contributory cause in disorders of CNS function
- infectious diseases acquired by the mother during pregnancy, e.g. cytomegalovirus, toxoplasmosis, influenza-type infections, rubella, etc.
- maternal exposure to toxic substances during pregnancy; e.g. due to employment in a chemical plant
- alcohol and nicotine abuse by the mother during pregnancy
- adverse psychological status of the mother-to-be: may have a negative effect on metabolism and hormone balance
- placental insufficiency, premature labor or bleeding during pregnancy, potentially resulting in fetal circulatory disturbances
- protracted second stage of labor; e.g. in breech presentation of the fetus
- arrested labor or coiling of the umbilical cord around the neck, leading to impaired fetal oxygen supply
- delivery by vacuum extraction or forceps
- premature birth with marked CNS immaturity
- meningitis and/or encephalitis in the infant and preschool child
- chronic illness in the child; e.g. metabolic diseases, diabetes mellitus, valvular heart disease, epilepsy, etc.

The process of sensory integration is powerfully influenced by the momentary individual emotional state. For example, we may focus our senses on a particular piece of information, anticipate this patiently or impatiently and be ready to analyze it and to react immediately. This anticipatory readiness to react may support the process of SI. However, if we have no motivation, if we are indifferent about how something tastes or smells, whether it thunders or rains, or how beautiful the sunset is, there is insufficient SI, no true sensory appreciation of the world about us and hence also no appropriate reaction.

However, there are also situations where sensory integration – from which we should in fact benefit – may even be harmful or detrimental to us. For example, because of the completed SI process, a previous bad experience with an orange that had gone moldy and tasted 'off' might mean that we would also refuse a perfectly good orange and that for a certain period, or perhaps for the rest our lives, we might experience aversion or even disgust at the mere sight or smell of an orange.

Clinical signs and symptoms

The possible existence of a sensory integration disorder may be suspected as a result of observing the child in everyday settings such as the home, playgroup or school. Children giving grounds for such suspicion may appear clumsy or awkward in general motor terms and tend to stand on the sidelines during activity games, or on the other hand often try to lead the group in order to conceal their own weaknesses. Some commonly display tactile defensiveness or balance problems, do not want to play on swings or avoid exposure to heights. Others appear to lack control in their movements, have little sensitivity to pain, require strong proprioceptive stimuli and are poor at assessing risk. These latter observations, for example, suggest a disturbance of tactile proprioceptive discrimination and of sensorimotor modulation.

Often children with a sensory integration disorder also suffer from delayed development and disturbed behavior with body perception disorders (see Case history below).

Diagnosis

History-taking can provide important clues to past events and to the child's social environment. We have also found it useful, even before the first appointment for treatment, to send the parents a questionnaire so that details of the child's history can be gathered in advance and then pursued specifically during the initial session. The following details appear to be particularly important: course of labor, development in infancy and preschool years, injuries sustained, family circumstances, social relationships in playgroup and school, leisure activities and exposure to electronic media (TV, PC, Game Boy, etc.) in hours per day. Supplementing these key data on the patient's history, the questionnaire may also comprise a second section with questions designed specifically to help assess the child's cognitive abilities and any special areas of note (specimen questionnaire Fig. 16.12). These questions, taken from educational psychology surveys conducted among parents, should help to sketch a preliminary cognitive profile. Moreover, this section of the questionnaire can be issued several times over the course of treatment (e.g. at intervals of 8 to 12 weeks) to document any positive results – but also relapses – in addition to verbal feedback provided by the parents.

The questionnaire offers the added advantage that children are spared endless repetitions of their personal 'list of shortcomings' during conversations between parents and therapist; this fosters a positive atmosphere in terms of communication.

Allopathic diagnostic procedures

Various social pediatric centers offer facilities for a detailed diagnosis to be made. Diagnostic observations and descriptions of the child from experienced occupational therapists and physiotherapists are also helpful. The medical diagnosis of SI disorders comprises various aspects:

- assessment of muscle tone regulation, vestibular function, coordination and proprioception
- evaluation of cranial nerve function, including acoustic and visual perception
- educational psychology assessments to test cognitive abilities and skills and cerebral processing activities
- reflex testing
- assessment of language development
- EEG and imaging techniques, as required in each individual case.

To diagnose a sensory integration disorder Ayres (1989) developed a series of 17 test procedures that were standardized in a representative sample of 4- to 9-year-old children in the USA. However, Karch et al (2003) have criticized these instruments, claiming that only very low reliability has been established for the two most important sensory integration tests; namely, those for postrotatory nystagmus and tactile sensation, and thus calling into question the validity of these test procedures.

Questionnaire for parents

Name of child: _____

Questionnaire completed by: _____ Date: _____

Put a cross through the numbered circle that best reflects the following statements.
0 = Not applicable 1 = Mild 2 = Marked 3 = Very severe

1. Has difficulty reading. 0 1 2 3
2. Has difficulty writing/spelling. 0 1 2 3
3. Has difficulty with maths. 0 1 2 3
4. Has difficulty understanding schoolwork. 0 1 2 3
5. Often appears not to listen when other people talk to him/her. 0 1 2 3
6. His/her attention is poor during lessons and homework. 0 1 2 3
7. Works slowly and is unable to complete schoolwork. 0 1 2 3
8. Has difficulty organizing tasks and activities. 0 1 2 3
9. Is often forgetful. 0 1 2 3
10. His/her sleep is disturbed. 0 1 2 3
11. Lacks self-confidence. 0 1 2 3
12. Lacks sufficient motivation to study. 0 1 2 3
13. Is often irritable and moody. 0 1 2 3

Figure 16.12 Parental questionnaire eliciting information on the child's cognitive abilities and any special areas of note

In addition, based on Ayres' theory and practice, specific observational diagnostic criteria have been formulated, which are designed to assist the diagnosis; for example the child's reaction to swinging, lathering with soap, and touch. Aside from these test procedures, a great many further tests have been proposed by other authors to assess sensorimotor development (Aksu 2002).

Osteopathic examination

As in all other functional disorders and pathologies, osteopathic examination in children with sensory disorders – a category that includes sensory integration disorders – also adheres to the principle of holistic assessment. It includes inspection with the child standing to gain an impression of the organization of the body in relation to gravity. Any asymmetries and rotational patterns are noted. This is followed by a dynamic examination of the locomotor system with the patient standing, seated and supine, as well as a gentle examination of the whole body, and specifically viscera and cranium with the help of involuntary motion (IVM).

The expectation that osteopathic lesions in the cranial region are more likely to be encountered in sensory disorders is certainly understandable and is justified to a considerable extent – it is no coincidence that various authors have unanimously attributed a high percentage of sensory disorders in children to cranial trauma during the birth process or in early childhood.

Frymann (2000), for example, basing her argument on the analysis of her study of learning disabilities in childhood, estimates that some 80% of learning and concentration difficulties in children are due to birth trauma involving the cranial region.

On the other hand, care must be taken to ensure that children with such difficulties are not considered merely in terms of their cranium. Practical experience indicates that reflex, biomechanical and biodynamic relationships in the body as a whole play an important role in the causation of sensory disorders.

The following case example is intended to help illustrate the relationships that emerge during the osteopathic examination.

> **Case study**
>
> Eight-year-old Tobias was brought to our practice by his mother because he was exceptionally reserved and shy. He was averse to making arrangements to play with his classmates, was awkward and anxious during PE lessons, and did not want to cycle or swim. An allopathic medical examination revealed considerable problems with vestibular regulation and coordination, as well as flaccid muscle tone.

By contrast, his scores in diagnostic psycholinguistic tests were in the upper part of the normal range and in some instances were actually above average.

Osteopathic examination revealed a right-sided SBS torsion, a reduced amplitude of IVM, compression of the sagittal suture and osteopathic lesioning of the atlanto-occipital joints. From the patient's history, these findings were attributable to the prolonged course of labor and the birth being ended with a vacuum extraction. Other noteworthy findings included a reduced excursion of the diaphragm, reduced motility of the caecum and osteopathic lesions at the lumbosacral junction and the right psoas muscle.

A marked improvement in the expression of IVM was already noted following treatment of the pelvis, diaphragm, psoas muscle and caecum during the first three sessions. As the fluid fluctuation in the body improved, it was possible to successfully release the cranial osteopathic lesions during ensuing treatments. In total, the course of the osteopathic treatment lasted for 1 year, during which period 12 sessions were necessary.

When the treatment was finished Tobias had not been transformed into a great athlete, but he became increasingly skilled at compensating for his problems. He grew more open, took the initiative to sing in a children's choir, and became increasingly adventurous in PE lessons. His hobby, however, became learning to speak Chinese!

Treatment
Allopathic medical treatment

SI therapy is delivered by specially trained occupational therapists and physiotherapists. The principal goal of treatment, according to Ayres (1979, 1984), is to use specifically targeted sensory input to address and promote disturbed basic functions and thus to improve the child's learning ability and general development.

Techniques such as massage with cream, therapeutic body brushing, and ball-pool games are used to treat the tactile defensiveness commonly encountered in these children; for example when playing, showering or hair washing. These methods are particularly suitable for children with combined tactile and proprioceptive disorders. In general, the treatment aims to address and engage as many of the child's sensory input channels as possible, and the child thus learns to respond more appropriately to sensory information.

In disorders of somatopraxis (i.e. processing of tactile and vestibular-proprioceptive sensory input), games involving bilateral coordinated movements are used to overcome these deficits. The child is instructed to perform tasks synchronously with both hands; for example, to paint two faces using the left and right hand simultaneously.

Karch et al (2003) have confirmed that the treatment techniques recommended by Ayres have enriched the practice of occupational therapy, and that they produce clearly discernible positive effects on motor skills, body posture control and secondary behavioral disorders, such as anxiety, insecurity or problems when relating to other children.

However, they think that SI therapy is not that effective in attention and concentration disorders in hyperactive children, in fine motor, graphomotor and visuomotor coordination disorders, and regarding learning difficulties in school. These critical comments concerning SI therapy suggest that this area is still largely virgin territory that needs to be occupied by other therapeutic approaches if children with sensory disorders are to be helped.

Osteopathic treatment

There can, of course, be no universal strategy for the treatment of children with sensory integration disorders. Similarly, it is not really possible to correlate a particular type of sensory disorder – be it a sensory integration disorder, a form of specific learning difficulty or ADHD – with specific osteopathic findings. The following remarks will therefore draw attention to just a few functional aspects and osteopathic lesions that are encountered with unusual frequency with sensory disorders.

Experience shows that working with the primary respiratory mechanism (PRM) can be very effective, and that such work should not be overly directive. Quite the opposite, in fact: having a definite goal in mind may have an inhibitory and restrictive effect on the treatment process (see p.186). Treatment approaches such as balanced ligamentous tension (BLT) (see p.183), fascial work or general osteopathic treatment (GOT) are also helpful.

At the start of treatment, in restless and hyperactive children in particular, it may be beneficial to begin with a GOT sequence (Druelle 2004). First, this may already achieve release for many locomotor apparatus osteopathic lesions and, second, the hyperactive child experiences intensive proprioceptive stimulation, receiving major input in terms of her own body. Starting the osteopathic treatment using this approach seems to eliminate or bring order to much sensory dysfunctional 'interference', and this manifests itself as the child becomes visibly more relaxed and respiration becomes deeper.

An important key in our view is the general improvement of hemodynamics, particularly in the cranial region. Frymann (2000), for example, in her study of children with learning difficulties, attributes the success of treatment to

improved venous and lymphatic drainage, which in turn leads to improved microcirculation of the neural system.

In our experience, the intracranial membranes often feel rigid on palpation with the help of IVM. An osteopathic study by Rütz and Röh (2002) appears to confirm this observation. They were working with children with ADHD and detected significant improvements in symptoms following reduction of intracranial membrane tension. Our own study (Goussel et al 2003) in children with auditory disorders revealed that the incidence of reduced motility of the reciprocal tension membrane (RTM) was 77%. This reduced motility adversely affected the venous drainage in the cranium (see p.358). Experience suggests that treating the intracranial membranes works very well. Afterwards, the IVM is often clearly more expressive and calmer. A previously fidgety child will gradually quieten down and is usually able to accept the treatment in a more relaxed way. Of course, the influence of the caudal pole of the reciprocal tension membrane should not be forgotten. Osteopathic lesions involving the sacrum and coccyx, as well as other osteopathic lesions of the spinal column, exert a major influence on the mobility and motility in the cranium.

Because of the neurotopography outlined above, possible osteopathic lesions of the occipital and temporal bones play a major role in sensory disorders, but these will be discussed in greater detail later in this section.

The frontal and parietal bones are also important because of their proximity to brain areas that are relevant for cognition. Osteopathic lesions in these areas may have hemodynamic and reflex effects on the somatosensory system of both the frontal and parietal lobes of the brain. The prefrontal cortex in particular plays a major role in motivation and the ability to concentrate.

However, these many references to cranial osteopathic lesions and their relevance for neurotopography should not cause us to lose sight of the body as a whole. In addition to the fascial relationships already referred to, visceral aspects may also be very important. Not infrequently we find that children with sensory disorders have problems involving the hepatobiliary system, which manifest themselves as disorders of biliary outflow and hepatic congestion. Osteopathic lesions of the small and large intestine are also commonly encountered.

Such functional visceral disorders will send information via the vagus phrenic nerves to the cranium where it becomes a permanent flood of input that irritates the ongoing integrative work of the CNS. Naturally, the causes underlying these visceral overload phenomena are complex:

• First, it must be remembered that the children we treat are still growing, and some may be pubescent; facts that place major metabolic demands on the internal organs, especially the liver, due to fluctuating hormone levels. In this context it must be noted that the liver plays a major role in hormone synthesis.

- Second, the child's sometimes less-than-ideal eating behavior is an additional possible cause. An imbalanced diet, frequent recourse to fast food, high sugar consumption, and usually inadequate fluid intake can place a heavy burden on the gastrointestinal tract. The consequence is intensive lymphatic activity, especially of Peyer's patches in the region of the terminal ileum and caecum. This high level of lymphatic information from the viscera may produce central overstimulation, possibly associated with integration disorders or hyperactivity. Symptoms of this kind usually respond well when dietetic suggestions are made to the parents and child. Osteopathic support for the visceral organs affected, including treatment of the diaphragms, is also beneficial for enteric and lymphatic reintegration.

Aside from puberty-related hormonal changes, other autonomic and endocrine imbalances may also be rooted in osteopathic lesions.

The diaphragms – which we know are special organizational features of the myofascial system – are of major importance for hemodynamics and for the circulation of body fluids because they may inhibit intercellular communication. In the treatment of sensory disorders it is therefore also immensely important to treat osteopathic lesions of the diaphragms.

Blood, lymph, cerebrospinal fluid (CSF), and intercellular and intracellular fluids are in a constant process of mutual interchange and thus we have permanent intercellular communication, which incorporates neurocrine, paracrine and endocrine components. This process includes all the nutrients, electrolytes, vitamins, hormones, neurotransmitters and neuropeptides present in solution. The blood vessels, lymph vessels and nerves can be thought of as specialized channels facilitating the direct and rapid transport of nutrients, metabolic end-products, hormones and neurotransmitters. Everything is designed to transmit information from 'one cell' to 'all other cells', irrespective of the current metabolic situation. Without these specialized channels, our body might be thought of as a sponge in which the movement of water and of the particles dissolved in it would be sustained by concentration gradients, colloid-osmotic pressure, electrical voltage potentials and embryological fascial patterns – in the sense of motility.

This picture can help us to discover and take account of a biodynamic level alongside the biomechanical and neuroreflectory level. Good exchange and optimal fluctuation of body fluids are important prerequisites for communication

between the brain and all other body organs. This is regulated and modulated by neurotransmitters, monoamines and neuropeptides. The true intelligence of the body, the power of self-regulation, lies in the unbroken continuity of blood, lymph, CSF, and intercellular and intracellular fluid. Accordingly, information contained in these fluids and originating from the viscera and the enteric nervous system is also immensely important for the CNS. Any visceral dysfunction disturbs balance and homeostasis in the CNS. In this context we also speak of a 'wet brain', a fluid intelligence, which may be found 'between the lines'; that is, between structures.

One final comment concerns children's leisure time. The downside of the much-vaunted 'communication era' in which we live is that children's leisure activities nowadays are often dominated by the electronic media – computers, TV, PlayStation and Game Boy. On the one hand this means that children experience a flood of sensory input, and on the other this electronic 'activity' leads to a sedentary lifestyle. It is an integral part of osteopathic treatment also to address this issue and to heighten awareness among parents and children. Our advice should be directed towards encouraging leisure pursuits that involve more physical activity; at the same time this will act as a desirable safety valve for tension and aggressive behavior. Seen in these terms, cognitive deficits may be rooted not only in the osteopathic lesions listed above, but also in the child's immediate environment, the family situation, and influences from school and leisure time.

Prognosis

The osteopathic approaches mentioned before may be helpful when addressing the complex subject of sensory disorders in children. In this setting osteopathy has in our opinion proved to be a very effective therapy. Sometimes we have seen decisive improvements in symptoms in just a few treatments, and occasionally a noticeable breakthrough is achieved after five to eight treatments. Usually, however, the treatment cycles tend to be rather lengthy, requiring considerable patience and time from all parties involved. Treatment may therefore extend over 1 or 2 years before notable progress is finally achieved. In this context the treatment intervals are usually fairly widely spaced, allowing periods of 3 to 5 weeks between treatments. Improvements in disorders of processing and sensation tend to occur over a prolonged time period. Because the process is associated with far-reaching changes in the CNS and places high demands on the brain in terms of neuroplasticity, the organism should be allowed time to integrate the impulses generated by the osteopathic treatment.

The best feedback on treatment is provided by assessing the rate and amplitude of the IVM, which is a representative of the vitality of the organism and hence its capacity for self-regulation. If the expression of IVM improves during treatment or is improved compared with the previous treatment, then this is an indication that the treatment has taken primary osteopathic lesions into account.

Central processing and sensation reflects a complex synergy between primary, secondary and associative brain centers. The sensory integration of all endogenous and exogenous input requires that the associative centers should function flawlessly. Tissue homeostasis is the prerequisite for physiological metabolic processes, and in the context of neural tissue this promotes optimal signal transmission at the synapses. We believe that osteopathy is able to contribute to the treatment of sensory disorders by promoting intercellular communication on the basis of improved blood circulation and fluctuation.

Bibliography

Aksu F: Neuropädiatrie, Diagnostik und Therapie neurologischer Erkrankungen im Kindes- und Jugendalter. Uni-Med, Bremen/London/Boston 2002

Ayres J: Lernstörungen, Sensorisch-integrative Dysfunktionen. Springer, Berlin 1979

Ayres J: Bausteine der kindlichen Entwicklung. Springer, Berlin 1984

Ayres J: Sensory integration and praxis tests. Western Psychological Services, Los Angeles, 1989

Doering W W: Sensorische Integration. Borgmann, Broadstairs (UK) 1990

Druelle P: Ganzheitliche Osteopathische Therapie (GOT). Sonntag, Stuttgart 2004

Fisher A G, Murray E A, Bundy A C: Sensorische Integrationstherapie, Theorie und Praxis. Springer, Berlin 1998

Frymann V M: Learning disabilities in childhood. In: The collected papers of Viola M. Frymann, Legacy of osteopathy to children. American Academy of Osteopathy, Indianapolis 2000

Goussel W, Guerassimiouk D, Markhoff J-P: Die therapeutische Wirksamkeit der osteopathischen Behandlung bei Kindern mit auditiven Verarbeitungs- und Wahrnehmungsstörungen. Diplomarbeit, Akademie für Osteopathie 2003

Karch D, Groß-Selbeck G, Pietz J, Schlack H G: Sensorische Integrationstherapie nach Jean Ayres, Stellungnahme der Gesellschaft für Neuropädiatrie. Monatsschr Kinderheilkunde 151, 2003: 218–220

Rütz M, Röh N: Entspannung der intrakranialen Membranen bei Kindern mit Hyperaktivem Verhaltenssyndrom. In: Osteopathische Medizin, Zeitschrift für ganzheitliche Heilverfahren. 3 (4), 2002: 22–26

SPECIFIC LEARNING DIFFICULTIES

William Goussel, Dina Guerassimiouk, Jens-Peter Markhoff

Definition

The specific learning difficulties encountered in many school-children are distinct sensory integration disorders that affect academic skills and abilities. Specific learning difficulties are defined in terms of three general characteristics:

- Without exception, they have their onset in infancy or childhood.
- There is impairment or delay in the development of functions that are closely associated with the biological maturation of the CNS.
- They have a constant pattern that is not characterized by the remissions and relapses typical of many psychiatric disorders.

A further important precondition in defining a child's weakness as a specific learning difficulty is to rule out the possibility of low intelligence or of global developmental delay; in other words, the child's general intelligence must be characterized by an IQ of at least 85.

In Germany the cut-off between normal ability and the need for a child to receive increased individual help is defined by an IQ of 80–85. According to WHO guidelines, the accepted minimum standard for a child to develop normally is an IQ of ≥70 (Schmid and Kühne 2003).

Specific learning difficulties are a major issue in the day-to-day school environment and elsewhere. Steinmacher et al (2000, 2002) and Esser (2003) estimate that specific learning difficulties are present in some 8–20% of all children in Germany. Similar numbers will probably apply to other European countries. This potentially means that difficulties at school and/or secondary behavioral problems could be evident in about 10–15% of all children (Steinmacher et al 2000). Early, sensitive diagnosis is therefore all the more important when planning therapeutic interventions in children with normal cognitive development but with specific developmental disorders. Such assessments should ideally be performed before the child starts school by an experienced pediatrician, a pediatric psychologist or in a center specializing in child development or social pediatrics.

According to Schulte-Körne and Remschmidt (2003), the international prevalence of dyslexia is 4–5%. In Germany 4.3–6.4% of adults do not attain the reading and/or writing skills of a year 4 pupil. Dyslexia affects boys two to three times more commonly than girls.

Etiology and pathogenesis

The causes of specific learning difficulties have not yet been satisfactorily established. A range of neurobiological factors are the most likely suspects for consideration (Schulte-Körne, Remschmidt 2003; see p.381):

- genetic disposition
- disorders of phonological awareness, i.e. of 'sound memory' and of the ability to analyze and synthesize sounds

- impairment of orthographic skill, which comprises verbal memory and the ability both to understand and recognize the rules governing syllabic construction and letter sequences and to grasp and retain the rules of grammar
- deficits in the area of perception and processing of visual and acoustic information.

Clinical signs and symptoms

Two specific learning difficulties are particularly important in school-age children:

- Difficulty in reading and/or writing, a condition known as dyslexia (Michaelis and Niemann 1995)
- Difficulty with arithmetic, a condition known as dyscalculia (v. Aster et al 2005).

Dyslexia primarily involves a disorder of acoustic and visual perception and processing, including short-term memory, sequential memory, phonemic differentiation and phonemic synthesis, dichotic discrimination, long-term memory and gaze control.

Dyslexia is encountered particularly commonly in school-age children. A recent study by Schulte-Körne and Remschmidt (2003) presents a very detailed description of the symptoms and diagnosis of this specific learning difficulty, as well as of its causes, its course over time and its treatment. In Germany dyslexia can only be reliably diagnosed in a child from the end of school year 2 onwards, with the aid of special reading and writing tests.

The differential diagnosis of dyslexia should consider general developmental delay or low IQ, visual and auditory deficits, neurological and psychiatric illness and, last but not least, possibly inappropriate teaching.

Sensory integration disorders in the following areas may be causes of dyscalculia: abstract logical thought, spatial and quantitative awareness, short-term and long-term memory.

Diagnosis
Allopathic diagnostic procedures

In order to detect a specific learning difficulty in a child, particular skills and abilities are assessed using a range of psychological tests, such as the Kaufman Assessment Battery for Children (K-ABC), Hamburg-Wechsler Intelligence Test for Children (HAWIK-III), Diagnostic Writing Test (DRT), Hamburg Writing Test (HSP), and the Neuropsychological Test Battery for Number Processing in Children (NUCALC), as well as positron emission tomography (PET). The areas assessed include:

- spatial and shape awareness
- mathematical thinking

- speed of perception
- acoustic or visual short-term memory
- ability to read and understand
- visuomotor coordination
- writing skills.

The criterion for a diagnosis of specific learning difficulty is met if the IQ for one individually tested ability is below the normal range and is at least 22 to 23 'intelligence points' lower than the general IQ of the particular child being tested.

The following example will illustrate this assessment practice more clearly: A child has a general IQ of 105. The normal range is 85–115, with a mean of 100. The child is therefore of average ability. However, on specific testing of acoustic short-term memory, the child achieves a score that is consistent with an IQ of 75. There is a considerable difference between the child's general intelligence and her score in terms of acoustic short-term memory. This child of otherwise average ability therefore has a specific learning difficulty in the area of acoustic short-term memory.

Osteopathic examination

Also in the case of specific learning difficulties, osteopathic examination is based on the holistic principle of osteopathy. For further details see p.383.

Treatment
Allopathic medical treatment

Treatment for specific learning difficulties is necessarily complex and involves both psychosocial and medical as well as educational measures (Aksu 2002, Schulte-Körne and Remschmidt 2003).

Psychosocial measures include educational counselling, psychotherapy, and the fostering of good parent–school cooperation through the agencies responsible for social services and the educational authorities.

Specific deficits in acoustic and visual perception can be addressed using an entire spectrum of medical treatment methods: ophthalmological and orthoptic correction as well as therapy to compensate for peripheral and central hearing disorders. Training of basic perceptual functions is a controversial area (Karch et al 2000, Schulte-Körne and Remschmidt 2003): training of non-language acoustic stimuli, gaze control training, stimulation using kinesiology, perceptual training using visual patterns and figure-ground discrimination.

The core element of educational efforts is symptom-related training designed to improve mathematical thinking, including mastery of counting strategies in dyscalculia, and to enhance phonological awareness and orthographic skills in dyslexia. Such training may be a component of integrated learning therapy; for example, a modality that is implemented by qualified integrated learning therapists.

Osteopathic treatment

Osteopathic treatment can make an important contribution in the area of specific learning difficulties. The key points have already been described in the previous section (see p.384) and will not be reiterated here.

However, it should be noted in particular that both intra-osseous and interosseous dysfunctions of the occipital bone often play a major role in children with specific learning difficulties. Because of the topographical location of the primary and secondary visual cortex, dysfunctions of this kind may have adverse repercussions for the processing of optical signals precisely in terms of difficulties with reading and/or writing. Sergueef (1995) reports that dysfunctions of the sphenobasilar synchondrosis and occipital bone are repeatedly encountered in children with learning difficulties.

A further important consideration in dyslexia is the location of the angular gyrus in the parietal lobe around the temporal sulcus. It is the central interface between the visual cortex in the occipital lobe and the sensory speech center and consequently has major importance for reading and writing. Two neuronal pathways lead from the sensory speech center, one to the auditory system and the other to the visual system. Dysfunctions of the temporal bones are believed to have an adverse effect on the performance of these processing centers, either as a reflex phenomenon or in hemodynamic terms. Sergueef (1995) recommends in dyslexia that special attention be directed to the temporal bones and the frontal bone.

In a study conducted by us in children with disorders of auditory processing and perception (Goussel et al 2003), we encountered the following phenomena: 87% of all children affected had an asymmetric expression of the IVM at the level of the body fluids; specifically, its expression was reduced in the left cranial hemisphere while being clearly detectable in the right cranial hemisphere. Simultaneously, in 90% of the children, we detected a preferred direction of motion for the left temporal bone in internal rotation and an intraosseous dysfunction of this bone.

Since the dominant hemisphere in right-handed people is on the left side, and the secondary auditory cortex in the dominant hemisphere is responsible for language understanding (Wernicke's area), it is reasonable to deduce that a dysfunction involving the left temporal bone could irritate precisely these local brain areas in the left temporal lobe (Sutherland 1990). All the patients in our study were right-handed!

In attempting to explain and in some way to understand this strong correlation between dysfunctions of the left temporal bone and disorders of auditory processing and perception in children, we discovered certain characteristics relating to the birth process itself: according to Pschyrembel and Dudenhausen (1986), by far the majority of normal births are a left occiput anterior presentation (LOA) (see p.59, 69), which after Sergueef (1995) accounts for 70% of all cephalic presentations. In this presentation, as the cervix dilates, the child's right parietal bone enters the pelvis first and thus finds itself in a relatively deeper position. As a result it tends to bulge more, whereas the left parietal bone tends to be more flattened due to pressure exerted by the maternal sacrum at the level of the promontory (Sergueef 1995; Fig. 16.13). In general it is true to say that, in the presentation described above, the left half of the cranium – especially the left temporal bone – is in danger of being subjected to mechanical stress.

Dysfunctions of this kind may arise if the mechanical forces exceed normal physiological limits and the compensatory forces in the neonate are exhausted. The pattern of birth described here may therefore be a model to explain the incidence of left temporal bone dysfunctions in the children in our study and, via a reflex effect on the left temporal lobe (Sutherland 1990), this finding may be linked with impaired auditory processing.

Prognosis

In our experience, osteopathy is able to make an effective contribution to the treatment of specific learning difficulties. At this point we should like to present the results of our pilot study, which confirmed the efficacy of osteopathy in children

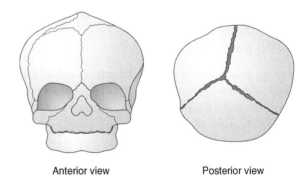

Anterior view   Posterior view

Figure 16.13 Possible deformation of the baby's cranium in the left occiput anterior (LOA) presentation.
With permission, Henriette Rintelen, Velbert

with disorders of auditory processing and perception. This was a controlled, randomized clinical pilot study with a main group treated by osteopathy and a control group treated by allopathic medical methods. After a treatment cycle lasting for between 10 and 15 months and comprising 11 to 14 osteopathic treatment sessions, the final ENT assessment no longer detected any severe or moderate disorders of auditory processing and perception in 88.9% of the children. By comparison, the success rate in the children in the control group treated with the conventional methods of allopathic medicine was significantly lower at just 33.3%.

Analysis of the parents' questionnaire yielded further interesting findings:

- On completion of the osteopathic treatment cycle 82.4% of the children had a better understanding of their school work and as many as 88.2% of the children were reported to be more attentive during lessons and homework.

- According to information provided by the parents, 76.5% of the children treated by osteopathy had improved in their reading and 64.7% had improved in their writing.

- The problem of seeming not to listen when addressed became less marked in 76.5% of the children – a fact that along with reading, writing and attentiveness also relates very directly to the area of hearing.

- The organization of tasks and activities had improved in 70.6% of the children, and the pace of working had accelerated in as many as 76.5% of the children.

This information, seen in tandem with the significant results of the ENT assessment, seems to indicate the extensive scope of osteopathy in supporting children with neuronal processing disorders so that they can use their cognitive potential in a manner that is appropriate to their situation.

In our opinion combined therapy, consisting of allopathic medical and psychosocial measures as well as osteopathy, is an optimal solution for helping children with specific learning difficulties via a range of different channels and mechanisms.

Bibliography

Aster M v., Kucian K, Schweiter M, Martin E: Rechenstörungen im Kindesalter. Monatsschrift Kinderheilkd 153, 2005: 614–622

Esser G: Basisdiagnostik umschriebener Entwicklungsstörungen im Vorschulalter für die pädiatrische Praxis. Kinderärztliche Praxis 4, 2003: 232–238

Goussel W, Guerassimiouk D, Markhoff J-P: Die therapeutische Wirksamkeit der osteopathischen Behandlung bei Kindern mit auditiven Verarbeitungs- und Wahrnehmungsstörungen. Diploma dissertation, Akademie für Osteopathie 2003

Karch D, Groß-Selbeck G, Rating D et al: Hörtraining nach Tomatis und 'Klangtherapie' Kinderärztliche Praxis 8, 2000: 533–536

Michaelis R, Niemann G: Entwicklungsneurologie und Neuropädiatrie. Hippokrates, Stuttgart, 1995: 106–124

Pschyrembel W, Dudenhausen J W: Praktische Geburtshilfe. de Gruyter, Berlin/New York 1986

Schmid RG, Kühne H: Diagnostik von umschriebenen Entwicklungsstörungen. Kinderärztliche Praxis 4, 2003: 220–230

Schulte-Körne G, Remschmidt H: Legasthenie-Symptomatik, Diagnostik, Ursachen, Verlauf und Behandlung. Deutsches Ärzteblatt 7, 2003: C333–338

Serguef N: Die kraniosakrale Osteopathie bei Kindern. Wühr, Kötzting, 1995

Steinmacher J, Jäger D, Starck M, Kupferschmid C, Bode H: Diagnostik von Teilleistungsstörungen im Rahmen der Vorsorgeuntersuchung U9. Kinder- und Jugendarzt 7, 2000: 676–679

Steinmacher J, Starck M, Fingerle J, Gräße A, Kupferschmid C, Bode H: Der Elefant beißt den Löwen, Diagnostik von Teilleistungsstörungen bei 5-jährigen Kindern. Kinder- und Jugendarzt 8, 2002: 638–642

Sutherland WG: Teachings in the science of osteopathy. Sutherland Cranial Teaching Foundation, Texas 1990

ATTENTION DEFICIT HYPERACTIVITY DISORDER (ADHD)

William Goussel, Dina Guerassimiouk, Jens-Peter Markhoff

Definition

In recent years the name 'attention deficit hyperactivity disorder (ADHD)' has come to replace the labels 'hyperkinetic syndrome' and 'hyperkinetic disorder', although both these older terms can still be found in the current scientific literature.

It will be useful at this point to cite the definition from ICD-10 (2004), Chapter V, for hyperkinetic disorder: 'This group of disorders is characterized by early onset, usually in the first 5 years of life, lack of persistence in activities that require cognitive involvement, and a tendency to move from one activity to another without completing any one, together with disorganized, ill-regulated and excessive activity. Several other abnormalities may also be associated with these disorders. Hyperkinetic children are often reckless and impulsive, prone to accidents, and find themselves in disciplinary trouble because of unthinking (rather than deliberately defiant) breaches of rules. Their relationships with adults are often socially disinhibited, with a lack of normal caution and reserve. They are unpopular with other children and may become isolated. Cognitive impairment is common, and specific delays in motor and language development are disproportionately frequent. Secondary complications include dissocial behavior and low self-esteem.'

According to ICD-10 (2004), a child must exhibit all three cardinal symptoms in order for a diagnosis of ADHD to be made: attention deficit, hyperactivity and impulsivity. DSM-IV identifies the existence of three types of ADHD:

- Combined type, in which all three symptoms are present
- Inattentive type, in which the attention deficit is very pronounced whereas hyperactivity and impulsivity are present in only very mild form, if at all
- Hyperactive-impulsive type, in which the attention deficit is only minimally apparent.

Both classification systems stipulate that for the diagnosis to be made, the ADHD symptoms must have been present for at least 6 months and in not fewer than two important life settings (e.g. in school and at home). Nevertheless, many authors believe that the cardinal symptoms of ADHD only become manifest in situations of constraint; for example at day nursery or in school lessons in response to the demands of nursery or teaching staff (Seile 1997, Döpfner and Lehmkuhl 1998).

Arriving at a diagnosis of ADHD is difficult and controversial. New studies and projects are repeatedly being conducted to research this problem. Martinius (2001) feels that while both classification systems provide detailed descriptions of the same symptoms, they do not refer to disease entities that have a known cause. Further on he writes: 'It is not these excellent systems, but rather a simplistic and incomplete understanding of ADHD that is responsible for what is now widely practised: attention deficit disorder (ADD) is used synonymously with hyperkinetic disorder and ADHD; because they have an *additional* attention disorder, children and adolescents with all conceivable – but very different – psychological problems and behavioral abnormalities are being labelled as having AD(H)D and – almost as a reflex response – being treated with methylphenidate'; that is, with Ritalin, Ritalin SR, Concerta, Equasym or Medikinet.

According to Schlack (2003) ADHD exists as a disease entity, for example in children with organic brain damage, but in his opinion the diagnosis has expanded to include several secondary ADHD-like behavioral abnormalities, which are merely the result of various defined developmental disorders and specific learning difficulties. In many cases, the people making the 'diagnosis' – teachers and kindergarten workers, psychologists, therapists and even physicians – fail to recognize the more or less clear functional causes of the attention deficit behind the external manifestations:

- visual and acoustic problems
- language difficulties and attendant communication disorders
- statomotor deficits characterized by clumsiness and a lack of play experience

- emotional disorders, e.g. depressive and/or anxiety disorders, poor school performance with experiences of failure due to specific learning difficulties such as dyslexia and dyscalculia
- low IQ levels that virtually rule out attentiveness
- stressful and adverse psychosocial conditions in the family, etc.

Under no circumstances, therefore, should the diagnosis be based solely on existing questionnaires for parents and teachers (Möller, Thoms 2002). For example, some physicians use the Parent-Teacher Conners Scales (Overmeyer, Ebert 1999), which are not adequate given the complexity of the diagnosis. Diagnostic checklists incorporating symptoms and research criteria according to ICD-10 and DSM-IV, as proposed by Döpfner and Lehmkuhl (1998), should be regarded as more appropriate and discriminating.

The controversies regarding definition and diagnosis have confirmed in us the belief that a single diagnosis of ADHD is not sufficient. Our proposal is to create two diagnoses: attention deficit hyperactivity disease (ADHD) and attention deficit hyperactivity syndrome (ADHS). In this way it will be possible to distinguish primary, cerebro-organic concentration disorders from those of secondary, functional origin. This solution is more likely to permit suitable treatment strategies to be tailored to each individual case.

Prevalence

The existing problems over diagnosis mean that there is a relatively marked lack of agreement in available figures relating to the epidemiology of ADHD, particularly since the statistical analyses are based on different age ranges. Thus, according to Brodehl et al (2003), some 500,000 children and adolescents in Germany between the ages of 6 and 18 years are affected by ADHD; this corresponds to a prevalence of about 5%. Schunke (2002) reported a prevalence of 4–6% in 6- to 16-year-olds, whereas Schubert et al (2004) noted a prevalence of 2–10% among all children in Germany. Prevalence rates of 3–10% for ADHD have been reported for children of elementary school age (Seile 1997). ADHD is seen in 3–10% of 4- to 10-year-old children in Europe and the USA (Schulte-Markworth 2003), and Hach et al (2000) have confirmed a prevalence of 2–9.5% for the English-speaking world. Various publications indicate that boys are affected by ADHD 2 to 9 times more commonly than girls (Hach et al 2000, Schulte-Markworth 2003). It appears certain that ADHD occurs at least twice as commonly in boys than in girls.

Etiology and pathogenesis

It has been suggested that the four factors listed below are causally involved in the etiopathogenesis of ADHD as a primary disease entity in its own right and not as a syndrome, and at the same time there is general unanimity that the pathogenesis is multifactorial (Overmeyer and Ebert 1999; Martinius 2001; Möller, Thoms 2002; Schunke 2002):

- cerebro-organic causes
- neurochemical disorders
- genetic factors
- food allergies.

Imaging and neurophysiological investigations of ADHD patients have revealed that functional inhibition in the area of the frontal brain, parietal lobe and parts of the corpus striatum and midbrain correlates with disturbed attention and increased impulsivity. Similar behavioral abnormalities, including hyperactivity, have also been noted in patients with frontal brain lesions.

Of remarkable interest is the observation (Overmeyer and Ebert 1999) that during an epidemic of lethargic encephalitis that raged between 1918 and 1923, affected adults were found to display symptoms of Parkinson's disease while affected children showed hyperactivity, attention deficits and impulsivity. It therefore seemed plausible that a dopamine function disorder or a dopamine deficiency, particularly in the basal ganglia as in Parkinson's disease, might be present as a causal factor in children with ADHD. In terms of its chemical structure, just like norepinephrine (noradrenaline) and epinephrine (adrenalin), dopamine is a catecholamine. And children with ADHD have in fact been shown to have abnormalities in the function of D_2 and D_4 dopamine receptors, increased expression of the dopamine transporter gene and an increased concentration of dopamine transporters in the corpus striatum, all of which were reduced in response to amphetamine administration and the resultant increase in synaptic dopamine concentration (Martinius 2001). The higher the concentration of dopamine transporters, the more dopamine can be bound and thus its activity can be blocked. However, these abnormalities have not been detected in brain regions that are even more important for the pathogenesis of ADHD, such as the frontal brain, reticular formation and parietal lobe (Martinius 2001; Paulus and Hammer 2002).

And it is not just the neurochemical catecholamine hypothesis for the causation of ADHD that has its weaknesses. The genetic theory for the pathogenesis of ADHD also appears to be too tidy and one-dimensional. The question can be raised as to whether psychological illnesses, including ADHD, are ever sufficiently straightforward and transparent for them to be explicable in terms of a functional abnormality of a single gene (in this instance, the dopamine transporter gene). As Martinius (2001) writes: 'As long as the general theory supporting a genetic pathogenesis of AD(H)D persists, parents can live with the burden of having been the one who passed the condition on – because they didn't know about it. And it remains uncertain whether one parent or both may have passed it on. On the other hand, awareness of a genetic disorder keeps them from worrying that the problem may have been produced by shortcomings in the way they raised the child. And so these etiological theories swing like a pendulum – now in one direction and now in the other.'

The idea that food allergies might cause ADHD is also very hotly debated. To date it has not been confirmed that phosphates, colouring agents, certain sugars and even food antigens have any causal significance in regard to ADHD (Möller and Thoms 2002). Hach et al (2000) concede that food allergies may be causally involved in only a very small proportion of children with ADHD.

Clinical signs and symptoms

The existence of the three cardinal criteria for a definition of ADHD (attention deficit, hyperactivity, impulsivity) does not always guarantee an accurate idea of the clinical picture of the condition. Five representative case reports follow here to illustrate the complexity and variability of the clinical picture.

1 Case study

Twelve-year-old Silke was referred to us with suspected ADHD by a social education worker. Silke was a Year 6 student attending secondary school and lived in a flat-sharing community. She lacked all motivation in school, busied herself with other things during classes, was easily distracted, and disturbed the lessons by interrupting, getting up from her seat and wandering around the classroom. Both with her classmates and at home she constantly provoked conflict situations in which she behaved aggressively and unpredictably. She was impulsive in her activities, conversation and play. In general, she was extremely troublesome and defiant. She is unable to stick to a single activity for longer than 10 to 15 minutes.

In terms of the girl's family history it should be mentioned that Silke's parents had been separated for about 3 years. She had one sister, 18 months older than her. When the parents separated, neither the father nor the mother wanted to take both girls and so they went to live for a year with an aunt on their mother's side. After one year the aunt decided to keep just one girl, the older sister. Silke was taken in by a foster family in which the relationships turned out to be extremely complicated, leading to a move to another foster family. Six months later there was another change when Silke moved into a children's home, and she had been living for 2 months in a flat-sharing community and attending a new school.

Neurological and motor assessment yielded inconclusive findings. The possible presence of ADHD could be affirmed on external grounds: attention deficit, ease of distraction, impulsivity, hyperactivity, and aggressive behavior. However, all these are merely outward signs. Reference to the patient's special personal history soon reveals the causes of Silke's behavior: parental neglect, loss of her sister and aunt, 'bad luck' with two foster families. Only very few psychologically stable adults would be able to cope with a set of circumstances such as this. Silke had a disorder of social behavior and emotionality, not ADHD. As a matter of priority she needed psychotherapy and a stable social environment.

2　Case study

Michael was 7 years old when he was referred to our practice at the suggestion of his class teacher. He was in Year 2 at elementary school and during lessons he often lacked concentration, was restless and easily distracted, but also sometimes lost in dreams. His behavior often distracted his classmates and was thus disruptive to lessons. Despite this, Michael was accepted in his class, popular even, and was a good friend and playmate. His behavior at home when doing school assignments was similar to that in school. In a play situation, especially when activities could be freely chosen, he was able to concentrate creatively over a longer period.

Psychological tests and specialist examination by an ENT physician revealed that Michael had a definite weakness in the area of acoustic processing and perception. In early childhood he had repeatedly suffered from otitis media and tympanic cavity effusions, which had been treated surgically by polyp removal, paracentesis and grommet insertion. Because of this auditory processing weakness Michael had difficulties understanding verbal instructions and explanations, and he rapidly lost the thread during lessons; this was the true main cause of his inability to concentrate, his ease of distraction, his poor performance in school and his dislike of school. Consequently, administration of methylphenidate would be totally inappropriate because this medication would not improve auditory perception and academic skills.

3　Case study

At 10 years old Daniella had no motor, language or neurological abnormalities. The girl was extremely dreamy in school and at home, slow and lacking in concentration. It seems as if she was living in a world of her own, although she was not autistic and had plenty of friends. Her teachers suspected that her academic performance could be very

much better than it was. On testing she was found to have an IQ of 105 (normal range 85–115), although specific skills testing to assess what she had learnt and her factual knowledge revealed a score of just 89.

Daniella's family was intact. Her parents were patient and loving and they were supportive of their daughter. She had no psychological problems and was not under pressure. The definitive diagnosis was 'ADS'. Careful individual adjustment of the girl's methylphenidate dose to 20 mg/day (10 mg in the morning and at midday) led to a marked change in Daniella's behavior: her poor concentration improved considerably and her performance in school went forwards by leaps and bounds.

4　Case study

Nine-year-old Marko was referred to us by his parents and his class teacher. He was in Year 3 at elementary school and was the second best pupil in his year. His parents were absolutely satisfied with his development and did not find him abnormal in any way. However, his class teacher reported that Marko was too lively during lessons. He very quickly finished virtually all his classroom assignments, but then had nothing to do so occupied himself with other things, and this distracted his classmates. For example, after having solved 15 maths problems, Marko would resist his teacher's instructions to do another 15 problems involving the same type of calculation because he perceived that as a punishment. Also he habitually asked too many questions during lessons and always wanted to be the first to answer. The teacher had diagnosed ADHD and wanted Marko to be put on methylphenidate. Marko's parents were very active, lively and contented people in their professional work, sport and everyday lives who felt happy and generated the same atmosphere in their family. Marko also had an 11-year-old sister and a 6-year-old brother.

A medical examination failed to reveal any conclusive findings, and in IQ tests Marko scored between 106 and 120 on a range of subtests and scales, a result that is in no way consistent with perceptual or specific learning difficulties. The premature diagnosis of ADHD was therefore not confirmed. Marko was a basically healthy boy who needed more challenging assignments to be given to him individually. Early advancement to the next class and more targeted assignments during lessons were other alternatives.

5　Case study

Philipp was brought to us by his parents when he was 9 years old. He was in Year 3 at school. According to his parents, Philipp had been a colicky, crying baby up to the age of 6 months. He showed very good motor and language development. The boy had always been inquisitive and active and played a lot outdoors, with a marked preference for activity games. In creative playing, e.g. Lego, he was very skilful and showed plenty of imagination, but only ever had patience for it for about 10 to 15 minutes. By the age of 5 Philipp knew all his letters, started to read, could write his name and found it very easy to learn things by heart. By that age he could already count to 20 and had mastered simple adding and taking away. He was stimulated by complicated questions that were far beyond his years; but he showed little patience in waiting for the answers, let alone listening through to the end.

When we first saw him, Philipp was always on the go, nimble and skilful with toys or a play idea, fast and slightly untidy when eating, and had problems falling asleep. People who knew him considered him highly gifted. However, his results in school did not live up to these expectations; he was only average and was unable to implement his good intellectual skills in practice. During lessons and homework assignments Philipp lacked concentration, he was over-hasty and superficial, impatient and easily frustrated. Lately, other behavioral abnormalities had also become noticeable: he got worked up easily, had problems using his strength appropriately, and was impulsively decisive and sometimes aggressive. Philipp himself was unhappy about his performance and his unusual behavior: 'Why aren't I like the other children? Why can't I stay calm when I work and play?'

ENT and ophthalmological examinations remained inconclusive. Neuropediatric examination did not disclose any unusual features in his development or any abnormalities. Further tests revealed no specific learning difficulties. On IQ testing (overall IQ) Philipp scored 113 and was in the upper part of the normal range, but on specific skills testing to assess what he had learnt and his factual knowledge he scored just 90. The prevailing atmosphere in the family was good; the boy was not under pressure and also had no psychological stresses to endure. The diagnosis was 'ADHD', and this was also substantiated by observing the boy during testing. Gradually titrating Philipp's methylphenidate dose to 15 mg/day rapidly produced a positive change in his behavior and school performance.

Differential diagnoses

The differential diagnosis of ADHD includes social behavior disorder, frontal brain syndrome, visual and/or auditory impairment, learning impairment (IQ < 85), mental retardation (IQ < 70), epilepsy, hyperthyroidism and possible pharmacological side-effects. The complexity of differential diagnosis is illustrated by the comorbidity list compiled by Döpfner and Lehmkuhl (1998) and by Schulte-Markworth (2003):

- In about 30–50% of cases of ADHD there are disorders of social behavior, including oppositional and aggressive behavioral disorders and emotional abnormalities
- Depressive illness is present in 10–40%
- Anxiety disorders are found in 20–25%
- General and specific learning difficulties are identified in 10–25%
- Tic disorders are evident in about 30%
- Disturbed family relationships or family interaction are also common.

The differential diagnostic process should therefore constantly consider whether the above conditions/illnesses are really concomitant illnesses or primary disease entities that cause attention deficit, hyperactivity and impulsivity.

Diagnosis

Allopathic diagnostic procedures

The diagnostic process includes taking a personal and family history, analysis of questionnaires from parents and teachers, psychological testing (see p.387) and neurological examination to exclude organic lesions, such as brain tumors that might provoke behavioral abnormalities.

Osteopathic examination

Also in the case of ADHD, osteopathic examination is based on the holistic principle of osteopathy. For further details see p.383.

Treatment

Allopathic medical treatment

Because ADHD is a multi-modal condition in terms of both its etiopathogenesis and its clinical features, and because the presentation of ADHD itself may encompass a wide range of functional disorders and impinge on several areas of life, most authors are agreed that the therapeutic measures adopted should also be multi-modal (Döpfner and Lehmkuhl 1998; Möller and Thoms 2002; Schubert et al 2004; v. Voss 2004). The following aspects are important if treatment is to be properly targeted:

- Psychological counselling and support for the parents
- Behavioral therapy for the child
- Psychological and social preventive measures: training in coping strategies for ADHD patients

- Pharmacological therapy; e.g. with methylphenidate
- Physiotherapy schooling perception to promote sensory integration

The implementation of particular measures and in what combination will be determined by the clinical picture in the individual case and, in the broadest sense, by the setting in which the child with ADHD finds himself or herself.

Various studies have shown that elimination diets (phosphates, colouring agents and sugars) are not a useful therapeutic option. In our experience, however, the restriction of sugar in the diet may be advisable to help balance physiological processes in the gastrointestinal tract and thus to achieve a generally positive effect on arousal processes in the CNS. According to Döpfner and Lehmkuhl (1998) and Möller and Thoms (2002), an oligoantigenic diet may be effective, although this appears to be hardly practicable as routine therapy.

Pharmacological therapy

Discussion centers most commonly around the use of psychostimulants such as amphetamine and methylphenidate, although these should only be administered in cases with a confirmed diagnosis of ADHD as a disease entity. The majority of authors believe that pharmacological therapy for ADHD should be the therapeutic modality of last resort when other attempted treatments have remained unsuccessful (Döpfner and Lehmkuhl 1998; Eckpapier 2003). However, it should also be added that amphetamines increase and stabilize the efficacy of other interventions, or make them possible at all in the first place (Döpfner and Lehmkuhl 1998). There are therefore some who believe that without the pharmacological approach, treatment for ADHD would not be successful (Overmeyer and Ebert 1999).

Amphetamines are indirect psychostimulants, a category that also includes methylphenidate (Ritalin, Equasym, Medikinet). Their mechanisms of action can be described as follows:

- They facilitate the release of neurotransmitters from the presynaptic vesicles of the nerve endings into the synaptic cleft.
- They inhibit mechanisms responsible for the back-transport of neurotransmitters from the synaptic cleft into the presynaptic vesicles of the nerve endings.

Both mechanisms serve to increase the concentration of neurotransmitters in the synaptic cleft and thus to improve the excitability of the postsynaptic receptors of contacting nerve cells. In addition, amphetamines increase receptor sensitivity for dopamine and norepinephrine (noradrenaline)

and to some extent they themselves act like these neurotransmitters. These mechanisms of action are believed collectively to result in stimulation of brain structures and optimization of their function.

Stimulation of the reticular formation and frontal brain is particularly important. Stimulation of the reticular formation non-specifically increases the activity level of cortical and subcortical structures necessary for creative and concentrated work. Stimulation of the frontal brain reinforces self-control and the capacity for self-criticism, for improving awareness of social responsibility, and for enhancing interest in the future and in past experiences.

The goal of starting a patient on methylphenidate, for example, should be to titrate to an individual, minimal effective daily dose because only in this way can the risk of pharmacological side-effects be reduced to a small residual level. During dose adjustment, regardless of the child's age – but generally not before completion of the 6th year of life – start with a single dose of 5 mg methylphenidate at breakfast. In the 2nd week, after having received feedback from parents, teachers or nursery staff, the physician will decide whether the daily dose should be increased, in each case by a further 5 mg at 1-week intervals. There are different regimens for spreading the dose through the day, such as at 07:30 and 11:30 or 07:30, 11:00 and 14:00; in any event it is inadvisable to take the medication after 15:00. The duration of treatment will be determined by the child's condition. However, it is recommended that an attempt be made to discontinue the treatment after about 10 months. Also, depending on the situation in the individual case, a break from medication at weekends and in the holidays may be experimented with.

The numerous side-effects of this type of medication occupy a central role in discussions concerning the administration of psychostimulants. Although many side-effects, such as loss of appetite and disturbed sleep, do not appear particularly dangerous and can be controlled to some extent by modifying the daily dose and the administration schedule for individual doses, side-effects such as disturbances of growth and sexual maturation cannot be taken seriously enough.

According to Huss (2004), graduated and individually prescribed daily doses of amphetamines do not generally produce any dependence. However, misuse of this medication can lead to dependence and addiction, particularly given that Paulus and Hammer (2002) have published evidence from headteacher reports indicating, for example, that methylphenidate 'dealing' is already happening in school playgrounds, a finding that renders any efforts to achieve a controlled dose absurd.

However, even where therapy is given correctly on the basis of careful, individually tailored dose adjustment, there are justifiable grounds for criticism: while the positive effect of amphetamines in ADHD is usually prompt, it is symptomatic or 'syndromatic' (Martinius 2001), rather like giving aspirin for a fever without knowing the cause. In other words, an improvement in concentration after amphetamine administration is not sufficient to confirm the diagnosis of ADHD as a disease with a known cause. Even in healthy individuals amphetamines exert a positive effect on symptoms such as exhaustion, tiredness and attention deficit.

Apart from psychostimulants, medication for the treatment of ADHD also includes tricyclic antidepressants and β-blockers, for example. However, these are used only very rarely, and generally only in patients who are refractory to treatment with psychostimulants (Overmeyer and Ebert 1999; Schulte-Markworth 2003).

Since March 2005 a new medicine has been licensed for the treatment of ADHD: Strattera contains the active ingredient atomoxetine hydrochloride, a highly selective norepinephrine (noradrenaline) reuptake inhibitor. This mechanism of action leads to the accumulation of norepinephrine in the synapses and thus to a potentiation of norepinephrine activity in various CNS structures, primarily in the system responsible for attention. Strattera belongs to the category of centrally acting sympathomimetic agents and is suitable for the treatment of ADHD in children from the age of 6 years onwards. Treatment may be continued into adulthood. The efficacy of the medication is comparable with that of methylphenidate; Strattera is given as a single daily dose with a continuous effect over 24 hours, there is no abuse potential and no special narcotics prescription is needed.

Osteopathic treatment

In our opinion osteopathic treatment also occupies an important place in the context of ADHD. The key aspects of osteopathic treatment have already been described in earlier parts of this chapter, see pp.384, 385 and 388 and will not be reiterated here.

However, we will take this opportunity to emphasize the importance of the intracranial membranes in terms of venous drainage in the neurocranium. Osteopathic lesions localized in this region can have adverse implications for cranial venous drainage. Here too we would draw attention to the anatomical fact that the great cerebral vein – which drains the diencephalon and hence the thalamus (which is responsible for impulse processing and selective impulse conduction) – empties directly into the straight sinus; that is into the venous sinus system of the intracranial membranes.

Osteopathic lesions in the area of the occipital bone are a common cause of disturbed venous drainage from the cranium. Both intraosseous lesions affecting the basilar part, lateral

parts and occipital squama, as well as interosseous lesions involving the sphenobasilar synchondrosis, the atlanto-occipital joint and the sutural articulation with the temporal bones around the jugular foramen may play a major role in children with perception disorders. In particular, osteopathic lesions in the region of the left jugular foramen may be important because of the principal direction of flow in the confluence of sinuses (see p.359).

We have detected osteopathic lesions of the atlanto-occipital joint in 70% of a population of children with disorders of auditory perception (Goussel, Guerassimiouk, Markhoff 2003).

The occipital bone – an important central cranial bone that is vulnerable to a variety of osteopathic lesions– may exert many different influences on:

- vital, autonomic centers of the brain stem and reticular formation
- the cranial nerve nuclei in the brain stem
- the fourth ventricle and CSF fluctuation
- the cerebellum and its important role in muscle tone regulation and the coordination of movements
- the hypoglossal nerve, which may be irritated by occipital bone compression, leading to speech disorders
- the primary and secondary visual cortex in the occipital lobe
- the basilar plexus, the drainage function of which can be disturbed by restrictions of the occiput–atlas–axis complex (OAA complex), especially condylar lesions
- the jugular foramen containing the glossopharyngeal nerve, the accessory nerve and in particular the vagus nerve with its visceral information and the jugular vein, which is the principal drainage vessel for venous blood from the neurocranium.

Sutherland (1990) pointed out that intraosseous lesions of the occipital bone are very frequently associated with compression of the atlanto-occipital joints and therefore they should be treated together. A compression of the OAA complex is often seen following mechanical stress during the birth process, and particularly commonly after caesarean section (see p.63).

The following report will illustrate the importance of the OAA complex:

Case study

Nine-year-old Marieke came to our practice with a diagnosis of ADHD. She appeared dreamy, slightly absent, was noticeably detached during the preliminary discussion with her parents and also showed very delayed reactions when spoken to. Her parents reported that the morning ritual of getting up lasted an extremely long time and that she was just as slow in the afternoon when doing her homework. Similar feedback was also received from her school.

During the osteopathic examination, Marieke's IVM was tentative in its expression and was notable for its lack of vitality. In addition, increased abdominal tone with mild hepatic congestion was found, together with compression in the area of the occipital bone and OAA complex.

During the following three treatment sessions attention focused primarily on the visceral problems, and on the release of intracranial membrane tension and decompression of the occipital bone. The expression of the IVM was slightly improved after each session but was still far removed from a state of fresh vitality. Also the parents' feedback was somewhat reserved regarding the success of treatment so far.

During the fourth session a clearly pronounced dysfunction (translation) of the occipital bone was detected – this had not previously presented itself in such obvious form. Accordingly, on this occasion a direct corrective technique was selected for occipital translation, which led (directly) to a marked improvement in IVM.

One week after this session Marieke's mother telephoned us to report that Marieke was now able to do her homework in a third of the time compared with previously, that her morning dawdling was a thing of the past, and that even her class teacher had commented to her how attentive Marieke had suddenly become during lessons.

Impressive though this development appears, it would certainly be wrong to attribute this positive change to the treatment of occipital translation as if it were the only causal factor. It is more likely that the previous sessions had prepared the way for this 'all-releasing' maneuver. In any event we can speculate what occipital release achieved: it may have improved venous drainage of the cranium via the basilar plexus and jugular vein, or interrupted possibly chronic facilitation of the superior cervical ganglion (which regulates the circulation of blood in the cranium), or improved longitudinal fluctuation of the CSF.

There is one osteopathic phenomenon that can be observed during concurrent treatment with methylphenidate: sometimes while this medication is being given, it feels as if tissue reactivity has become slower or more rigid and that improvements from a previous session are lost again until the next session. In such circumstances there are grounds to suspect a certain sluggishness of the self-healing mechanism that may be of pharmacological origin.

Prognosis

Since the mid-1980s it has been known (Martinius 2001) that while 10% of children with ADHD no longer display this condition as adults, 65% still have symptoms of attention deficit and hyperactivity in adulthood. In their adult years, several of these patients also have additional psychiatric disorders. When they reach adulthood, 20% of children affected with ADHD experience problems that are chiefly social in nature, including drug problems and various disorders of social behavior.

Pharmacological therapy with amphetamines has been shown to bring a slight improvement in the prognosis, but according to Martinius (2001), complex therapy and the early assessment and reduction of risk factors have markedly greater significance in this respect.

Hyperactivity or an attention deficit alone has a favourable prognosis if the child is well integrated in a group of children of the same age. In this context the therapeutic effect of sports clubs and youth groups should be emphasized. However, the situation is completely different if the affected child also has a number of associated behavioral abnormalities, for instance aggressiveness or communication problems.

In our opinion osteopathy is of considerable value in the setting of ADHD; firstly, in our practice we have so far gathered very positive experiences in the treatment of children with ADHD, and secondly, methylphenidate is not a harmless medicine without side-effects. Consequently, any other treatment approach that has good results without identifiable side-effects is justified per se.

As regards the pharmacological therapy of ADHD with methylphenidate, this does not exclude concomitant or parallel osteopathic treatment. Here too (see p.385) long-term therapy has proved to be highly effective and of lasting benefit. Osteopathic treatment cycles over 1 to 2 years, with treatment every 3 to 5 weeks, have shown good results. In any event, for the benefit of all parties, it is useful to do away with any therapeutic vanity or fear of contact so that all those involved in therapy can benefit from interdisciplinary exchanges and cross-fertilization of ideas concerning the current state of treatment.

Bibliography

Brodehl J, Gritz K, Mau M et al: Konsensus der Kinderheilkunde und Jugendmedizin zu ADHS. Kinder- und Jugendarzt 5, 2003: 374–375

Döpfner M, Lehmkuhl G: Die multimodale Therapie von Kindern mit hyperkinetischen Störungen, Teil I, Indikation und medikamentöse Interventionen. Der Kinderarzt 2, 1998: 171–181

Döpfner M, Lehmkuhl G: Die multimodale Therapie von Kindern mit hyperkinetischen Störungen, Teil II. Der Kinderarzt 3, 1998: 331–334

Eckpapier der Bundesgesundheitsministerium, Bundesärztekammer, Fachgesellschaften und Elternverbände. Deutsches Ärzteblatt 7, 2003: C320

Hach I, Ruhl U, Knölker U: Frontalhirnsyndrom und/oder Aufmerksamkeits- und Aktivitätsstörungen im Kindes- und Jugendalter. Monatsschr Kinderheilkunde 148, 2000: 45–49

Huss M: ADHS und Sucht. Kinderärztliche Praxis (Special ADHD issue), 2004: 42–44

ICD-10, International Statistical Classification of Diseases and Related Health Problems, 10th revision, World Health Organization, Geneva 2004

Martinius J: Aufmerksamkeitsdefizitstörung, hyperaktiv, verhaltensgestört oder was? Pädiatrische Praxis 59, 2001: 397–406

Möller C, Thoms E: Hyperkinetische Störungen bei Kindern und Jugendlichen. Pädiatrie 8, 2002: 186–191

Overmeyer S, Ebert D: Die hyperkinetische Störung im Jugend- und Erwachsenenalter. Deutsches Ärzteblatt 19, 1999: C897–C900

Paulus F, Hammer R: Pharmakotherapie mit Ritalin oder Medikinet bei so genanntem AD(H)S. Motorik 2, 2002: 78–81

Schlack HG: Aufmerksamkeitsstörung und andere Modeerscheinungen. Kinderärztliche Praxis 4, 2003: 217

Schubert I, Köster I, Ihle P, Lehmkuhl G: Häufigkeit und Behandlung der Hyperkinetischen Störung im Kindes- und Jugendalter. Kinderärztliche Praxis (Special ADHD issue), 2004: 10–16

Schulte-Markwort M: Rastlos, aber nicht ratlos. Pädiatrie hautnah 2, 2003: 78–82

Schunke H: Psychostimulanzien bei ADHS richtig einsetzen. Kinder- und Jugendmedizin 1, 2002: 50–51

Seile H: Aufmerksamkeits- und Hyperaktivitätsstörungen bei Kindern, Ursachen und neue Akzente bei der Behandlung. Report Psychologie 22, 1997: 872–883 v.

Voss Hv: Relevanz der Pharmakotherapie bei ADHD mit Methylphenidat nach dem OROS-System. Kinderärztliche Praxis (Special ADHD issue), 2004: 36–39

EPILEPSY

Robyn Seamer

Diagnosis of epilepsy has a profound effect on a child's life. Orthodox medical treatment, while beneficial in many cases in reducing numbers of seizures, can also cause long lasting damage as the side-effects of the current drugs used often outweigh the benefits derived. Osteopathy can be an extraordinary tool in supporting a child's path to health because it has the ability to observe, and in some cases remove, the precipitating factors that can lead to seizures in a child predisposed to epilepsy.

Definition

Epilepsy is derived from the Greek word 'to seize upon' and is a medical term to describe chronically, recurrent, cerebral cortical seizures. Seizures are brief malfunctions of the brain resulting in excessive synchronous electrical discharges in the cortical neurons. The term seizure encompasses a range of paroxysmal events, both epileptic and non-epileptic. Epilepsy involves chronic seizure activity while non-epileptic seizures are transitory events.

Classification of epilepsy

Evaluation of a patient with epileptic seizures is determined by seizure type and epileptic syndrome. Seizure type describes the site of origin in the brain, while the epileptic syndrome describes the etiology or cause.

Epileptic seizures types are subdivided into 'partial' and 'generalized'. (Adams 1997)

1. Partial (focal) seizures: activity originates from a single focal area in one hemisphere of the brain.

- Simple Partial Seizures: No impairment of consciousness.

  Motor signs:

  – **Tonic:** a stiffening of the affected muscle.

  – **Clonic** or sudden shock like series of jerks, shaking.

  – **Tonic-clonic:** Jacksonian; seen as a 'march' of involuntary movement through a series of muscles. Benign childhood epilepsy usually occurs between the years of 5–9 years of age with nocturnal seizures. 'Epilepsy partialis continua' involves repeated rhythmic clonic movements of one muscle group (Jacksonian seizure).

  Sensory signs: tingling or numbness sensations from a sensory cortex lesion

  – Auditory signs of buzzing or hearing voices are a sign of a superior temporal lobe lesion.

  – Gustatory symptoms of salivation or thirst follow a lesion in the temporal lobe.

  – Olfactory hallucinations of usually foul smells are a result of an inferior medial temporal lesion.

  – Visual sensations of flashing coloured lights or sparks when the lesion is near the striate cortex of the occipital lobe.

  Autonomic Nervous System pathways affecting viscera.

  Psychic symptoms affecting thought processes; e.g. obsessional ideas.

- Complex partial seizures; involve impairment of consciousness.

  – Beginning as simple partial seizures then progressing to an impairment of consciousness; temporal lobe seizures.

- Partial seizures evolving to secondary generalization.

  – Simple partial seizures evolving to generalized seizures.

  – Complex partial seizures evolving to generalized seizures.

  – Simple partial seizures evolving to complex partial seizures, then evolving to generalized seizures.

2. **Generalized seizures:** the discharges probably originate from deeper midline structures, thus affecting both hemispheres simultaneously and strongly from the start

of the seizure. These seizures can be non-convulsive or convulsive.

- Non convulsive absences (petit mal seizures).

- Convulsive: myoclonic, tonic, clonic, atonic and tonic-clonic (grand mal) seizures.

Epilepsy syndromes are classified by etiology and are divided into:

- Partial seizures:

  - Idiopathic: of unknown cause, e.g. benign partial seizures (benign rolandic epilepsy)

  - Symptomatic: of underlying brain damage/ disease, e.g. temporal, frontal, parietal or occipital lobe epilepsy

  - Cryptogenic: with no obvious cause. There is neither a metabolic problem, nor a clear structural problem with the brain. However an underlying cause for the seizures is suspected, usually because the child is developmentally delayed or has abnormal neurological findings.

- Generalized epilepsies:

  - Idiopathic: benign neonatal seizures (5-day convulsions), benign myoclonic infantile epilepsy, pyknolepsy, impulsive petit mal (juvenile myoclonic epilepsy), grand mal epilepsy on waking.

  - Symptomatic: myoclonic encephalopathy of early infancy, epileptic encephalopathy of early infancy with burst suppression (Ohtahara syndrome)

  - Idiopathic and/or symptomatic: lightning/nodding/salaam attacks (West syndrome), Lennox-Gastaut syndrome, epilepsy with myoclonic astatic seizures, epilepsy with myoclonic absences.

- Epilepsies with no classifiable focal or generalized cause: such as neonatal seizures, severe myoclonic epilepsy of infancy, ESES (electrical status epilepticus during slow sleep, epilepsy with persistent spike wave discharges in synchronized sleep), aphasia-epilepsy syndrome (Landau-Kleffner syndrome)

Special syndromes: Occasional seizures (febrile seizures, seizures from sleep withdrawal, after consuming alcohol or drugs), infrequent seizures, epilepsies with specific forms of attack triggers, chronic progressive epilepsia partialis continua of infancy.

Etiology and pathophysiology

Epilepsy has its origin usually in multiple causes. Usually a genetic disposition and external factors come together.

Hopkins (1987) approached the etiology of epilepsy by looking at the predisposition or susceptibility to epilepsy and the precipitating factors that initiate seizure activity.

When investigating predisposition, three critical periods can be identified along the developmental path:

- Genetic: It is possible to inherit a low seizure threshold.

- Developmental brain abnormalities: During the embryological development of the brain the neuronal migration may follow an abnormal path, leading to a range of neurocutaneous, metabolic and chromosomal disorders. This may present as a low IQ and severe learning difficulties.

- Acquired structural brain abnormalities are developed after birth and may be due to

  - prenatal insults from extreme prematurity or hypoxic-ischemic injury
  - prenatal infections
  - postnatal infections
  - prolonged febrile or other seizures
  - trauma
  - tumors
  - metabolic causes like hypocalcemia, hypoglycemia or vitamin B6 deficiency
  - neurodegenerative disorders
  - vascular disorders.

The following precipitating factors can initiate a seizure in the above predisposed or susceptible child.

- toxic and metabolic causes: hypoglycemia, hypocalcemia, hyponatremia, hypoxia, overdose of drugs or their withdrawal

- reflex causes: flashing lights, sounds, (from a computer or TV, or being startled and shocked)

- sleep wake cycle alterations involving sleep deprivation

- fever

- infections

- stress.

An epileptic seizure occurs when relatively large clusters of neurons discharge excessively and abnormally, during which process there is a paroxysmal depolarization of the nerve cell membrane.

To determine the predisposition and precipitating factors, an osteopath can assess through palpation and sensing the quality of the interrelationship between structure and function.

Trauma or disease mechanisms are superimposed upon the child's physiology leading to compensatory adaptation. In certain cases, trauma at birth, or in infancy, can lead to small areas of cortical scars, which are surrounded by irritable epileptogenic foci that trigger the seizures in the developing CNS (Adams 1997). In certain cases, this can give symptoms years later with the increased growth of the cerebral hemispheres, as there are limits to the extent of adaptation to which the nervous system can accommodate. Any extra compensatory adaptation by the body through further injury, as well as the above precipitating factors, can increase the stress response or allostatic state in the body (McEwen 1998) and thus trigger seizures. By diagnosing the cause of the allostatic state, the osteopath is able to support the child in her effort to diminish the overloaded compensatory response and restore a normal homeostasis.

Paradoxical or asynchronistic motion of the CNS, dura or bone and an inability of the body to express the fluid drive to disengage these layers as one synchronous unit of function can present as precipitating factors, affecting the allostatic load on a child predisposed to epilepsy.

Clinical signs and symptoms

The sort of seizure depends on the area of the abnormal neuronal activity in the brain, with the symptoms pointing to the affected area. A seizure may manifest in the form of involuntary movements with or without change of consciousness. There may be only, or additionally, changes of the senses (seeing, hearing, smell), of behavior or perception. The symptoms when affected by a seizure differ depending on the age of the child.

- A newborn with her immature CNS and developing myelination presents, when having neonatal seizures, with movements such as eyelids fluttering, eye deviation, fixed open stare, sucking, chewing; there may be posturing of a limb or bicycling movements of the legs.

- An infant aged 1 month to 3 years may have infantile spasms, where initial myoclonic jerks of the head or arms lead to flexion or extension of the whole body.

- A child of 4 years and older, having more advanced cerebrocortical organization, more advanced myelination of cortical efferent systems and interhemispheric commissures, would present a more organized tonic-clonic seizure with the ability to become a generalized seizure as seen in grand-mal (Volpe 1989).

Differential diagnosis

The differential diagnoses to be considered are:
- breath-holding: cyanosis, loss of consciousness, loss of muscle tone
- vascular conditions: migraine
- seizure-like movement disorder: tics, chorea, tremor, dyskinesias

- syncope: sudden loss of muscle tone and posture, loss of consciousness, vertigo, nausea, muscle spasm
- affective psychological seizures.

Diagnosis

Accurate history taking is the essential prerequisite for making a diagnosis, and one should obtain the clearest possible description of the course of the seizure.

Allopathic diagnostic procedures

An electroencephalogram (EEG) is used to confirm the area involved and diagnose the type of seizure by recording differences in electrical potential at various points on the scalp. It is thought that the thalamus and high brain stem reticular formation are responsible for the synchrony, or entrainment, of the neurons to collectively produce rhythmic brain-wave patterns such as alpha and beta rhythms and also sleep spindles (Adams1997). As a result the thalamus has been referred to as the 'pacemaker' of the brain. Subtle seizure types such as blinking or fixed stare are rarely seen with an EEG. Tonic seizures such as stiffening have variable evidence on EEG, while the tonic-clonic repetitive jerking usually shows EEG changes (Volpe 1989).

Laboratory tests for epilepsy include a full blood count, ESR (erythrocyte sedimentation rate), CRP (Cross-reacting protein), blood glucose, urea, electrolytes and calcium levels. Liver function and plasma glucose tests are also used when investigating a patient presenting with seizures. Systemic acidosis is a common result of convulsive seizures. Almost all convulsions produce a rise in serum creatine kinase activity. Therefore a blood test immediately after a seizure will help the differential diagnosis between seizure and fainting, as long as the faint did not involve extensive muscle injury, which can also produce an increased serum creatine kinase (Adams 1997).

A lumbar puncture is sometimes performed to rule out bacterial meningitis. Magnetic Resonance Imaging (MRI) or Computerized Tomography (CT) scan may be required if there are clinical grounds to suspect a structural lesion of the brain such as subtle subcortical swellings or if a slow wave focus is seen on an EEG.

Osteopathic diagnosis

The prerequisite for osteopathic diagnosis is a thorough examination of the whole body, including the head. When palpating IVM and the effect of primary respiration on the child, you may be able to feel the function within the tissues of the CNS, dura, CSF and bone, as well as sensing dysfunction when it is present. While palpating for a diagnosis, care is always required to avoid looking too closely as this can irritate an overactive CNS and ANS and provoke a seizure. During a seizure, the bio-electric field is over stimulated and is perceived through palpation as a vibration, or a buzz, similar to static or frictional electricity. It is felt generally close to the epileptogenic focus and from that agitation, a crescendo follows similar to an electrical storm. Diagnosis can be made observing the Tide's ability to pass through the different layers.

A mechanical irritation can be felt at the tissue layers of bone, meninges and CNS. Inertia, or lack of fluid drive, can follow trauma or infection. Paradoxical asynchronous motion between these tissue layers can also be palpated.

A metabolic imbalance, such as hypoglycemia or from the side effects of the drugs, is sensed in the fluid. This is palpated as a sense of inertia or a general bogginess in the tissues with no sustaining fluid drive.

The bioelectric field can also lesion, presenting a feeling of over excitability that is not synchronized with the tidal forces passing through the body.

Epilepsy may be affected by one or more of these layers and fields; hence the importance of developing accurate palpatory diagnostic skills as this will influence the treatment and its clinical outcome.

Treatment

Avoidance of triggering precipitating factors is important. For example, a balanced sleep–wake cycle may be necessary. Teenagers should try to have plenty of sleep and avoid alcohol. If suffering from photosensitive epilepsy, the child should not use a computer or watch television. Correct eye protection from the sun should be worn outside in summer.

A ketogenic diet has been found to be effective in managing epilepsy. As the diet is low in carbohydrates and high in fats, ketone acids are released into the blood. The resulting acidosis has been found to have an anticonvulsive effect. This is a very strict diet and it needs medical supervision and daily urine analysis. Research by Hemingway (2001) found that 'three to six years after initiation, the ketogenic diet had proven to be effective in the control of difficult-to-control seizures in children. The diet often allows decrease or discontinuation of medication. It is more effective than many of the newer anticonvulsants and is well-tolerated when it is effective.'

Allopathic medical treatment

Before starting treatment with anti-epileptic drugs (AEDs) with severe prolonged or frequent seizures, it is necessary to weigh the impairments from the seizures against the drawbacks of medical treatment. Some drugs are more effective for particular types of seizure, thereby emphasizing the need for a correct diagnosis.

Usually one drug is initially administered and then the dosage is slowly increased over a period of months until the seizures respond to the drug. It should be noted that overdosing on AEDs can also cause seizures to increase.

Some times several anti-epileptic drugs are used, but this polypharmacy is best to be avoided. The dosage of monotherapy should, if necessary, be as high as possible until adverse effects appear. Polypharmacy usually follows, in the effort to control seizures. Adams (1997) states that these drugs have adverse effects, when interacting with each other, by releasing active metabolites that can produce toxicity. Unfortunately in the desire to eliminate the seizure pattern quickly in serious cases, polypharmacy is often applied. This makes it more difficult to observe and thus eliminate the drug that may possibly aggravate the condition.

Anti-epileptic drugs have a wide spectrum of side-effects. They range from depression to aggression, memory alteration, psychosis, ataxia, confusion, visual disturbances (diplopia or blurred vision), amnesia, vomiting, anorexia, dyskinesia, liver and kidney damage. These iatrogenic side-effects have serious implications as they can lead to greater disability than the original symptom of epileptic seizure. The overall benefit of the drug has to be weighed up against the possible risk of delaying the child's development as well as impairing the function of various organs. Some of these drugs can take a long time to finally be metabolized by the liver and excreted by the kidney.

Surgery is used in 20% of uncontrolled cases of epilepsy:

- A focal resection, usually in the temporal lobe, can be used to remove the proven focal source of the seizures.

- In larger focal areas either a callosotomy is performed, where neuronal pathways of the corpus callosum are disconnected, or a hemispherectomy where the whole hemisphere is removed. Unfortunately seizures can still return, possibly due to scar tissue creating another epileptogenic focus (Adams 1997).

- Recently, the less invasive approach of an electrical device called a vagus-nerve stimulator (VNS) implanted under the skin of the chest has been seen to be effective in controlling seizure activity (Schacter et al 2003).

Osteopathic treatment

The aim of osteopathic treatment would be to assist the body in re-establishing its intrinsic homeostatic balance by diminishing the allostatic state or stress load (Willard 2000). Removal of the precipitating factors that trigger the seizure activity will allow natural homeostatic mechanisms of the body to restore normal physiological function.

Still, in the late 19th century, talked about anatomical malpositions from the atlas to the diaphragm, following a fall or injury, being responsible for many seizures. He restored 'blood and nerve circulation to the impoverished spinal cord from the medulla to the diaphragm'. Still instructed to keep the patient drug free as he said he had more difficulty removing the toxic effects of the drugs than the mechanical cause of the epilepsy.

In 1947, Fryette's study of 13 adults found a restriction of motion around T2 to be the causative factor of epilepsy. Fryette also only worked with drug free patients, as he found the toxic elements of the drugs impeded his treatment. Seizure activity initially increased until the toxicity was removed from the body; all 13 patients became seizure free.

Osteopaths usually find that a diagnosis of epilepsy has been made and medications of AEDs have already been prescribed before the patient comes for treatment. Therefore it is of benefit to work together with a pediatric neurologist in helping to find the AED that is giving the best tissue response. This can be assessed osteopathically by placing a drop of the drug on the patient's tongue and monitoring the response of the tissues in regard to motion, vitality and potency. If there is a response of IVM expansion off the midline, the drug is improving the tissue vitality. However, if there is a contraction in the tissues, then that drug is best avoided.

It is possible to work with AEDs providing they are not proving to be too toxic. If there is still some inherent motion which is both moving longitudinally and sustains motion from the midline moving along a lateral/transverse axis, then the body has the vitality to cope with the drugs. If however there is only lethargy or a boggy feeling in the tissues and no vitality available, the drugs may have iatrogenic side-effects by dampening down the body's ability to self-correct. A change in dosage or drug may then be advisable.

Children respond very well to the gentle, unthreatening approach of osteopathy in the cranial field, using balanced membranous tension (BMT). BMT can be approached through either

- direct action: when the tissues are taken directly by the osteopath to a point of balance and held on a slight barrier until resolution occurs, or an

- indirect approach: when the osteopath applies a functional modality of keeping away from any form of barrier and following ease until the local area being treated synchronizes with the whole body.

The choice of approach in epilepsy would depend on the case being treated. A child with uncontrolled seizures would react unfavourably to any form of direct action or feeling of containment or barrier. If there is too much focus or intention of diagnostic thought during examination or treatment, the unstable activity in the CNS can be activated by the stress response of the autonomic nervous system and could trigger another event. Parents should be warned that this may happen. This treatment reaction is an indicator to the osteopath to adjust the treatment approach for the following visits. The child may not be able to sustain a long treatment and short frequent sessions may be more beneficial. Constant respect and listening to the tissues is required throughout the examination and treatment.

The safest treatment would be to work using an indirect approach.

- BMT motion permitted: Avoiding barrier, following the feeling of ease at the tempo of the motion in the lesion. There is always some form of motion in a somatic dysfunction, be it ever so small. By observing and following this ease in the tissues, the local feeling of motion gradually expands to encompass the whole body. In this state of suspended balance called neutral, the whole body is free to be shifted by thoracic respiration or primary respiration. A therapeutic process emerges during the stillpoint that follows, as the body's own intelligence makes decisions on a cellular and metabolic level and attempts to return to normal homeostatic function throughout the whole body.

- BMT motion present: Sometimes paradoxical motion in tissue layers requires, from the osteopath, the skill to work with tissue, fluid and potency as a unit of function. Then it is necessary to find a fulcrum, a 'doorway' to a new state of balance that replicates the suspended automatic shifting fulcrum of a healthy system. This new fulcrum has a quality of a neutral state of balance which, when established in dysfunctional and paradoxical tissue motion, has the ability to resynchronize the motion of the whole including bone, CNS, CSF and dura. This resynchronization in turn will support biomechanical exchange within all the fluids of the whole body (Jealous 2001).

Case study

A 4-year-old girl was brought for osteopathic treatment. She had been diagnosed with complex partial epilepsy and developmental delay in cognitive skills, motor control and in psychosocial behavior, including lack of eye contact or speech.

Her past history revealed an uneventful birth and normal development, but at 1 month old, a lumbar puncture was performed for suspected meningitis. After this event, developmental delay was observed.

A rapid onset of seizures occurred while making her first attempts to walk at 2 years old. Two anti-epileptic drugs were prescribed and later a third was added. Seizure activity increased 1 year later when she finally managed, at 3 years old, to walk unaided.

Osteopathic examination: revealed an axial compression, especially in the cranial vault, cranial base and CNS. There was restricted motion in the nerve roots and surrounding dura at the level of the 3rd lumbar vertebrae, the site of the lumbar puncture and paradoxical motion between the CNS and cranium and L3-4.

Osteopathic diagnosis: The predisposing factor of the seizures may have been due to the high temperature of the suspected meningitis; an infection which could have created an epileptogenic focus in the developing CNS, leading to symptoms appearing 2 years later with the increased growth of the cerebral hemispheres. The child's attempts to walk may have been one of the precipitating factors of the epilepsy. The scar tissue around the dura at L3-4 resulting from the lumbar puncture comprimized neurotrophic flow to the lower limbs and increased stimuli to the CNS through the increased activity at L3-4 from walking. The toxicity of the metabolites from the polypharmacy of the anti-epileptic drugs also aggravated the seizure activity, as they were not eliminated effectively from the liver and kidneys.

Osteopathic treatment: was addressed at supporting the metabolic function of the liver and kidneys. The shock in the tissues around the site of the lumbar puncture was resolved and synchronized motion was restored within the cranium, L3-4 area and CNS. An immediate improvement of her cognitive skills and psychosocial development and general well-being was observed. The girl started to speak, have eye contact and interactive play, with improved concentration and diminished aggressive behavior. However, although seizure events decreased considerably in number and severity, they were still present.

Two months later her medication was lowered to one AED instead of three. This included the removal of one medication which seemed to have aggravated her condition as she had been taking this for 2 years. The child's seizures then ceased.

Prognosis

Prognosis would depend on the vitality of the tissues and whether the child could sustain, or even improve, on the changes made during the treatment. Intervals of at least 3 to 4 weeks can be left between appointments when treatment is progressing well and the child is sustaining the treatment

changes. If the child, however, continues to return with a similar diagnostic picture, weekly intervals between treatments are indicated and further investigations into AED or other precipitating factors should be made.

As this case history illustrates, epilepsy is a challenging neurological condition for the child, the parents and practitioners. Each child has their own unique, individual physiological and psychological response to treatment, be it medication or osteopathy. Osteopathic assessment of the child's vitality and tissue response can offer an invaluable aid in preparing the treatment plan and monitoring the child's ability to manage the proposed treatment. Depending on the severity of the seizures, the child may require osteopathic treatment alone, or in collaboration with the ketogenic diet, medication or the more recent success of the Vagal Nerve Stimulator. Such cooperation between osteopaths and pediatric neurologists can provide a combined understanding of treatment approaches and enhance the future therapeutic outcome for epilepsy.

Bibliography

Adams R, Victor M, Ropper A: Principles of neurology. McGraw-Hill, 1997, 25–33, 313–343, 539

Carreiro J E: An osteopathic approach to children, 1st edn. Churchill Livingstone , Edinburgh 2003, p. 11

Fryette H: Second dorsal lesion, a causative factor in epilepsy. Academy of Applied Osteopathy Year Book, 1947, 121–123

Hemingway C et al: Pediatrics. 108 (4), 2001: 898–905

Hope R A, Longmore J M, Hodgetts T J, Ramrakha P S: Oxford handbook of clinical medicine. 3rd edn. Oxford University Press 1997, pp 450–451

Hopkins A: Epilepsy: the causes and precipitation of seizures. 1st edn. Chapman and Hall, London 1987

Jealous J: Interactive audio text – balanced membranous tension, Nos.1&2, 2001

McEwen B S: Stress, adaptation and disease. Allostasis and allostatic load. Annals of the New York Academy of Sciences 840, 1998: 33–44

Schacter S C, Schmidt D: Vagus nerve stimulation. 2nd edn. Martin Dunitz, London 2003

Still A T: Osteopathy in research and practice. 1st edn. Still, Kirksville Mo. 1910, p 248–249 (Reprinted by Maidstone College of osteopathy, Kent, UK)

Volpe J J: Neonatal seizures: Current concepts and revised classification. Pediatrics, 84(3), 1989: 422–428

Volpe J J: Neurology of the newborn. 3rd edn. W B Saunders, Pennsylvania 1995,p 80, 190

Willard F: Homeostasis, allostasis and osteopathic education. Abstract, European School of Osteopathy UK. International Conference July 2000

Website

www.jamesjealous.com

HEAD PAIN IN CHILDREN

Timothy Marris

In this chapter I will be discussing head pain from the perspective of the child. However, adult pathophysiology from the osteopathic perspective will also be of relevance to the reader. Consequently most of this chapter will be just as pertinent to adult as well as child patients.

It is not possible to discuss the subject of head pain completely, but I would like to give ideas and tips for the osteopath confronted with a child suffering from head pain.

It has to be said at this point that, unlike adults or older children, very small children or babies won't be able to tell you nor describe their symptoms. This may be an obvious statement but its significance is profound. You will only be getting the symptoms 'second hand', usually from the mother. Although emotionally very close to their offspring, the parents can only at best guess the symptoms the child is experiencing. In many situations there are neither visual clues nor clinical signs, so the necessity for a very detailed case history and careful palpatory examination has to be emphasized. Do not rush these aspects of your initial consultation, even if pushed for time.

Definition

Head pain is usually described as a sharp sensation with or without throbbing in a specific location. The patient is normally precise as to its location. Head pain can be anywhere in the head.

Headache is medically defined as pain in the head that is located above the eyes or ears, in the back of the head (occipital region), or in the upper neck. However the common definition by patients would be more described as being less sharp and more diffuse. Headache can be continuous or throbbing in character. It is less localized than a sharp pain. Headache, as the term is used by patients in the UK (this may vary in other countries), would normally only describe symptoms of the suboccipital region or neurocranium, not the face (viscerocranium).

Migraine is a headache occurring in intervals that are combined with neurological and autonomic dysfunctions. An aura may precede the migraine attack.

Etiology and pathology

Although, by the general public, headache is considered a relatively minor symptom, its pathophysiology is very variable both in causation and hence in seriousness.

In this section I will review different tissues and structures that may cause head pain symptoms. Firstly it will be impossible to describe all possible tissue pathologies that may cause head pain. I will attempt to give the reader an *insight* into tissues from an *osteopathic* perspective linking the clinical and palpatory aspects of our science.

Tissue and tissue states are discussed in no special order of significance. I will mention bone tissue, meningeal tissues, fluid states, the CNS and connective tissues, relating all these to head pain. The student of cranial osteopathy will recognize this '5 phenomena' of IVM approach to the subject which I hope will assist an easier assimilation of the discussion in the earlier chapter (see Ch.8, pp.162, 163).

It should always be borne in mind that symptoms are rarely from just one event or from one tissue but often a series of events leading to a reduction in tissue tolerance, resulting in symptoms. This is nearly always true in adults but can often also be the situation with children. Although each tissue will be discussed separately for the sake of clarity, it should always be considered a part of the dynamic whole.

Causes of headaches

Headaches can be caused by:

- transferred pain from the eyes (see below), ears (otitis media, see Ch.13), nose, sinuses (sinusitis, see Ch.13), teeth, pharynx, temporomandibular joint (see below), cervical spine
- increased intracranial pressure – tumors (see below), hydrocephalus, abscess, trauma, benign intracranial hypertension
- ocular defects – myopia, hyperopia, astigmatism
- vascular disturbances – arterial hypertension, migraine
- nerves – neuritis (e.g. trigeminal neuralgia)

or the origin may be:

- meningeal – meningitis, leukemia, bleeds
- osseous – osteitis, osteomyelitis, fracture
- psychogenic – fear, depression.

Eye problems

Orbital tension head pain or headache is quite a common complaint. Usually the patient complains of tension at the back of the orbit on one or both sides. As each orbit comprises seven separate bones (frontal, ethmoid, lacrimal, maxilla, sphenoid, palatine and zygomatic), it is not unusual for there to be some osseous tensions between one or more sutures of each orbit. Also some of the ocular muscles have a specialized tendon ring for their origin. This ring attaching to the frontal, sphenoid, ethmoid and maxilla may add to the osseous tension. The zygomatic bone is a protective bone for the face against trauma, so it can easily be a source of imbalance to orbital mechanics. For obvious reasons, each orbit has to work in harmony with its partner; any imbalance between the two orbits can result in tension and head pain. When making an assessment, it is important to evaluate each of the constituent seven bones of each orbit plus how each orbit works, in or out of harmony with the other.

Floaters

Floaters are associated with a clouding of the vitreous body by imbalance in the vitreous humor (VH). If there is tension in the sclera wall of the eye this may cause 'ripples' in the VH and so refraction is imperfect.

Temporomandibular joint (TMJ)

(See Ch.18.)

This highly specialized joint is probably the most used joint in the whole body, as speech and nutrition are its purpose in life. The mandible, however, is very susceptible to trauma, taking up the whole of the lower face. Falls on to the chin, the lower cheek or, sadly, school fights can be causes of trauma to the TMJ. Dental work requires the TMJ to be open for sustained periods and may stress its muscles and ligaments. If dental occlusion is not appropriate (see Chapter 18) it can be a common cause of microtrauma to the TMJ. Cervical posture also has a strong relationship to this joint via the occiput and temporal bones, which may cause chronic dysfunction.

Tumors

Any space occupying lesion within the skull has serious consequences. As the neurocranium is an enclosed space, any developing tumor will raise the intracranial pressure. The tumor being of a higher density will also have the effect of causing displacement of healthy CNS tissue, which has a very low density. This displacement results in compression against other higher density tissues (membrane and bone) so causing damage to the CNS. If the tumor is adjacent to a cranial nerve, this too can be displaced and or damaged.

Bone tissue

In the head region bone is primarily a tissue involved with protection and stability. The mandible is an exception, as it has in addition the special function of mastication.

Childbirth

In babies and children the significance of childbirth cannot be overestimated (see Ch.5, Normal labor). Birth is possibly one of the most traumatic events of our whole life. The sequels of strain to bone tissue may result in reduced plasticity and tolerance to further stresses from life events. As already stated, a baby will not be able to complain of suffering head pain; all she is able to do is express her distress with her behavior (usually crying)! Childbirth is an extraosseous force resulting probably in intraosseous strain. As the child grows, ossification between the constituent parts 'locks in' these strains holding them within the bone itself to create intraosseous strain.

Trauma

As a child grows she becomes more adventurous and naturally wants to explore her surroundings. From the time when an infant can crawl, trauma is likely to occur (mothers cannot have eyes in the back of their head). When the first footsteps happen the number of falls increases and head trauma becomes a greater risk. Again, even a mother cannot know all of the falls their young child has experienced, and certainly will not remember them all. It is often up to the palpating hands of the osteopath to explore the history in the living tissues. Sport and games in older children are also common causes of trauma. Remember that some older children may have participated in activities that they do not want their parents to know about! They may not tell you all the detail of their activity in front of their parents. Careful practitioner skills are necessary and sometimes even asking a parent to leave the room for a few minutes can be helpful. Do be mindful of the medico-legalities of treating children without the parents' consent, so ask for the parents consent to be alone with the child and give reasons why you wish to discuss aspects of their history in private.

Membranous tissue and the reciprocal tension membrane

For osteopaths familiar with the cranial concept the phrase 'the membranes' is often used as a shortcut to mean:

- the dural membranes or dual meninges – cranial and spinal

- both the endosteal layer and the meningeal layer

- plus the reflections or infolding – the falx cerebri and tentorium cerebelli

- plus the little and often forgotten falx cerebelli.

It should also be pointed out that the external periosteum *functionally* and embyologically is also dura. From our embryology we know that the bone develops after 'the membranes' in utero as the bone stiffener to the membranous coat or filler to use a 'sandwich' analogy. Thus at cranial sutures the external periosteum of the bone is continuous with the endosteal dura on the interior of the skull. It is one and the same tissue because the osseous bone developed later (i.e. membrane pre-existed the bone).

Dissemination of force

Being composed of white fibrous tissue, these dural collagenous structures are designed to transmit and disseminate any force applied to them. This fact helps us to understand the types of symptoms which may occur from strain and stress to 'the membranes'. Unlike bone which is denser, the membranes will always be trying to *spread* their stresses away from the focal area of a lesion. Consequently the patient is more likely to complain of an area rather than a point of pain or tension.

Swelling and localized bleeds

However, if a trauma occurs to the head, the response will be inflammation. Edema occurs, plus bleeding if blood vessels are damaged. This fluid build up will cause pressure and distension of the periosteum. As described above, the periosteal layer and endosteal dural layer are one and the same tissue, passing through the sutures as if wrapping the bone (see Fig. 16.14). Blood and/or extracellular fluid (often termed the extracellular matrix) in the subperiosteal space or in the endosteal dural lining of the bone cannot pass over sutures to adjacent bones. This will localize the pain from tissue distension to the location of that traumatized bone.

If the swelling from a fluid build up lies on both sides of a suture then either there is separate damage on either side, or the swelling is deeper than the endosteal layer within the skull. This second scenario clearly has greater pathological significance and has to be referred appropriately.

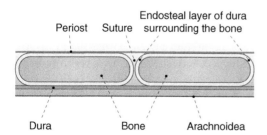

Figure 16.14 Dural envelopes enclose the bone and prevent a sub-dural hematoma from spreading over the suture. Bleeds stemming from fractures therefore do not extend over the suture; they are bounded by the dural membrane.
With permission, Henriette Rintelen, Velbert

Symptom expression

Where there is no significant swelling, the nature of membranous symptoms is more diffuse than bone. The function of the RTM is to disseminate force and hence maintain stability and protection. A common expression used by patients when relating membrane-caused symptoms is 'it feels like a tight band' especially when indicating a line across the mid-occiput. Babies and young children may often hold their hands to an area of the skull where they feel discomfort. I (at the time of writing) have a patient who is only 8 weeks old and he often has his hands behind his head holding the occiput region – even when breastfeeding. I do not advocate any one such finding or description in a case history as sufficient to make a diagnosis, but such clues should not be ignored and are valuable data for further questioning and examination. The description of symptoms associated with membranous tissues can include nausea, throbbing, dull ache, dull pain if of a lesser severity, to severe pain and irritability.

Infection of the meninges

Infection of the meninges – meningitis – whether stemming from bacteria or viral infection, usually produces a high fever. After the febrile state has dissipated, the patient often has increased susceptibility to headache or head pain. To the trained osteopath, a patient who has had an infection of the meninges and high fever can often exhibit palpatory changes in the quality of the membranous tissue. Mostly such membranes feel dried out: 'cooked' is a common osteopathic expression for such membranes. Such a florid description may not be classical medical terminology but it is an excellent palpatory description since the tissues feel as if they were left in a hot oven for a long time. Just as food when cooked in an oven changes its structural state, so too do the meninges from the 'cooking effect' of a very high fever.

Desiccation

Dried up or desiccated tissues are by definition less well lubricated. When the intracellular fluids and extracellular fluids are reduced in volume, then the diffusion of nutrients into cells and the elimination of toxins out of cells is also less efficient.

Reduced mobility

Remember the RTM is or should be in continual motion. Dry tissues are 'tacky' and more likely to adhere to adjacent tissues. Also remember that to the palpating trained fingers, that this 'dryness' is both intra- and extracellular. The overall result is that the membranes have reduced ability and tolerance for their main designed purpose of offering protection and stability to the central nervous system.

Central nervous system (CNS)

CNS symptoms

The CNS is not well known for being a cause of pain, as it does not have sensory nerves to its own tissue. However, we are all familiar with the effects of CNS 'pain' with reference to our psyche. Anxiety states, depression, hyperactivity and restlessness are all expressions of CNS 'pain and discomfort'. It is with reference to such symptoms in babies and children that I will address the CNS. This is not meant to be a guide to child psychology, a subject which I would not be qualified to discuss. However, by outlining some findings and principles, we should be guided to greater understanding of our patients and so find 'a way in' with regard to a diagnosis and treatment.

Trauma to the CNS

In traumatic states the CNS, although afforded protection by bone and the meninges, nevertheless becomes shaken and disorientated. Any trauma to the CNS, even if not sufficient to cause a bleed, will shock the delicate CNS tissues and result in a 'protective shut down' scenario. Here the patient feels dazed and has difficulty in concentrating. The CNS is not able to function like in its normal state and requires rest and reduced stimulation – time for recovery. Both chronic vasoconstriction and toxic shock into the CNS tissue from vascular bleeds result in a change in tissue quality. To the osteopath experienced in the 'cranial field' such tissue changes are exhibited as compression states (localized or general), often accompanied by the tissues feeling irritable. Sometimes a high frequency 'quivering' is palpated when the CNS tissue is unable to find a stable fulcrum for its motion.

Blood vessels: arteries and veins

Head pain, especially if 'throbbing' in nature, often involves blood vessels. Most well known in this context is migraine. The pathology is related to sudden changes in the vascular tone of the middle meningeal artery. Lack of sleep, fever or stress (physical or mental) can cause migraine.

The middle meningeal artery (m.m.a.) enters the skull through the foramen spinosum of the sphenoid bone and crosses over to lie on the squama of the temporal bone as it fans out over the interior surface of the anterolateral aspect of the cranial vault. It is probably no coincidence that the crossing point between the greater wing of the sphenoid

and the temporal squama is at the functional and anatomical point of the 'sphenosquamous (SS) pivot'. This location is the point of bevel change of the SS suture. This point of bevel change is the point of least motion of the suture and of greatest protection to the artery.

If there is any history or palpatory finding of trauma to the pterion region, the ability of the SS suture to express IVM will be disturbed and may irritate the m.m.a. Any degree of facilitation of the m.m.a. at either the SS suture or the foramen spinosum may predispose the patient to migraine. Certainly patients with history of unilateral migraine should be carefully examined in respect to the above, *but not* forgetting to be holistic in examination and diagnosis.

Head pain or headache can occur when the venous drainage is compromized. It cannot be over emphasized that 90% of venous blood exits the skull at the jugular foramen and that this foramen lies between the occiput and temporal bone, within the occipitomastoid suture. Sadly this suture, because of its complex anatomy, can become restricted or 'locked' very easily. Reduction of the IVM of this suture may reduce its capacity for venous drainage, thus hindering the venous flow throughout the whole skull.

The diploic veins pass within the table of the cranial vault. Any trauma to the vault could interfere with the flow of venous blood and create localized congestion. These veins do anastomose and so alternative routes will be found for the venous blood, but venous congestion over the trauma area would still occur.

The anterior end of the superior and inferior sagittal sinuses have to flow uphill. The venous pressure in the sinuses is extremely low. IVM significantly assists the flow in these areas. Reduced IVM causes reduced venous flow in the sagittal sinuses. Venous congestion from any cause can lead to increased toxicity and headaches or dull head pain.

Biomechanical causes

Soft tissue tensions from outside the skull may result in tissue changes in the cranium and be a cause of headache or head pain.

Postural tension from any cause will result in changes to the balance of the suboccipital area. Changes in muscular tone (usually increased tone) will refer to the occiput, and via the attachment of the dura mater at the occiput, C2, and sacrum, also to the meninges. Suboccipital headache in adults is a common finding and it benefits extremely well from osteopathic treatment; however in young children this is rarely found as their posture is still developing and naturally modifying. In mid to late teenage years their posture is becoming more permanent and so such an etiology is more likely.

Although distant from the skull, the sacrum and the coccyx have an intimate functional relationship to the cranial base. The meninges have their final attachments to the sacrum and coccyx. Any disturbance to sacral or coccygeal function will reflect through the meninges to the suboccipital area and neurocranium. Heavy falls onto the pelvis, being kicked in this area at school, or any other injury to the pelvis has to be considered with reference to head pain. Treatment to the head without the necessary treatment to the sacrum, coccyx and pelvis can be fruitless and very frustrating.

Sadly, whiplash is becoming increasingly common as our roads become more congested. Following a road traffic accident it is necessary to consider how the children were sitting in the vehicle. Most seats face forwards but in some vehicles the rear seats may face sideways and young babies have rear facing car seats. These factors will have a significant effect of the whiplash forces on the patient.

From which direction did the force come? Was it a 'head on', 'side impact' or 'rear impact'? In my experience side impact or lateral whiplash injuries are the most complicated to treat as the body is less able to compensate for rapid movements in such a direction. Do bear in mind that the driver will not always give accurate information.

Clinical signs and symptoms

Migraine is an acute headache with unilateral, frontal, throbbing pain that can last for a couple of hours. Migraine can be bilateral and non-throbbing in children before the onset of puberty. The headaches are accompanied by nausea, sometimes up to vomiting, and sensitivity towards light and noise. Autonomic reactions such as pallor, tachycardia, feeling cold, sweating, trembling, watering of the eyes, urge to urinate or diarrhea are possible. An aura (focal neurological sign) may precede the headache attack as well as blurring of vision, disturbances of the visual field, warped perception, paresthesia, motor paralysis or speech problems. The headaches often pass with rest and sleep. During the migraine intervals there are no symptoms.

Tension headache is a continuous diffuse or fronto-ocippital localized pain. Often a feeling of a ring around the head is described. They usually appear from the age of 10 years onwards, especially in the afternoons and evenings. Stress and depression also can cause tension headaches. Sleeping does not ameliorate the pain.

If the headaches are related to eye problems, patients may complain of pain in or behind or around one or both orbits. The following symptoms can occur: pain in or behind or around the eye, visual disturbances, bulging of the eye (exopthalmos) or pressure in the eyeball.

Headaches during otitis media (see Ch.13) are associated with pain and tenderness localized to the temporal region. The character of the pain is either local or diffuse, tender not sharp and increases with the inflammation of the tissues. Pressure applied to the antitragus of the ear as well as a pull on the ear lobe increase the pain. Otitis media is often accompanied with (high) fever. The headaches are a result of the inflammatory process of the mucosa.

Sinus pain (see Ch.13) is marked by a dull pain of the forehead and the maxillary region. The pain usually intensifies when the head is held down. The child often can identify the affected area of the maxilla or the forehead.

Headaches stemming from the temporomandibular joint show acute pain and discomfort over the area of the joint(s), although the patient may complain of clicking with or without pain, on opening of the mouth. Imbalance of muscles and ligaments, if chronic, can lead to chronic headache over a wide range of the same side of the head due to the wide origin of the temporalis muscle especially, but also the other muscles of mastication.

Any irritation from tumor pressure will produce symptoms associated with the relevant cranial nerve. Consequently the importance of cranial nerve examination should not be underestimated (see p.136), and its findings considered with careful diagnostic thought. The nature of any cranial nerve or CNS dysfunction can give vital clues as to the anatomical location of any pathology, which along with palpatory clues will be vital information. Depending on the localization of the tumor, symptoms such as fits, nausea and vomiting, cerebellum signs, behavioral changes, visual disturbances, nystagmus or endocrine disturbances may occur.

Bleeds can produce mild to severe headaches associated with nausea and vomiting. The patient's consciousness is often disturbed. In 25% of cerebral bleeding, fits will occur.

Head pain resulting from biomechanical causes such as soft tissue tensions and postural problems may present themselves anywhere in the head but mainly begin in the suboccipital area.

Head pain or headache may result from whiplash to the cervical spine resulting in a translocation of the mid-cervicals with reference to the upper and lower cervical spine. Careful osteopathic diagnosis is required. Lumbar whiplash, where the pelvis is thrown against the lap seatbelt and back down into the seat again, also occurs from road accidents. Changes to the sacrum have a significant effect on the cranium.

Diagnosis

Warning: Any prolonged, persisting headaches should ring your 'alarm bells'. A thorough case history taking usually gives the necessary diagnostic clues.

Acute onset

Acute onset is common after trauma or with fever resulting in pathological (major/minor) changes to the bones, meninges, or vascular system.

Trauma

With children, minor trauma is inevitable as they are having falls frequently, many of which will not be observed by the parents. You need to ask the child whether she has had any falls which she felt were unusually painful or where she fell in a harder manner. Remember that the memory of a young child soon fades so that if the trauma was not recent, her description may be hazy.

If the parent saw the incident happen you can be more specific with your questions

- How far did the child fall?
- What did the child fall onto?
- If the child was hit by something: what was it, what was it made of?

Answers to these questions will give clues to the degree of potential tissue damage which resulted from the trauma.

Fever

With fever the child may have a headache before other symptoms appear, as the meningeal tissues respond to the changes in body temperature. Often an initial symptom of this type of headache would be irritability. Examples of headache from fever can be associated with sinusitis or otitis media.

Slow onset, chronic headaches

Head pain or headache where there has been no obvious time of onset or causation that the mother or child may be aware of, has to be considered very carefully. Of vital importance is detecting if the cause may be serious pathology such as a tumor. Chronic causation may, however, be from mechanical soft tissue causes, such as spinal postural problems referring symptoms into the head from the cervical spine and occiput. The pathological causes will generally display differing signs and symptoms to mechanical etiology.

You should consider the following thoughts and questions as part of the differential diagnostic screening process, in order to decide to treat with osteopathy or refer to a medical specialist (see also p.150).

Fracture or bleed

If there is intense head pain following trauma, especially if associated with throbbing, there may be a fracture or vascular damage. Refer to a specialist or hospital medical practitioners for X-ray and further medical screening.

Tumor

Enquire about the following signs or symptom changes, which can be associated with tumors:

- Weight change. Has there been any significant or unexplainable weight loss? Tumor development can be associated with weight loss for no particular reason. You will need to ask about the child's appetite and see if it has changed during the time of weight loss. With a young child this can be tricky, as especially toddlers can appear to 'live on air' and not eat much yet still thrive.

- Loss of vitality. Has there been an unaccountable, significant loss of vitality and energy of the child? Children, especially in normal circumstances, are brimming with a vitality and energy that as adults we can only envy! A chronic loss of this vitality and energy without an obvious causation will naturally be observed by the parents. Serious pathology such as tumor generally depletes the body energy so this can be important diagnostic criteria.

- Personality change. Depending on the location, tumors may result in personality changes or strange/uncharacteristic behavior from the child.

- Visual disturbance. Has there been any visual disturbance such as double or tunnel vision? Should a tumor develop with close proximity to the visual pathway, then visual disturbances may result. Depending on the location, the vision may be disturbed in different ways. Damage to the visual cortex of the occipital lobe in the brain will give different symptoms to pressure on the optic chiasm. The occipital lobe may cause altered vision to either the left or right field of vision, damage to the optic chiasm may lead to tunnel vision. The topic of visual disturbances is a complicated subject and beyond the scope of this chapter. If the child has shown any of the above signs or symptoms refer to a medical practitioner because these may be associated with space occupying lesions.

- Raised intracranial pressure. Has there been vomiting and/or nose bleeds continuing since the onset? Raised intracranial pressure results from space occupying lesions such as tumor or bleeding within the neurocranium. The raised pressure leads to these symptoms so they should be carefully considered. If the patient has or had 'clear fluid' draining from the nose since trauma, or if vomiting or nose bleeds developed and are still persisting at the time of your consultation, refer the patient for medical examination immediately. If raised intracranial pressure is allowed to persist then permanent damage may ensue to cerebral tissue and may be life threatening.

Allopathic diagnostic procedures

Careful neurological examination is required for good diagnosis. Clearly there is the need for a good clinical examination, especially testing the cranial nerves. Other signs such as skin coloration, pulse rate and strength will give clues as to possible causation. Shock, for example, will lead to pallor and low pulse rate and lowered blood pressure. A combination of a good history along with good observation and clinical tests will prove invaluable to you in these cases.

The fundus of the eye and the ear-nose-throat area and the mastoid are examined as well as the sinuses. These are then X-rayed and an ultrasound scans are made if necessary. In some cases an EEG is undertaken.

A CCT scan and an MRI are made to rule out any space claiming or degenerative processes.

Osteopathic examination

Palpation of the bones

Healthy bone

In utero and for the first 2½ years, bone is expressing greater softness and fluidity than at any other time in our life. Unlike adults, babies and very young children do not have sutures between bones. The bones of the skull are 'floating in a membranous and cartilaginous sea'. The vault bones are 'sandwich fillings' between the 'dural slices of bread'. The reason I used these very un-scientific terms is because they are good palpatory analogies of healthy infant bone in the skull. William Garner Sutherland, the osteopath who developed of cranial osteopathy, likened baby vault bones to a 'soft shelled egg.' Healthy bone, especially in the young is soft, tender and fluid in its quality when palpated by the trained osteopath.

Depending on the degree of acuteness or chronicity, bone tissue will reveal 'its secrets' to the osteopath in different ways.

Acute trauma

If *very* recent (for example if palpating a child very soon after a fall) the experience may be that of the bone being in a state of inertia and shock. Sometimes your palpating fingers experience the bone in a state of dynamic 'flux' where it is already trying to resolve the trauma. This can feel like 'swirls and unwinding' motions. In the case of recent trauma the bone may not feel harder. There may be some extra softness from swelling and edema.

Warning: Any localised crepitus at the point of pain may be from a fracture, in which case referral is necessary for X-ray and further medical examination. In this case do not give any local osteopathic treatment!

Chronic trauma

Make a careful note of any area of bone tissue which feels harder or denser than the surrounding softness of children's bone. In simple terms, where you feel extra hardness in bone, you are palpating the local shock response in the tissue from a chronic trauma. Here the softness from any inflammatory response (edema) will have dissipated and the intraosseous osteoblastic response is palpated.

Clearly any trauma beyond a very mild incident can lead to head pain and the child complaining that her head hurts. Any symptoms which last more that half an hour or so will usually be remembered by the mother. Usually if children cry following a fall, this persists for a short while and then they 'forget about it', as their attention is moved onto another interesting aspect of their life. It is the persistent complaint of pain in the head that causes 'alarm bells to ring' for both the parent and practitioner.

Interosseous lesions

Interosseous strains can have the effect of locking sutures (if they are already fully formed). The practitioner should be diligent to palpate the skull for sutures which are not moving comfortably. Again, with experience, the practitioner will be able to ascertain the chronicity of a suture not moving well.

Intraosseous lesions

With intraosseous strain the forces are primarily acting within the bone itself. The effects of intraosseous strains in terms of symptoms are often secondary to their effects on other tissues. Can intraosseous strains be a primary cause of head pain? If very strong forces have been absorbed here, then the answer must be yes; however in many cases there is the presence of intraosseous trauma which may not be a local source of symptoms, although a major etiological factor. With adults, for example, most have intraosseous compression of the sternum and of the sacrum, with very few actually complaining of pains *within* these bones. Usually, if at all, their complaints would be from adjacent structures. With babies and young children, one can only at best guess their symptoms. The comparison with adults can only give clues, not the truth.

Palpation of CNS

For osteopaths who have not yet built up their palpatory database with regard to the CNS, altered CNS tissue states are differentiated by 'what it is not'! On palpating your patient's skull you may note a heaviness or irritability or lack of IVM, but may not be able to understand which tissue is the primary cause. If this is your experience with some patients, ask yourself:

Does it feel primarily like bone tissue or could the lesion be primarily in the membranous tissue or fluid based?

If the answer to these questions is a clear 'no' then it is likely that the primary tissue problem lies in the CNS.

It is important to always remember when palpating the CNS: you are palpating a tissue which is highly sensitive and is the 'home' of the patient's consciousness. Consequently it is vital that you match the delicacy of the tissue tone with your palpation. Any difference between the tissue tone and the palpation tone of your fingers will be interpreted as 'unwanted interference' not 'harmonious empathy' by the patient. The result of the unwanted interference will be that the patient (consciously or unconsciously) tenses the body and makes it harder to palpate anything, plus this may result in the causation of headache or head pain – the opposite of what we try to achieve for our patients!

However, sensitive and mindful palpation of the CNS is very beneficial diagnostically to the osteopath and rewarding to the patient – a skill worth developing indeed.

Differential palpation of CNS

Different palpatory states and sensations will gradually emerge, the more you become familiar with palpation of the CNS.

Traumatic shock

Trauma will tend to express as either a locked 'shut down' on palpation or it will feel 'lost at sea', as if the tissues are trying to find some mechanical stability and fulcrum, having been 'shifted off center' from their comfort zone. Although an important role of the meninges is to prevent or dampen this effect, with more severe trauma this disorientation occurs. The severity and chronicity of the trauma can be ascertained in such patients with developing osteopathic skill.

Psychological shock

In my experience these tissue states reflect the CNS expression through the psyche. When the CNS feels irritable and unsettled, the patient is often unsettled, anxious or irritable as described by the parents. When the CNS feels 'locked' the patient may act as if still in a mild shock. If the CNS feels dull, as if there is no electrical charge then the patient may express depressive symptoms. Always remember that as osteopaths, we are not psychologists unless separately trained as such, but we do have 'thinking fingers' and are able to help the CNS express its full function. How does the CNS express its function: through our thinking, our mood and emotions, and our state

of being – our consciousness. Osteopaths help to improve tissue quality and hence life's expression.

Treatment

Allopathic medical treatment

It is necessary to keep track of the efficiency of the treatment by noting this in a headache diary.

Patients with migraine should avoid known trigger factors such as cow's milk, chocolate, citrus fruits, stress and chronic emotional tension. Biofeedback techniques and relaxation techniques (progressive muscle relaxation, autogenic training) can reduce the frequency of the attacks. During a migraine attack, stimulus reducing methods (dark and quiet room, cooling the forehead, sleeping), antiemetics and analgesics can be applied. In exceptional cases ergotamine may be given. As prophylactic treatment in cases of more than two or three migraine attacks per month, β-blockers are used.

Osteopathic treatment

On purpose I have not delineated a precise treatment regime for any condition discussed in this chapter. My reasons being that it would be non-osteopathic to do so! Any treatment has to reflect many different findings and any diagnosis should always be attempting to address the primary cause. Of greater benefit to the reader would be comments on tissue tone and the practitioner's 'empathy' with the tissues.

The more we are able to totally empathize with our patients' tissues the greater the information and treatment responses will result. Most adverse treatment reactions result from not 'reading' the tissues and their requirements. It is very easy in our desire to help our patients to try too hard and make greater changes than are appropriate at that moment in time. Always beware of doing too much, too soon. Allow your thinking fingers to match the tissue tone as exactly as possible and follow the story they wish to tell. Ask questions of the tissues whilst your fingers are in this total empathic state as to what is the primary cause and how the tissues would choose to be treated. You may be surprised as to what answers reveal themselves. If no answers seem to become clear, choose a treatment principle and feel if it seems appropriate, 'listening' for positive or negative responses. If the response is positive, carry on, if the response is a feeling of the tissues 'shutting down' then try another treatment principle.

Questions to be 'asked of the tissues' are:
- Is this dysfunction different to the overall pattern of the head?
- Is this dysfunction recent or longer term?

- Are there any other sutures restricted from secondary effects?

In young children and babies I would strongly advocate disengagement and direct action treatment principles being applied (see p.165). In such patients the skull is small and there is little space between structures. Exaggeration and compression principles may easily compromize delicate tissues and not produce the desired benefit. Fluid techniques (but not CV4 as it involves compression) are also very good with babies and young children for the same reasons.

When treating children over 8 years of age a CV4 may be utilized, but not within 10 to 14 days of head trauma. Head trauma, as already discussed, may have resulted in fracture or vascular damage. For this reason it would not be advisable to give compression to the occiput and fourth ventricle. If such a technique is appropriate, treatment via the sacrum is possible.

Always remember when treating children and babies that their physiology is much more dynamically changing than ours. Growth itself is a form of treatment. Consequently children, and especially babies, require less osteopathic input in order to make good therapeutic change. Do not overtreat. Stop before the tissues start to feel irritable.

Otitis media

(see Ch.13)

Restoration of good temporal and sphenoidal physiology can help improve middle ear drainage and hence reduce the frequency of infection and consequent pain to the child.

Sinusitis

(see Ch.13)

Many young children have nasal congestive states, and osteopathic treatment to restore good function of the upper and mid face brings much benefit to these patients. Treatment enhances the venolymphatic drainage of the face and so reduces the swelling of the mucosa of the nose and throat.

Temporomandibular joint (TMJ)

(see Ch.18)

The TMJ responds well to osteopathic treatment. Besides the cranial function, the posture of the patient should also be considered and treated if necessary as the TMJ is closely linked via muscles and the spine to the rest of the body.

Bleeds

It should be clear that localized treatment to the site of trauma may not be appropriate on the initial consultation. In such a situation I would focus on treating the associated shock and

other areas, working locally after a few days. Any bleeding from the eye should be referred for medical examination.

Eye problems

The muscles coordinating the mobility of the eye should be balanced. Any irregularity in the mobility of the cranial bones of the orbit should be addressed to make sure that cranial nerve entrapment is avoided and venous and arterial blood can flow freely.

Acuity problems should be referred to an ophthalmologist/optician; however, osteopathic treatment to rebalance the orbits can be very beneficial. I would recommend osteopathic treatment before an optical evaluation so that any prescription prescribed is based on well treated and hence well-functioning orbits!

Any patient who is undergoing treatment for increased ocular pressure can gain benefit from skilled simultaneous osteopathic care. You need to bear in mind that the treatment you give has to be ancillary to that of the ophthalmologist and not be the primary treatment. Raised ocular pressure is serious and if left unchanged may result in blindness from damage to the retina; it therefore has to be treated by the appropriate medical physician. Osteopathic care is able to help the physiology of the orbit mechanics, thus helping drainage of the aqueous humor through the Canal of Schlem.

Exopthalmus (bulging of the eye) may be from thyroid imbalance (e.g. Graves disease) or from pressure of a tumor and should be referred to a medical specialist. If after specialist examination no tumor was found, osteopathic care may assist the hormonal balance of the body. The osteopath should check for mechanical tensions located around the body of the sphenoid and pituitary fossa, or in the fascial tissues around the thyroid gland. In my experience, mechanical stresses do affect glandular secretions from the thyroid and should not be ignored.

Good orbit physiology is paramount for the treatment of floaters. Skilled 'thinking fingers' from a trained cranial osteopath can help assist these patients in addition to treatment given by their medical colleagues.

Biomechanical causes

Headaches stemming from biomechanical causes react well to osteopathic treatment. As mentioned before, the whole body condition has to be considered and osteopathic treatment applied as suggested (see p.161).

Prognosis

Head pain in children and babies is a rewarding field of practice for both patient and practitioner. Some aspects require significant osteopathic expertise, others less so. Aspects where severe pathology may be of risk have been indicated and should be heeded with appropriate medical referral. However do not let this prevent you from applying appropriate osteopathic care. Carefully applied osteopathy can give great benefit to all patients even if that patient is undergoing treatment elsewhere. When a patient is having treatment from a medical specialist, osteopathy can play a supportive role, enabling the body to respond better to the medical treatments and recover faster. The skill is in the appropriate choice of osteopathic input!

Bibliography

Devinsky O, Feldmann E, Weinreb H J: Neurological pearls, Davis, Philadelphia 2000

Sutherland W G: Teachings in the science of osteopathy, Rudra Press, Sutherland Cranial Teaching Foundation, Texas 1990

The aim of this chapter is to explore the application of osteopathic principles and treatment of infants with genetic conditions, using Down syndrome and achondroplasia as examples. It is intended as an illustration of an osteopathic approach to any patient with a genetic syndrome. At the same time it is an invitation to us all within the profession to 'dig on'. Osteopathy in the cranial field is a very helpful approach when treating children with these conditions. As with all aspects of osteopathy in the cranial field, a detailed working knowledge of embryology is essential for the therapeutic 'pictures' we use.

A mother telephones to enquire: 'Can you help my child with Negar's syndrome?' You explain that this is not a syndrome you have come across and ask for more information. You discover that this parent, having searched on the internet, is well researched and up to date on this particular clinical picture. It is not a common condition and it is highly unlikely that there will be anything to find in osteopathic literature. What do you reply?

Fairly regularly we get requests similar to this in everyday practice and we need to find an answer. There is enough anecdotal evidence of the treatment of various genetic disorders within osteopathic circles to encourage us to respond positively.

Negar's syndrome is a very rare syndrome of which the principal clinical features are abnormalities of palatal development with a hypoplastic mandible, leading to facial disfigurement, speech problems and consequent difficulties with self-confidence. With the careful application of osteopathic principles and treatment, this child suddenly starts to improve. Perhaps his mandible is developing, it certainly looks as if it is, both to the practitioner and the mother. His speech is definitely improving and with it his confidence in his communication skills both at home and at school. Maybe this was about to happen anyway, without osteopathic treatment? That we can never know. As a lot of genetic conditions, like this syndrome, are rare, this precludes the possibility of proper controlled trials. However, it is our purpose here to encourage ourselves to explore and confer to expand our knowledge base of osteopathic practice, albeit 'anecdotal'.

In discussing both Down syndrome and achondroplasia my overriding concern is to challenge the assumption that we, and the parents of our patients, come across; that is, that particular symptoms are a part of the condition and therefore to be accepted. For example that neurodevelopmental delay is a result of the chromosomal abnormalitiy in Down syndrome, or that compromized airways are an inevitable consequence of Down. Another common assumption is, for example, that joint and back pain are an inevitable result of the bone dysplasia in achondroplasia, or that upper respiratory tract congestion is due to the skull abnormalities in achondroplasia.

We could add many more to this list, but these are a few I have selected in order to illustrate a recurring theme. My experience is that many symptoms of genetic conditions may be helped by appropriate osteopathic treatment and need not be accepted as an inevitable part of the syndrome.

DOWN SYNDROME

Definition

Down syndrome is the most common chromosomal abnormality. It affects 1 in 650–700 newborns. In most cases it is due to a third chromosome 21 being present in all body cells (trisomy 21). Children with Down syndrome are found in all ethnic communities.

We are quite likely to see children with Down syndrome in our osteopathic clinic. This may be due to the fact that successful treatment for a variety of symptoms in Down syndrome children is probably talked about among parents and self-help groups.

Etiology and pathophysiology

In most cases (95%) there is a numerical chromosomal abnormality: in trisomy 21 you find a chromosome three times. The child has an extra chromosome present in all body cells, with a total chromosome count of 47 instead of 46. This is due to chromosomal disjunction during the process of meiosis, and is more common the older the parents get. The incidence is 0.0005% in mothers at the age of 20,

1–2% in mothers under 35, and 3% in mothers aged over 40. The age of the father seems to be also relevant if he is older than 40. Other than that no causative factors are certain.

In about 4% of Down syndrome cases the cause is a structural chromosomal abnormality: an unbalanced translocation (often between chromosomes 14 and 21). In translocation two chromosomes break and reunite, exchanging the broken off bits. This process is independent of the age of the mother. The total chromosome count, the sum of the genome, stays the same and is still 46. In about 60% translocation is a new event. In the other cases it is present in a parent, but balanced; that is, the amount of the genetic material is not changed. This is called a balanced translocation. This parent is healthy, but the risk of having a child with Down syndrome is high. Depending on where the translocation is, and whether the father or mother carries it, the risk of having another child with Down will vary between 5 and 100% (Handoll 1998). When a child is found to have trisomy due to translocation, it may be worth doing a karyotype analysis of the parents (Rossi 1989, Nelson 1990).

In about 1% mosaicism is found (Nelson 1990). Usually two cell-lines with a different number are found; for example some cell-lines display trisomy 21, but others are normal. This is due to non-disjunction in the process of mitosis during early fetal development; it is independent of the age of the mother. These children often have a wider range of abilities.

Clinical signs and symptoms

Face and head

The typical craniofacial appearance includes brachycephaly, a flat occiput, a flat face, a small midface, upturned nose and epicanthal folds (Fig. 17.1). The maxilla and mandible are often small and therefore the tongue appears protruded without being larger itself. The palate is high and narrow, the mouth often open. This may dispose the child to recurrent upper respiratory infections. It also may make speech more difficult; children with Down often need speech therapy. They are also more likely to develop problems with their teeth, owing to disharmonic growth. Orthodontic treatment is often necessary.

Cranial base

The cranial base is shorter on its anteroposterior (a/p) axis as a result of the poor development of the sphenoid bone. The occipital squama can be steep and angled sharply in an upright direction, giving the characteristic flattened appearance to the back of the head. The angle of the whole cranial

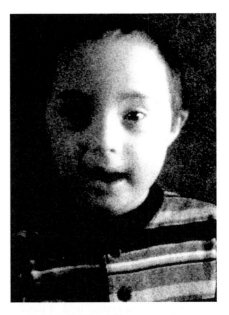
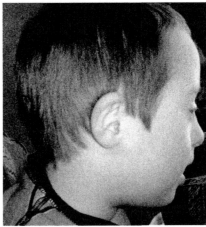

Figure 17.1 A child with Down syndrome. With permission, Donna Paget, Bath

base tends to be more vertical. This can narrow the space of the suspended nasopharynx, thereby reducing the airways. Airway resistance and consequent lack of oxygen saturation is commonly a problem. This aspect is vitally important to the osteopathic treatment rationale. The foramen magnum can be small and ellipsoid in shape.

Cranial vault

At the time of birth there is little difference in vault size between a child suffering from Down syndrome and a normal child. But after birth, especially during the 1st year of life, the rate of vault growth in the Down syndrome child will begin to drop below the norm. Thereafter head circumference will stay on a graph fairly constantly about 4 to 5 cm behind normal growth until the age of around 14. At this point it will stop growing and remain at about the size of a normal 3 to 4 year old child. The width of a Down syndrome child's skull will be close to the normal, but the marked lack of growth in length is highly significant and becomes of interest to us when we look at ways we might help with cranial base development.

Sinus spaces

The sinus spaces will normally develop after birth, culminating in huge growth spurts at the age of 12 to 14 years. Because a child with Down syndrome has a skull development deficient in growth, these spaces remain very compromised. This particularly affects the frontal and ethmoid bone, the two maxillae, and also the sphenoid body itself. If we can improve development of these air spaces by osteopathic treatment it is going to have enormous benefits for a child struggling with poor and inadequate function of the airways and respiratory tract, be that from developmental narrowing or repeated infection.

Ears

The ear lobes may be small and dysmorphic. There may be abnormalities leading to degrees of hearing impairment and therefore disturbed speech development. Some problems will lie more on the side of the nervous system and can deteriorate with age. Others are due to the actual size of the cochlea and the numbers of receptor cells in the spiral ganglion. The stapes are not always of normal size.

Eyes

The eyes may show a tendency for strabismus or nystagmus. Brushfield spots (white dots in a light iris) may be found. Glaucoma or coloboma may be a feature.

Internal organs

Organ malformation is common. Heart problems like a septal defect are found in about 40–50% of children. In the digestive system stenosis or atresia may be present, for example Hirschsprung disease, atresia of the duodenum or pancreas anulare. Affected children have therefore often had serious operations at an early age.

Hernias are more common, and a tendency for constipation has been observed. There is a tendency for malignancy (leukemia), in boys hypogonadism and later infertility. Women are mostly fertile.

Musculoskeletal system

As newborns and in infancy these children often suffer from muscular hypotonia. Walking may appear clumsy, possibly due to this hypotonicity. Affected children can take a longer time to gain stability in the development of postural reflexes, which could lead to slower integration of proprioceptive stimuli in the cerebellum. For example, it can take them a longer time to gain a sitting position, as they lack the necessary tone to save themselves if they fall (parachute reflex).

Virtually all Down syndrome children are smaller than peer age children. Hands and feet may show typical signs, like an increased distance between the first and second toe The hands are also short and plump; the middle phalanx of the fifth finger may be shorter and joints may be hypermobile.

Neurology, psychology, development

An important deficiency in Down syndrome involves the function of the CNS, which is underdeveloped. Dendrites of the cortical neurons have been shown to be abnormal, and the anterior commissure may be small. As the child grows, developmental delay, learning difficulties and often a low IQ (of about 50) become more obvious. Intelligence is often, but not always retarded. The range of abilities can be very wide. Abstract thinking may be missing, but manual and other abilities (e.g. swimming) can develop. Therefore, simple work at home or in a protected work environment may be possible.

These kids are usually of a cheerful and affectionate disposition.

Diagnosis

During pregnancy there may have been bleeding in the first or second trimester, or other signs of the danger of a miscarriage. The mother may also have noted the child moving less, an early sign of muscular hypotonia.

Important for diagnosis are the typical dysmorphic signs, muscular hypotonia and developmental delay.

Allopathic medical diagnosis

If Down syndrome is suspected, the diagnosis is confirmed or excluded by chromosomal testing. As often malformed organs may be present, heart, abdomen and eyes are examined thoroughly.

Treatment
Allopathic medical treatment

This includes operations for heart or intestinal malformations, early physiotherapy, often orthodontic treatment, speech therapy, and advice and support for parents.

Osteopathic treatment

When treating children I have found working with osteopathy in the cranial field of prime importance, although I am certain that this is not the only approach that can be beneficial to our patients. Particularly useful can be the approach according to Jealous (see www.jamesjealous.com), which includes among many other areas of interest an understanding of the value of the dynamics of embryology and its relevance to our diagnostic and therapeutic osteopathic approach to our patients. The work that Jealous presents on the dynamics of facial development is hugely helpful, along with the understanding of the blueprint for health that embryology can give us.

Some of the principal clinical features to highlight when thinking about osteopathic treatment are: airway problems and tongue protrusion with the associated oxygen deprivation, hypotonia and mild to moderate developmental delay. It may be also important to treat the after-effects of surgery with osteopathic treatment.

Obviously, there is a lot of complexity and detail in the full clinical picture. I want, however, to stay with the main thrust of my argument that many of these symptoms will be accepted as part of the syndrome by many professionals and parents alike and therefore left untreated. I and many of my colleagues suggest that appropriate osteopathic treatment can help change some of these symptoms by improving blood supply and drainage (both venous and lymphatic), particularly intracranial, by improving the patency of the airways and upper respiratory tract, and by restoring function to the thoracic cavity.

Typical changes in the cranial base

Handoll (1998) explored in detail the pre- and postnatal development of the cranial base in Down syndrome. Between week 6 and 12 of fetal life, the baby reaches a critical stage of development. At this point, development in a fetus with Down syndrome will begin to slow down. Among other effects, the growth of the cranial base is limited, leading to shortening on an a/p axis. This shortening of length on an a/p axis is one of the most striking findings in examining the head of a child with this syndrome. Conversely, when the child responds well to treatment, as a practitioner you feel a change in this length and with it a change in many symptoms. If you can get to a point in treatment when it feels as if the sphenoid bone and the whole of the cranial base can 'breathe' on its longitudinal axis, then you know the body physiology has a better chance of working.

It will be helpful at this point to remember some important stages of the prenatal development of the cranial base and, in particular, the sphenoid and its sphere of influence. First things first: the body of sphenoid will gradually condense out of the mesenchyme at the rostral tip of the notochord. The notochord is playing a vital role in inducing the

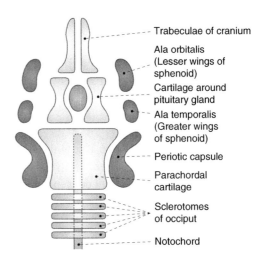

Figure 17.2 A schematic illustration of the mesenchymal and cartilagenous fields contributing to the formation of the chondrocranium in the first trimester.
With permission, Henriette Rintelen, Velbert

development of the neural tube. It continues to play this role within the developing sphenoid as many structures converge: the forebrain and midbrain, pituitary fossa and gland, all dural septae and many cranial nerves (CN I–VI). You can watch the complex shapes and contours of the ossifying sphenoid gradually appear as a response to these developmental processes.

The schematic representation in Figure 17.2 shows the various mesenchymal and cartilagenous fields that will form the platform of the cranial base during the first 12 weeks.

Of importance here are what will become the attachments of the dural membranes. The trabeculae will form the ethmoid and provide attachment for the falx cerebri. Remember here that the attachments of the falx cerebri blend slightly more posteriorly in the newborn onto the anterior body of the sphenoid itself. This is clinically significant. The lesser wings will form within the alae orbitales and provide attachment for the anterior dural girdle or anterior dural septum, which is much larger in the neonatal cranium than in an older child or adult. The two borders of the posterior dural septum or tentorium cerebelli will attach onto the body of the sphenoid and form the anterior and posterior clinoid processes around the sella turcica, itself orientated towards the end of the notochord within the sphenoid body.

It is important to spend time on the details of these developing structures in order to grasp the dynamics of what we often refer to as the five pointed star. Having an appreciation of this 'star' and using it diagnostically and therapeutically gives us a useful tool in the treatment of any children, but in particular in the treatment of a child with Down syndrome.

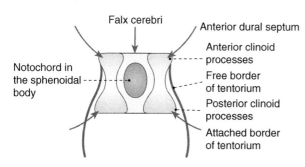

Figure 17.3 A schematic representation of the insertions of the reciprocal tension membrane to the various parts of the sphenoid, all orientating to the notochord in the center.
With permission, Henriette Rintelen, Velbert

Here the relationships of the compartments defined by these structures becomes even more crucial. The diagramatic illustration of this star shows it to be both simple yet profound (Fig. 17.3).

I refer you, in this context, to Carreiro's book *An osteopathic approach to children* (2003) for an illustrated guide to these structures. The dissections carried out by herself and Professor Willard on neonates allow us an inspirational view of fetal anatomy without which our understanding could not be so informed.

In Figure 17.3 you see the dural membranes represented by lines. The falx cerebri, the anterior dural septum along the lesser wings of the sphenoid and the tentorium cerebelli with its fixed and free border are shown. All these lines converge on the pituitary, the body of the sphenoid and, within it, the tip of the notochord. At birth, these membranes are prominent and lend strength to the adaptive tolerance of the bony cranium. Sometimes this tolerance is challenged and some effects of the birth process remain in the tissues, placing complex demands on such an important area. This is particularly important in children with Down syndrome. In normal development, the pre- and postsphenoid will ossify by the 8th month of intrauterine life. Therefore it gains a greater degree of stability and can compensate better for the forces experienced at birth. In a Down syndrome child the union of pre- and postsphenoid remains cartilagenous until the first months of infancy, thus making the cranial base more vulnerable to unphysiological strain patterns, both vertical and lateral strains. This fact makes it all the more important to check these children osteopathically after birth, no matter the type of delivery. The best chance we can give these children is to relieve them of any potential birth strain to an already compromised cranial base.

The sphenoid and the rest of the cranial base needs to be given every chance of developing on its a/p axis to give it as much length as possible. The physiological implications of

this could be enormous when we consider the function of the pituitary gland and its communication with other hormonal relationships. Down syndrome children, for example, often have problems with thyroid function. In addition, other closely related structures close to the tip of the notochord are interesting in this respect. I would like to mention especially the third ventricle, hypothalamus and the control of such functions as appetite.

Facial structures and airway problems

What you often see in the face of a Down syndrome child is an open mouth with mouth breathing, a protruding tongue and a runny nose. What you cannot see without further investigation are chronic sinus infections, middle ear infection and congestion and consequent hearing loss. These chronic infections often lead to repeatedly prescribed antibiotic treatment and a cycle of poor immune response. These are symptoms, however, that we can often help. They are related to the anatomical and physiological variations in development; that is, a high palate, shortening of the nasal septum, narrowing of the nasal antrum, and the small mandible.

They are definite developmental anomalies. In the 4th week of embryonic life, the branchial arches are formed as the head flexes down and the heart and diaphragm move to their respective locations. The branchial arches are 'rolled up' between the developing brain and the heart. Various forces are active in the further development of the face over the next 8 weeks, which coincides with the period of metabolic disturbance in Down syndrome. Because of this, many structures can be affected: ethmoid, nasals, maxillae and mandible. There is poor sinus development in the frontal bones, sphenoid, ethmoid and the maxillae. The tongue often protrudes, not because it is necessarily too large, but because the mouth is too small. With appropriate osteopathic treatment we see that tongue control might be improved. Therefore it is worth putting the effort and perseverance into training it. As tongue control improves, the added bonus is that it provides the most vital stimulus to sinus development – nose breathing. These vital changes in face shape have been reported by many osteopaths (Handoll 1998). Hearing can improve too, often avoiding the need for grommet insertion. The implications of this for speech and therefore social development are obvious.

Influencing hypotonia and developmental delay

The most crucial point is perhaps that a restriction of airways will compromise oxygen saturation in a situation where the developing nervous system most needs it to prevent further neurodevelopmental delay, and to increase muscle tone. Handoll (1998) quotes research papers that suggest that prolonged cerebral hypoxemia, with associated blood and tissue pH changes, is a significant obstruction to the postnatal developmental synaptic pathways. There was seen to be a related absence of axonal plexus in the hippocampal area in prolonged metabolic and cardiorespiratory disturbances.

The implication here for osteopaths is that the more we can improve oxygen supply to the developing nervous system, the more we can hope that some aspects of neurodevelopment will be helped. The oxygen supply for the CNS might, for example, be improved not only by helping circulation in the cranium with cranial work but also by optimizing excursion and function of the thorax, and therefore breathing patterns.

Strains after surgery

Congenital malformation of organs are common in Down syndrome. It is therefore important to mention that children who have undergone surgery can be left with unresolved strains in the abdomen, thorax, ribcage or cervical musculature. Perhaps the head turns more easily one way and this becomes the favoured orientation to the world. Sometimes it can literally feel as if the sternum does not 'match' the midline, as if it has not been sewn up to meet its opposite side. These patterns of strain can be helped with treatment to help resolve the tensions in the sternum, ribs and their attachment at the costochondral junctions, such as after open heart surgery with a heart defect.

> **Case study**
> John was brought for assessment at the age of 7 weeks. He was born vaginally with no complications at 37½ weeks after a good pregnancy. Although he was hypotonic, he had no heart abnormalities. The principal osteopathic finding was a flattened interparietal occiput with reduced anterior-posterior dimension across the cranial base. John had slight difficulty with nose breathing and early indications of a middle ear problem. On the second visit he had weeping from the right ear and was being treated with external antibiotic drops by his GP. This area of function, along with a tendency to chest infections, became an important focus for his treatment programme. Figure 17.1 shows the hypotonic appearance with mouth open, tongue beginning to protrude and the flattening at the back of the head.

On account of his osteopathic treatment, John now has good maxillary development with excellent tongue control. He nose breathes most of the time. With the occasional use of hearing aids he has avoided the insertion of grommets and his speech has slowly developed. The back of his head has changed shape with increase in his a/p dimension. The facial profile is relatively good. These changes were achieved over a period of 18 treatments in 7 years, more of these sessions being concentrated in the first 2 years. Thereafter, treatment was timed with growth spurts and seasonal considerations – autumn and winter being times of increased risk of respiratory tract infections.

Prognosis

Life expectancy may be an issue for parents confronted with a diagnosis. Mortality can be as high as 12% in the first year, which is primarily due to congenital heart complications. In a study in Europe in 1997, attainment of good self-help skills like self-feeding and mobility were found to be pointers to life expectancy of 50+, whereas with poor skills this could be reduced to 40. The study found 88% of children with Down syndrome alive at 1 year and 82% alive at 10 years.

As with all children with genetic conditions, the prognosis is going to depend on the severity of the accompanying malformation of organs. Much can be done osteopathically for facial development, tongue control, nose breathing, airway patency, hearing and consequently speech and social interaction. Part of such success is due to increased muscle tone, improved expression of motion through the face and improved respiratory tract function. After surgery it is absolutely necessary to check the function of the ribcage or abdomen, and treat if necessary.

ACHONDROPLASIA

Definition

Achondroplasia is an autosominal dominant disorder. Its cause is a genetic defect of the short arm of chromosome 4, which in 80–90% happens by spontaneous mutation. It affects endochondral ossification at the epiphyseal cartilage plates, particularly of the long bones. It is the most prevalent type of bone dysplasia.

Achondroplasia is the most common form of bone dysplasia and affects mainly the proximal parts of the limbs. The trunk usually has normal proportions leading to a disproportion in size between trunk and limbs. An achondroplasic adult might not expect to grow beyond 130 cm (4ft 4in), unless there has been surgical intervention, like limb lengthening.

In achondroplasia the endochondral ossification is disturbed, but the membranous ossification is normal. This leads to the characteristic skull abnormalities with a vault that is larger than the cranial base and face.

The prevalence is 23/100,000 births, and it is therefore a rare disorder. In the UK about 30 babies are born each year, mostly to parents of normal stature with no history of the condition on either side of the family.

Etiology and pathophysiology

The genetic defect impedes the change from proliferating to maturing cartilage, because the chondrocytes produce 'wrong' collagen of type 1, not type 2, in the zone of maturation. Mineralization of cartilage is still possible, but resorption of cartilage is slowed. Therefore, the disturbance of growth affects the growth plates.

Clinical signs and symptoms

The long bones of the proximal parts of the limbs are shortened, with the trunk being of normal proportions leading to a disproportion and short stature.

Children with achondroplasia also have varying degrees of developmental skull abnormalities. Typical changes of the cranium involve the occiput and other bones of the cranial base as they are formed in cartilage. The whole cranial base, but especially the occiput can be small and irregular in shape, affecting the shape and contents of the posterior cranial fossa. The foramen magnum may be smaller and misshapen. If the posterior cranial fossa is compromized, there may be also difficulties in the circulation of cerebrospinal fluid, with a degree of hydrocephalus. This is however mostly asymptomatic. The cause is usually the growth of the foramen magnum not keeping up with the growth of its content, and closure of the foramen of Magendii leading to hydrocephalus.

Since the membranous ossification is not affected by the defect, the vault bones grow normally. This asymmetrical growth of the cranial vault and base leads to an obvious difference in growth of the middle face and vault, with a smaller face and a normal sized vault.

Because of the underdevelopment of the maxillae, the mandible appears larger. In comparison with the face the cranial vault appears distended, with a large forehead. The nose is small and the nasal bridge depressed (Fig. 17.4).

As the child gets older, a tendency for a marked kyphosis of the dorsals and lordosis of the lumbars may appear, with the abdomen protruding. The vertical height of the bodies of the vertebrae may be shorter and the vertebral arch may be shorter, leading to a smaller spinal canal.

You may find a flattened and widened pelvis with a narrow a/p entrance. Coxa vara with a short neck of the femur and small head is common, as is a flat acetabulum. There may be a tendency for bow legs, as the fibula is relatively long, and you may find genua vara and crura vara.

The thorax appears flat, often bell-shaped because of delayed ossification at the interface between cartilage and bone at the ribs. The pelvis is small and appears rectangular, with typical cone-like areas pulled out at the ilium.

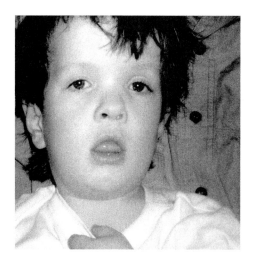
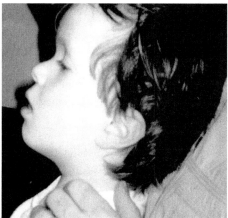
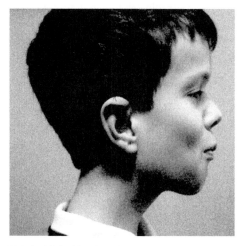

Figure 17.4 A child with achondroplasia. With permission, E leen Rodger, B th

Typical changes to the hands include isodactylism and brachydactylism. Joints may be less mobile; for example a reduced extension at the elbow joint is common. Metacarpals, metatarsals and phalanges are plump and short.

Achondroplasia is a purely physical condition affecting growth of bone. It has no mental implications; intelligence is normal and sometimes also quite high.

Diagnosis

The clinical picture is obvious. Diagnosis can usually be made at birth.

Allopathic medical diagnosis

X-rays show typical changes in pelvis and spine. The vertebrae are smaller and malformed.

Treatment

Allopathic medical treatment

Operations may sometimes be performed to improve leg length or the axes of the legs. Limb lengthening is however a painful and prolonged process and can lead to complications of pin site infection; therefore these days it is not a common procedure.

Another operation which may sometimes be necessary later on in life is decompression of a narrow spinal canal. In hydrocephalus a shunt may have been inserted.

Osteopathic treatment

Osteopathic treatment may achieve visible changes in posture, with a less protruding abdomen indicating a better balance of body cavities (thorax/abdomen). Back pain and pain in the extremities may be greatly reduced. Early cranial treatment may lead to visible and functionally significant changes in head shape. Improvements in upper airway function can also be important, leading to less vulnerability to infection.

Some of the common features of achondroplasia will be discussed from an osteopathic point of view. Many symptoms have a functional component and are therefore amenable to treatment. In addition, the earlier that treatment can begin, the better are the chances of avoiding some longer term complications.

Back pain and spinal problems

Back pain is a common symptom in achondroplasia. There can be a structural reason for this pain in that spinal stenosis can occur along the whole length of the spinal canal. It may cause neurological complications, affecting the legs with weakness, numbness, pain, and even interfere with bladder and bowel function.

Also the postural patterns that many child achondroplasics have can create structural problems. Lumbar lordosis and thoracic kyphoscoliosis are prominent, and often severe, but they can change with carefully applied treatment. Positive changes in the whole balance and functioning of the abdomen and thorax can be achieved.

Especially important are here changes in the lumbosacral angle and in the thoracolumbar curves, and the sternum, which tends to be small and depressed, affecting ribcage function and the diaphragm. The function of the diaphragm, with its crural attachments to the anterior longitudinal ligament of the upper lumbar vertebral bodies, might play a particularly important role in this picture.

Sleep apnea

Efficient thoracic respiration is vital for good oxygen saturation and the delicate balance of oxygen supply to the brain. Breathlessness and sometimes sleep apnea can be additional complications.

This form of apnea happens as the child sleeps and can lead to unsatisfactory oxygen saturation levels in the brain. It registers alarm through the respiratory centers in the third and fourth ventricles. Sleep apnea not only leads to restless sleep, headaches and general lethargy, but can also affect the developing CNS at crucial stages. The cause of the sleep apnea lies partly in the hypotonicity and overrelaxation of the pharyngeal structures.

Headache

With achondroplasia there is often raised intracranial pressure with a degree of ventricular dilation, which is picked up on MRI scans. Often there are no symptoms except headaches. Because the endochondral proliferation is disturbed, asymmetry of the cranial base is common. The occiput tends to be small and distorted, sometimes to the point of affecting the shape of the foramen magnum. The cranial vault, which grows normally, will accommodate this by expanding to give a characteristic look to the head. It is interesting to see how such a cranial base has recovered after the birth process. How could this malformed occiput manage the forces of labor? If the four parts of the occiput are more vulnerable to distortion, can we help them with osteopathic intervention soon after birth? Obviously great care also has to be taken in assessing any degree of spinal cord compression through the foramen magnum and the upper cervical complex.

How can CSF circulation and absorption be improved? Possibly by improving functioning of the aqueduct of Sylvius, between the third and fourth ventricle, a common site of CSF flow obstruction. Osteopathic treatment could also have some positive effect on the performance of the foramen in the fourth ventricle, the foramina of Magendie and Luschka.

These foramina allow passage for the CSF from the ventricular system through to the subarachnoid space. In a study regarding hydrocephalus in achondroplasia carried out by Steinbok (1999), it was postulated that the pressure in the cerebral venous system that normally absorbs the CSF was too high and was inhibiting absorption. He suggested that the pressure could be too high as a result of a blockage to the flow of venous blood at the base of the skull, that region which is known to be very small in children with achondroplasia. In his study, Steinbok inserted small catheters into the venous system via the groin and injected dye; he could show that there is a narrowing of the jugular veins at the base of the skull. This conclusion of the study and reasoning will be very familiar to any osteopath who has studied the works and thinking of Sutherland, with particular reference to the importance of the jugular foramen.

Upper respiratory tract congestion and infection

Mention has been made already of the changes in the frontonasal angle and the small nose in children with achondroplasia. This leads to a reduced airway patency. Added to this is a tension in the attachments of the falx cerebri, part of the reciprocal tension membrane described by Sutherland, to the ethmoid bone. Contained within the ethmoid bone are the ethmoid sinuses, which need physiological motion to achieve good drainage of the mucous secretions. Any reduction in motion can lead to poor drainage and stagnation. Reduced motion expressed through the facial bones also affects the maxillae, also containing vital sinus spaces with secreting mucous membranous linings. If the ability to take in air through the nose and throat is compromised, it will lead to mouth breathing. Mouth breathing, in turn, is known to reduce the stimulus for the actual development of the maxillary bones themselves, affecting the postnatal development of the whole of the mid-face. This further complicates the picture and can lead to perhaps unnecessary orthodontic intervention in early adolescence because of the consequent overcrowding of the teeth.

We can also include at this point the middle ear and its vulnerability to infection and congestion. In the development of the embryo the middle ear cavity develops as a direct outgrowth of the nasopharynx and is therefore lined with the same continuous mucous membrane. Infection can track in either direction. Children with achondroplasia often have degrees of hearing loss associated with chronic serous otitis media. In my experience, hearing in some of the children treated with osteopathy has improved, making surgical intervention and insertion of grommets unnecessary. Improved drainage down the eustachian tube and function of the

nasopharynx will explain this symptom relief. Improved hearing leads to better speech development and all the positive knock-on social effects that follow.

Case study
Malcolm, a 4-year-old boy with achondroplasia, complained about breathing problems.

The osteopathic examination of his whole body showed a narrow, poorly functioning thorax, a distended, protruding abdomen and consequent lumbar lordosis. The boy suffered severe sleep apnea with very poor oxygen saturation. Nightly he had to insert an endotracheal tube to ease his airways and improve oxygen intake. This he did himself. Although it was a painful procedure, he found, even at the age of 4 that it was easier and more comfortable if he did do it himself. He had no other pain but had a constant stream of perspiration on his brow and face, indicating raised sympathetic nervous system tone. In the past he had had middle ear infections with perforations. Grommets had been implanted but had fallen out.

Treatment was started cautiously to help first with the ribcage dynamics. More balanced interchange function was gradually achieved between the different body cavities. Respiration improved, abdominal protrusion lessened and the bulging forehead started to recede. In osteopathic palpation of the cranium it was possible to feel the change in size and pressure of the ventricular system. As the pattern within the cranium was allowed to change, there began some facial development with the maxillae beginning to expand. Hard work was put in by the boy and his family to break the habit patterns formed around mouth breathing.

After 6 months and 11 treatments he was able to dispense with the endotracheal tube. This was a big and significant milestone for everyone! We knew then that his brain was beginning to get the regular supply of oxygen it needed.

Malcolm developed his speech now more consistently, being helped by the improved tongue function. The maxillae developed well and this aided better breathing, tongue control and overall facial development. Although the boy has been left with a degree of neurodevelopmental delay, his overall health has improved.

This case concentrates on the symptom picture of upper respiratory tract problems. It should, however, be mentioned that also back and limb pains of children with achondroplasia can be helped considerably.

Prognosis

Children with achondroplasia have a normal life expectancy. However, complications may lead to higher mortality in all age groups.

After osteopathic treatment I have seen some significant structural and functional changes both in the children that have come to my practice and also from photographs sent to me by other practitioners or satisfied parents.

CONCLUSION

This chapter has been an attempt to illustrate possible osteopathic approaches to children born with genetic disorders. It is impossible to discuss all disorders, especially as, due to research, their numbers increase almost by the day.

This should, however, not keep us from applying osteopathic principles and striving to understand anatomical and physiological nuances, based on which we could help these children. The main thrust of my discussion is that time and again we will come across situations where symptoms have been accepted as part of a particular condition. Such symptoms often involve pain, disability and other factors compromising health. In my experience these symptoms can often be relieved, depending of course on the individual case.

Bibliography

Association for Spina Bifida and Hydrocephalus GB (ASBAH): Hydrocephalus and you. 42 Park Road, Peterborough PE1 2UQ, UK

Carreiro J: An osteopathic approach to children. Churchill Livingstone, Elsevier 2003

Handoll, N: The osteopathic management of children with Down's syndrome. British Osteopathic Journal 21, 1998: 11

Hull D, Johnston D: Essential pediatrics. 3rd edn. Churchill Livingstone, New York 1994

Nelson: Essentials of pediatrics. W B Saunders, Philadelphia 1990

Newsletters of the Restricted Growth Association UK

Rossi: Pädiatrie. 2nd edn. Thieme, Stuttgart, 1989

Steinbok P: Hydrocephalus in achondroplasia, LPA Today, 1999

18 Orthodontics

Ariane Hesse

NOMENCLATURE AND MORPHOLOGY
Dental formula and intraoral terminology

The dental formula mostly used in Europe is described in the following paragraph. The first number (1–4 or 5–8 for the deciduous teeth) of the dental formula (Fig. 18.1) denotes the relevant quadrant, the second number the relevant tooth. Sequential numbering of the teeth always starts at the center between the middle incisors and moves outward from 1–8, or 1–5 for the deciduous teeth. For example: the first left lower molar is called 36 (pronounced 'three six', not 'thirty-six'). The first right upper deciduous incisor becomes 51 (pronounced 'five one'). Figure 18.2 gives a directional guide to terminology within the jaw.

Occlusion and centric relation

The contact of the teeth in the bite is called occlusion. The situation with the most possible occlusal contacts, the maximum intercuspidation, mostly corresponds to the habitual occlusion.

A cranioventral and not laterally shifted position of the condyles is defined as centric relation, which is attained only through neuromuscular control, independent of dental contacts.

In centric relation the tissues of the physiological condyle–disc relationship are loaded with adequate physiological forces. To achieve the centric relation, the habitual neuromuscular pattern should be deprogrammed. (Bumann 2000). Out of this neuromuscular-determined mandibular position an early tooth contact can arise when the dental arches close together with the lower jaw consequently sliding into its habitual occlusion. If this initial sliding occurs within a range of 0.5 to 1 mm, it is within physiological limits – provided there is no lateral deviation. A certain leeway in the centric relation creates more space for compensatory maneuver (Ramfjord 1983).

Common malocclusions

In the beginning of the 20th century Angle described a classification of the occlusal positions which is still used today (Angle classes I, II and III, see Fig. 18.3). Class II, the distal occlusion, is divided in subdivisions one and two. The whole classification is defined by the articulation of the cusps of the first molars in the sagittal plane:

- Neutral occlusion or Class I occlusion: the mesiobuccal cusp of upper 6 is within the transverse fissure of the lower molar.

Permanent dentition

Upper jaw (maxilla)

Right | 18 17 16 15 14 13 12 11 21 22 23 24 25 26 27 28 | Left
48 47 46 45 44 43 42 41 31 32 33 34 35 36 37 38

Lower jaw (mandible)

Deciduous dentition

Upper jaw (maxilla)

Right | 55 54 53 52 51 61 62 63 64 65 | Left
85 84 83 82 81 71 72 73 74 75

Lower jaw (mandible)

Figure 18.1 Dental chart to name the teeth. Front teeth numbers 1 and 2, canines number 3, premolars numbers 4 and 5, molars numbers 6–8.
With permission, Henriette Rintelen, Velbert

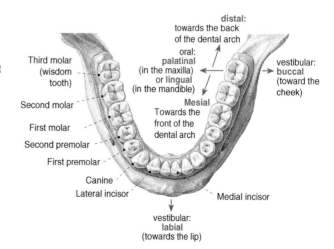

Figure 18.2 Topographical intra-oral terminology.
With permission, Sobotta: Atlas der Anatomie des Menschen. Publisher: R. Putz and R. Pabst, 21st edn. Elsevier/Urban & Fischer, Munich/Jena, 2000

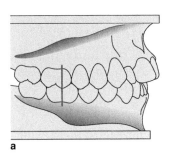
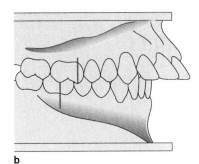
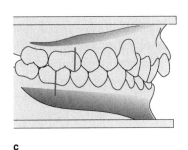
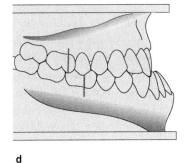

Figure 18.3 The Angle classes to distinguish between occlusal positions **a:** Class I. **b:** Class II₁. **c:** Class II₂. **d:** Class III.
With permission, Kahl-Nieke: Einführung in die Kieferorthopädie. 2nd edn. Urban & Fischer, Munich/Jena, 2001

- Disto-occlusion or Class II occlusion:
  - Class II₁: distal occlusion with protrusion of the upper incisors, the mesiobuccal cusp of upper 6 lies in front of the transverse fissure of the lower molar.
  - Class II₂: distal occlusion with retroinclination of the upper incisors, often associated with a deep bite.
- Mesial occlusion, prognathism of the lower jaw or Class III occlusion: the mesiobuccal cusps of the upper molar lie behind the transverse fissure of the lower molar. Pseudo-Class III: the mandible is normal, the maxilla is underdeveloped. Extreme forms of class III need treatment in the form of a combination of orthodontics with orthodontic surgery.

The Angle classes can be associated with all further malpositions of the teeth, such as crowding, rotation, torque or tipping or lateral displacement; to dental malformations such as hypoplasia, gemination, aplasia or hyperdontia; and with vertical or transverse discrepancies.

- Vertical discrepancies: As well as a deep bite (Fig. 18.4) there is an open bite (Fig. 18.5), which can occur both frontally and laterally and signifies a loss of contact between the upper and lower teeth.
- Transverse deviations: This includes lateral cross-bite and nonocclusion (Fig. 18.6).

DEVELOPMENT OF DENTITION AND THE JAW

Intrauterine development of dentition

Without going into detail of the embryologic craniofacial development, some significant contexts are described

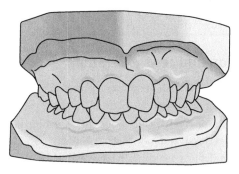

Figure 18.4 Deep bite. The upper incisors overlap the lower incisors by more than 2–3 mm.
With permission, Henriette Rintelen, Velbert

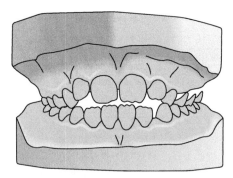

Figure 18.5 Frontal open bite. There is no contact between the upper and the lower teeth.
With permission, Henriette Rintelen, Velbert

which are important to the further understanding of this chapter.

The maxilla develops from a median process of the frontal bone and the two lateral maxillary processes. Whereas the

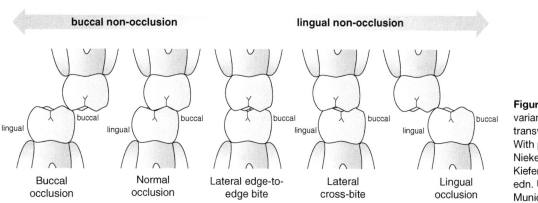

Figure 18.6 Occlusal variants in the transverse plane. With permission, Kahl-Nieke: Einführung in die Kieferorthopädie. 2nd edn. Urban & Fischer, Munich/Jena, 2001

process of the frontal bone forms the primary palate around the 5th week, the lateral maxillary processes are still in a vertical position on either side of the tongue. In the 7th to 8th week the tongue descends and the lateral processes of the maxilla become horizontal until they touch and form a common epithelium, which is then replaced by connective tissue. Palatal closure initially starts posteriorly from what will later become the incisive foramen; for about another 3 weeks the anterior part closes, depending on a further descent of the nasal septum and the median development of the lateral processes of the maxilla.

The development of the mandible is initiated by the spreading of the mandibular nerve. The Meckel cartilage sets the blueprint for ossification; together with the malleus and incus this cartilage forms the primary temporomandibular joint (TMJ). In the 8th week first jaw openings are performed with the help of the tensor tympani muscle (Sperber 1992). The development of the definitive TMJ does not begin until the 10th week, from temporal and a condylar cells independent of the Meckel cartilage, which then ceases to contribute to the actual development of the mandible. A large mandibular angle with a short ascending ramus and a small articular process are characteristic for the embryologic mandible.

Because the maxilla and mandible differ in the course of their growth, the relation of the jaws change within the uterus, from an embryonic retrusion of the mandible via an edge-to-edge bite to a mandibular protrusion; a prenatal growth of the maxilla causes this protrusion to develop into a second embryonic retrusion. Temporary transverse cross-bites can develop because space is becoming increasingly restricted. Mostly they correct themselves spontaneously after birth (Kahl-Nieke 2001).

In the development of the teeth, the ectoderm is responsible for the formation of the enamel, the neural crest cells for the dentine and pulp tissue. The tooth cement and the periodontium originate from the mesenchym.

Odontogenesis begins about 30 to 40 days after conception with epithelial thickenings on the maxillary and mandibular

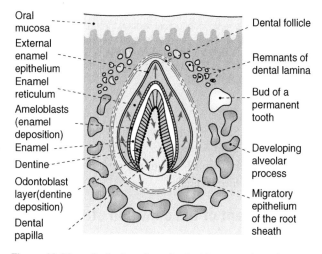

Figure 18.7 Longitudinal section of a deciduous tooth under development showing the direction of growth of the various dental tissues.
With permission, Henriette Rintelen, Velbert

processes which unite to the dental lamina. Ectodermal eversions of the dental lamina become the enamel organ, which develops via a bud and cap stage into the bell stage. In this phase, between the external and internal enamel epithelium there is a reticular tissue with star-shaped cells in a liquid matrix. Ameloblasts of the internal enamel epithelium are responsible for the formation of the enamel. The enamel organ encloses the dental papilla of the neural crest cells; both together are enclosed within small mesodermal dental follicles. At the junction of the dental papilla and the internal enamel epithelium, odontoblasts form for the development of dentine (Fig. 18.7). After tooth eruption intradental osteopathic treatment is possible because of the liquid precursors of enamel and dentine.

An epithelial lamina arises at the junction of the external and internal enamel epithelium. It encloses the papilla more and more and thus contributes to root formation. The dental follicle provides the basis of the tooth cement which surrounds the root. Adjacent mesenchymal tissue differentiates itself in association with the tooth cement into the periodontal collagen

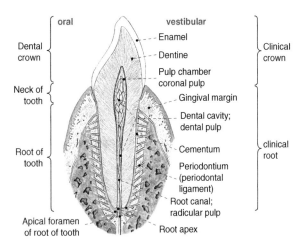

Figure 18.8 Schematic longitudinal section through an incisor with the tissues enamel, cementum, dentine and pulp (pulpa dentis). With permission, Sobotta: Atlas der Anatomie des Menschen. Publisher: R. Putz and R. Pabst, 21st edn. Elsevier/Urban & Fischer, Munich/Jena, 2000

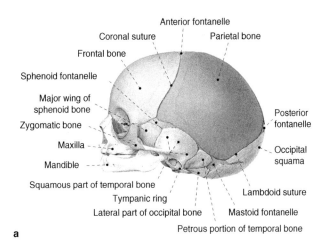

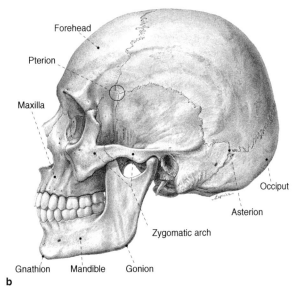

Figure 18.9 The extent of growth-related changes in the mandible is made clear by comparing a lateral view of a child's cranium **a:** with that of an adult cranium **b:**
With permission, Sobotta: Atlas der Anatomie des Menschen. Publisher: R. Putz and R. Pabst, 21st edn. Elsevier/Urban & Fischer, Munich/Jena, 2000

fibres (Fig. 18.8). While the deciduous teeth are developing (their mineralization begins in the 17th week), the permanent teeth emerge further orally out of the permanent tooth ridge and the molars further distally.

Development of the dentition after birth

At birth the physiological mandibular retrusion is about 4 mm. A functional stimulus for remodelling the initial retrusion is provided by feeding as the baby is moving his mandible forward in a milking motion (Hotz 1970). This process comes to an end at the time of the first dental eruption at around 6 months.

Between the 2nd and 3rd year eruption of the deciduous teeth is completed. During later development, gaps form between the front teeth, and these gaps are important in providing the extra space needed for the permanent teeth. The deciduous dentition period merges into the early mixed dentition phase with the eruption of the 6-year molars and the shedding of the front teeth. A pause of 18 months to 2 years in the eruption of the permanent teeth usually follows. This is succeeded by the late mixed dentition phase with the eruption of the canines, premolars and the 2nd molars, which is completed on average in the 12th year. The wisdom teeth often follow between the 17th and 22nd years, unless they are impacted because of lack of space or abnormal position. Wide variations between individuals are common during the mixed dentition period. In general girls are 3 to 6 months earlier than boys.

With the eruption of the molars, bite openings are physiological. The distance between the base of the maxilla and that of the mandible increases. The first physiological bite opening takes place during the eruption of the deciduous teeth, the second when the 6-year molars appear and the third with the shedding of the premolars and the eruption of the second molars.

In general there is vertical growth of the mid-face and lower face with a lengthening and broadened ascending mandibular ramus, a smaller mandibular angle and a functionally driven development of the fossa and the condyle in the TMJ (Fig. 18.9). From the 6th year onwards, until the eruption of the premolars and canines, the mid-face and lower face are largely determined in growth by the developing teeth.

Without going into detail about the complex growth processes in the face (they are described in detail by Enlow

1989), the concept of growth partners of Enlow (1989) is especially important from the osteopathic point of view. 'This is only intended to state that the growth of one cranial or facial part corresponds with certain other structural and geometric partners in the face and the skull. The maxillary and mandibular arches are growth partners, as are the anterior cranial fossa, the maxilla and the palate and also the middle cranial fossa and the ascending mandibular ramus with the pharyngeal space.'

Etiology of malocclusion

'From this I deduce that a malocclusion is the effect rather than the cause.' (Magoun 1962).

'The bone itself does not grow at all; its growth is induced through the matrix of soft tissues which encloses the entire bone. The genetic and functional determinants of bone growth are found in the soft tissues. Growth is not programmed in the calcified parts of the bone. The plan for the design, construction and growth of the bone lies in the interplay of muscles, tongue, lips, cheeks, skin, mucous membrane, connective tissue, nerves, blood vessels, airways, pharynx, the brain in its entirety, the glands, etc.' (Enlow 1989).

Osteopathic view

Magoun (1962) describes the following important causes of malformations of the jaw and dysfunctions of the stomatognathic system.

Starting with intrauterine cranial development, trauma during pregnancy or birth can impair the form or the growth development of the cranial bones in their membranous or cartilaginous precursor. Also non-physiological tension of the reciprocal tension membrane can be a major factor. Magoun names in particular (1962):

- restricted intrauterine space, as with twins, tumours or a deformed pelvis – can compress the fetal skull and deform it.
- changes in the skull at birth due to excessive forces of labor with the child being in an unfavourable presentation, improper use of instruments, an excessively rapid or lengthy labor.
- falls and trauma after birth, which can impair growth or function at a period of rapid development.

Early treatment of the membranes and of the precursors of the later cranial bones can stop or prevent later effects on jaw development. Even developmental dysfunctions of the jaw, such as mouth breathing (see below), result from the processes outlined above and are not the primary causes of an anomaly.

Transverse compression compromises the function of the nose and sphenopalatine ganglion so that it weakens immunity and thus increases susceptibility to allergies and other diseases of the nasal passages.

Persistent movement patterns of the skull over a long period will also affect growth and jaw development. The following examples are listed in the literature.

- An external rotation of the temporal bones is followed by a displacement of the mandibular fossa posteriorly and thus to a mandibular retrusion (Magoun 1962, Jecmen 1995, 2001).
- Conversely, an internal rotation of the temporal bones can also be associated with a forward displacement of the mandible, even to a class III relationship.
- A hyperflexion of the SBS leads to a broad maxilla with retrusion of the front teeth and mandibular retrusion, i.e. Angle's classification II$_2$ (Jecmen 1996) via the connection between the sphenoid bone, the palatine bone to the maxilla and by the occiput–temporal bone–mandible connection.
- An extension in the upper quadrant (e.g. in the case of a sphenoid in a high vertical strain) can be expressed as a narrow maxilla with protruding front teeth (Jecmen 1996).
- Torsions and side-bending rotations are manifested as jaw asymmetries, sometimes even as a lateral cross-bite, or unilateral displacement of a canine due to crowding in that half of the maxilla which is more in external rotation, and also with midline discrepancies.

Orthodontic view

The literature on dentofacial orthopedics also cites traumatic labor as a cause of jaw malformations (Bahnemann 1992). Disorders such as hyperdontia, hypodontia and impaired tooth shape, can to some extent be genetic in origin as well as class-III and class II$_2$ malocclusion.

Caries with premature loss of tooth substance or even the loss of the deciduous teeth can lead to migration of the permanent teeth, crowding, tipping and rotations of the teeth. To prevent malocclusion good dental care of the deciduous dentition is therefore mandatory.

One other important area is that of myofunctional dyskinesias. These are malfunctions of the stomatognathic muscles and are involuntary in nature. If they are the cause of a malocclusion they are termed primary; as a reaction to malocclusion they are secondary.

Visceral swallowing is the term for the persistent early childhood swallowing pattern past the 4th year of life. In toothless babies, the tongue lies between the alveolar ridges, the tip of the tongue lying in front. The oral muscles and the contact between tongue tip and lips stabilize the mandible during swallowing. As the deciduous dentition develops, the act of swallowing develops over time into somatic swallowing, in which the teeth touch each other, the tongue lies within the mouth behind the dental arches and rolls down dorsally, and the lips form an unforced seal. If this transition does not occur, the tongue is pressed between the teeth. As the dental arches do not close the oral cavity, the lips have to take over and this is manifested as an increased activity of the orbicular muscle of the mouth. As people swallow about 1800 times in 24 hours, a massive pressure is exerted on the teeth each time, both from the tongue and from the lips and cheeks. Possible consequences are an open bite, which can be lateral or frontal depending on the site of the tongue (Fig. 18.10), also an unnaturally narrow jaw, formed by the external compression of the soft tissues and the lack of the stimulus of tongue pressure on the transverse development in the maxilla.

The sucking of thumbs, fingers, dummies or other objects can cause an open bite and can deform the jaws, particularly the maxilla. If children can drop this habit by the end of the 3rd year, self-correction often occurs. A shield lying in the buccal parts of the oral cavity has often proved useful in the transition of giving up sucking a dummy or the thumb as it does not impair the position of the teeth and at the same time trains lip closure (Fig. 18.11).

Further myofunctional habits are sucking, biting and pressing the lips; sucking or biting the cheeks; or increased activity of the mentalis muscle. It must be especially emphasized that a lack of a competent lip seal is followed by insufficient nose breathing and habitual mouth breathing. Characteristics are a slightly open mouth and hypotonic cheek and lip muscles, which compress the jaws to the consequence of narrow arches and crowding. The tongue lies either behind the lower incisors or is flat and retracted. Cross-bites or distal occlusion can develop (Fig. 18.12). Often the habitual mouth-breathing is associated with visceral swallowing. In addition, as the accessory muscles of respiration are insufficiently used, a postural weakness in the head, neck and shoulders occurs. As the air

in inspiration does not reach the nasal mucosa the cleansing effect of the ciliary epithelium and of the immunoglobulin A on the mucosa is deficient. The immune response is transferred to the pharynx and the bronchi. Instead pathogenic bacteria can grow on the nasal mucosa and start a vicious circle of nasal infections and increased susceptibility to allergies. (Hotz 1970, Garry 1995, Kahl-Nieke 2001). Further consequences which have been described are sleep disturbances, fatigue on waking, impaired attentiveness and reduced oxygen levels in the blood (Annunciato 2002). Besides habitual mouth-breathing, constitutional mouth-breathing has been described in the literature: exhibiting narrowed nasal passages accompanied by enlarged adenoids and tonsils. The clinical symptoms are otherwise identical to the picture described above.

Dysostoses, some syndromes and developmental anomalies are a further etiological factor in malocclusions. The syndromes include Apert, Down and Pierre-Robin and the dysostoses can be cleidocranial, craniofacial, mandibulofacial, mandibular or otomandibular. Other anomalies are oculoauricular dysplasia, facial hemihypertrophy, cleft lip, cleft jaw and cleft palate.

Without going into further detail about this very broad topic, a few characteristic features of jaw development in

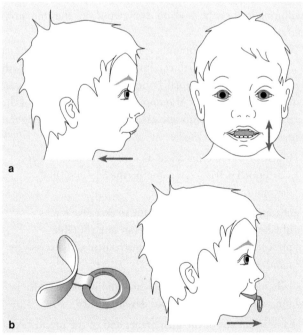

Figure 18.11 a: Increased overjet in the deciduous dentition due to mandibular retrusion and sucking and lip habit; **b:** the insertion of an appliance for the external oral cavity leads to a forward thrust movement of the mandible, the lower lip pressure is reduced and the body of the dummy cannot be embedded.
With permission, Kahl-Nieke: Einführung in die Kieferorthopädie. 2nd edn. Urban & Fischer, Munich/Jena, 2001

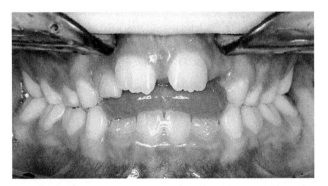

Figure 18.10 Open bite with tongue thrust due to a persistent visceral swallowing pattern.
With permission, Kahl-Nieke: Einführung in die Kieferorthopädie. 2nd edn. Urban & Fischer, Munich/Jena, 2001

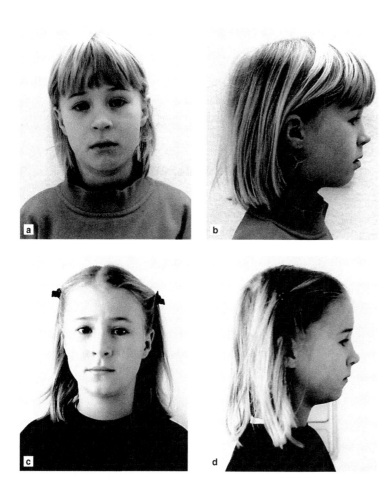

Figure 18.12 a, b: Girl 8 years of age with left-sided cross-bite and habitual mouth breathing before treatment. **c, d:** Result after correction of the cross-bite followed by myofunctional treatment from a speech therapist to correct the swallowing pattern and to develop a good lip seal.
With permission, Ariane Hesse, Hamburg

Down syndrome will be mentioned here. The general muscular hypotonia also extends to the orofacial region. Without treatment, this results in an open mouth with mouth breathing and a hypotonic and seemingly over-large tongue. The palate is underdeveloped transversely and sagittally, with the development of a step shape leaving no room for the tongue. The relative underdevelopment of the maxilla causes a pseudo-prognathism of the mandible to develop. Usually, the eruption of the permanent teeth is delayed and there can be hypodontia. The narrow maxilla also predisposes to massive crowding. For many children, a functional Castillo-Morales therapy using special functional appliances, with interdisciplinary collaboration between the orthodontist, the physiotherapist and pediatrician, can alleviate the symptoms and even bring about a habitual lip seal. This therapy should start in early infancy.

TEMPOROMANDIBULAR JOINT DISORDERS

The normal physiological relationship between the mandibular fossa, the condyle and the disc in the TMJ is shown in Figure 18.13. The disc should be situated at a 12 o'clock position on the condyle. The pain-sensitive dorsal bilaminar zone, with the

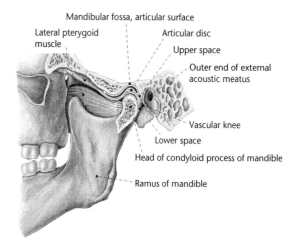

Mandibular fossa, articular surface
Lateral pterygoid muscle
Articular disc
Upper space
Outer end of external acoustic meatus
Vascular knee
Lower space
Head of condyloid process of mandible
Ramus of mandible

Figure 18.13 Temporomandibular joint with bilaminar zone (sagittal section, lateral view).
With permission, Sobotta: Atlas der Anatomie des Menschen. Publisher: R. Putz and R. Pabst, 21st edn. Elsevier/Urban & Fischer, Munich/Jena, 2000

stratum superior, stratum inferior and the genu vasculosum with its good nerve supply, are not compressed.

Magnetic resonance images of children aged between 2 months and 5 years show this picture with a low probability of disc displacement (Isberg 2001). Between the 8th and 15th year the proportion of asymptomatic and symptomatic disc displacements rises to about 6%. Asymptomatic displacements are about twice as common in women as in men; this applies both to adolescents and to adults. In patients with TMJ symptoms such as clicking, pain or limitation of movement, and a radiologically-confirmed disc displacement, women are 4 to 6 times more commonly represented than men. According to Isberg, there is a peak in the development of displacements, one at puberty in both girls and boys and another in the 3rd and 4th decades in women. Potential predisposing factors are an increased laxity and the presence of certain collagens in the tissues. Trauma and deep bites can play a part but the precise multifactorial mechanisms have not yet been fully explained.

Even in children and adolescents inflammations of the joint capsule and of the bilaminar zone (capsulitis) and myopathies can occur. A functional compression in the TMJ with the above symptoms can be caused by the absence of the vertical dimension in deep bite or the dorsal position of the mandible when the upper incisors are retruded.

A transverse discrepancy with, for example, a cross-bite or other reasons for early tooth contacts can cause a muscular displacement of the mandible, with the lateral pterygoid muscle functionally shortened on one side. Although there are no other clinical symptoms apart from a deviation or deflection in mouth opening, this should be noted and treated by orthodontists in respect to further growth development, not only in the jaws but also in the whole body.

PRINCIPLES OF TREATMENT IN ORTHODONTICS

In planning treatment, a case history is taken and the following clinical records: examination of the bite and oral cavity; a survey of dyskinesias; an assessment of swallowing pattern and of tongue function, mandibular movements and speech, a manual examination of the TMJ and the muscles of mastication. Positional asymmetries in general and orthopedic tests for the function of the pelvis have started to be a regular routine for more orthodontists than previously. Also included are plaster models of the jaw, frontal and profile photos, a panoramic view of both jaws and a lateral cephalometric radiograph; the information provided by this last includes the sagittal relations between maxilla and mandible, between the jaws and the base of the skull, the position and inclination of the front teeth. It provides information about the expected growth pattern and thus about the expected changes in growth. This is done by a cephalometric analysis measuring various angles and stretches on the radiograph and relating them to one another. As the radiographs are taken from some distance (1.5 m), and in a defined position, the X-rays

are approximately parallel. This allows the comparison of the cephalometric analysis of one patient during his treatment.

There are two distinct main principles in dentofacial orthopedic treatment: functional dentofacial orthopedics and orthodontics. They can be applied individually and in isolation, or in combination, and have their specific indications.

Functional dentofacial orthopedics

Functional dentofacial orthopedics is understood as the functional reshaping of the structures of soft and hard tissues of the stomatognathic system by utilizing growth.

It mainly employs removable bimaxillary appliances which are inserted between the maxilla and mandible, thus changing their spatial interrelationship. Protruding the mandible creates a larger vertical and, if necessary, a readjustment of the midline, while the appliance is worn; new neuromuscular patterns create functional forces used in the remodelling of tissues. These functional forces act directly on the sutures, base of the jaws, alveolar processes and the teeth. Muscle tension can be influenced by shields and loops, thus changing the alveolar and skeletal growth.

All devices in dentofacial orthopedics also influence the motion patterns of the cranium. For example moving the mandible forward exerts traction on the temporal bone, which rotates more internally so that the mandibular fossa is displaced further forward. How far this mechanism is efficient in the correction of a Class II relationship has not yet been investigated. A vertical adjustment of this device can also affect the position and function of C1 and thus the vertebral column.

The best-known appliances, apart from the classic Andresen/ Häupl activator, are the Bimler bite trainer, the Stockfisch Kinetor, the Balters Bionator, the Klammt elastic-open activator, and the Fränkel function regulator, which shifts the active elements mainly into the vestibular space between lips, cheeks and teeth. Meanwhile, principles of functional dentofacial orthopedics are also incorporated into single appliances (e.g. the Twin-Block) or in fixed mechanisms (Herbst hinge, Jusper Jumper, SUS spring, and similar).

Orthodontics

In orthodontics active mechanical forces are used to change the tooth position or the size of a jaw. A profound understanding of the biomechanics of orthodontic appliances is mandatory. The difference between functional orthodontics and dentofacial orthodontics can be explained from the example of jaw stretching. Whereas in functional orthodontics the jaw is expanded indirectly through the development of growth by modified soft tissue function, in dentofacial orthodontics the jaw is expanded directly by mechanical means. Amongst other reasons, a dentofacial orthodontic mechanism is needed for the direct correction of torsion, rotation or positional changes of the teeth within the jaw. The therapeutic devices employed are removable appliances, such as the Schwartz appliance, and fixed appliances, such as the Multiband-Multibracket systems. The advantage of fixed appliances in comparison to removable ones is that they can move the teeth bodily through the bone; that is, they can bring about parallel displacement or modify the position of the root of the tooth.

To enable these mechanisms to function, each movement needs a point of resistance for stability, or, as orthodontists call it, anchorage. The teeth or groups of teeth which take on the anchorage are the more immobile part in the system of treatment. This leads to a reduced space for movement within the socket, which is manifested throughout the skull as a relative limitation of movement. This is fully justified if the patient's functional condition allows for good compensation before the appliance is incorporated. This disadvantage can be warded off to some extent by concomitant osteopathic treatment (see p.433) and small modifications of the appliances. In the long run the benefit of a good function in occlusion in accordance to the function of the whole body is an important factor to ensure free and living motion of the skull. In many patients orthodontic mechanics may be the only possibility to come to a satisfactory result.

In some cases when the task of anchorage is extremely difficult, extraoral appliances may be used. The best known is the headgear with a face bow fixed on molar bands or a removable appliance. The external force pulls either from the cervical neck or more situated in a vertical pull from the vertex of the skull. As the force of the cervical headgear acts via the palatine bones and the sphenoid and via the occiput directly on the SBS, it should only be used with the greatest caution, and if no other form of anchorage is available.

In mandibular prognathism, a face mask, which is supported either on the chin (Délaire mask) or on the zygomatic arch (Grummons mask) has proved useful. At the first sight this seems to be a troublesome treatment, but it makes sense if the goal is to avoid surgical treatment later as it is very effective and helps to open the mid-face bones.

To make a fixed multi-bracket appliance more mobile, wire loops can be inserted or the wire may be cut down to two or three segments. Removable appliances for the maxilla can be separated in the middle and kept together with a coffin spring, which allows sufficient leeway for extension and flexion of the maxilla. For osteopathic use especially, Nordstrom (Smith 1998) has developed the Advanced Light Functional (ALF), an appliance made out of very thin wires. This is particularly helpful in resolving limitations of movement of the skull which also manifest themselves positionally in the jaw. A multibracket appliance is usually indicated after this for finishing adjustment of the teeth.

Start and progress of treatment

The start of dentofacial orthopedic or orthodontic treatment depends on the clinical records, the goal of treatment, the appliances planned and, very essentially, on the motivation of the patient and her family. If a functional orthopedic approach is to be taken, it is advisable to start in the 2nd phase of mixed dentition. Where marked dysfunctions are to be treated, an earlier start may be considered (i.e. approximately at the age of 9–11 years). If the plan is to use fixed appliances only, it is usually necessary to wait until the second dentition has fully erupted. Many orthodontists follow a two-phase process. First, the relationship between the jaws is changed and space is created if needed with functional removable appliances. In the second phase the occlusion is adjusted with a multi-bracket appliance. The outcome of treatment should always be maintained by appliances worn at night after the active treatment has been completed. In adults a lifelong retention is mandatory.

Early treatments before 9 years old are always indicated if the position of the teeth considerably impairs function or if the malocclusion will be more difficult to be corrected with advanced growth. This applies to frontal and lateral cross bites, especially if they force the mandible into a muscle dysfunction, and also for extreme retrusions of the jaw. With regard to the total period of treatment, early treatments should always be limited in time. Starting early is also indicated for mandibular prognathism, cleft lip, alveolar or palatal cleft patients, Down syndrome and other syndromes.

If there are myofunctional habits such as sucking, visceral swallowing or mouth breathing, consideration should be given to recommending treatment with a speech therapist or an ENT specialist before orthodontic treatment.

One variant of early treatment – build-ups on the deciduous molars – is described at p.433, as this procedure is directly connected with an osteopathic procedure.

Extracting deciduous teeth can sometimes help to control the eruption of the permanent teeth. The removal of permanent teeth to create space cannot always be avoided and remains as controversial as ever. An extraction further back in the dental arch (wisdom teeth, 2nd molars) has the advantage to secure the natural jaw size in growth. For some years new kinds of biomechanics in fixed appliances have been developed that enhance skeletal growth in the alveolar process, so that extractions can be avoided more and more.

Finally, attention should be given to the combination of orthodontics and orthognathic surgery. These complex treatments are carried out for severe malocclusions (such as Class III, open bite) and for certain treatments in adulthood and should always be accompanied by, and followed up with, osteopathy.

TEAMWORK BETWEEN THE OSTEOPATH AND ORTHODONTIST

Orthodontic treatments are often associated with considerable positional changes of the jaw and thus with craniofacial changes. This presents both an opportunity and a risk for the function of the body as a whole. Sometimes considerable advances in osteopathic treatment can be made by an orthodontic intervention; for example the correction of a lateral cross bite or a deep bite. On the other hand if changes in the orthodontic field are not integrated in the overall function of the body, restrictions and malfunction can be the consequence.

If the involuntary movement in the cranium can express itself unrestrictedly, possible temporary stresses from orthodontic appliances can be sufficiently compensated. It is therefore sensible to check this before starting the orthodontic treatment.

Tests that offer an insight in the functional interweaving between the occlusion and the body function are the key for a successful teamwork between both disciplines.

Test procedures

The following diagnostic procedure has proved helpful in assessing the effect of the occlusion on the body's static state and function.

In the first step, the clinical assessment of posture is performed in an upright standing position, then the quality and expression of the PRM, SBS movement pattern, tension of the RTM, position of C1, sacroiliac joint function, leg length in the supine position or any other clinical findings the osteopath thinks helpful are evaluated. In the second step, the occlusion and position of the TMJ is changed by inserting a cotton roll on both sides of the mouth between the rows of teeth. The patient then swallows and walks a few steps, thus reorienting his neuromuscular system to the new bite position and to the altered situation of the TMJ. The examination is repeated with the altered bite position. If pre-existing limitations of movement have been removed and asymmetries reduced, the bite has a decisive influence on function as a whole. The problem is then described as descending. The situation is an ascending one if the altered position does not bring about a functional or positional improvement. Osteopathic treatment with any change in the occlusion will be sufficient. This test was first developed by the chiropractor Meersseman and is named after him.

For getting more accurate records concerning the vertical dimension of the occlusion, midline correction and anterior-posterior position of the lower jaw, thin pieces of dental wax or paper strips can be used. Similarly, occlusal splints, functional orthopedic appliances or the habitual occlusion can be tested for their effects on the PRM and on other functions. The testing process in detail is as follows.

In habitual occlusion: The initial assessment is made without occlusal contact by asking the patient to close her lips lightly while leaving some space between the teeth. Then ask her to close her jaw and swallow and to walk a couple of steps. With the patient in a supine position you can flex and stretch the legs for pelvic movement with teeth in habitual occlusion. Swallowing and pelvic movement are necessary to transfer the neuromuscular program of the occlusion to the body. How have the initial records changed?

- Splint or functional orthopedic appliance: The splint or the appliances are inserted after the initial records, followed by re-orientation of the system by swallowing and pelvic movement. The initial tests are repeated.

- New mandibular position: By inserting wax plates or paper strips the vertical is changed until an improvement in function is palpable. The height can be different on each side, left and right. Does the finding improve if the skeletal midline is also adjusted or the mandible is pushed forward? With retrusion of the upper front teeth: what happens if the patient 'thinks' his upper incisors forward?

Anatomical–physiological correlations

The way these tests work can be explained on an anatomical and physiological basis.

- Through intercuspation the occlusal surfaces stimulate proprioceptive information to the periodontium of the teeth. In a full dentition the occlusion can be regarded as a joint with 16 surfaces.

- A new more forward position of the mandible exerts a traction on the TMJ, its ligaments and muscles (masseter, temporal and lateral pterygoid). By the concomitant change in proprioceptive information in these tissues a possible pathologic influence for a functional compression of the joint may be interrupted.

- The neurological information described above passes through the maxillary and mandibular divisions of the trigeminal nerve. This nerve does not only receive information from various cranial nerves (VII, IX, X, XI and XII), but is also connected with afferent branches from the cervical spine within the sensorius principalis nucleus (Bumann 2000).

- Biomechanically, habitual occlusion determines the position of the mandible in the TMJ and the base of the skull, independent of the muscles, and also determines the position of the maxilla. In dentistry very little attention has yet been paid to the latter. The case history below describes this correlation and its implications. The position of the maxilla influences the sphenoid bone directly through the palatine bones, as the position of the mandible relates to the occiput via the temporal bones. Thus the SBS can be supported or disturbed by occlusion.

- The following hypothesis is put forward by the American dentist Gerry Smith: All vertebrae have three supporting surfaces, the lateral articulations and the vertebral body. Only the atlas has two supporting surfaces through the condyles. Occlusion can be seen as the third supporting surface (workshop 1999).

- From the orthopedic point of view the TMJ can also be seen as the 'top joint of the head' (Kopp in Ahlers 2000).

A practical example will make these theoretical reflections easier to understand.

Case study
A 14-year-old boy came to my practice with severe backache in the sacrum and lumbar spine. He had a dysfunction of the left sacroiliac joint which could not be treated by osteopathy alone; this and a lateral side-bending rotation of the SBS to the left, associated with a low position of C1 on the left, were corrected merely with a vertical elevation of the bite by two strips of paper inserted on the left side of the dental row. This unilateral elevation erased the side-bending of the maxilla and the base of the skull, and C1 became balanced as well, together with the sacroiliac joint. This slight unilateral elevation was transferred to the permanent dentition by bonded acrylic build-ups and accompanied by osteopathic treatment. The patient was almost free of symptoms after only 2 weeks of the 6-month course of therapy.

The acrylic build-ups were successively ground down, starting with the molars, so that the posterior teeth could extrude into the new level.

Occlusion-related correlations

Unilateral tooth loss reduces the support of the maxilla. The bone tilts and consequently so does the sphenoid bone. The skull generally compensates by torsion or side-bending rotation and corresponding adjustments in the vertebral column. This occurs temporarily in children in the second phase of tooth eruption in the premolar and molar region. With the new teeth in occlusion the skull becomes balanced again.

If the vertical is too low in a deep bite, the vertical for the atlas is often lacking, so that the vertebra cannot position itself symmetrically. A vertical elevation creates the space which makes this possible. While a splint tends to be used for adults, functional orthopedic appliances are used for children. However, with bite elevation care should be taken to ensure that the membranes can cope with the change. If it is too much a strong dural tension will develop, which leads to a general limitation of the expression of the PRM. It is sometimes necessary to elevate the occlusal plane in several steps to allow the membranes to adapt. This can also be supported by adjunctive osteopathic treatments. With small children needing orthodontic therapy, the vertical can be corrected by acrylic build-ups on the deciduous molars. Over time, the 6-year molars grow into the new level. This procedure has also proved helpful with children with frequent attacks of middle ear inflammation. The increased vertical creates a greater inclination of the eustachian tube, allowing for better drainage (Dean 1994).

Retruded front teeth can force the mandible into a more dorsal position than is good for the patient. If the retrusion is accompanied with a deep bite, as in Angle's Class II$_2$, the mandibular condyle is higher up in the mandibular fossa. This can lead to painful compression of the pain-sensitive bilaminar zone of the TMJ. Also, the two temporal bones are held in external rotation. In the upper jaw the premaxilla is in a relatively dorsal position, thus hindering the free movement of the maxilla and the mid-face. If the patients only imagine their front teeth further forward, there is often a spontaneous improvement in expression of the PRM. This is an indication to protrude the front teeth orthodontically.

Cross-bites can cause a lateral strain by forcing the mandible to one side and the maxilla to the other (Fig. 18.14). Lateral cross-bites are usually associated with asymmetries in body statics, as the functional asymmetry of the base of the skull is projected on further downwards. During and after correction of the malocclusion, osteopathic monitoring and treatment is necessary to integrate the craniofacial changes into the body function and to remove habitual muscular compensations which are no longer needed once the cross-bite has been corrected.

Besides cross-bite, an early tooth contact with a side shift of the mandible can cause a lateral strain in the habitual occlusion. Often, buccal pre-contacts on the lower teeth or on splints are responsible.

In an open bite the lateral support as a whole is missing and an extremely wide variety of compensatory patterns can develop. If in testing the open bite is temporarily bridged with paper strips or wax, there is often a remarkable functional or static adjustment.

These mechanisms occur in children just as they do in adults. On the other hand, because children have a greater

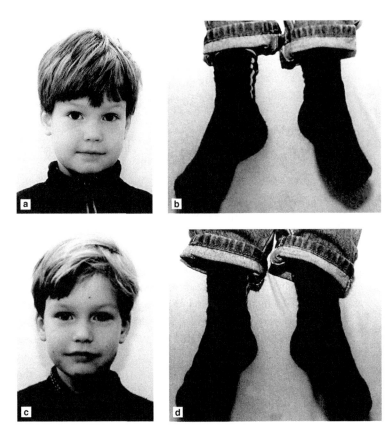

Figure 18.14 a: A 4-year-old boy before treatment, with lateral cross-bite on the right and a midline shift of the mandible to the right. In the SBS he shows a lateral strain on the left in occlusion with descending effect on the cervical spine and the pelvis; **b:** the pelvic tilt is also manifested in the difference in leg lengths; **c:** the same boy after treatment; **d:** with the insertion of the bite plane, the difference in leg length has also disappeared. With permission, Ariane Hesse, Hamburg

ability to compensate, they usually show no pain symptoms or less marked pain symptoms. For prophylactic reasons, however, these mechanisms should be attended to by the orthodontic treatment. It requires interdisciplinary collaboration, in which the osteopath plays an important role in both diagnostic procedures and treatment.

Osteopathy accompanying orthodontic treatment

The following procedures have been proved helpful in practice:

- Releasing the SBS before the construction bite for a functional orthopedic appliance and subsequent control of it.

- Treatment of the membranes and mid-face with special attention to the vomer, zygomatic bone and palatine bones after inserting a new appliance, eventually with the appliance in situ.

- Treatment of the premaxilla up to its junction with the frontal bone in connection with positional changes on the upper front teeth.

- To avoid a fixation of the sphenoid in all movements of the molars in a caudal direction, treatment of the palatine bones in regular sequences. This is mandatory if a headgear is being used.

- With rigid anchorage arches on the maxilla, with problems with individual teeth or groups of teeth, an intraosseous

treatment is helpful. Treatment of the individual tooth is particularly important here. It can be done by treating the ligaments of the periodont. However, it is also possible to treat the tissues of the teeth, like the pulp, dentine and enamel, intradentally with reference to the embryonic tooth organ in its bell stage. For this, one should first make contact with the tooth hanging in its ligaments. Then follow through the different tissues, by visualizing the bell stage of the embryologic development and addressing the growth potential of the tooth as a whole. This treatment approach can also support dental treatment in traumatic injuries to the deciduous and permanent teeth.

Thus osteopathy can help orthodontic treatments to be carried out with the least pressure on the tissues as possible and can contribute to the integration of the occlusion in to the function as a whole. Orthodontics can frequently assist in decisively improving the baseline conditions for a free expression of the PRM.

Bibliography

Ahlers M O, Jakstat H: Klinische Funktionsanalyse. dentaConcept, Hamburg 2000

Annunciato N: Fortbildungsaufzeichnungen: Neuroanatomie der Formatio Reticularis und des Limbischen Systems. Hamburg 2002

Ash M, Ramfjord S, Schmidseder J: Schienentherapie. Urban & Schwarzenberg, Munich 1995

Bahnemann F: Anthropologische Grundlagen einer Ganzheitsmedizin. Haug, Heidelberg 1992

Bahnemann F: Der Bionator in der Kieferorthopädie. Haug, Heidelberg 1993

Bumann A, Lotzmann U: Funktionsdiagnostik und Therapieprinzipien. Thieme, Stuttgart/New York 2000

Dean R: A possible connection between the temporomandibular joint and middle ear symptoms in children. Cranio-View 3(3), 1994: 47–55

Enlow D: Handbuch des Gesichtswachstums. Quintessenz, Berlin 1989

Garry J: Upper airway compromise and musculo-skeletal dysfunction of the head and neck. Self-published, Fullerton, Calif. 1995

Hotz R: Orthodontie in der täglichen Praxis. 4th edition, Huber, Berne 1970

Isberg A: Temporomandibular joint dysfunction. Isis Medical Media 2001

Jecmen J: Understanding malocclusion. Cranio-View, Cranio-View 4(2), 1995: 9–32

Jecmen J: The temporal bone as it relates to occlusion. Cranio-View 10(3), 2001: 14–19

Kahl-Nieke B: Einführung in die Kieferorthopädie. 2nd edn. Urban & Fischer, Munich/Jena 2001

Magoun H: Osteopathy in the cranial field. 3rd edn. Sutherland Cranial Teaching Foundation, Texas 1976

Magoun H: Osteopathic approach to dental enigmas. Journal of the American Osteopathic Association 62, 1962: 110–118

Ramfjord S, Ash M: Occlusion. 3rd edn. Saunders, Philadelphia 1983

Schreiber E: Der Einfluss osteopathischer Behandlungen bei Patienten mit Okklusionsstörung und kieferorthopädischer Versorgung. Diploma dissertation for the title of doctor of osteopathy, Hamm, August 2000

Schumacher G-H: Anatomie für Zahnmediziner. 3rd edn. Hüthig, Heidelberg 1997

Smith G: Alternative treatments for conquering chronic pain. CD Version 1.3. self-published, Langhorne, Pa., July 1998

Sperber G, Arnold W H: Embryologie des Kopfes. Quintessenz, Berlin 1992

19

Speech therapy

Sigrid Graumann-Brunt, Noori Mitha

Disorders of language development are often found in young children. A very large investigation of 6-year-olds, taking place between 1986 and 1991, showed that in only 53% was it possible to rule out an articulation disorder (Graumann-Brunt 1999). Moderate abnormalities were still found in 22% of the children, serious ones in 4%, and this was without taking any account of deficits in grammar and vocabulary. These findings show that developmental language disorders are a problem in a large group of children, and coping with them has become a matter of general concern.

WHAT DO WE MEAN BY LANGUAGE?

Sigrid Graumann-Brunt

Mass studies (for an explanation of this term, see: Reulecke and Rollett 1982) concentrate on expression and consequently the quality of articulation, because pronunciation is a key stimulus in assessing linguistic interactions. We perceive the non-standard production of speech sounds as of primary significance; Bierkens (1968) even cites lisping as a classic example of a typical key stimulus. However, these key stimuli can lead us astray because they are apt to divert our attention from more important matters. The content of an utterance is more important than whether pronunciation is standard or speech fluent. Language, the most important means of human communication, serves to transmit content and requires much more than just accepted standards of articulation. Besides grammar and vocabulary, research interests in language therefore cover questions of pragmatics, psycholinguistics and sociolinguistics (Funkkolleg 1987) and other areas, including genetic drift. On the other hand, the ability to speak comprehensibly is so important that 'the presence of language, and thus the communicative function of language depend on the presence and functioning of the physics and physiology of speech sounds' (Pètursson and Neppert 1991).

We generally give little thought to the prerequisites for the functioning of our 'physics and physiology of speech sounds', or indeed to grammar and vocabulary. Certainly this is also because language is omnipresent in our modern world and it is so hard to imagine our everyday life without language that we take its presence for granted. We are hardly ever aware that

the ability to use language is quite a special attribute. Its many and various modes of expression can be expanded infinitely; it can develop and adapt and is a living thing. Pinker (1994) says that this 'remarkable ability of our species' enables us to 'shape events in each other's brains with exquisite precision'. A transfer of this sort is not bound by time and space. Language can bring life to earlier moments, and to places which are not present; through it, we can share other people's experiences and perceptions – even those of people long dead – and take on their painstakingly acquired knowledge and transmit it to other people, even to those yet unborn. Through language we communicate information from one person to another. Language therefore always contains a social component, even in the most academic of discussions. It is always an interaction between two people, a transmitter and a receiver, who debate the content. Although the individuals always see a topic of conversation differently because of their personal preconceptions and experiences, they have the option of using language to bring their different points of view closer together, to make themselves 'understood' to each other.

Making oneself understood through language is always an enormous achievement, physically, intellectually and socially. Pascher (1984) says that it draws on the highest functions of the human brain. The question of the nature of the cortical structure of grammar and of the mental lexicon of words has often been studied. The large number of reported cases with localized brain lesions justifies the presumption that a 'language center' exists (Pinker 1994). While the generation of grammatical structures is attributed to 'Broca's area', there are indications that the representation of individual words is scattered in various locations across the cortex, although verbs seem to lie closer to Broca's area. Some findings (Pinker 1994) and theories (McClelland and Elman 1986) suggest, however, that it is premature to regard this representation as being confined exclusively to one area.

THE PRODUCTION OF SPOKEN LANGUAGE

Sigrid Graumann-Brunt

The known facts about the cortical representation of speech sounds are as follows. Broca's area is cited as the center for their initiation, control and coordination (Pètursson and Neppert 1991). However, although motor aphasias have been diagnosed when there are lesions in that area, one cannot conclude from this fact alone that all the control processes involved in generating speech sounds operate there. On the basis of various case reports, it is presumed that there is another 'secondary motor language center, which lies in front of the upper part of the general motor center' and which can complement or even take over the functions of the Broca center in producing speech sounds (Pètursson and Neppert 1991). It is quite possible that this is where movements are coordinated to produce speech sounds. Another area, Wernicke's area, which is close to the ear, at the end of the Sylvian fissure, makes an essential contribution to recognizing sounds: the arcuate ligament serves to connect Wernicke's and Broca's areas. However, areas which represent functions contributing to language production are also found in other places in the cortex (Pinker 1994). Some interesting findings about the processing of vowels and consonants in the hemispheres also suggest that European language families are lateralized differently from the Austroasian/Japanese language families (Pètursson and Neppert 1991). However, these statements refer rather more to perception and cannot therefore simply be applied to language production.

Facial movements during the production of speech sounds have been described in detail by Wängler (1981), and reference is therefore made here to him and to Scholz (1982). They describe, with the utmost precision, the tasks of the active parts: 'mandible, tongue (front, center and back), lips, soft palate (including hyoid and epiglottis) and the passive parts: teeth, alveolar ridge and hard palate (Wängler 1981) – in producing all the sounds in the German language. Wängler does not count the vocal folds as tools of speech, although it is only through their vibrations that voiced sounds can be made. For some time, the question of the control and function of the movements of the vocal folds was hotly debated and made the subject of experiments (Sonninen 1996). Husson's idea, which sparked off the dispute, was that there is a cortical control of the movement of individual muscle fibres in the vocal folds, but this idea was ultimately discarded. Today, an explanation of the processes of phonation takes into account the effect of physical laws (suction or Bernoulli effect) with decreased pressure (closing the vocal folds) and increased pressure (the vocal folds part explosively) during speech (Pètursson and Neppert 1991).

Considerations about the nature of the control of speech movements led to the assumption that this followed a programme which contained entire 'movement complexes'. The organs and functional systems involved in forming sounds coordinate their activity independently. This theory seems plausible, 'as speaking is such a complex series of movements that it is inconceivable that each of the muscles which are moved is specifically and individually innervated. It is far more likely that each relevant programme is merely called upon and released for action. The individual muscles are not independent in these actions. They monitor and control one another, sometimes subordinating themselves and their functions to the greater process in its entirety' (Neppert and Pètursson 1986). The fact that demands are being made on primary systems, such as breathing, digestion and locomotion, to perform a secondary function adds to the complexity of the process. Although this form of regulation is economical, the failure of individual organs can lead to considerable difficulty in this mutual monitoring and control. In the autonomic region there is a 'double burden' during speaking, through the control of the basic autonomic functions on one hand and of secondary function in sound production on the other. This can cause speech to break down, especially in emotionally charged situations.

These demands on the systems involved in language production are made on the listener as well as the speaker because the smooth functioning of movement complexes is a prerequisite for listening as well as for speech. The sounds which reach the ear are indeed the most important sensory elements in decoding spoken language, but the listener also uses the speaker's facial movements to decode what is being said. Moreover, far more sensory areas are involved in decoding speech than might be apparent at first glance. There are indications that the listener imitates the speaker's actions (Graumann-Brunt 1999, Herrmann 1985). The speaker's eye in turn fixes its gaze on the listener and the speaker can detect, through eye contact, whether his interlocutor has 'understood' him. Thus, the process of communication uses other senses as well as hearing – vision and proprioception – and, the prerequisite for this, the vestibular sense.

LANGUAGE DEVELOPMENT

Sigrid Graumann-Brunt

Language and child development

Language development in childhood, as it is now understood in modern developmental psycholinguistics, is not an isolated process, but part of a comprehensive overall development. 'The acquisition of linguistic structures is integrated into a universal developmental plan consisting of sensory, motor, cognitive, emotional and socio-communicative functional areas which have a mutual effect on one another' (Grohnfeldt 1986). Pascher (1984) described the development of language as exceptionally complex. He said that 'it depends for its timely physiological development on the seamless interlinkage of other brain processes, which reach maturity in their turn: central processing of sensory impressions, development of intellectual abilities, of psychomotor function, of cerebrality and laterality. They mold the development of the child's personality in the many and various interactions between the child and its immediate and wider personal and social dependence and areas of reference.'

Zollinger (2002) looked at the development of language from the point of view of language use and the understanding of language as a 'connection between the personal and objective world' in a 'triangular relationship' between the child, the interlocutor and the object of negotiation. Here, the connection between language development and the child's overall development is made especially clear by the dependence of the content, nature and meaning of the conversation on the stage of the child's development. She described in great detail the connections between the course of development in the practical-gnostic, symbolic and sociocommunicative area and that of language from the 9th month of the child's development; for further information, please refer to her (Zollinger 2002).

However, important prerequisites for the use of language are created at a much earlier stage in a child's development. An investigation of disorders in the use of language will uncover delays or impairments in the course of neurophysiological development. For instance, communication is impaired if poor control of eye movements – which in turn may be caused by inadequate maturation of the equilibrium – make eye contact difficult; or if the act of grasping cannot be performed independently of the direction of vision, thus rendering impossible the handling of objects while communicating simultaneously. Impairments to the production of speech sounds due to delays in neurophysiological development also play an important part. This will be dealt with in more detail later.

Diagnostic procedures

Accordingly, an examination of the stage of neurophysiological development must be part of any thorough diagnostic investigation. This is not yet the rule at present and no appropriate diagnostic methods for younger children are currently available. The following remarks on diagnostic procedures therefore relate to the traditional method of ascertaining language development.

Teumer (1986) and Grohnfeldt (1986) classified the evaluation of the stage of neurophysiological development under 'adjunctive diagnostic procedures'. They include in this an analysis of motor function, of visual perception and of social competence. Language development in the narrower sense is viewed on the phonetic-phonological level (speech

sounds); the semantic-lexical level (vocabulary); the syntactic-morphological level (grammar) and the pragmatic level (understanding of language), the four sub-groups of linguistic diagnosis. Within this framework, the active and passive aspects of the linguistic level are examined separately, and, if necessary, prosody, fluency and voice are examined also. This simple diagnostic system, with a division into a core area of language and concomitant aspects of the child's development as a whole, allows an efficient processing of the data in practice (Bierkens 1968). Another advantage of this classification is that it makes the investigator sensitive to the possibility of abnormalities in other areas, besides the fact that the articulation is not age-appropriate, and that these areas often need a second look. However, it is not exactly easy to find a method of testing deficits, for example in grammar (syntax, morphology), which is at once discriminating and economical (Borstel 1984).

Factorial analysis has shown that in children from 4 years old upwards the area of articulation can be assessed independently of the other three areas of diagnostic linguistics. In a joint factorial analytical treatment of items from the areas of vocabulary (adjectives, verbs), morphology (comparative forms) and practical understanding of a task, no statistically significant correlations were found with the articulatory items (for the formation of speech sounds) under scrutiny (Graumann-Brunt 1999). The correlations between each of the three areas first mentioned were closer (Graumann-Brunt 1999). Therefore, an isolated finding about the stage of articulation can give no indication of performance in other areas of diagnostic linguistics.

Several investigational procedures exist to assess vocabulary, grammar and articulation in children 4 years old and upwards (Neumann 1982). However, it is practically impossible to use standardized tests to examine children below 4 years of age. Analysis of the quality of communicative behavior is a complicated procedure for all age-groups and is therefore often disregarded. The items that are easier to test and which relate to the passive understanding of a task do not offer enough information about communicative ability. Figure 19.1, which shows some items for testing articulation, vocabulary, grammar and understanding of a task, is taken from a linguistic diagnostic screening procedure for preschool children (Corinth and Graumann-Brunt 1992). For the articulation, vocabulary and grammar (here, morphology only) items to be tested pictures should be used; for the activity tasks, toys.

DEVELOPMENTAL STAGES IN LANGUAGE
Sigrid Graumann-Brunt

In the practice of speech therapy, linguistic diagnosis cannot assess language utterances – or utterances which are at least

ARTICULATION (PHONATION)

Wheel	Suitcase	Bird	Glasses	Bag	Sun
Hair	Book	Fork	Bone	Scissors	Mouse
Lamp	Four	King	Crown	Pig	

VOCABULARY

Adjectives:	dirty	bent	short	square	light blue
Verbs:	to jump in	to sell	to show	to read	

GRAMMAR (COMPARATIVES)

longer	dirtier	higher	more

UNDERSTANDING LANGUAGE (TASKS)

Put the ball in the hoop [or tire] and take the horse out.
Before you give me the hoop, roll the ball over to me.
Move the car all the way around the hoop and then put it inside it.
Take the car out of the hoop, then roll the ball to me and then put the horse in the hoop.

Figure 19.1 Items used to check articulation, vocabulary, grammar and the understanding of tasks.

language-like – before a certain age. However, parents, relatives and people in a position of trust (Wöhler 1980) are able to form a picture of the stage of a child's language. Parents are delighted to hear a child's first sounds and, soon after, his first syllables, and to respond to them. But when does language development really begin? Is it when a baby first babbles or does it begin only with one-word sentences or later still? Long before a child produces his first linguistic utterances, developmental processes within him are laying the foundations for future language utterances.

The first seeds of the organs and systems later used in language are found at the embryonic stage. The foundations of the later tools of speech are laid down in the early stages of pregnancy, with the primordium of the alimentary tract, and thus of the mandible also. Although the mandible, lips, oral cavity and tongue should primarily be classified under the alimentary system, they later count equally as tools of speech. The soft palate and larynx originally have a protective function, but these also serve, secondarily, to produce language. The organs of respiration, the autonomic nervous system and the pattern of movement also have this dual function; they all have a primary function, and a secondary one in producing speech sounds.

In this early period, the foundation for language development is laid; not just through the organs which are later used secondarily for spoken language but also by means of reflex systems which later exert their effect on the development of language. In the intrauterine period and the first 6 months after birth these include the early childhood reflexes, which serve to pave the way for, and develop, various functional systems. These include the tonic labyrinthine reflex, with which

the vestibular basis is laid for the later control of movement via proprioception. The tonic labyrinthine reflex forwards is produced by a forward movement of the head across the level of the spine. It leads to a flexion of the entire body including the extremities (fetal flexion, earliest form). The tonic labyrinthine reflex backwards causes the body to stretch when the head moves back (Goddard 1996). Lateral movement patterns, such as the fencer's pose, here understood to be identical to the asymmetric tonic neck reflex according to Goddard (1996), are also observed in the uterus. But the preparations for the first food intake, through oral reflexes (rooting and sucking) and the regurgitation of undigested food also serve, at the same time, to prepare for speech.

In the time spent in the uterus, during labor (when the tonic labyrinthine reflex backwards becomes active) and in the first 6 months after birth, the early childhood reflexes form, mature and are ultimately inhibited. By the end of the 6th month of life the development of these early functional systems, which are basal and controlled by the brain stem, should, by and large, be coming to an end. The homologous, horizontal and lateral patterns of movement give way to diagonal patterns. However, remnants of the early childhood reflexes are often retained, and can then appreciably disturb the more complex reaction patterns which supersede them, while at the same time being constructed upon them. This can also affect the production of spoken language.

Here, one must also mention the initial building of autonomic reactions which are later involved in the production and processing of language. Parasympathetic reactions in the form of the withdrawal reflex appear as early as the 5th–7th week of pregnancy. The first sympathetic startle reactions have been observed in the 9th week (Moro reaction). An initiation of a sympathetic reaction will always precede speech as a social interaction associated with much movement, alternating with parasympathetic incursions depending on the structuring of the language actions. The control of autonomic respiration is also prepared for even in the prenatal phase when the foundations for autonomic functions are laid.

The fetus certainly also perceives changes in the mother's autonomic system, just as he perceives, through his vestibular system, the changes in her bodily posture and activity while speaking. Similarly, acoustic stimuli also become clearer to him as pregnancy progresses. The fetus experiences prosody while still in the womb. The fetus can hear throughout the final three months of pregnancy (Eliot 1999). However, when investigating the onset of the ability to hear, one must distinguish between conduction through bone and tympanic membrane and conduction through another element (perhaps an organic substrate). According to Pawlik (1976), investigations by Henry have found clear indications of factors which can be classified under these three modes of hearing, including specific frequency ranges. Here, one cannot presume from the outset that all component areas of hearing are initiated and subsequently all develop simultaneously. This also means that there are probably qualitative differences between the acoustic perception of an unborn child that of a newborn child, and that of an older baby.

0–6 months

The newborn child comes into the world with his own 'blueprint' for language. Pinker describes the ability to use language as an instinct (1994). However, another speaking person and a number of other prerequisites are needed before language development can be set in motion. It is impossible to specify exactly how large the timescale is for its initiation. However, a few examples indicate that the chances of acquiring complete command of language are reduced if language development begins very late. This might be because there is a sensitive phase which is limited in time, but it could also be that there are other demands made on an individual as he grows older which leave too little energy and time to develop language.

The symbiotic relationship between mother and child does not end at birth, and only gradually leads to the distance which is needed for communication. Zollinger (2002) describes the relationship during the first 2 months as a 'dual unit' or 'symbiosis'. This does not mean that the baby could not distinguish his mother from himself and from other people; but on the psychological level he learns that she always knows his feelings, which are aroused by changes in his needs and states of tension, and can give them a meaning.

Language utterances do indeed play a part here, because the sounds the child produces are answered by the caregiver. The stock of sounds available to a baby, however, is much more comprehensive than that which an older child possesses. The newborn child is at first a universal phonetician; in other words, he can distinguish phonemes from phonetic systems which the adults around him cannot differentiate. He can, however, also distinguish the sounds which specifically belong to his mother-tongue as such (Ingram 1989). Thus, in the first phase after birth there is an adaptation to the stock of sounds produced by the language community to which the child will belong. This process of adaptation can later be observed in the reduction of consonantal clusters to single sounds, as in the transition from 'tsch' to 'sch'.

Newborns and infants express their needs through wailing, crying, gurgling; that is, through actions controlled by the brain stem. The first language-like utterances are vocalized (voiced). The ability to imitate speech sounds is already marked. The baby's perceptual abilities develop very fast. At as early as 3 to 4 months he reacts to trial subjects who speak to him and then also turns his head to the source of the sound. It is of great diagnostic significance that even deaf babies babble, but that these utterances are less varied than those of other children, and that deaf children form fewer sounds as they grow older. Special attention must therefore be paid if babbling begins quite late, is infrequent and not very varied, or if the occurrence of babbling actually decreases over time.

6–10 months

A decisive change occurs at about the age of 6 months. This is also the time when the primitive reflex movements should disappear. When the baby babbles, he plays aimlessly with types of sound, sometimes even polysyllabic, and listens to his own babbling – the prerequisite for imitating his parents' language. While he already reacts when others speak, he does indeed use his voice to draw attention to himself but still communicates through wailing and simple gestures. The child is now starting to discover for himself the objects round about. At this time, the child is mainly getting to know his own body (on this, see Zukunft-Huber 1998).

During this time, neuronal connections are still being constructed. Long distance connections are not complete until 9 months. The number of neuronal connections in the cortex peaks between 9 months and 2 years (Pinker 1994). Actions with objects can be repeated, varied and transferred. According to Zollinger (2002), the lines of development for the interaction with the primary caregiver and those of actions with objects run parallel during the 1st year of life. 'If the child is busy with an object, it cannot draw a person into its play, and if it is in a direct exchange with a person, the objects recede into the background.'

10–12 months

At 10 to 12 months the child is no longer a universal phoneticist; the variability of the sound quality becomes specific. The child begins to form individual words associated with a particular situation but these words still lack the quality of sentences. He still communicates with the aid of gestures and eyes. By crawling and moving on his belly the child acquires a physical independence, enabling him to regulate, by himself, his closeness to and distance from his primary caregiver. He learns that things continue to exist beyond his field of vision (Zollinger 2002). Around the end of the 1st year of life the child first begins to interconnect the world of people and the world of objects. He can avert his gaze from an object and 'speak to' his primary caregiver with his eyes. This eye contact with the object in mind is also termed referential or triangular. According to Zollinger (2002) this first eye contact is the real origin of language in a child. A 'triangular relationship' arises between the child, a second person and an object, the 'primordial form' of a conversation.

12–18 months

From 12 months the child is in the holophrastic phase, the one-word phase. He understands single words and also repeats some of them spontaneously. Above all, the meaning of the words comes to life when he says them himself. Now, quite unlike 2 months ago, the child can give the words a communicative dimension with the quality of a sentence, especially if they are directed at a person and contain an intention.

The child develops an initial understanding of language and points to things. He reacts to commands to fetch things, but will only give what he is holding in his hand at that very moment. There is already a passive understanding of words. He can understand language if he acts appropriately. However, he cannot yet use words alone to communicate something. Language is therefore still largely bound to actions. The child communicates his refusal to carry out commands by shaking his head or turning away.

By the time the child is 12 months old, he should be able to understand simple commands. He must also be able to keep his mouth closed, swallow his saliva, babble syllables, imitate sounds and lick a spoon.

18–24 months

From 18 months the child makes a massive leap forward in his vocabulary. He acquires a new word every 2 hours on average (Pinker 1994). Moreover, he notices that his words are also understood and have an effect; the child discovers the representational and communicative function of language. Now he also starts to communicate intentions and feelings. Whatever the cultural milieu in which the child is growing up, he will form similar two-word sentences (Pinker 1994) and name everyday objects and actions. The development of language from the first two-word sentences to complete sentences can take place within a few months, whereby differences due to the child's social milieu become increasingly evident from the age of 16 months (Graumann-Brunt 1999).

Now the child is able to refuse actions by saying 'no', refers to himself by name, recognizes the word for 'you' and discovers that every object and action has its corresponding word. The child takes an interest in words for objects and actions and notices that actions are not always bound to a concrete object. By 21 months, 95% of children have spoken their first word.

24–36 months

From 24 months onwards the child begins to discriminate in his use of words. He begins to string words together to form what are still but the rudiments of a sentence (infinitive form). He can now understand absurd commands. An initial understanding of spoken language, of non-situational utterances, develops, such as 'Where is the dog?' The child uses language to describe situations and events. Questions are formed with 'What's that?' and 'Where?' to grasp relationships between people, things and events.

The most important achievement of the 3rd year of life is the word for 'I' (Zollinger 2002); this word cannot be acquired by direct imitation.

Language acquires great importance for further cognitive and social development. The child expands his world by understanding language and conquers it by producing language, but he cannot as yet gauge how much he has to say to make himself understood. This is why conversation with children this age is still a 'once only giving and taking'. The child's vocabulary continues to increase considerably. A 2-year-old child should have 50 words at his command, including some names and several adjectives. He should be able to express his wants through language. The consonants 'b', 'p', 'm', 'f', 'w [ɯ]', 'n', 't' and 'd' should be audible in words he speaks and he should be able to produce more than eight clusters of sounds. The child must be able to chew solid food.

36–48 months

From 36 months onwards the child can hold conversations, although still in the simplest form. The interlocutor can now, however, attach a question to the child's answer and in this way 'give back' the 'subject of conversation' to the child. At round about 3 years of age the child should be able to use the article (in German language), ask questions ('Why?') and at any rate be able to form sentences of several words.

Inflectional endings, functional words and prepositions are used correctly 90% of the time. Complex sentences with subordinate clauses are formed correctly, for the most part, and the rules of grammar and word order are adhered to. In morphology there are overgeneralizations (e.g. 'many' instead of 'more'). The difference between 'r' and 'l' is worked out, 'k' and 'g' are increasingly formed in the standard fashion, and 't' and 'd' are differentiated.

From 48 months onwards

At 48 months the child follows syntactic rules and uses a complex grammatical structure. Adjectives and verbs are used selectively. As regards morphology, all essential forms are laid down. He can form the comparative, use prepositions and form tenses. He can also understand and carry out tasks. This is when the rationalization of language begins. It is widely known that 4-year-old children already have the grammatical structure of adult speech at their disposal (Bee 2000). However, various studies point to the influence of the social milieu on differences in the developmental stage, and these differences can be as great as a year (Oevermann 1971). From the age of 4 years onwards structures already acquired are perfected and the child's vocabulary continues to grow. The production of speech is accelerated and increased. The impression of a wide gulf in linguistic competence between a 4-year-old and a 10-year-old is attributable to the content which the child addresses, the interests of younger children being very different from those of older children. Also, those around the child are mainly interested in the spoken sounds, which are not yet formed in the standard fashion, and are less interested in the correctness of the grammar.

The sounds 'r' or 'R' (r = rolled 'r', R = guttural 'r'), 'l', 'f', 'w[ϖ]', 'ch [ξ]' and also 'k' and 'g' are not yet consistently pronounced correctly; 'sch [Σ]', 's' and some consonantal clusters are mostly replaced or omitted. The sound which is the last to be formed correctly is 's' which as many of 22% of children reaching 7 years of age consistently pronounce incorrectly. That means that one cannot expect a correctly pronounced stock of speech sounds until the child has turned 7 years old. With regard to the development of pronunciation in children under 4 years of age, there is a lack of standardized data in German-speaking countries (Szagun 1986), so that reference is usually made to literature in English, although one should not automatically assume that the latter can be just as accurately applied to the German-speaking world. The extent to which German children aged 4 to 7 are

able to accurately pronounce German speech sounds has been the subject of a very large study in which consonants were tested in a variety of settings. The study mentioned at the beginning, which was carried out on a total group of 1648 preschool children (Graumann-Brunt 1999), showed a clear structure with six factors:

- Factor 'r' and '[R]' and 'l'
- Factor 'ch [ξ]', 'f' and 'w [ϖ]'
- Factor 'k' and 'g'
- Factor consonantal clusters
- Factor 'sch [Σ]'
- Factor 's'.

The difficulties in articulation ascertained from these factors proved to be age-related, in the order shown here. The factor 'sch [Σ]' was generally the one most subject to variance, and the factor 's' was the most clearly demarcated. The 'ch [ξ], f and w [ϖ]' factor was remarkably informative with regard to the quality and quantity of pronunciation difficulties in articulation and therefore justified a later search for a common difficulty in the production of the sounds classified under this factor.

NORMAL DEVELOPMENT OF SPOKEN LANGUAGE

Sigrid Graumann-Brunt

The development of the stock of sounds in the mother tongue, in German, generally takes the child an exceptionally long time, 7 to 8 years. It is known that a child's ecological circumstances, his emotional state, habitual structures, and also his physical state and special features in his psychophysical processes, play a part in the course of language development (Graumann-Brunt 1999).

The development of the production of speech sounds (a part of the development of language) is particularly closely linked to the development of movement. It is easy to see why the motility of the facial organs (lips, tongue, soft palate, vocal folds) is a fundamental prerequisite for the process of speech. Also, the task of breathing has always been regarded as a constituent element in speaking. However, the extent to which synergistic elements from the torso play a part in the production of speech sounds is as yet less well known. The following is therefore an explanation of the connections which are of interest here between the production of speech sounds and sound-specific synergists. By forming a 'string', a number of different muscles (Tittel 1994) make a decisive contribution to facial movements. That means that special attention must be paid to the synergists when treating pronunciation disorders in children because the caudal parts of the body which act in synergy often show delays in their predisposition and ability to function. This is especially evident in the pelvic and abdominal areas.

In producing the 'sch [Σ]' sound the rectus abdominis muscle becomes active. It appears that full maturity for the fine control needed for this sound, including the inhibition of other muscles, is not generally reached until the age of 5 years. Of children approaching 7 years of age, 30% still make errors in forming the 'sch [Σ]' (Graumann-Brunt 1999). One of the reasons for this might be that the rectus abdominis muscle has to control exhaled air at the same time as it supports the production of the 'sch [Σ]', and thus has to undertake different forms of movement simultaneously.

In forming the 's' sound, the serratus anterior is tensed while the ribcage tilts frontally. This results in a slight upwards and downwards movement of the head, through which the tip of the tongue draws upwards to the alveolar ridge. At the same time, the top part of the rectus abdominis must be activated for the specific tensing of the tip of the tongue to form the 's'. Although the lower parts of the rectus abdominis are involved in controlling exhalation, unlike the upper part they are not involved in forming sounds. That means that the intramuscular differentiation must function perfectly to produce a standard 's'. By and large children do not seem to be in a position to do this until they are 6 years old, and even by that age only 33% are as yet able to produce a perfect 's' sound (Graumann-Brunt 1999).

Occasional non-standard forms of the 'ch [ξ]', 'j [φ]', 'f' and 'w ['ϖ']' sounds can still be found in about 70% of 4-year-olds, but in only around 6% of children just below 7 years of age. In the production of these sounds, as with the 'h', a tensing of the back muscles can be found, originating from the pelvis. The forming of the voiced sounds 'j [φ]' and 'w [ϖ]' requires further movements in the back because the closure of the vocal folds to produce voiced sounds is economically initiated by a slight, scarcely perceptible traction from the pelvis. A movement of the multifidus muscles in the back might also occur during speech for forming the intonation.

The sounds 'k' and 'g' present problems of their own, as can be seen from the factorial analysis. To produce these sounds, it is necessary to tense the pelvic floor and form a closure by means of the back of the tongue and the palate. However, the diaphragm must remain relaxed throughout, as otherwise a mixture of 'k' and 't', or 'g' and 'd', will be produced. In forming 'k' and 'g', the lower parts of the rectus abdominis are synergistically active, while the upper part does not participate in this tension. It makes sense that the 't' and 'd' sounds, in which the diaphragm is tensed, are formed in standard fashion earlier, as their production is not decisively disturbed by additional tensing of the pelvic floor. Regarding the 'k' and 'g' group of sounds, 28% of 4-year-olds and 12% of children just below 7 years of age still make errors (Graumann-Brunt 1999). The standard production of these sounds seems to progress more slowly than that of the 'ch [ξ]', 'j [φ]', 'f' and 'w [ϖ]' sounds (Graumann-Brunt 1999).

70% of children just below 4 years of age still make errors with consonantal clusters, and 30% of 6-year-olds still do. From the results of the factorial analyses, there seems to be a special difficulty in forming consonantal clusters, independently of the consonants. With the factor of consonantal clusters, there is probably a problem with coarticulation. In the articulatory continuum, the sounds are intermeshed, which means that movements for several future sounds have to be built up at the very same moment that sounds are being spoken. Here, the organs involved are accelerated at different rates, rapid simultaneous movements are not possible, and a simultaneous start, conclusion and progression of the movements cannot be achieved. A problem with speed might have been brought to light by this factor. However, there may also be problems with differentiation involved here, because an inserted vowel ('belau [β ≅ λαY]' instead of 'blau [βλαY]') is known to make the critical consonantal clusters easier to deal with.

IMPAIRED DEVELOPMENT OF SPOKEN LANGUAGE

Sigrid Graumann-Brunt

Delayed or impaired language acquisition

Non-standard linguistic utterances are more readily tolerated in young children than in adults or older children (van Riper and Irwin 1958). '"Baby language" reflects the language of the young child in the first 2 years of life. Until nearly 3 years of age, it is taken for granted that any deviant articulation is a temporary form of behavior attributable to the process of acquisition' (Graumann-Brunt 1999).

There has been much discussion about when a non-standard articulation is a delay, and when it constitutes an impairment. (In labelling, 'temporary' is distinguished from 'structural'. See Scholz on this subject [1970]). Jakobson (1964) presumes that there is an impairment if slowed phonological development, as it is, 'sets'. Ingram uses the term 'impairment' if non-standard 'earlier' sounds persist, even though 'later' sounds are already being correctly pronounced (1989). In fact, in the above study a few findings from a group of children with articulatory insufficiency of the third (highest) degree do in fact bear out Ingram's assumption (Graumann-Brunt 1999). However, they do not supply enough information on which to base a prognosis in an individual case. Other studies, such as longitudinal and cross-sectional studies from English-speaking countries offer only a few points which can be used in practice. Therefore, if articulation is non-standard, it is not possible at present to call an impairment a lasting one until after the age of 7 or 8 years, and even later if development is generally delayed. However, if the number of deviant articulations is above average for the child's age-group in more than one area (see p.443), the child is at risk of an impairment. In this case one should investigate whether therapeutic intervention is needed.

Non-standard grammar can be regarded as an impairment as early as the age of 3 years, and by the age of 4 years at the latest, because one can expect the development of grammatical structures to be completed quite early as a rule (see above). A simple indication of deficits in this area is the absence of comparative and superlative forms or oddities; for example, in the position of words in the sentence. Delays in vocabulary acquisition must be differentiated according to the type of word. The vocabulary of nouns depends on the child's social milieu, and is therefore not very informative in preschool children. Verbs and adjectives give better indications here for checking whether the vocabulary development is at an age-appropriate stage.

Incipient and chronic stuttering

Problems with forming speech sounds also occur with stuttering (van Riper 1982). With incipient stuttering, unlike chronic stuttering, non-standard production of speech sounds is more often observed. This is why a careful distinction must be made between incipient and chronic stuttering.

Van Riper made a particularly intensive study of the phenomenon of stuttering and its therapy (1982), for which he collected findings from a variety of fields from all over the world. He paid particular attention to chronic stuttering, which is seen mainly in older adolescents and adults. If one follows the multimodal approach (van Riper 1973), in chronic stuttering the self-image and the dominance of the symptoms of stuttering, which sometimes affect the entire personality, are the focal point of the therapeutic approach. Not until avoidance behavior has been broken down and the stuttering has reappeared in its original form does one start work on articulation itself.

Van Riper (1973) derived the treatment of incipient stuttering mainly from the therapeutic approach for adults, regarding the child's overall development as less important. Research findings about chronic stuttering cannot, however, necessarily be applied to the initial situation. In his theory of stuttering, van Riper leaves no room for examining the link with the development of movement, which is now thought to be

especially important. However, he did point out some important connections between stuttering and impaired movement (1982). In Germany, work on movement has also been regarded as relevant to the therapy of stuttering; traditionally, the aim has always been to improve movement (Teumer 1989, Sommer 1982), on empirical grounds. However, so far the nature of this connection has not yet been specified.

There is little doubt that stuttering is multifactorial in its causation and that there are very different causative complexes and thus types of stuttering. It is also known that there is an important hereditary component. Despite the many studies, mainly in English-speaking countries, about the etiology of stuttering, which have also brought to light a number of neurological peculiarities, too little is known as yet about its nature and causes (van Riper 1973). The many empirical findings have not so far produced any really satisfactory advances in the therapy of stuttering children. The important factors which have been found for the appearance of the symptoms of stuttering include autonomic stress of all kinds (resulting from the ecological circumstances of the affected person, sleep deficit, illnesses, accidents, etc.), and this previously led to the assumption that stuttering was essentially psychological in origin. However, in children stuttering does not occur only under stress, but can also appear at particularly quiet times and can just as well be ever present. However, it often occurs only periodically at the beginning. It is therefore difficult to give a prognosis of the course it will take.

There is known to be a connection between stuttering and problems with articulation (van Riper 1982). In the third phase of van Riper's multimodal behavioral therapy for adults and older children, work is done on the speech movements (1986). If one turns one's attention from the precise examination of facial movements in stuttered speech sounds to stuttering in very young children, one finds a relative high incidence of the types of deficit that occur in problems with articulation.

With incipient stuttering, there are only a few specific problems with forming speech sounds. The dysfunctions also arise with other forms of impairment. However, in stuttering they reinforce each other and compound the difficulties in producing speech sounds until a re-start becomes necessary because the process has broken down. The following paragraphs describe problems involved in forming speech sounds which have been observed in incipient stuttering but which have also been observed with delays in the development of speech sounds.

Breathing during speech

Breathing problems in conjunction with dysfluent speech have been a subject of discussion for a long time (van Riper 1982,

Hubatch 1982). In some cases 'alternating breathing patterns' with an irregular alternation between abdominal and chest breathing (high breathing) is observed when the diaphragm moves out of line. The switch from one mode of breathing to the other while speaking will invariably cause a change in the way speech sounds are produced during the exhaling phase. A number of problems ensue from this. For example, when the 's' sound is formed, the pattern of movement with chest breathing is different from that with abdominal breathing. The two patterns are incompatible, and this impairs movement, particularly in the chest and head areas. With breathing disorders of this kind, one of the things to be borne in mind is the possibility of impairment to the function of the vagus nerve from locked vertebral segments in the upper cervical region in early childhood; another being persistent sensitivity following injuries, for instance to the clavicle, in accidents. The presence of a unilateral or bilateral restriction of the mobility of the diaphragm should also be borne in mind when there are breathing problems during speech.

Pulse fluctuations during speech

In practice there are indications of withdrawal reactions on occasions for speaking, especially in the case of 'elective mutism' disorder (mutism or silence with no detectable organic cause once speech has been acquired, in certain situations, such as at school or with adults). Irregular breathing is another symptom which occurs here. When a pulse oximeter with a finger sensor is used to monitor the pulse and percentage oxygen saturation in patients with this diagnosis, at the very moment when the patient is unable to speak, bradycardia is observed. The causes of this outwardly almost imperceptible bradycardia are unknown. It could be one of several probably multiple triggers with physiological conditioning (fixed at the subcortical level).

Marked increases in the pulse rate with violent fluctuations during communicative situations have often been observed in patients with developmental delays of all kinds and etiologies.

Immature vestibular system and defective proprioception

Many problem clusters in the sphere of perception are attributable to a defective maturation of the vestibular system. With auditory, proprioceptive and visual sensory impressions, the perception required to process the stimulus from its point of origin is only possible through a spatial system of reference with a fixed origin, three dimensions, directions and interval distances. Such a system of reference is in turn dependent on our processing vestibular impulses correctly. It is reasonable to

assume that an unstable vestibular system means greater effort is necessary in processing sensory impressions because the real and indispensable referential system has to be re-established and stabilized each time after movements. That means a considerable effort is necessary during speech because of the constant changes in body position which this requires. The cause of such problems could be a retardation of neurophysiological development, for one of many reasons, such as an asymmetry in the upper cervical region.

Impaired development of the diagonal pattern of movement

Persistent residual reactions from early childhood reflexes, with homologous, horizontal or lateral patterns, disturb the development of the diagonal patterns, which must be available for the development of fluent speech. Pelvic rotation is then also generally impaired. The earlier patterns cannot be controlled at will, are difficult to inhibit and take a long time to eliminate. They thus impair the various delicate diagonal patterns that proceed at immense speed during the act of speaking (Graumann-Brunt 2000). Asymmetries in the upper cervical area and a laterally divergent course of development are quite often seen in children with this problem. Immature eye muscles, blocks in the iliosacral region or a general immaturity may also be present.

Persistent inhibition of forward mandibular movement

Among the movement patterns which produce spoken language and which are particularly affected by developmental impairments are those of the mandible. With mature, efficient speech they have an important task. The following description of mandibular movements presupposes that language production is associated with abdominal breathing.

Before speech begins, the mandible is slightly lowered. It can thus be moved along past the upper incisors. During speech, it is generally engaged in continuous (minimally lateralized) downward, upward, forward and backward movements, and in combinations of the basic movements (Lippert 1995). For instance, shovelling movements occur with the German diphthong 'au [αY]'. The forward movement of the mandible during speech – especially easy to observe when the word 'ich [IX]' is formed in standard fashion – is required to form the various sounds or syllables efficiently. It is more or less marked, depending on the syllable, and varies. There is also a loop-like downward movement followed by upward movement at the end of a spoken entity. However, a very young child is not yet developmentally ready to perform these forward and backward mandibular movements in speech.

Only as the capacity to chew solid food grows does it become more possible to integrate more differentiated mandibular movements into the process of speech.

If the mandible cannot be moved forwards successfully, early forms of speech persist, with a reduced radius of action of the tongue. Syllables with the vowels and consonants: 'i', 'u [Y]', 'ü [Ψ]' and 'ö' and 'f' and 'w [ϖ]' are particularly affected. In an extreme case of dysfunctional mandibular motility, the result is muffled speech, with little pleasure in speaking and poor social acceptability.

The shape and position of the mandible relative to the maxilla are important in carrying out movements in the course of speech. Attention must also be paid to conditions in the cranial area, such as the position of the sphenoid, the functioning of the temporal muscle (intramuscular differentiation, tension level), of the pterygoid muscles, of the sphenomandibular ligament (which has an important role when the mouth is first opened) and of the temporal bone (because of the stylomandibular ligament). It is as important to take account of the functional readiness of the cranial nerves, especially the inferior alveolar nerve, the mental nerve, the mylohyoid nerve and the masseteric nerve, as of that of the vascular and fascial connections (Liem 1998). It must be remembered that asymmetries in the head and neck region can exert an influence on the forward movement of the mandible. The possibility of a pelvic ring block should also be borne in mind with impairments in the forward movement of the mandible. In this connection, a relative flattening of the physiological lumbar lordosis is often found.

Dysfunctions of the rectus abdominis muscle

The control of exhaled air occurs synchronously and in rhythm with the shaping of the prosody, intonation and accent. It is done by the rectus abdominis muscle, and for this abdominal breathing is a prerequisite. To form the intonation, accent and the pauses between the words the air must be discharged sequentially, with sufficient power, speed and variability. In very young children the muscle is initially lacking structure, has little strength and lacks the fine motor function required for the process of speech.

In the 'sch [Σ]' sound, the rectus abdominis also acts as a synergist in a string of muscles that leads to the tongue. For the 'sch [Σ]' sound, the intermuscular distinction between the rectus abdominis and the serratus anterior is important. If it is not achieved, a mixed sound is produced, between 'sch [Σ]' and 's'. The dual function of the rectus abdominis, on the one hand to control exhaled air and on the other its synergistic task in forming the 'sch [Σ]', explains why the

'sch [Σ] factor' was subject to so much variance, from other sounds tested, in the aforementioned study (Graumann-Brunt 1999).

If 'cluttering' is diagnosed, or if a non-standard formation of the 'sch [Σ]' is found by the age of 6 years, a dysfunction of the rectus abdominis should be considered. Often there are also persistent residual reactions of the early childhood tonic labyrinthine reflex. In that case, the extremities flex inwardly in response to a stimulus in the abdominal region.

Dysfunctions of the muscles of the back

The following description of movements in the muscles of the back presupposes that speech production is connected with abdominal breathing.

The muscles of the back are also involved in the production of speech sounds. Movements for the formation of syllables with the consonants of the 'ch [ξ], f and w [ϖ]' (including the 'h') factor, which proved particularly troublesome, run from the pelvis to the head. The glottal closure when the vocal folds start to vibrate (primarily, probably a part of the retching complex) is also linked to a movement rising upwards from the pelvis.

If the rigid connection of head to spinal column from early childhood development is still present, the pelvis stiffly follows movements of the head. There are also problems in the opposite direction, which is that the head cannot swing freely in response to pelvic movements. Any muscle tension in the back takes a long time to unwind and thus blocks preparation of the next links in the speech production chain. If speech production cannot continue quickly enough, speech breaks down and then stuttering occurs. Involuntary attempts to counter this problem by tensing the head and neck, with a reduction or inhibition of head movements, lead to further new difficulties during the act of speaking. This problem is most evident with interrogatives at the start of a sentence. Starting a question requires preparation for movements which lead, for example, to the production of the sound 'w [ϖ]', preparation for the first closure of the vocal folds and for the start of intonation and thus the initiation of several different strings of movement in the back with a high degree of differentiation necessary.

The causes of problems in the back are multiple. Besides functional impairments in the development of movement (Zukunft-Huber 1998), there are genetic and prenatal, perinatal and postnatal factors to consider, and also accidents and previous illnesses (see also Bauer 2002). Head size and shape, as well as peculiarities in the postural structure of the body, can also cause difficulties in the development of the movement pattern in the back. When the synergistic movements in the back are impaired in the production of speech sounds, there is often a tendency to walk on the balls of the feet and on tiptoe, which is often observed and indicates static immaturity.

Dysfunctions of lip movement

The following description of lip movements presupposes that the production of speech sounds is connected with abdominal breathing.

An inability to satisfactorily form the sounds 'p' and 'b', which are seldom formed in non-standard fashion, but also an inability to form 'f' and 'w [ʊ]' satisfactorily, means the child might be considered to have a dysfunction of the orofacial muscles. A connection with dysfunctions of the musculature at the back of the pelvic floor region, especially of the external anal sphincter, which acts synergistically with the lip muscles, should be checked for.

Remaining traces of the early childhood rooting and sucking reflex can considerably impair the functioning of the ring of the lips. Remnants of the rooting reflex cause hypersensitivity in the facial area. The sucking movements, which now occur as a reflex to stimuli in the facial area, are slow to break down and also impede the outward stream of exhaled air by generating an inwardly directed suction effect. An activated sucking reflex leads to a stalemate situation in the formation of speech sounds and a subsequent brief spell of inhalational speech.

In this situation, the speech movements are often contracted, the ring of the lips lacks elasticity, and the lip environment stiffens. The result is unclear pronunciation with problems in forming the vowels. It must be remembered that the lips are exceptionally widely represented in the cortex (Lippert 1995) and that any impairment in their mobility, however slight it may seem, must be regarded as significant.

Activation of the diaphragms

The following description of movements in the diaphragms presupposes that the production of speech sounds is connected with abdominal breathing.

To form the plosives 'k', 'g', 'p' and 'b' effectively, it is necessary to tense the pelvic floor temporarily. For 't' and 'd' the diaphragm is briefly tensed. Four-year-olds often have appreciable problems forming 'k' and 'g'. Here, it is thought that the cause of the difficulties in forming 'k' and 'g' may be a defect in the proprioceptive differentiation between the diaphragm and the pelvic floor. Inadequate differentiation of muscle movements in the pelvic area or an asymmetry in this area can also impair the progress of speech. An overflow caused by immaturity (Goddard 1996) is especially problematical, because the 'k' is followed by an aspiration through

'h' and that in turn by an impulse for a renewed vibration of the vocal folds, also from the pelvic area. All three movement patterns contain contributions from synergists from the lowest region of the back; the power, precision and speed in the movement of the muscles of the pelvic region are of great importance in generating 'k' and 'g' sounds. Too little power input in the anterior region of the pelvic floor results in a weak 'k' and 'g'. An immaturity in this region is associated with a protracted relaxation of the pelvic floor, which leads to interlinkage delays in the course of speech (most noticeable in the syllable 'ka'), which may be irrecoverable, thus resulting in a stutter. A block of the pelvic ring is often found with this problem.

In the case of diaphragmatic dysfunction the articulation of 't' and 'd' is inadequate. In some cases an indistinctive 'k' and 'g' are produced. In these cases, the listener drawing upon his psychophysical processing and corrective procedures for decoding, may well perceive the 'k' as 't' (Pètursson and Neppert 1991), so that the diagnosis is not easy. If a child is still unable to form 't' or 'd' up to standard having reached the age of 4 years, an investigation of the functional efficiency of the diaphragm and rectus abdominis muscle should be undertaken.

Upward movement of the tip of the tongue

The following description of movements in the tip of the tongue presupposes that speech production is connected with abdominal breathing.

The 's' is the last sound to be formed in a standard fashion. Younger children form it with the tip of the tongue touching the bottom teeth; the mature speaker, forms it with the tip of the tongue touching the alveolar ridge of the upper incisors. For the sounds 'n', 'l', 'r', 't' and 'd', it is also necessary to raise the tip of the tongue. Closer examination of this pattern of movement shows that the muscular movement of the tip of the tongue is supported by an upward movement of the head, followed by a downward movement similar to the start of a nod. The tongue then moves upwards easily. Synergists from the chest area give support. The synergistic assistance afforded by the serratus anterior muscle is well known (tilting movement of the ribcage).

Problems arise here when there are retained residual reactions of the early childhood tonic labyrinthine reflex backwards. The cause of the impairment to the progress of speech movements is then a reflex tension reaction in the back, which follows the backwards inclination of the head during the sequence of movement in raising the tip of the tongue for the aforementioned sounds 's', 'n', 'l', 'r', 't' and 'd'. However, if this slight nodding of the head is not done to avert the disturbing tension in the back, considerable muscular effort will be needed to raise the tongue while speaking: an impossible task under the circumstances. The result is indistinct pronunciation, especially of the 's' sound. Due to its high frequencies it is readily perceived as non-standard.

If there is a locked segment in the thoracic spine, impeding the synergists, the sequence of movements for creating the above sounds is hindered by a restricted radius of action and a loss of speed. The sounds 'n', 'l', 'r', 't', 'd' and 's' are then formed 'economically', which again causes problems in the control systems.

If the intramuscular differentiation within the rectus abdominis muscle is not fully developed, either, in its control function of regulating exhalation, the tip of the tongue cannot perform its 's' specific task. The prerequisite for producing the 's' sound is a special skill in forming a groove with the tip of the tongue, with synergistic support from the uppermost part of the rectus abdominis muscle. For several reasons, therefore, the movements for the 's' require a high degree of intermuscular and intramuscular differentiation (this also means the ability to inhibit; McClelland and Rumelhart 1986), precision and skill. This is surely the reason why the 's' is the last of the German sounds to be formed correctly.

Therapeutic options

There are very many indications that the dysfunctions of synergists in the torso can appreciably impair the forming of speech sounds. In most cases of abnormalities in the development of speech sounds, one or more of the dysfunctions described is apparent. Whether the delay will become an impairment depends, in each individual case, on how far dysfunctions can be remedied, existing compensatory mechanisms deactivated and learning processes reacquired. Jacobson's view (1969) that impaired pronunciation is a result of 'frozen' developmental processes, and Ingram's conclusion (1989) that impairments retain 'earlier' departures from the norm, fall in line with the belief that deficits in an infant's muscular function systems persist later on. Work on the underlying deficits in the muscular and functional systems affected is therefore strongly advised in the case of a delay in the forming of speech sounds. When treating incipient stuttering, it is also very important to pay attention to the connection between articulatory difficulties and persisting dysfunctions affecting motility.

A timely intervention is recommended to eliminate structures that are delaying development, like those which arise from blocks in the upper cervical region at a prenatal, perinatal or postnatal stage. Individual muscle areas with dysfunctions should be relieved of blocks and activated. Further measures, such as the maturation and inhibition of residual reactions from earlier reflexes and paving the way for the

diagonal patterns, are also almost always necessary. This must be followed by a reorganization of compensatory social and habitual structures that have already been set in place, and of other aspects of the personality such as loss of self-esteem or harmful misconceptions.

An account of the part played by ecological, habitual, organic and individual psychophysical assimilation processes has been left in the background here because the focus of interest was the physiological processes involved in the development of standard speech sounds. Attention is drawn to the relevant literature on this (Oevermann 1971, Major 1974, van Riper 1982, Graumann-Brunt 1999, Bee 2000, Zollinger 2002).

In any attempt to improve the quality of speech sounds, however, it must never be forgotten that the ultimate purpose of speech is not the perfection of its outward form but the communication of essential content from one person to another.

Bibliography

Bauer J: Das Gedächtnis des Körpers. Frankfurt am Main, Eichborn 2002

Bee H: The developing child. 9th edn. Boston, Allyn and Bacon 2000

Bierkens PB: Die Urteilsbildung in der Psychodiagnostik. Johann Ambrosius Barth, Munich 1968

Borstel M: Differentialdiagnostik auf sprachlichen Ebenen nach linguistischen Prinzipien. In: Pascher W, Bauer H (eds): Differentialdiagnose von Sprach-, Stimm- und Hörstörungen. Thieme, Stuttgart 1984

Corinth B, Graumann-Brunt S: Sprachheilbilderbuch. Self-published 1992

Eliot L: What's Going On in There? Bantam Books, New York, 1999

Funkkolleg: Sprache 1. Eine Einführung in die moderne Linguistik. Fischer, Frankfurt am Main 1987

Goddard S: A teachers window into the child's mind. Fern Ridge Press, Eugene/OR, USA, 1996

Graumann-Brunt S: Ausgewählte Probleme bei der Konstruktion eines Prüfverfahrens der Diagnostik sprachbehinderter oder von Sprachbehinderung bedrohter vier- bis sechsjähriger Kinder zur Erfassung deren Lautbestandes am Beispiel des Hamburger Lautprüfverfahrens (HLPV). Dissertation, Hamburg 1999

Graumann-Brunt S: Auswirkungen von KISS auf Sprache. Lecture paper, Salzburg 2000

Grohnfeldt M: Diagnose von Sprachbehinderungen. Marhold, Berlin 1982

Grohnfeldt M: Störungen der Sprachentwicklung. Marhold, Berlin 1986

Herrmann T: Allgemeine Sprachpsychologie. Urban & Schwarzenberg, Munich 1985

Hubatch LM: Early receptive and expressive speech abilities of high risk children with a history of prematurity and respiratory distress syndrome. Dissertation Abstracts international 43(6): 1806-B AAT 8225940. Evanston, Ill., Northwester Univ. 1982

Ingram D: Phonological dObility in children. Whurr, London 1989

Jakobson R: Child language, aphasia, and phonological universals. The Hague, Mouton, 1964

Liem T: Kraniosakrale Osteopathie. Hippokrates, Stuttgart 1998

Lippert H: Anatomie Text und Atlas. 6th edn. Urban & Schwarzenberg, Munich 1995

Major S T: Parental Ratings of Speech Abilities in Preschool Children. Dissertation Abstracts International 34(9): 4737-B AAT 7407780. Evanston, Ill., Northwestern Univ. 1974

McClelland J L, Elman J L: Interactive Processes in Speech Perception: The TRACE Model. In: McClelland J L, Rumelhart D E, PDP Research Group (editors): Parallel distributed processing – explorations in the microstructure of cognition. Vol. 2: Psychological and Biological Models. A Bradford Book MIT, Cambridge Mass. 1986

Neppert J, Pètursson M: Elemente einer akustischen Phonetik. Buske, Hamburg 1986

Neumann B: Sprachbehindertenpädagogische Diagnostik. In: Knura G, Neumann B (eds): Pädagogik der Sprachbehinderten. Handbuch der Sonderpädagogik, Vol 7. Marhold, Berlin 1982

Oevermann U: Schichtenspezifische Formen des Sprachverhaltens und ihr Einfluss auf die kognitiven Prozesse. In: Roth H (eds): Begabung und Lernen: Deutscher Bildungsrat Gutachten und Studien der Bildungskommission des Deutschen Bildungsrates. 4th edn. Klett, Stuttgart 1971

Pascher W, Borstel M, Hambeck-Gaumert G, Kegel G, Spiecker-Henke M: Sprachentwicklungsverzögerung und Artikulationsstörungen. In: Pascher W, Bauer H (editors): Differentialdiagnose von Sprach-, Stimm- und Hörstörungen. Thieme, Stuttgart 1984

Pawlik K: Dimensionen des Verhaltens. 3rd edn. Huber, Berne 1976

Pètursson M, Neppert J: Elementarbuch der Phonetik. Buske, Hamburg 1991

Pinker S: The language Instinct, William Morrow & Company, New York 1994

Reulecke W, Rollett B: Pädagogische Diagnostik und lernzielorientierte Tests. In: Pawlik K (editors): Diagnose der Diagnostik. 2nd edn. Klett, Stuttgart 1982

Scholz H-J: Sprachwissenschaftliche Aspekte. In: Knura G, Neumann B (eds): Pädagogik der Sprachbehinderten. Handbuch der Sonderpädagogik. Vol 7, Marhold, Berlin 1982

Sommer M: Spezielle Probleme der Leibeserziehung bei Sprachbehinderten. In: Knura G, Neumann B (eds): Pädagogik der Sprachbehinderten. Handbuch der Sonderpädagogik. Volume 7, Marhold, Berlin 1982

Sonninen A: Reflections on European Voice Research. Open Symposium in Honor of Aatto Sonninen, Helsinki 1996 *http://www.let.uu.nl/-Gerrit.Bloothooft/personal/onderwijs/Zangstem/Reflections%20. Entnommen am 27.1.2004*

Szagun G: Sprachentwicklung beim Kind. Urban & Schwarzenberg, Munich 1986

Teumer J: Zum Beispiel Albert Gutzmann. Marhold, Berlin 1989

Teumer J et al: Informelles Prüfsystem Sprache. Unpublished manuscript, Hamburg 1986

Tittel K: Beschreibende und funktionelle Anatomie des Menschen. 12th edn. Urban & Fischer, Munich/Jena 1994

van Riper C: The nature of stuttering. Prentice-Hall, Englewood Cliffs, N.J. 1982

van Riper C: The treatment of stuttering. Prentice-Hall, Englewood Cliffs, 1973

van Riper C, Irwin JV: Voice and Articulation. Prentice Hall, Inc. 1958

Wängler H H: Atlas deutscher Sprachlaute. Akademie, Berlin 1981

Wöhler K: Soziologische Aspekte der Frühförderung von Behinderten. Zeitschrift für Heilpädagogik 31(5) 1980: 285–296

Zollinger B: Die Entdeckung der Sprache. 5th edn. Haupt, Berne 2002

Zukunft-Huber B: Die ungestörte Entwicklung ihres Babys. Trias, Stuttgart 1998

OSTEOPATHIC TREATMENT OF LANGUAGE DISORDERS

Noori Mitha

Diagnostic considerations

As already described in detail in the earlier parts of this chapter, speech demands the harmonious coordination of extremely diverse areas. The following are particularly important in the formation of language and are therefore investigated with special care in osteopathic diagnostic procedures:

- Optimum mobility of the cranial bones, good intraosseous motion, a well balanced tension of the reciprocal tension membrane, an unrestricted fluctuation of the cerebrospinal fluid and an unhindered motility of the central nervous system are important in ensuring that there is no impairment to the neurological prerequisites for speech; namely the function of the relevant cranial nerves: V, IX, X and XII, and of the speech center.

- The arterial blood supply and venous drainage of the brain must be guaranteed in order to enable optimum functioning of the areas of the brain relevant to language – Broca's (motor language region) and Wernicke's (sensory language region). Other language regions and associative connections needed for speech are also distributed throughout the brain (Willard 2004).

- How is the child's oral cavity constructed? Are there any dental malpositions or changes in the mandible or maxilla which might make speech difficult? The free movement of the mandible is a prerequisite for the formation of various sounds. If the maxilla and mandible do not match in size or shape (e.g. in prognathism or an extreme overbite) articulation can be more difficult.

- Is there a good muscular basis for the development of speech? Do the muscles of the lips, tongue and floor of the mouth work together? How symmetrically oriented are the muscles involved in upright posture, such as the erector spinae and the rectus abdominis, and what is their tone? What is the tone of the diaphragm and of the pelvic floor? Do these two diaphragms work well together to support breathing? A good alternation between tension and relaxation of the pelvic diaphragm and the abdominal diaphragm is a prerequisite for clear speech.

- Is the musculoskeletal system freely mobile? Does the thorax adapt freely to various body positions, to enable breathing and articulation to be accomplished correctly? Is the cervical spine free from lesions, to enable unrestricted movement of the head, and thus also to optimize the function of the neck and laryngeal muscles?

- A further important precondition for the acquisition of speech is good hearing. Does the middle ear drain properly? A hearing impairment, as with polyps or a chronic glue ear, can delay the learning of speech.
- Does the child's auditory processing work well? Can the child hear and understand speech? This is one of the main prerequisites for learning correct speech.
- The autonomic nervous system can play an important part in speech. Overexcitement leading to an increased sympathetic tone can, for instance, intensify stuttering and promote indistinct speech.

Therapeutic approaches

The osteopathic approach to treating speech impairments is holistic, as with all pathologies. This is most clearly demonstrable in stuttering.

Definition

Stuttering is an impairment to the flow of speech. It generally first appears at the age of 3 to 5 years and can manifest itself in various ways: from repetition of consonants at the start of a word or a sentence to repetitions of individual words and entire sections of sentences. 'Blocks' can occur, which can manifest themselves as anything from a 'hanging on' to one consonant to the associated movements of entire groups of muscles.

In many children between the age of 2 and 4 years a stumbling mode of speech is perfectly normal (in up to 80%). This is explained by later maturation of the nervous system, or by the fact that thought and speech must first harmonize with each other. Stammering is also no cause for concern until the child reaches 3 years of age. These transitional phases generally fade spontaneously. In only about 2% does this dysfluency of speech consolidate into a stutter. In a small proportion this can develop into a chronic stutter (in about 1% of the population).

Etiology

Stuttering has a multi-factorial causation. There is a high incidence in certain families, which points to a genetic predisposition. The circumstances of the first years of life and of language development then determine whether or not this predisposition manifests itself. Neurological disorders can also underlie a stutter. It is four times more common in boys than in girls.

Psychological influences can intensify a stutter but are rarely causative.

Conventional therapy

Stuttering is treated with speech therapy, breathing exercises and psychotherapy (generally behavioral therapy). The parents are often included in the treatment.

Osteopathic treatment

In people who stutter the flow of speech is disturbed, especially in situations of tension. The osteopathic approach is therefore to help the child to relax more and become more confident. This needs a comprehensive examination and diagnostic procedures, and the resulting treatment is targeted towards any lesions which might be found (p.450). Every lesion which is eliminated improves the child's confidence in his own body. The strength needed to compensate for the lesion is now once again at the child's disposal. He becomes less distracted by his physical problems and can therefore concentrate better on his speech.

A treatment which balances the autonomic nervous system can help the child achieve a greater inner calm. This can alleviate the emotional pressure which is often associated with language disturbances.

Muscle energy techniques (MET), Sutherland's peripheral balanced ligamentous tension techniques (BLT) and work with involuntary motion all have a place in this field.

Collaboration between speech therapists and osteopaths

Osteopathy and speech therapy complement each other well. By working together in this way, the duration of speech therapy can often be shortened. Good communication between the two professional groups is in this case essential. For instance, it is helpful if speech therapists draw the attention of the osteopaths giving treatment to important areas for this specific language impairment. Osteopaths in their turn may discover further causes from their diagnostic procedures and thus contribute to a comprehensive view of the patient. Osteopathy often treats areas which are inaccessible to speech therapists. Nevertheless, osteopaths should always bear in mind that the speech therapy is the basic therapy; the osteopathic treatment is adjunctive and supportive, and is given at longer intervals.

I have had good experiences in treating children with speech problems about every 6 weeks, after starting with shorter treatment intervals. This adjunctive treatment should extend over a long period, about a year. Speech therapy is generally given about once or twice weekly.

Case study

Tobias was 5 years old and had very indistinct speech. His speech therapist advocated additional osteopathic treatment. Nothing unusual was reported about the pregnancy. He was born after a labor of less than 6 hours, very fast for a first birth.

The general motor development was slightly delayed. Tobias had mild sensorimotor perceptual impairments and a general muscular hypotonia, for which he attended psychomotor gymnastic sessions. As a young child he had often had middle ear infections and tympanic effusions, which greatly restricted his hearing and necessitated the insertion of grommets. His speech was indistinct and 'thick'. Tobias had been receiving speech therapy for 2 years. His soft palate did not close properly and the lingual frenum was too short. Tobias was a friendly and alert child and otherwise healthy. The other organ systems were unremarkable

Osteopathic findings

Tobias was evidently a mouth-breather and had a slightly puffy face, which indicated a problem with lymphatic drainage. The osteopathic examination showed a functional pelvic torsion with an intraosseous compression of the sacrum.

Other findings were: anteriority of the left occipital condyle, a lesion of C3, a restricted occipitomastoid suture on the left, an increased dural tension and generally reduced muscle tone in the mouth area. The temporal bones showed intraosseous compressions, particularly of the petrous parts. The cranial restrictions and the compression of the sacrum were probably attributable to the rapid labor, which had left the child little time to adapt to the pressure of expulsion. The frequent middle ear infections were certainly a contributory cause of the intraosseous compression of the temporal bones.

Osteopathic treatment

During the first treatment, the lesional areas were worked upon. One particular aim of the treatment was to improve Tobias's upright posture along the spine. Here, the biodynamic approach, keeping the midline in mind, was particularly helpful. It also seemed very important to improve the mobility of the SBS and improve the tone in the floor of the mouth. This was achieved by balanced membranous tension techniques at the relevant cranial sutures. The floor of the mouth was also treated by balanced tension.

When Tobias attended for his 2nd treatment 3 weeks later, his mother reported that the speech therapist had noticed an unequivocal improvement in Tobias's speech and had asked whether he had visited an osteopath in the meantime.

At this examination and treatment, an improvement in venous-lymphatic drainage was noted. There was now only a minimal residual restriction at the left occipital condyle. This time, intra-oral work was included, on the palatine bone and the vomer, which Tobias accepted very well.

Further treatments are to follow for another year, at 6-week intervals, with the aim of treating the muscular hypotonia and to achieve a beneficial effect on the perceptual disorders.

Bibliography

Illing S, Classen M: Klinikleitfaden Pädiatrie. Urban & Fischer, Munich/Jena 2003

Willard F: Teaching documents. Lecture, Hamburg 2004

Internet addresses

www.stotter-infoseiten.de
www.medicine-worldwide.de

20

Vaccination

Manuela Da Rin

The subject of vaccinations is of vital importance in the life of a child and has led to controversial debate all over the world as to their necessity, safety and effectiveness. Knowledge of the immune system and research of vaccination procedures reveal that there are myriad responses, as each child is an individual, with individual needs. Osteopathy can address these individual requirements and therefore has also a prominent role to play within this debate.

The immune system has the ability to differentiate between self and non-self. It provides the body with defence against substances collectively termed 'non-self' and translates this information into a signal for an immune response. These substances are either derived from external sources such as bacteria and viruses or from abnormal cellular processes within the body, as in tumor cells. The immune system is designed to make high level comparisons which then enable specificity, memory and associative recognition. This is performed by antibodies that have specific recognition abilities to provide this self and non-self discrimination. The immune system recognizes, remembers and produces antibodies against millions of antigens also called foreign agents (Cotman et al 1987).

THE IMMUNE SYSTEM

There are two types of immune system:

- Humoral immunity, which involves the formation and secretion of antibodies by B lymphocytes, which mature in the bone marrow. All humoral antibodies are immunoglobulins (Ig), consisting of five basic types (IgA, IgD, IgE, IgG and IgM). They are the major defences against antigens, such as bacteria and viruses.

- Cell mediated immunity is a specific type of immune response controlled by thymus dependant T lymphocytes, which react directly with foreign cells.

Innate Immunity

Innate immunity, also called inherited immunity, is determined by genetic factors. It is present from birth and lasts throughout life.

Both the immune and lymphatic systems begin to develop at approximately the 5th to 6th week of fetal age (Larsen 1998). The lymphatic system is immature at the time of birth and continues to undergo changes until approximately puberty. Hence the neonate is more vulnerable to attack from bacteria, viruses and fungi than the older infant. The defence mechanisms are still immature and therefore some organisms, which are non-pathogenic in the older child, can cause serious infection in the neonatal period. In the preterm infant, these defences are even less mature, so that serious consequences of infection are more likely.

Naturally acquired passive immunity

Until about 3 to 4 months of age, the baby has only a limited capacity to produce antibodies in response to infection. Therefore some IgG from the mother is transferred via the placenta in the last weeks of pregnancy to protect the child in the first months of her life. This is called 'naturally acquired passive immunity'. IgG is the most common immunoglobulin to be found in the serum and in the extravascular spaces. IgG is also the only class of immunoglobulin that crosses the placenta. This immunity does not stimulate the baby to make her own antibodies and lasts only as long as the original antibodies persist. It gives the infant protection from viral diseases such as measles, mumps, chickenpox and rubella for 4 to 6 months, as long as the mother has immunity following exposure to these infections.

The infant's level of both IgM (the first immunoglobulin to be made by a virgin lymphocyte B cell when it is stimulated by antigen) and IgA (found in secretions such as tears, saliva, colostrum and mucus, providing local mucosal immunity) is low (Mayer 2004).

Antibodies against such bacteria as *Escherichia coli*, group B streptococcus, *Hemophilus influenzae* and *Streptococcus pneumoniae* are not usually transferred by passive immunity, which may partly explain why these organisms in particular are more likely to infect the newborn baby.

Colostrum affords some protection against infection by providing the infant with substances such as IgA, lysozymes, lactoferrin and lymphocytes. Later on, the breast milk reduces the proliferation of unwanted organisms in the gut.

This is due to the acidity produced by the breakdown of the excess lactose in the large bowel, which favours the growth of harmless lactobacilli and inhibits the more pathogenic *E. coli* organisms. Breast milk is an excellent nutrient that also gives the baby some protection against infection. It contains lactalbumin, proteins which influence the infant's bowel bacterial flora; namely lactoferrin, vitamins, minerals, enzymes (especially lipase, lysozyme) and IgA (Hull 1996).

Artificially acquired active immunity

Infectious diseases are caused by specific microorganisms. In 1796, Edward Jenner created the smallpox vaccination. The term vaccine is derived from 'vacca', the Latin word for cow. Jenner injected people with cowpox, a disease affecting the udders of cows, to protect them against smallpox. Cowpox vaccinations became popular in Western Europe, but devastating outbreaks of smallpox in the latter half of the nineteenth century led to the prohibition of Jenner's methods. The skills of Louis Pasteur initiated the present ideas and methodology of immunization via vaccination (Chaitow 1994).

Vaccines provide an 'artificially acquired active immunity'. They contain weakened amounts of the disease and stimulate the immune system, which then produces antibodies that defend the body from non-self substances called 'antigens'. These antibodies remain in the body and are able to remember and recognize the antigens that caused the particular disease.

Vaccination has two objectives:

• Increasing individual resistance to disease.
• Increasing 'herd/group immunity' by creating a critical mass of disease resistant individuals.

The herd immunity offers a degree of protection to susceptible individuals. Although a minority may still be prone to infection, an infectious disease cannot survive in the group if sufficient individuals are resistant.

VACCINATIONS: PRO AND CONTRA

The majority of medical doctors consider vaccines to be the most important tool in protecting public health. When childhood vaccination was introduced, babies were offered single dose vaccines. Thus the efficacy of the vaccine against the disease was easier to assess. Today, children are usually being given multiple vaccines in each inoculation. Mass vaccination with multiple vaccines is believed to be safe and effective in controlling disease and improving individual and public health. Simultaneously, ethical and legal arguments challenge the right of government health officials to force vaccination on everyone. In the middle of this scientific, legal, and

political debate is a growing pharmaceutical industry with billions of dollars invested in new vaccine development. Doctors are increasingly questioned by concerned parents about the safety of vaccines. This has led to official investigations and medical practitioners having to report within 6 to 30 days (depending on the country) any adverse reactions after the administration of any vaccine to the VAERS, Vaccine Adverse Event Reporting System (Institute of Medicine 1997). This variation of time notification illustrates the difficulty in assessing accurately adverse vaccine reactions. Not all reactions are immediately evident following vaccin-ation. Inactivated antigens (killed bacteria) such as in the diphtheria, pertussis and tetanus (DPT) vaccination will have side-effects occurring within a few days, such as local tenderness, erythema and swelling at the injection site, low grade fever and behavioral changes (drowsiness, unusual cry). However, live, attenuated (weakened) virus vaccines such as measles, mumps and rubella (MMR) will multiply for days or weeks and can create 'vaccine-associated' disorders within 30 to 60 days (Wong 1997).

Professional advice and reliable information from pro and con-vaccination view points are necessary. Parents are obliged to make a choice with the awareness that situations can occur when unvaccinated children contract the disease. Conversely, children, although vaccinated, can still contract the disease, as the antibody titer (a measurement of the amount of antibodies in the blood) may drop early; this is usually not checked after the vaccination. In this case, the illness is usually less severe. Another reason is probably genetic adaptations in bacteria, as in the pertussis bacteria. For example, it was found in 2000 that in 50–60% of pertussis cases in Germany the person had been vaccinated. Furthermore, vaccines pose the risk of an allergic reaction, either to the preservatives in the vaccines, or to the foreign protein of the pathogen used for the vaccine.

Adjuvants and stabilizers

The addition of adjuvants enhances the desired immune response to vaccines. The chemical nature of adjuvants, their mode of action and their side-effects are highly variable. According to Gupta et al (1993), some of the side-effects can be ascribed to an unintentional stimulation of different mechanisms of the immune system, whereas others may reflect general adverse pharmacological reactions which are more or less expected. The seriousness of their adverse effects is dependent on the strength of the hyperactivation of the immune system (Scheibner 2000, 2001).

The most common adjuvants for human use are aluminium hydroxide, aluminium phosphate and calcium phosphate.

Other adjuvants are based on oil emulsions, products from bacteria, endotoxins, cholesterol, fatty acids, aliphatic amines, paraffinic and vegetable oils.

Stabilizers in the vaccine may also play a role in the undesired adverse side-effects. This raises important questions about the safety of the preservatives and antiseptics. Diodati (1999) stated that 'alcohols such as ethanol, methanol, isopropyl, and 2-phenoxyethanol (used in conjunction with aluminium hydroxide adjuvant) are used to inhibit the growth and reproduction of micro-organisms in the live or attenuated (killed) biological component of the vaccine. Alcohols are highly toxic and can cause [a] myriad [of] problems including: general malaise, acidosis (causing shallow respiration), hypoglycemia (low blood sugar), hyperlipidemia (e.g. elevated levels of fats, triglycerides, and cholesterol in the blood), central nervous system depression, gastrointestinal damage, coma'. Formaldehyde and mercury, such as ethylmercury, also called 'thimerosal', were used in the past as preservatives in vaccines, but have been eradicated in most countries in order to fulfil the Worldwide Pharmacopoeia safety standards.

Triplevaccine: diphtheria, pertussis, tetanus (DPT)

The triple vaccine against diphtheria, pertussis and tetanus is usually given at 3, 4, 5 and 11–14 months of age.

Diphtheria

Pathophysiology

Diphtheria is now a rare but severe infection which affects the upper respiratory passages, especially in the young. The infecting organism, *Corynebacterium diphtheriae* multiplies in the nose and throat and produces a powerful and dangerous toxin which is carried by the bloodstream to other part of the body. The toxin kills the mucous membrane lining of the pharynx and upper air passages, so that a grey membrane is formed and the surrounding tissues swell. This can obstruct the larynx and in extreme cases, tracheotomy is necessary to enable the child to breathe (Brown 1991).

Complications

The main complication is myocarditis with damage to the valves, but also the nervous system and kidneys may be affected.

Treatment

Treatment is with medication such as penicillin or erythromycin. These antibiotics eliminate the bacteria but do not neutralize the toxins secreted by these bacteria. Therefore an antitoxin is given simultaneously.

Complications after vaccination

Complications or severe symptoms may develop after diphtheria-containing immunization, including seizures; fever above 41°C; difficulty breathing, other signs of allergy, shock, collapse; or uncontrolled crying that lasts for more than 3 hours at a time.

Pertussis

Pathophysiology

Pertussis is caused by the *Bordatella pertussis* bacteriium, spread by droplet. The catarrhal stage, with a runny nose and slight cough, is followed by the convulsive stage with longer and intense coughing attacks, especially at night. This dry hacking cough is paroxysmal and is followed by the characteristic whoop which is caused by trying to breathe in through partially closed vocal cords. During the attack, more or less pronounced cyanosis may develop; after the attack there is often retching and vomiting. Attacks may also be stimulated by eating or drinking. Babies are often spared the typical coughing attacks but may suffer from short spurts of interrupted breathing (sleep apnea).

Complications

Babies under 6 month of age are more likely to develop complications such as encephalitis or pneumonia. Babies who are breastfed usually get enough antibodies to protect them against a severe form of the illness if their mother has had pertussis or has been vaccinated against it (Hirte 2001).

Treatment

The allopathic choice of treatment is antibiotics against the bacteria, which is usually clinically not very helpful, as the symptoms might still persist.

Depending on the child's health and vitality, osteopathic treatment has been seen to accelerate the recovery process, so that the child is symptom free within a week instead of the usual 3 to 4 weeks; thus reducing the risk of complications such as pneumonia.

Complications after vaccination

Fever and local swelling is rare with the new acellular vaccines. Fits after the vaccinations are not as common as was stated in the past. It has been estimated that 1/1,000,000 children may have complications such as encephalitis following the vaccination.

Dr Odent's research (1994) detected some negative side-effects on health such as asthma following pertussis vaccination and the associated diphtheria and tetanus vaccines (DPT). Conversely, he detected positive effects of no asthma episodes following the same DPT injection when given in conjunction with BCG, Bacille Calmette-Guérin, live attenuated anti-TB vaccine. Dr Odent (2000) therefore emphasized the requirement for more information documenting the interactions between vaccinations.

Contraindications to the vaccination

Contraindications for this vaccination are progressive neurological disease and fits. The Oxford Handbook of Clinical Specialty (1997) warns medical practitioners to not use pertussis vaccination if there is a history of epilepsy in the family.

Tetanus

Pathophysiology

Tetanus is a severe life-threatening illness due to an anaerobic bacterium *Clostridium tetani*, highly resistant to disinfectant. The bacteria enters the body through a wound then releases a toxin 'tetanospasmin' which travels from the peripheral nerves to the spinal cord, where it impairs inhibitory synapses. This causes muscle rigidity, spasm and sympathetic overactivity (Brown 1991). Mortality occurs in one third of the cases.

Treatment

Antibiotics to eliminate the bacteria, Intensive Care management – injecting high doses of hyperimmune globulins, additionally muscle relaxants to reduce the risk of laryngospasm, sedation and if necessary, artificial respiration.

Vaccination

Tetanus vaccination is part of the triple vaccine, DPT, given initially at a very early age of 3 months old. If parents wish to give the child an individual vaccine, it would be beneficial to delay the vaccination to a later stage when the child is beginning to crawl and walk. At this time, there is a risk of contracting the disease by being exposed to the possible toxin in rust and soil. Tetanus vaccination is undoubtedly highly effective and has long lasting effects. The risk of adverse reaction is low (Odent 2000).

When the DPT vaccine is reduced to a single vaccine, such as tetanus only, the antigen load and the amount of adjuvants are minimal (Odent 2000).

Complications after vaccination

Important complications are unusual and allergies are rare. Most allergic reactions are due to extreme hypersensitivity to the tetanus toxoid component. If scheduled program of vaccinations has been supplemented over a short period of time, due to an emergency booster following a recent injury, there may be fever, swelling of the joints and lymph nodes.

5x and 6x Vaccines

Multiple vaccinations are now including five or six antigens in one session: diphtheria, tetanus, pertussis, polio, Hib and hepatitis B. This multiple vaccine is given at 3, 4, 5 and 11–14 months.

One advantage of multiple vaccines is that children get fewer painful injections, less adjuvants and stabilizers with their vaccination. It appears, however, that multiple vaccines may not be so effective in building up a level of antibodies that last.

Studies have been indicating that multiple vaccines may bring more side-effects. In 1997, Dr Osman Mansoor was demonstrating in New Zealand that after DTP/Hib-vaccinations, babies showed a high pitched cry 10 times more often than after the DTP combination. A study done by Aventis in 2000 showed more local reactions such as fever, irritability and drowsiness after the 6x vaccine Hexavac than after the 5x vaccine Pentavac (Hirte 2001).

In September 2005, the European medicines agency EMEA ordered as a preventative measure to withdraw the 6x vaccine Hexavac from the market, as the long term protection (5–10 years) against hepatitis B was not sufficient. This is an example illustrating that in multiple vaccines, the individual antibody titer may be too low.

In the near future, more research studies are needed to assess the interactions of 5x and 6x vaccines and their long term effects. When complications occur after multiple vaccines it is difficult to determine which might be the causative factor, and therefore more complex to decide whether and how to proceed with the vaccination program.

Poliomyelitis

Pathophysiology

Polio is caused by entero (gut) viruses, which first infect the intestine. Contagion occurs via droplet and contact. Three antigenic types (types 1, 2, 3) are known. Worldwide infections with polio have been steadily decreasing, even in third world countries.

In most cases the infection is asymptomatic. About 50% of the infected individuals develop minor illness with flu-like symptoms, vertigo, vomiting, headache and constipation. Less than 1% of the infected will suffer from the neurological form of the disease: either a meningeal form without paralysis or paralytic polio. Paralysis initially affects the legs, then other muscles, and induces muscle pain. Nerve and muscle atrophy, as well as coordination problems, may also occur.

Complications

Death by paralysis of the respiratory musculature is a rare complication. In some cases the paralysis is not reversible and leads to a partial disability. Long-term effects may present as a shorter leg, contractures or scoliosis.

Treatment

A specific treatment is not possible. Artificial respiration may be needed. Physiotherapy is useful to avoid pneumonia and contractures.

Vaccination

There are two types of vaccine, which contain forms of the three major strains of the wild polio virus:

- The Sabin vaccine is a live attenuated virus vaccine and is given orally (OPV). It is supposed to confer life-long immunity. The recipients can excrete the vaccine virus for a number of weeks through the mouth and feces. This led to the theory that it could pass on the immunity to non-vaccinated individuals, thus raising the herd immunity (McTaggart 2000). However, in some cases, the attenuated virus vaccine genetically alters in the gut, transforming into its virulent form. This vaccine can lead to complications of the neurological system, and should not be given to immune-compromized individuals, since it can then lead to poliomyelitis. The potential side-effect of the Sabin vaccination is called vaccine associated paralytic poliomyelitis (VAPP), a reaction that happens in about 1: 800,000 cases of oral vaccination (Hirte 2001). Since the 1990s there have been more vaccine associated cases of polio in the USA and Europe than true polio. Some of these cases were due to alleged contact polio, where family members became infected through contact with a vaccinated person in their family.

- For this reason a vaccine with 'dead'/inactive polio virus (IPV) is recommended: the Salk vaccine. It is injected under the skin; in the bloodstream antibodies are created, which will block the virus before it reaches the central nervous system. Although the IPV stops paralytic polio, it does not raise the antibodies in the intestines; hence it does not give the child a 'gut immunity'. So, theoretically, this vaccinated child could catch the wild virus, but would not produce paralytic symptoms on account of the antibodies present in the blood. But the infant could, however, still pass on the virus to someone else who lacks the polio immunity (McTaggart 2000). The Salk vaccine

does not produce vaccine-associated poliomyelitis and also gives better and longer immunity than the oral vaccine (McTaggart 2000). Used as a single vaccine it usually shows no side-effects; but as it is mostly used in multiple vaccines, it is hard to identify potential side-effects. Hirte (2001) recommends polio vaccination after the 1st year of age, when the central nervous system is more mature, as the polio virus has a special resonance with the CNS.

Complications after vaccination

Rare vaccine-associated poliomyelitis. Local irritation or swelling,

Hib

Pathophysiology

Haemophilus influenzae type B is found in the pharyngeal area of healthy individuals, usually in 2–5% of the population. It rarely leads to severe illness in the adult. The Hib bacterium is encapsulated, which makes it difficult for the relatively undeveloped immune system of young children to recognize and respond to it. This is why Hib tends to lead to more severe illness in infants, especially laryngitis, meningitis, pneumonia and endocarditis. About 90% of Hib infections happen to children under the age of 5, and 60% in the 1st year. A Swedish investigation showed that breastfed children have a significant lowered risk of being affected by Hib (Hirte 2001).

Complications

Due to the damage to the CNS following meningitis, about 4% of the affected children will be disabled, 3% will be hard of hearing (Hirte 2001).

Treatment

If diagnosed in time, these illnesses can be treated with antibiotics, but even so, 2–5% of this type of meningitis is terminal.

Hib vaccination

Since 1990, a Hib vaccination with a non-active vaccine containing parts of the bacterial capsule is used. It is recommended for children under the age of 5, because after that age a Hib infection is very rare.

The number of Hib infections has been greatly diminished since the introduction of the vaccination. The vaccination, however, does not give 100% protection, especially if given in combination with other vaccines. Dr Kondler-Budde showed in 1999 that the level of antibodies is less than half after a 5x vaccination compared with single vaccination.

As Hib meningitis has decreased in the last 15 years, meningitis caused by other bacteria, especially pneumococcus, have increased, and the overall incidence of bacterial meningitis is only very slightly lowered (Hirte 2001). The Pediatric Infectious Disease journal (1992) has made a connection between this increasing prevalence of penicillin-resistant pneumococcal meningitis and Hib vaccination.

Complications after vaccination

Local swelling is rarely observed.

Hepatitis B

Pathophysiology

The hepatitis B virus is transmitted by blood (blood transfusion, unsterile syringes) and sperm (sexual transmission) and causes infection of the liver. If their mother is a carrier, babies can be infected at birth. In this case the newborn should be vaccinated after birth to develop hepatitis B immunoglobulins. Apart from these exceptions, a baby or a young child is unlikely to contract the virus.

At the beginning of the disease there is usually arthralgia and skin changes, followed by icterus (jaundice), decoloring of feces, lack of appetite, uncharacteristic abdominal symptoms and hepatomegaly.

With neonatal infection, symptoms usually start at the age of 4 to 6 months, progression is unfavorable and prognosis worse.

Complications

There may be a fulminant hepatitis (active liver failure), chronic persisting hepatitis or chronic carrier status. Late complications are liver cirrhosis and liver cell carcinoma.

Treatment

There is no specific therapy. Chronic hepatitis may be treated with interferon alpha; however there are no existing studies concerning children.

Vaccination

Hepatitis B vaccination has been available since the 1980s and was originally only recommended for high risk groups, such as relevant hospital staff. In Germany since 1995 this vaccine has also been advised for babies in an attempt to eradicate hepatitis B. The reason for this is not because babies are high risk but because they are already following a vaccination program – and young adults would not necessarily have preventative immunization.

The efficiency of this vaccination is under scrutiny, as a study published in the Journal of Infectious Diseases (164, 1992:7–8) showed that 10% of volunteers vaccinated failed to produce antibodies.

Complication after vaccination

In rare cases, there are raised liver enzymes or gastrointestinal symptoms.

Classen, director of the American institute Classen immuno-therapies Inc. in Baltimore suggests that the hepatitis B vaccine can cause a number of autoimmune diseases such as insulin-dependant diabetes (McTaggart 2000). Hirte (2001) claims that the risk of children developing severe side-effects is three times higher than of getting hepatitis B. He recommends hepatitis B vaccination only to high risk groups and not children and teenagers.

Measles, mumps and rubella vaccination (MMR)

Pathophysiology

The measles, mumps and rubella vaccination is an attenuated (weakened) virus and is usually given first at 11–14 months of age and then at 15–23 months.

Mitchell and Tingle (1998) found that one year after the first MMR vaccination of 134 healthy one year old infants, 16.4% and 22.4% of vaccinees lacked demonstrable IgG antibodies to measles and mumps respectively, while IgG rubella antibodies were present in all cases. They suggested that earlier administration (at age 18 months) of the second dose of MMR may be more desirable than revaccination at school entry.

An antibacterial drug such as neomycin is used as one component of the mumps, measles and rubella (MMR vaccine). Neomycin has been reported to interfere with the absorption of vitamin B6 (Teasdale 2002), and vitamin B6 uptake error can cause mental delay. Therefore it is being discussed whether there is the possibility of an adverse reaction from this stabilizer. This may play a role in the observation of some children developing autistic characteristics following MMR vaccination.

Parents raised concern that within a week of MMR injection, their child would show marked personality changes, regressed milestones and behavior, such as lack of eye contact. However, this is not the norm. It is important not to conclude that all children are at risk when being vaccinated. In the UK, with the media raising controversy over MMR vaccines and potential side-effects, a few medical practices have offered the choice of single dose vaccination. Long term future studies would then be able to determinate the efficacy and side-effects of one individual vaccine and its lasting cover in a more specific manner, rather than trying to determine the effect of multiple vaccination at once.

Measles

Pathophysiology

Measles is a highly infectious disease. It is due to a paramyxovirus which affects the respiratory system and the skin. The incubation period is of 11 to 14 days.

The prodromal period is of 3 to 5 days duration, characterised by a low-grade fever, dry cough, non-purulent conjunctivitis with photophobia. Koplik spots, grain of salt-like-spots in the buccal mucosa are pathognomonic. They generally fade as the macular rash appears, starting around the ears and eventually spreading down the body.

Complications

Most common are bacterial secondary infections like otitis media or pneumonia. Feared is the measles encephalitis which appears in 1:500–2000 cases, clouds the awareness, leads to fits and neurological focal symptoms, is lethal in 30%, with defects healing in 20% of cases. A very rare complication (1:10,000–50,000) is the subacute sclerosing panencephalitis (SSPE) which is almost always lethal.

Treatment

Treatment is symptomatic and involves antipyretics (drug that reduces fever) and bed rest.

Complications after vaccination

In 10% of cases, there are vaccine induced measles which are attenuated and not contagious, with slight exanthema, mostly of the trunk, and fever up to 39°C.

Possible side-effects to the vaccine such as fever, headache, convulsion and behavior changes, sometimes 6 to 11 days following vaccination. The incidence of measles-vaccine-induced encephalitis occurs in 1:200,000. Martinon-Torres (1999) observes that neurological disorders secondary to the measles component of viral triple vaccine are not frequent, but rare cases might develop minor neurological signs. It may therefore be possible that such reactions, which may lead to developmental delay detected later in life, are under-reported.

Mumps

Pathophysiology

Mumps is usually a mild infectious disease of childhood, due to an RNA paramyxovirus that attacks one or both salivary parotid glands and is spread by droplet infection. Prodromal symptoms include headache and sore throat, followed by painful swelling of a salivary gland, often the parotid gland. The other parotid or another salivary gland is usually affected after a few days.

Complications

A meningeal irritation is common (up to 50%), 1–2% get meningitis. Encephalitis is rarer, but prognosis is worse concerning long term after-effects. Boys after puberty may get orchitis, a very painful testicle inflammation. In 30% of incidents there is testicle atrophy, which is the most common cause of acquired infertility.

Treatment

Treatment is symptomatic.

Complications following vaccination

There may be unspecific slight symptoms; very rarely meningitis or encephalitis, but not leading to permanent damage.

Rubella

Pathophysiology

Rubella is caused by the rubella virus, an RNA virus with 14 to 21 days incubation. The patient is infective for 5 days before and 5 days after the day the macular rash starts.

Rubella is a mild infection that sometimes escapes detection as it resembles chronic childhood symptoms, such as runny nose, sore throat and mild fever. Characteristically lymphadenopathy is manifested as enlarged lymph nodes in the neck. The macular rash consists of small spots which are slightly raised, close to each other but not confluent, start at the head (behind the ears) and may persist for 3 days.

Complications

These are very rare. Rubella is mostly threatening to pregnant women who have neither been vaccinated nor acquired immunity by contracting the disease earlier, as it may cause congenital rubella syndrome (CRS) in the 6th to 10th weeks of pregnancy. This may lead to birth defects such as brain dysgenesis, impaired hearing, microphthalmus, heart malfunction and serious psychomotoric developmental problems.

Treatment

This is symptomatic, with antipyretics and bed rest.

Rubella vaccination

Rubella vaccination of children is mostly aimed at protecting pregnant women from the risk of contracting rubella.

Studies have shown, however, that children with CRS have been reportedly born to mothers who had been vaccinated against rubella (McTaggart 2000). The lasting cover of the rubella vaccine has been shown to be variable. A study made in 1973 showed that 80% of all army recruits who had been vaccinated against rubella still contracted the disease 4 months later (McTaggart 2000).

It seems, therefore, that the natural protection is more effective that the artificial protection given by vaccination (Joncas 1983). In pregnant women it is useful to check the rubella titer early on in pregnancy and to immunize passively if necessary with hyperimmune globulin.

Complications after vaccination

In 10–15% of infants, slight fever, swelling of lymph nodes and slight rash occur. If the first vaccination happens in puberty or later, in approximately 25% there is some form of slight arthralgia.

Chickenpox

Pathophysiology

Chickenpox is a primary infection with the varicella-zoster virus. These persist, dormant, in the posterior root ganglion along the spine after symptoms of the primary infection wear off. Shingles (herpes zoster) is a reactivation of this dormant virus. Chickenpox has a long incubation period of 11 to 21 days and is highly contagious. It is spread by droplets.

Fever, headache and achy limbs are followed by the characteristic rash, which can present first, especially in the face and scalp. It then appears in crops over the whole body, mostly concentrated over the trunk. The palms and soles of feet are usually spared. Mucous membranes such as in the mouth, the tongue, pharynx, larynx, and trachea can be involved, also genitalia and rectum.

The rash starts as fine macules and papules, which change within a day to vesicles which contain a clear fluid full of virus, and pustules before finally crusting. These skin lesions are very itchy, and scratching leads to excoriations (superficial skin abrasion) and later scarring. All variations can occur at the same time. Crusting generally arises from the middle, giving it the typical umbilical appearance. Once overall crusting occurs, the child is no longer infectious.

After contracting chickenpox, lifelong immunity follows. The virus, however, stays in the body and may be reactivated after years, especially if immunity is suppressed, leading to herpes zoster. Varicella-zoster virus is carried by 95% of adults.

Complications

The most common complication is a bacterial superinfection of the pustules, pneumonia, bronchitis, otitis media; rarely neurological diseases like cerebellitis, encephalitis and cerebral infarction. In immunocompromised children it may become hemorrhagic.

Non-immune pregnant women should avoid contact with affected persons, as within the first 20 weeks the virus can cross the placenta causing congenital chickenpox and leading to cerebral cortical atrophia, microcephaly, mental retardation and limb hypoplasia. Following contact of an unprotected individual with ill persons, passive immunization with hyperimmune globulin is possible.

Treatment

Is symptomatic and antipyretic. If very itchy a local zinc tincture may be used. Keeping cool and bathing with camomile has a soothing effect and reduces the skin irritation. Sometimes antihistamines are given. Trimming the child's nails can lessen damage from scratching. In very serious cases intravenous therapy with acyclovir is considered.

Vaccination

Chickenpox vaccination is current in USA and has been recommended by STIKO (official German vaccination plan) since 2004. The aim is to reduce the number of the illness occurrences due to chickenpox (750,000 per year in Germany, 651,000 cases of varicella in GB in 2003 and approximately 400,000 cases per year in 2005 in the US). Until recently, this vaccination was only recommended for high risk groups. Children at risk include children with leukemia who are having chemotherapy, which depresses the immune system, or children and adults taking steroids for asthma or suffering from cystic fibrosis.

Critics debate whether the chickenpox vaccination is now exposing healthy children to the risk of potential vaccine side-effects for the benefit of this small risk population, as for the majority of the population this is a mild disease.

The live chickenpox vaccine virus itself is contagious; evidence shows that it can incubate in the body, causing shingles in later life. In one study, 11 children developing a rash after the vaccine were found to have the shingles virus (McTaggart 2000).

One concern about the chickenpox vaccination is that injecting a live virus into babies and children might lead to the virus becoming latent in the nervous system, which could reactivate many years later and lead to herpes zoster/shingles, resulting in painful blisters on the skin along the nerve infected by the virus.

A study on adults showed that 27% of a Merck-studied group who received 2 doses of Varivax still developed chickenpox 2 years later (Watson et al 1993; McTaggart 2000). The artificially acquired active immunity given by this vaccine might create a population of adults at greater risk of getting the disease than if they had had chickenpox as children, thus developing a naturally acquired active immunity.

Complications after vaccination

The vaccine does have side-effects, such as fever (in 15% of vaccinated children), irritability, fatigue and nausea (McTaggart 2000).

Possible causes of reaction to vaccines

Each vaccine has an individual history of safety and effectiveness. The vaccine is injected directly into the blood, bypassing the normal portal of entry and may create a brief inflammatory response.

The Australian scientists Scheibner and Karlsson are concerned that the interaction between vaccines might play a role in creating a non-specific stress or general adaptation syndrome (GAS) as described by Selye (1984). The GAS includes three stages: the alarm stage when the body is under acute attack and mobilizes all its defences; the stage of adaptation or resistance, when it seems to relax and seemingly accepts the intruding noxious substance; and the stage of exhaustion, when the body again tries to rid itself of the intruder. In 1991, Scheibner and Karlsson assessed the stress-induced breathing pattern. This pattern is defined as a low-volume breathing of 5–10% of the volume of normal 'unstressed breathing'. It occurs in clusters such as three to six shorter episodes within 10 to 15 minutes, when a child is incubating illness or teething or following 'insults', such as exposure to cigarette smoke, fatigue, overhandling by visitors, or vaccination needles. They demonstrated that babies' breathing after DPT injections revealed a pattern of flare-ups of stress-induced breathing. This follows closely the dynamics of adrenocortical activity in an individual under stress as observed by Selye. Scheibner concluded that the cumulative effect of harmful stress that some babies may endure from birth and the eventual injection of vaccine will, in some cases, cause attenuation of immune response, distress and tissue damage.

The lasting cover will vary from one vaccine to another. Vaccination commits immune cells to the specific antigens involved in the vaccine. Its clinical benefits have been questioned by Kalokerinos (1974). Following a DPT vaccinations campaign in Australia in the 1970s, he observed that the immune cells of aboriginal children became incapable of reacting to other infections. The immunological reserve of these children appeared to have been reduced, causing an overall lowered resistance. He was devastated when he witnessed that every second child died after the DPT shots. He concluded that the nutrition of the aboriginals at the time was deficient in vitamin C and gave each child 100 mg vitamin C per day per month of age. The result was staggering, as mortality ceased following vaccination.

Contraindication to vaccination

- Moderate or severe illness with or without a fever is a contraindication to any vaccine. This can lead to difficulty in following the vaccination program of 3, 4, 5 months for some infants who have repetitive illnesses.
- An anaphylactic reaction to yeast (Hep B), egg (MMR) or a previous vaccine contraindicate further dosage of that vaccine (Wong 1997).
- Live vaccine must not be given when the child suffers from primary immunodeficiency disorder or if the child is taking steroids, equivalent of >2mg/kg/day of prednisolone (Collier et al 1997).

Alternative vaccination plans

The seriousness of possible childhood disease is a determining factor in planning vaccination. Administrating single dose vaccines given at intervals would enable parents and practitioners to monitor possible side-effects. Otherwise, a shorter list of vaccines could be given to the child at one time. Assessing the disease and the age at which the child is most 'at risk', one may decide to delay the start of the vaccination program, thus benefiting from an increased maturity in the child's immune system.

The components of the widely used combination DPT (p.455) may be also given individually and at a specific age. Diphtheria vaccine is not essential as it seems to be rare in the well-immunized western countries and the risk of contracting this disease is extremely low. Pertussis vaccine is suggested to be given in early age, at about 3 months, for bottle fed babies. The susceptibility for severe illness with the pertussis vaccine is lessened after the age of 6 months. Tetanus vaccine has been shown to be very effective. It will be required later, when the child is crawling and walking, as it is then that there is more susceptibility to this threatening disease.

Odent's data (2000) showed that children who were vaccinated with pertussis at the same time as tuberculosis (BCG) did not suffer from asthma, hence showing some benefit in combining vaccines. This research illustrates the complexity of combined and single vaccination schedules and the long term effect on health.

The Salk polio vaccine, with the inactivated polio virus is advised, especially when the child is exposed to a public swimming pool.

MMR vaccination can be given after 1 year old, by which time the immune system of the child is more effective. Side-effects of this triple vaccine have been mentioned (pp.459, 460) and single dose vaccines are available in UK.

Hepatitis B vaccine may be considered for high risk groups; for example when there is drug addiction or exchange of needles.

Hib vaccination is recommended for children under the age of 5 years, because after that age a Hib infection is rare. However, Odent warns that this vaccine has had many adverse reactions.

Vaccination: yes or no?

A healthy child who acquires and benefits from a robust immune system will be in a favorable position to develop a natural immunity to illnesses and therefore have a good ability to overcome the contracted illness.

Care should be taken in the decision to vaccinate children with underlying dispositions such as eczema, allergies, asthma, epilepsy or gastrointestinal disorders. A healthy environment of sufficient light, living space, good water and sanitation, a healthy diet and life conditions will provide strong foundations for a sound immune system. Children who benefit from this environment will develop a naturally acquired immunity and therefore may not need to be immunized against all the vaccine-preventable illnesses.

If the child appears to have a weak constitution, the general tendency may be to vaccinate. Goldberg (2005) from South Africa observes that 'impoverished children, living in an unhealthy environment, will be less able to fight infectious diseases and therefore may need to be fully immunised'. He suggests that the child might benefit from a homeopathic remedy called Thuja D30 taken 3 days before and after vaccination, as homeopathy seems to lessen potential adverse reaction to vaccination.

As mentioned before, a useful strategy would be to shorten the list of vaccines the child will receive at any one time. Ultimately, there is always the option to delay the vaccinations until the child's development has stabilized and is less vulnerable to a vaccine reaction.

RELEVANT OSTEOPATHIC TREATMENT

As early as the 1870s osteopaths used their knowledge to help the body self-regulate and self-heal in overcoming disease and epidemics. Vaccination understanding was then in its early stages; penicillin was not discovered until around the Second World War.

Dr Fulford, a student of Dr Sutherland, taught a lot about newborns and children and the importance of the first breath

for the immune system. Birth is a miraculous event; a newborn, who was suspended in a fluid capsule inside the uterus for 9 months, suddenly encounters gravity and experiences a full deep first breath of air. At birth, on entering this new world, the child's ignition system must fire up in order to charge the 'battery of life' and charge the pulmonary, visceral, postural and psychological system (Jealous 2001). The successful completion of that first breath will enable circulatory, pulmonary and neurotrophic changes to take place and this will subsequently influence the future of the baby's health and immune system.

As an osteopath, the first endeavour is to assess and find healthy motion. A useful and effective approach with children would be to sit quietly, hands afferent, sensing without interfering. The osteopath gains clarity and information about the patient by waiting until the tissues reach a state of balance. Diagnosis can then take place in the assessment of the quality and amplitude of longitudinal and transverse motion. This motion reflects the fluid drive ability to charge the whole system, like a battery, and influences the vitality of the immune system.

After vaccination, a child may develop psychological disturbances like behavior changes or tantrums as well as physical problems like cough, eczema, psoriasis or juvenile arthritis. In this instance, the immune system has been compromised by the vaccine and overreacted. The toxicity of the vaccine can also affect the self–non-self interaction and in extreme cases lead to autoimmune symptoms. A noticeable decrease in amplitude of the transverse and longitudinal motion during inhalation phase of primary respiration is present when the immunity is compromised.

Osteopathic treatment can support the function of the thoracic diaphragm and the lymphatics via the cisterna chyli and the thoracic duct. The physiological centers along the reticular formation close to the 4th ventricle within the CNS regulate respiratory and cardiovascular rhythms and play a key role on behavior and alertness, as it provides neural integration to the limbic and hypothalamus circuit. When osteopathic treatment allows a state of balance to move from the local area to the whole body, a functional perceptual shift is made and a balanced state of awareness of self and non-self can return. Many osteopathic clinical situations demonstrate that the child, when treated, can regain a sense of the whole with a 'spark in the motor' enabling the immune system to restore its function and identity.

CONCLUSION

There appears to be no simple answer either way in this vaccination debate. Each child has an individual response to the vaccines or the disease itself. Individually, one must consider two options: going through an illness with a risk of possible complications, or vaccination with its possible side-effects.

Factors which parents can influence are: a healthy environment of sufficient light, living space, good water and sanitation and a healthy diet. Surrounding their child with love in a happy environment will also help to provide a strong foundation for a sound immune system. The child will then be in an optimum situation to obtain a naturally acquired active immunity. If the child contracts one of the illnesses which in principle could have been avoided by vaccination, advice can be sought from holistically orientated health practitioners about broad-based management of the condition. Treating the child holistically will reduce the risk of complications.

When concern is raised about a specific virulent pathogen, vaccination has a complementary role to play by providing an additional artificially acquired active immunity. This immunity will last as long as the antibodies or memory cells persist and is variable from one vaccine to another.

Osteopathy can enhance the immune function. It may support the body in restoring a sense of the whole; by redefining the importance and ability of recognising self and non-self, which is vital for a successful immune response.

Bibliography

Brown J A C , Bennett H: Pears medical encyclopaedia, Sphere Books, London 1991, pp 191, 628

Chaitow L: Vaccination and immunization: dangers, delusion and alternatives. C W Daniel, UK, 1994: 107–110

Collier J, Longmore M, Scally P, Oxford handbook of clinical specialties, University Press, Oxford 1997, p 208

Cotman et al: The neuro-immune-endocrine connection, Raven Press, New York 1987, pp 1–3

Diodati C: Immunization: history, ethics, law and health, Integral Aspects 1999

Fulford R.: Dr. Fulford's touch of life. Pocket Books, New York 1996

Goldberg R: Awaken to child health 8: Immunisation 2005

Gupta R K, Relyved E R, Lindblad E B, Bizzini B: Adjuvants – a balance between toxicity and adjuvanticity. Vaccine 11(4), 1993: 293–306

Gustafson T L, Lievens A W, Brunell P A, et al: Measles outbreak in a fully immunized secondary school population. New England Journal of Medicine 316, 1987: 771–4

Hirte, M.: Impfen- Pro und Contra, Knaur München 2001

Huang X, Yuang J, Goddard A et al: Interferon expression in the pancreases of patients with type I diabetes. Diabetes. 44(6), 1995:658–64.

Hull D, Johnston D: Essential pediatrics. 3rd edn. Churchill Livingstone, London 1996, pp 76, 157

Institute of Medicine, Vaccine Safety Forum, Board on Health Promotion and Disease Prevention. Vaccine Safety Forum: summaries of two workshops. National Academy Press, Washington DC 1997

Jealous J S: The biodynamics of osteopathy in the cranial field, an interactive audio text. An introductory overview, balanced membranous tension. No2, Ignition system 2001

Joncas J H: Preventing the congenital rubella syndrome by vaccinating women at risk. Canadian Medical Association Journal 129(2), 1983:110–2

Kalokerinos A: Every Second Child. Thomas Nelson, Melbourne 1974

Larsen W J: Essential of human embryology. Churchill Livingstone, Edinburgh 1998, p 141

Mark A, Bjorksten B, Granstrom M: Immunoglobulin responses to diphtheria and toxoid after booster with aluminium-adsorbed and fluid DT-vaccines. Vaccine 13, 1995: 669–73

Martinon-Torres F, Magarinos M M, Picon M, Fernandez-Seara M J, Rodriguez-Nunez A, Martinon-Sanchez J M: Self-limited acute encephalopathy related to measles component of viral triple vaccine. Revista de Neurologia 28(9), 1999:881–882

Mayer G: Microbiology and immunology on line, 2004

McTaggart L: The vaccination bible, a 'What Doctors Don't Tell You' publication, London 2000, pp 57, 73, 125, 127

Mitchell L A, Tingle A J, Decarie D, Lajeunesse C: Serologic responses to measles, mumps, and rubella (MMR) vaccine in healthy infants: failure to respond to measles and mumps components may influence decisions on timing of the second dose of MMR. Canada Journal Public Health. 89(5), 1998:325–328

Odent M: Vaccinations, prevention of diseases can be a cause of ill health. Primal Health Research Center, London, 8(3), 2000: 1–8

Odent M , Culpin E, Kimmel T, Pertussis vaccination and asthma: is there a link? Journal of the American Medical Association 272, 1994: 592–3

Pediatric Infectious Disease Journal newsletter (USA): Relationship between prevalence of pneumococcal meningitis and universal hemophilus influenza vaccination. PIDJ 18, 1992: 6

Scheibner V: Adverse effects of adjuvants in vaccines, Nexus 8(1), 2000 and 8(2), 2001

Selye H: The stress of life, McGraw-Hill, Montreal, 1984

Still A T: The philosophy and mechanical principles of osteopathy (1902) ed. Osteopathic Enterprise, Kirksville, Mo. 1986

Sutherland W G: Contribution of thought. Sutherland Cranial Teaching Foundation, Idaho, 1967 p 233

Teasdale C A: There are so many parts to the whole picture to consider. 17 February 2002, www.whale.to/v/bmj7.html

Watson B M, Piercy S A, Plotkin S A, Starr S E: Modified chickenpox in children immunized with the Oka/Merck varicella vaccine. Pediatrics 91, 1993:17–22

Wong D L: Whaley and Wong's essentials of pediatric nursing. 5th edn. Mosby, Mo. 1997 pp 318–321

Internet addresses

www.birthworks.org/bwodent.html

www.immunecentral.com

www.jamesjealous.com

www.syringahealth.co.za

www.whale.to/vaccines/scheibner.html

www.whale.to/vaccine/adjuvants.html

www.whale.to/v/quotes5.html

Appendices

Glossary

Noori Mitha, Eva Moeckel, Susan Turner

The definitions and descriptions of these words are intended to make it easier for the reader to understand the texts in this book. We have taken pains to do justice to the terms which Sutherland coined. However, certain terms can be interpreted in different ways.

Automatic

Works by itself; mechanical functioning.

Automatic shifting suspension fulcrum

This is Sutherland's term for a functional area at or near the anterior end of the straight sinus, around which the reciprocal tension membrane (RTM) organizes its motion. His students also called this area the 'Sutherland fulcrum'.

Balance

The normal state of equilibrium of action and reaction between two or more parts or organs in the body.

Breath of life

A biblical quotation often used by Sutherland, in order to emphasize that he was not referring to the breathing of air. 'And the Lord God formed man of the dust of the ground, and breathed into his nostrils the breath of life; and man became a living soul' (Genesis 2, 7).

Extension

See under *Inhalation, primary*.

Fetal distress

Physical distress in the unborn child due to oxygen deficiency.

Flexion

See *Inhalation, primary*.

Fluctuation

The movement of a fluid body located within a natural or an artificial cavity. The phenomenon of cerebrospinal fluid (CSF) fluctuation within the craniospinal cavity was observed by Sutherland. He was careful to distinguish his observation of its fluctuation from other generally used references to the circulation of the CSF. He described the fluctuation as an ebb and flow, similar to a tidal motion: 'A movement coming in during inhalation and ebbing out during exhalation' (Sutherland 1990).

Fluid drive

Directing a fluid wave from one part of the body to another with a very gentle impulse. It is generally carried out from the most distantly situated diagonal.

Fluid fluctuation (as a therapeutic principle)

An inherent therapeutic principle used by the body, in which the fluid (most commonly referring to the cerebrospinal fluid) moves in either a longitudinal or an alternating lateral direction. This principle of alternating lateral fluctuation can also be induced as a therapeutic maneuver by the osteopath.

Fulcrum

Mechanical still point around which a lever turns. It is the still leverage point which contains the kinetic potential or potency for the motion of the lever. The concept of the still point which gives rise to a new cycle of organized physiological motion has been extended to apply to the principles of treatment (see also *automatic shifting suspension fulcrum*).

General osteopathic treatment (GOT)

A system of examination (diagnostic procedure) and treatment. The GOT influences a dysfunction through the treatment of the body as a whole. This is achieved by rhythmic, circular movements which influence efferent reactions through the afferent tracts in the spinal cord.

GOT improves the mobility of the joints and tissues and helps harmonize the central nervous system (CNS) and the autonomic nervous system. This enables a regenerative and healing collaboration between the individual bodily systems. A further aim of GOT treatment is to relax the body and normalize disturbed reflex activity.

GOT brings about a stabilization of the body through an enhanced tissue tone and mobility. The balance of natural movement between the body cavities is improved. Lymphatic and venous return and gaseous exchange are also optimized.

Inhalation, primary

Primary respiratory motion or involuntary motion is expressed in the body as a three-dimensional shape change. This takes place in two phases. On the bony, membranous and fascial level, the midline structures express this motion as flexion and extension and the bilateral structures as external and internal rotation. Within the CNS and the cerebrospinal fluid the two phases are termed primary inhalation and primary exhalation. Inhalation therefore corresponds to flexion and external rotation and exhalation to extension and internal rotation.

Involuntary motion (IVM, IM)

The rhythmic, three-dimensional shape change of the body as response to primary respiration. (See: Inhalation, primary)

Lamina terminalis cerebri

Terminal plate, velum terminale. A thin layer of nerve tissue which extends upwards from the optic chiasm and forms the anterior wall of the 3rd ventricle. Originally it is the anterior closure of the embryological neural tube.

Lateral or vertical strain

A shearing strain at the sphenobasilar synchondrosis (SBS) in a vertical or lateral plane. Though this is defined as a pattern of the SBS, it is expressed through the whole cranium and its effects are felt throughout the body. These strain patterns are referred to as 'unphysiological' in that they are normally induced by trauma and involve a discontinuity in the cranial base midline.

Ligamentous articular strain

See *Strain*.

Membrane

Is often used as a synonym for the dura mater and the reciprocal tension membrane, except where explicitly stated otherwise.

Membranous-articular strain

See *Strain*.

Mobility

Ability to move. In the cranial area, mobility relates to a motion which occurs in reaction to an extrinsic stimulus, as in the description in Sutherland's hypothesis of the cranial bones, of the sacrum between the iliac bones, and of the reciprocal tension membrane. Sutherland distinguished between motility

(see *Motility*) and mobility for teaching purposes, to help the students develop their palpatory abilities and to distinguish the tissue qualities of the five components of the primary respiratory mechanism.

Motility

Describes an inherent motion, which arises spontaneously from within. Examples are the inherent motility of the brain and spinal cord and the inherent fluctuation of the cerebrospinal fluid. Cells also have an inherent motility.

Motion permitted

Any motion pattern which the tissues will readily accept on motion testing.

Motion present

The term for any motion pattern of the body which can be perceived on palpation in the inhalation phase. It is the effect of primary respiratory breathing through all tissue layers.

Molding

Adaptation of the child's head and body to the birth canal, during which process the cranial bones may overlap slightly.

Potency

The inherent power within the body to restore health as expressed in organized rhythmic motion. This term was coined by Sutherland. He spoke of 'potency' around us and in our bodies. Potency is often perceived on palpation as a living quality of potential for therapeutic change. This living quality differs appreciably from the static inertia in dysfunctional tissues. During a still point the body comes into harmony with the omnipresent potency for health.

Primary respiration

Expresses itself in the body as involuntary motion in the sense of rhythmic three-dimensional shape change; see *Inhalation, primary, Involuntary motion* and *Rate*.

Primary respiratory mechanism

This term was used by Sutherland to describe his concept of a physiological process. The human body is called a primary respiratory mechanism (PRM) as it can express the effect of primary respiration as involuntary motion (IVM).

Sutherland described five aspects of the PRM: the fluctuation of the cerebrospinal fluid, the function of the reciprocal tension membrane, the inherent motility of the CNS, the articular mobility of the cranial bones and the involuntary mobility of the sacrum. However, involuntary motion is not restricted to these five aspects but is expressed in every cell of the body.

Rate

Three different rates are observed with primary respiration:

- the cranial rhythmic impulse (CRI) has a rate of 8–14 cycles/minute
- the middle rate has an expression of 2.5 cycles/minute
- There is also a slow rate of 6 cycles/10 minutes, which is often termed 'long tide'. It was first described by Rollin Becker.

These different rates coexist, with one rate usually predominating. The rates are interrelated, like a harmonic in music.

Reciprocal tension membrane (RTM)

Sutherland coined this term to describe the mechanical function of the specializations of the inner layer of the dura mater, which can be seen as an interosseous membrane for the cranium and spine. It guides, limits and integrates the involuntary motion of all the cranial bones and the sacrum, since the spinal dura merges into the cranial dura. It is termed 'reciprocal' because all the parts are interdependent and influence each other. Essential to the concept of the RTM is that every part is free to shift around the automatic shifting suspension fulcrum (also called Sutherland fulcrum). If any part is restricted this forms a fixed fulcrum, which distorts the involuntary motion of every other part of the RTM from cranium to sacral part. This often has negative physiological consequences.

Respiratory center

An area in the medulla oblongata which has the task of integrating afferent information and thus controlling the action of thoracic (secondary) breathing.

Sacral sag

A condition which Sutherland described in which the sacrum is fixed in a caudal position, often with the sacral base anterior, and unable to rise cephalad in the primary inhalation phase. He observed that this may often have a global effect of fascial drag throughout the body. In his view it could contribute to hormonal disturbance, as in postnatal depression.

Spark in the motor

One of the ideas which Sutherland pursued was that of the brain as a motor or a self-charging battery, in which the inhalation phase corresponded to the positive charge and the exhalation embodied the negative charge. Anne Wales commented that a fluctuating body of fluid within a closed container within an electromagnetic field constitutes a battery. She went on to refer to the human body as having its electromagnetic field within the electromagnetic field of the earth. Another analogy that Sutherland used for the brain was the 'motor of respiration'. Just as an engine needs ignition, the spark is an analogy to describe the initiation and maintenance of the inherent motility of the CNS.

Sphenobasilar synchondrosis (SBS, sphenobasilar junction)

The junction between the sphenoid and the occiput in the area of the clivus is a synchondrosis. This means that there is first hyaline cartilage between the two parts of the joint, which is later remodelled into cancellous bone. This transformation is generally complete by the 25th or 30th year of life. Sutherland believed that cancellous bone formed in this way retained a certain measure of flexibility throughout life.

Still point

The expression of involuntary motion becoming still. Here, the body gathers itself to carry out a therapeutic change. A still point is a resting phase between two patterns and initiates a new cycle in which a new, better organized pattern of health follows. A still point can vary in therapeutic depth and potency.

Strain

An injury or change in a structure which is based on overuse or the effect of trauma. Sutherland emphasized that every strain which affects a joint also affects the associated connective tissues. He termed strains in the cranial bones and in the dural membrane 'membranous articular strains'. The strains which affect joints which are surrounded by ligaments were termed by him 'ligamentous articular strains'.

Sutherland fulcrum

See *Automatic shifting suspension fulcrum*.

Tide

Sutherland used this term to describe the inherent fluctuation of the CSF. He also spoke about the 'tide within the tide', the 'breath of life', stated to be the driving force within the tide. The concept 'tide' was expanded to describe a universal motion. To make this clearer, Sutherland used the analogy of the body as a house at the bottom of the ocean with its doors and windows open. The house is completely open and the ocean can flow through it unhindered.

Transmutation

Changing of one shape, nature, or substance into another.

Literature

Liz Hayden

PREGNANCY

- Nathanielz P: Life in the womb – the origin of health and disease. Promethean, New York 1999
- Verny T: The secret life of the unborn child. 2nd edn. Dell Trade, New York 1988

BIRTH

- Chamberlain D: The mind of your newborn baby. North Atlantic Books, Berkeley, Calif. 1998
- Hacker N, Moore G, Gambone J: Essentials of obstetrics and gynecology. 4.edn. Elsevier, Philadelphia 2004
- Llewellyn-Jones D: Fundamentals of obstetrics and gynaecology, vol 1. Faber & Faber, London 2004
- Odent M: The scientification of love. 2nd edn. Free Association Books, London 2001
- Odent M: Primal health. Clairview Books, London 2002

PEDIATRICS

- Green: Pediatric diagnosis. W B Saunders, Philadelphia 1998
- Kelnar C, Harvey D, Simpson C: The sick newborn baby. 3rd edn. Baillière Tindall, London 1995
- Nelson: Essentials of pediatrics. W B Saunders, Philadelphia 1998

PEDIATRIC OSTEOPATHY

- Carreiro J: An osteopathic approach to children. Elsevier, Edinburgh 2003
- Frymann V: Collected papers of Viola Frymann, American Academy of Osteopathy, Indianapolis 1998
- Sutherland W: Teachings in the science of osteopathy. SCTF, Texas 1990

- Sutherland W: Contributions of thought. SCTF, Texas 1998

OSTEOPATHY

- Arbuckle B: The selected writings of Beryl E. Arbuckle. 2nd edn. American Academy of Osteopathy, Indianapolis 1994
- Becker R: The stillness of life. Stillness Press, Ore. 2000
- Becker R: Life in motion, 4th edn. Stillness Press, Ore. 2006
- Deoora T: Healing through cranial osteopathy. Lincoln, London 2003
- Feely R (ed): Clinical cranial osteopathy. Cranial Academy, Idaho 1988
- Fulford R: Dr. Fulford's touch of life. Pocket Books, New York 1996
- Lee P: Interface. Stillness Press, Ore. 2005
- Magoun H: Osteopathy in the cranial field. 3rd edn. Journal Printin, Kirksville, Mo. 1976
- Sutherland W: Teachings in the science of osteopathy. SCTF, Texas 1990
- Sutherland W: Contributions of thought. SCTF, Texas 1998

INVOLUNTARY MOTION

- Frymann V M: A study of the rhythmic motions of the living cranium, Journal of the American Osteopathic Association 70, 1971: 928–945
- Mosalenko Y et al: Periodic mobility of cranial bones in humans, Human Physiology 25 (1), 1999: 51–58
- Mosalenko Y, Frymann V M, et al: Slow rhythmic oscillations within the human cranium: Phenomenology, origin and informational significance, Human physiology 27(2), 2001: 171–178

- Mosalenko Y Frymann V M: Wave phenomena; circulatory dynamics, Lecture: PRM Research Symposium/SCTF continuing studies program, Bloomingdale, Ill 2003
- Nelson K E et al: The cranial rhythmic impulse related to the Traube-Herring-Mayer oscillation, comparing laser-Doppler flowmetry and palpation, Journal of the American Osteopathic Association 101(3), 2001
- Sergueef et al: Changes in the Traube-Herring wave following cranial manipulation. American Association of Osteopathy Journal 11(1), 2001:17

Websites

Liz Hayden

- Osteopathic center for children in London: www.occ.uk.com
- Osteopathic center for children in San Diego: www.osteopathiccenter.org
- Osteopathic center for children in Hamburg: www.osteopathische-kindersprechstunde.de
- Sutherland Cranial Teaching Foundation: www.sctf.com
- Sutherland Cranial College: www.scc-osteopathy.co.uk
- Birth: www.midwiferytoday.com
- Books: Osteopathic Supplies Ltd.: www.o-s-l.com

Self-help groups

Liz Hayden

- Active Birth Center, 25 Bickerton Road, London N19 5JT, Tel: 0171 561 9006
- Association for Breastfeeding Mothers, Sydenham Green Health Center, 26 Holmshaw Close, Sydenham, London SE26 4TH
- Association for Spina Bifida and Hydrocephalus (ASBAH) 42 Park Road, Peterborough, PE1 2UQ, Tel: 0845 450 7755, http://www.asbah.org
- Association of Radical Midwives (ARM) 62 Greetby Hill, Ormskirk, Lancashire L39 2DT, Tel: 01695 572776
- Contact a family – Support group for families with disabled children, www.cafamily.org.uk
- Foresight – Preconceptual Advice, 178 Hawthorn Road, Bognor Regis, West Sussex PO21 2UY, Tel: 01243 868001, www.foresight-preconception.org.uk
- La Leche League, Spencer Lester, PO Box 29, West Bridgford, Nottingham NG2 7NP http://www.lalecheleague.org
- National Childbirth Trust, Alexandra House, Oldham Terrace, London W3 6NH, www.nct.org.uk
- Restricted Growth Association, PO Box 4008, Yeovil, BA20 9AW, www.restrictedgrowth.co.uk

Associations in Europe

Liz Hayden, Eva Moeckel

- European Federation of Osteopaths (EFO), www.e-f-o.org
- Austria: Österreichische Gesellschaft für Osteopathie (OEGO), Vinzenzgasse 13/9, 1180 Wien, Tel: 0043 69911906887, www.oego.org
- Belgium: Belgian Society of Osteopathy(SBO/BVO), Rue rempart des moines, 57100 Bruxelles, Tel: 0032 69214612, www.osteopathie-be
- Germany: Verband der Osteopathen Deutschlands (VOD), Untere Albrechtstr 5, 65183 Wiesbaden, Tel: 0049 6119103661, www.osteopathie.de
- Greece: Greek Register of Osteopaths, M Boulenger-Papadimitriou, Irodotou st 19, 10674 Athens, Tel: 0030 17229790, www.osteopathy.gr
- France: 1) Union Federal des Osteopathes de France (UFOF), 13, Rue des trois capitans, 26400 Crest, Tel: 0033 475257904, www.osteofrance.net; 2) Registre des Osteopathes de France (ROF), 8, Rue Thales, 33692 Merignec Cedex, Tel: 0033 556188044, www.osteopathie.org
- Italy: 1) Associazione Diffusione Osteopatica (ADO), Via Paolo Emilio 57, 00192 Roma, Tel: 0033 490682577, www.adoitalia.it; 2) Registro degli Osteopati dÌtalia (ROI), www.roi.it
- Ireland: Irish Osteopathic association (IOA), www.osteopathy.ie
- Luxemburg: Association Luxembourgeoise des Osteopathes (ALDO), c/o J.Buekens Tel: 00352380638, www.osteopathie.lu
- Netherlands: c/o Muts, Postbus 10013, 1001 EA Amsterdam, Tel: 0031 206827788
- Poland: www.osteopatia.pl
- Portugal: 1) Association et Registre Portugais des Osteopathes, c/o A.Lucas, Rua Joaquim Bonifacio 21, 1150195 Lissabon, Tel: 00351 21 315 1143; 2) Federacao Portuguesa Osteopatas (FPO), www.osteopatiaemportugal.com
- Spain: Registro de los Osteopatas de Espana (ROE), c/o Bustos Juli, C.Diputacio 273, 08007 Barcelona, Tel: 0034 932158485, www.osteopatas.org
- Switzerland: Swiss Register of Osteopaths, Case postale 171, 1162 St-Prex, Tel: 0041 21 8065454, www.osteopathy.ch
- **United Kingdom:** General Osteopathic Council (GOsC), 176 Tower Bridge Road, London, SE1 3LU, Tel: 0044 (0) 207 357 6655 Email info@osteopathy.org.uk, www.osteopathy.org.uk

Training in pediatric osteopathy in the UK

Liz Hayden

- Osteopathic Center for Children: 15a Woodbridge Street London, EC1R 0ND, Tel: 0207 490 5510
- Sutherland Cranial College (SCC): PO Box 91, Chepstow, NP16 7ZS, Tel: 0044 1291 689908, www.scc-osteopathy.co.uk

Index

References in *italic* indicate pages where a topic can be found only or mainly within a Figure.

A

abdomen
  'abdominal' pain in preschool child, 216, 257
  acute pain, 153
  anatomy of intestinal viscera and abdominal cavity, 261–2
  auscultation, 120–1
  and chronic respiratory distress, 153
  motion of posterior abdominal wall, 192–3
  observation, 120
  osteopathic diagnosis of the abdominal cavity, 216–17
  palpation, 121–2, 270
  percussion, 121
abdominal gas, 120, 121
abdominal masses, 122
abdominal muscles, 122
abducent nerve (CN VI), 126, 137, 140, 145
abuse *see* child abuse
academic development, 98
accessory nerve (CN XI), 138, 173
acetabulum, 124, 125, 188, 189, 324
Achilles reflex, 129
achondroplasia, 103, 418–22
acid maltase deficiency, 361, 364
acromioclavicular joint, 120, 131, 132
acromion process, 130
ACTH (adrenocorticotropin hormone), 51
adenoids, 281–3
  hypertrophy, 202
ADHD (attention deficit hyperactivity disorder), 389–96
adjuvants, 454–5
adolescents

case history, 98–9
  practice considerations, 10–11
adrenal glands, 34
adrenal medulla, 81
adrenaline *see* epinephrine
adrenocorticotropin hormone (ACTH), 51
Advanced Light Functional (ALF) appliance, 431
aftercare, 349
alcohol
  case history, 99
  in pregnancy, 36, 73, 83
  toxicity of alcohols, 455
aluminium hydroxide, 454
aluminium phosphate, 454
alveoli, 28, 74, 116, 294, 297, 301
  inflammation, 302
  unfolding, 52
amniocentesis, 16, 38–9
amniotic fluid, 16, 29, 30, 31, 38–9, 215
  calculation, 55
  oligohydramnios, 68
amniotomy, 56
amphetamines, 394
amygdala, 353
anal examination, 122
analgesics, given during child labor, 55, 57, 245
anemia, in pregnancy, 20
anencephalus, 82–3
anesthesia
  childbirth and, 57–8
  endotracheal, 65
  epidural, 22–3, 55, 57–8
  hypotonia and, 361
  spinal, 58
  treatment after epidural, 26

angina, 116
angular gyrus, 355, 357, 388
ankle, 133, 187, 188
  mortise, 187, 188, 209
anlage
  CNS, 81
  heart, 82, 85
  skeletal, 340, 341, 342
  twins, 32
anorexia, 154
ANS *see* autonomic nervous system
antenatal checkups, 15–16
anterior dural girdle (anterior transverse septum), 49
anterior knee pain, 338
anti-epileptic drugs (AEDs), 400, 401
antigravity responses, 108
antiseptics, 455
anxiety
  anxiety disorders with ADHD, 393
  examining the anxious child, 100
aortic arch, 120
Apert syndrome, 428
Apgar score, 50, 55, 364, 368, 369, 378
apical impulse (AI), 117
apnea, 114, 304, 420
appendicitis, 120, 122, 153
aqueduct of Sylvius, 420
arachnoidea, 81
ARAS (ascending reticular activating system), 351
arms, 110, 132
  muscle tone, 126
  treatment in infants of interosseous membrane, 199
arterial blood supply, 356–8
arterial hypotonia, 58
arthrocentesis, 347

diabetes mellitus, 35, 48, 154, 240, 363
Diagnostic Writing Test (DRT), 387
diagonal pattern of movement, 446
diaphragm
    activation and dysfunction in speech
        production, 448
    crurae, 192–3, 273, 296
    diaphragm lift, 25
    embryogenesis, 83
    emotional effect of diaphragmatic
        tension, 300
    mobility, 23, 192–3, 269
    palpation of thoracic diaphragm, 122
    pumping function for lower
        extremities, 20
    releasing with pneumonia, 303
    structure and function, 296
    treatment in infants, 194–5, 273
diarrhea, 262–6, 267, 269, 271, 273
    with dehydration, 154, 263
    with gastroenteritis, 254
    with otitis media, 284
    with vitamin deficiency, 155
diazepam, 76
    rectal tube, 150
diencephalon, 82, 352–3
diet
    avoidance of migraine triggers, 410
    babies, 238–41
    with breastfeeding, 252, 255
    constipation and, 270
    diarrhea and, 264
    ketogenic, 400
    low allergen, 252
    in pregnancy, 18, 20, 33
    and sensory integration disorders, 385
    toddlers and schoolchildren, 240–1
digastricus muscle, 137
digestion
    coordinating mechanisms of, 261
    incomplete lactose digestion, 250
    malabsorption syndromes, 263–4
    maldigestion, 263
diphtheria, 455
    single vaccine, 461
diphtheria, pertussis and tetanus (DPT)
        vaccine, 455–6
disengagement, 166
divided awareness, 160
diving seal reflex/response, 245, 377
doll's eye sign, 91
dorsiflexion, 133
Down syndrome, 413–18
    adjusted growth charts, 103
    congenital heart disease and, 117
    diagnosis, 102, 110
    hypotonia, 361, 429
    jaw development, 428–9
    malocclusions, 428

sphenoid bone, 175, 416, 417
    unreliability of serum testing, 16
DPT (diphtheria, pertussis, tetanus)
        vaccine, 455–6
drawing, 135–6, 229–31
Drehmann sign, 156
drugs
    anti-epileptic drugs (AEDs), 400, 401
    breastfeeding difficulties after, 27
    as cause of malformation, 35
    developmental delay from mother's use
        of, 369
    drug-based treatment of premature
        child, 76
    with early contractions, 21
    given during child labor, 22–3, 55,
        56–7, 297
    hypotonia and, 361
    in IVF, 37
    medication during pregnancy, 36, 76
    pharmacological therapy in ADHD,
        394–5
    polypharmacy, 56, 400, 402
    risk of embryonic malformation, 83
    see also individual drugs
ductus arteriosus, 75–6
duodenum, 258, 272
    duodenal atresia, 120, 272, 415
dural membranes, 50, 72, 175, 180, 203,
        404–5, 416–17
    dura mater, 49, 57, 79
    dural arrangement of infant cranium,
        203
    see also reciprocal tension membrane
dwarfism (achondroplasia), 103, 418–22
Dynamic Listening System, 147
dynamic systems model of posture
        control, 374
dynamic systems theory and brain
        organization, 374–5
dysarthria, 134, 377
dyscalculia, 387
dyskinetic cerebral palsy, 376–7
dyslexia, 386, 387, 388
dysplasia
    achondroplasia, 418–22
    bronchopulmonary, 74
    of the hip see developmental dysplasia
        of the hip (DDH)
dyspnea see respiratory distress
dystocia, 59–62

E

ears
    active drainage of the middle ear, 286
    auditory tube, 279–81, 284
    clavicular dysfunction and ear
        infection, 198

    in Down syndrome, 415
    ear drum (tympanic membrane),
        142–3, 146, 284
    examination, 111, 141–3
    glue ear (chronic seromucinous otitis),
        139, 143, 286–7
    organ of equilibrium in inner ear, 31,
        137
    otitis media, 89, 143, 145, 157, 283–6
    tympanic nerve, 279
    tympanic ring, 147, 204, *426*
    see also hearing
ears, nose and throat (ENT):
        otolaryngology, 277–91
eating disorders, 154
eclampsia, 21
ectoderm, 80, 81, 83, *85*, 168
    in tooth development, 425
EEG (electroencephalogram), 215, 370,
        382, 399, 409
elbow, 131, 132
    treatment in infants, 199–200
'elective mutism' disorder, 446
embryo transfer (ET), 37
embryonic development, 32, 79–86,
        341, 416
    anlage see anlage
    of the auditory tube, 279
    embryogenesis of bone and muscle,
        168
    embryogenesis of diaphragm, 83
    embryogenesis of heart, 83
    embryogenesis of rectum, 83
    embryogenesis of spine, 200
    of the gastrointestinal tract, 257–60
    of the lower respiratory system, 293–4
embryos
    care of the mother, 15, 16
    embryological development see
        embryonic development
    embryonic folding, 83–5
    pre-implantation diagnosis, 37
    protection law in Germany, 37
emesis gravidarum, 17
emotional abuse, 101
emotional awareness, 225–8, 232–3
emotional traumatization
    effect on babies of prenatal trauma,
        39–40
    embryonic, 32
    with 'underinflated first breath', 298
emotions
    diagnosing and treating emotional
        factors, 223–8
    emotional relief, 300
    importance of parental affection,
        ambivalence or rejection, 38–9
    lungs and, 300
    orchestrated by solar plexus, 274

Printed and bound by CPI Group (UK) Ltd, Croydon, CR0 4YY

08/06/2025

01896878-0003